At a Glance

Radiographic Technique, Radiographic Anatomy

Radiographic Pathology

Pocket Atlas of Dental Radiology

Friedrich A. Pasler, DDS, PhD
Professor Emeritus
Department of Radiology
Dental Institute
University of Geneva
Geneva, Switzerland

Heiko Visser, Dr. med. dent., MSc Physics
Professor
Dental School
University of Göttingen
Göttingen, Germany

Foreword by Thomas M. Hassell, DDS, Dr. med. dent., PhD

798 illustrations

Thieme
Stuttgart · New York

Library of Congress
Cataloging-in-Publication Data

Pasler, Friedrich Anton.
[Taschenatlas der zahnärztlichen Radiologie. English]
Pocket atlas of dental radiology / Friedrich A. Pasler, Heiko Visser.
p.; cm.
"This book is an authorized and revised translation of the German edition published an copyrighted 2003 by Georg Thieme Verlag, Stuttgart, Germany" – T.p. verso.
Includes bibliographical references and index.
ISBN 978-3-13-139801-7 (alk. paper) – ISBN 978-1-58890-335-8 (alk. paper)
1. Teeth–Radiology–Atlases. 2. Skull–Radiography–Atlases. I. Visser, Heiko, 1956 - II. Pasler, Friedrich Anton. Taschenatlas der zahnärztlichen Radiologie. English. III. Title.
[DNLM: 1. Radiography, Dental–Atlases. WN 17 P282t 2007a]
RK309.P6338 2007
617.6'07572–dc22
2007009515

This book is an authorized and revised translation of the German edition published and copyrighted 2003 by Georg Thieme Verlag, Stuttgart, Germany. Title of the German edition: Taschenatlas der Zahnärztlichen Radiologie.

Translated by: Professor Thomas Hassell, Associate Vice Chancellor for Research, School of Graduate Studies, NC A&T State University, Greensboro, NC, USA

Rüdigerstrasse 14, 70469 Stuttgart, Germany
http://www.thieme.de
Thieme New York, 333 Seventh Avenue,
New York, NY 10001, USA
http://www.thieme.com

Cover design: Thieme Publishing Group
Typesetting by OADF, Holzgerlingen, Germany
Printed in Germany by APPL, aprinta druck, Wemding, Germany
ISBN 978-3-13-139801-7 (TPS, Rest of World)
ISBN 978-1-58890-335-8 (TPN, The Americas)
1 2 3 4 5 6

Important note: Medicine is an ever-changing science undergoing continual development. Research and clinical experience are continually expanding our knowledge, in particular our knowledge of proper treatment and drug therapy. Insofar as this book mentions any dosage or application, readers may rest assured that the authors, editors, and publishers have made every effort to ensure that such references are in accordance with **the state of knowledge at the time of production of the book**.

Nevertheless, this does not involve, imply, or express any guarantee or responsibility on the part of the publishers in respect to any dosage instructions and forms of applications stated in the book. **Every user is requested to examine carefully** the manufacturers' leaflets accompanying each drug and to check, if necessary in consultation with a physician or specialist, whether the dosage schedules mentioned therein or the contraindications stated by the manufacturers differ from the statements made in the present book. Such examination is particularly important with drugs that are either rarely used or have been newly released on the market. Every dosage schedule or every form of application used is entirely at the user's own risk and responsibility. The authors and publishers request every user to report to the publishers any discrepancies or inaccuracies noticed. If errors in this work are found after publication, errata will be posted at www.thieme.com on the product description page.

Some of the product names, patents, and registered designs referred to in this book are in fact registered trademarks or proprietary names even though specific reference to this fact is not always made in the text. Therefore, the appearance of a name without designation as proprietary is not to be construed as a representation by the publisher that it is in the public domain.

Preface

In medicine and also in dentistry, clinical inspection and palpation represent the first steps in a comprehensive examination of the patient's status quo; inspection and palpation also provide the data upon which each clinician must base her/his decisions concerning the necessity for additional, supplemental diagnostic procedures to solidify a final diagnosis and appropriately target treatment planning.

Within the concept of a thorough pre-treatment examination, the images that can be produced through the use of ionizing radiation almost always play a critical role in providing visual information that cannot be garnered by clinical examination alone. In today's modern dental practice, examination of the teeth and their supporting osseous structures with out the use of radiographic imaging is unthinkable. Indeed, radiography, magnetic resonance imaging, scintigraphy, and sonography have become indispensable components within our diagnostic larder, to name only the most important tools at our disposable.

The use of ionizing radiation for the preparation of two-dimensional images of the teeth and osseous cranial structures has been with us for over 100 years, and we have learned the importance of protection for both patient and auxiliary personnel against the dangers of excessive radiation exposure. Both the profession and those in industry have expended all energies in the search for techniques and technologies that minimize radiation exposure while providing images of the highest diagnostic quality. We are quickly approaching what appear to be the limits.

It is therefore incumbent upon us all to, quite simply: *Avoid the necessity for re-takes!* This will involve *in every case* a well thought out examination strategy, a well considered minimal radiation dose, and also perfect radiographic technique (patient positioning, central ray targeting, proper settings).

This *Pocket Atlas of Dental Radiology* will find its niche in the education and training of students of dentistry, dental hygiene, radiographic technology, and for dental assistants and medical radiology assistants. This book is also meant for practicing dentists, and those engaged in all of the various dental specialties. It provides important advice and clinical tips concerning the basics of radiographic technique and quality control, radiographic anatomy, and radiographic diagnosis. The book provides comprehensive information about both conventional radiography as well as digital imaging in all of its contemporary incarnations, always with a sharp eye toward means for minimizing radiation exposure for each and every patient.

Radiography cannot fulfill every demand for a comprehensive and all-inclusive documentation of each patient's clinical/pathological/anatomical condition, because the images reveal only a "slice in time" in the patient's life and disease process. Today's radiographic image says little about what things looked like yesterday (or last month), and nothing at all about what things will look like tomorrow (or next month). The radiograph can say little or nothing about clinical findings, and the patient's age and gender may influence any "conclusions" drawn from the radiographs.

The authors are grateful for the intense communication and participation of Thieme Publishers as this book traversed its conception and ultimate birth. Especially the input by Dr. Christian Urbanowicz and other Thieme colleagues are worthy of praise and thanks. We are grateful also to the many colleagues who contributed their practice-based radiographs as illustrations in this book.

F.A. Pasler
H. Visser

Foreword

For over 100 years, dentists have been "shooting x-rays" to enhance their clinical examinations of patients who present with pain or pus or otherwise apparent pathological alterations of dental and/or head and neck osseous structures. Throughout the decades, techniques changed little, and practice-based radiographic equipment remained for the most part unchanged also. "Wet film" developing has persevered as the gold standard, despite its limitations, difficulties, and demands.

This new book—*Pocket Atlas of Dental Radiology*—is a refreshing breath of new air for the dental professions. The book is presented in such a way, and in such a format, that it will be welcomed by students of dentistry and dental hygiene, and by dental assistants who are licensed to take radiographs. Periodontists, oral and maxillofacial surgeons, and perhaps especially dental implantologists will benefit greatly by having this excellent "pocket" reference at hand in the operatory as individual patients' requirements demand special projections for the elucidation of special problems.

The Pasler/Visser volume provides the most current, state-of-the-art information concerning techniques and equipment for producing images of diagnostic high quality, while limiting to the Nth degree exposure to ionizing radiation, for both the patient and the auxiliary personnel who are tasked with taking the radiographs.

The book is exquisitely organized to make reading or referencing easy for the clinician who needs a piece of knowledge at a moment's notice. The format is user-friendly, with text on the left side and illustrations on the right side. No flipping back and forth!

The treatment of the latest advances in digital imaging is excellent and up-to-date. Everyone expects that intraoral digital radiography will be the "thing of the future" in dentistry, and the authors provide useful guidance for those dental practices that are getting ready to move into the digital age. Tips about equipment and training of personnel are well chosen and on-point.

The chapters on radiographic appearances of a myriad of head and neck pathological conditions exceeds what is presented in most traditional textbooks on oral/dental radiology, venturing into the radiology of oral pathology. The authors take a two-pronged approach in this regard: Here is how to perform the procedure clinically, and here is how to evaluate the resultant image. A fresh approach, indeed!

The illustrations and diagrams are well selected to illustrate every point of the text, and are reproduced vividly by the publisher's highly qualified technicians.

For a new, small book to successfully address the state-of-the-art in oral/facial radiology is a milestone. Clinicians and educators will welcome this contribution by Pasler and Visser.

Thomas M. Hassell, DDS, Dr. med. dent., PhD

Contents

Radiographic Technique, Radiograpic Anatomy, Image Processing

Radiographic Technique, Radiographic Anatomy, Image Processing

Panoramic radiography, also known as orthopantography (OPG) or panoramic tomography, makes it possible to depict in a single image a complete representation of the jaws, teeth, temporomandibular joints (TMJ), and the alveolar lobes of the maxillary sinuses. The extraordinary capabilities and possibilities provided by the panoramic radiograph give dentists the opportunity to record and analyze all components of the masticatory system and their interrelationships. Within these parameters, the panoramic radiograph forms the basis of a logically conceived and relatively low-radiation strategy for diagnostic examinations.

Fig. 1a Principle of the tomographic technique. These diagrams illustrate the basis of linear attenuation (blurring): **AB** = path of the radiation source, $\mathbf{A_1/B_1}$ = counter-orbiting path of the image receptor (film), **SE** = plane of the tomographic slice, **SW** = angle of the slice, **U** = desired detail in the targeted layer (black dot that will be in sharp focus), $\mathbf{U_1}$ = undesired detail outside the target layer (gray dot and blurred figure on the image receptor). This will be more or less completely attenuated depending upon its distance from the plane of focus. The thickness of the slice depends upon the selected slice angle. A small angle (short path, blue) will image a thicker plane than will a larger angle (longer path, red). If the layer in focus is thicker than 5 mm, the procedure is referred to as zonography, and if less than 3 mm, tomography.

Fig. 1b Attenuation methods for tomography. **a** linear, **b** circular, **c** elliptical, **d** hypocycloidal and **e** spiral attenuation with contra-rotating image receptor motion. The method of spiral attenuation (with the longest pathway) provides the best results with the thinnest layers in focus and the least amount of volume artifacts, especially in skull radiographs.

Fig. 2a Principle of panoramic radiography (orthopantography). The radiation source (right) and the image receptor holder (left) move in the clockwise direction around the skull, while the image receptor (IR) itself moves in the opposite direction behind the secondary slotted diaphragm. The central ray falls upon the counter-orbiting image receptor, having first passed through the primary slotted diaphragm, then through the vertical slot nearest the image receptor. According to the original version by Paatero, the central ray is guided in an elliptical track over three pivotal points from **C** over **B** after **A**. It would be better to think of these three pivotal points as three vertical axes of rotation within a flat bundle of rays.

Fig. 2b Midline of the slice thickness. With modern radiographic equipment, the shape of the slice can be adapted (±) according to the patient's age and shape of the jaws. The thickness changes from about 9 mm in the anterior region up to approximately 20 mm in the region of the temporomandibular joints. This imaging procedure can be categorized as zonography with different depths of field in different segments of the jaws. Structures outside of the plane are not completely eliminated, so that a summation effect from the third dimension may lead to improper interpretation of the two-dimensional radiographic image.

Fig. 3a Object distortions in panoramic radiographs. In this example of the anterior region of the mandible, it becomes clear that objects **in front of** the plane are not sharply depicted and are *reduced* in size, while objects **behind** the plane are also not sharply depicted but are *expanded* in size. A metal sphere positioned in front of the plane of focus, for example during implant simulations, appears blurred and vertically oval in shape, while a metal sphere behind the plane appears blurred but laterally oval.

Fig. 3b Principle of the slot-technique. Conventional skull radiographic techniques are associated with an inevitable pattern of scatter radiation. The slot-technique provides clearer images, but at the cost of higher radiation exposure. The skull can be effectively scanned vertically or horizontally with narrow, continuously applied "lines" of radiation, via focus-near (primary) diaphragms and secondary diaphragms slotted nearer the image receptor. The panoramic radiograph described by Paatero is therefore actually based on the slot-technique, in that it is an elliptoid-shaped zonography with varying depths of field.

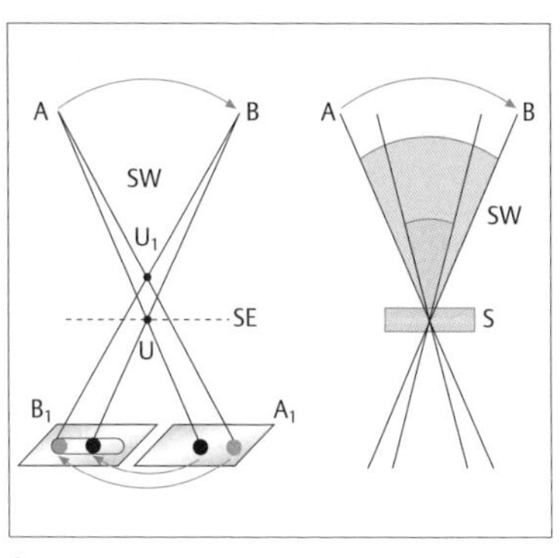

1 a

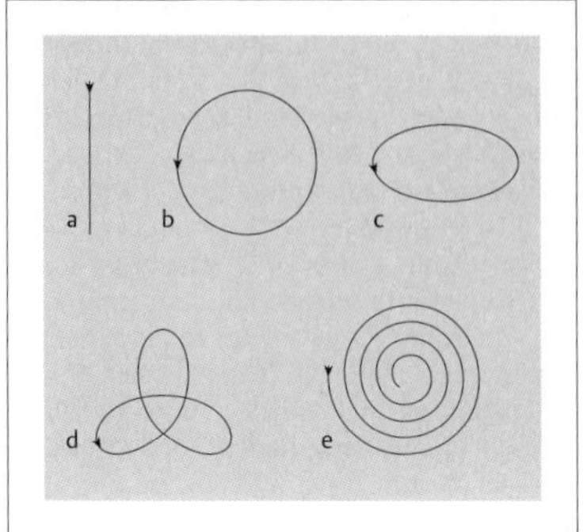

1 b

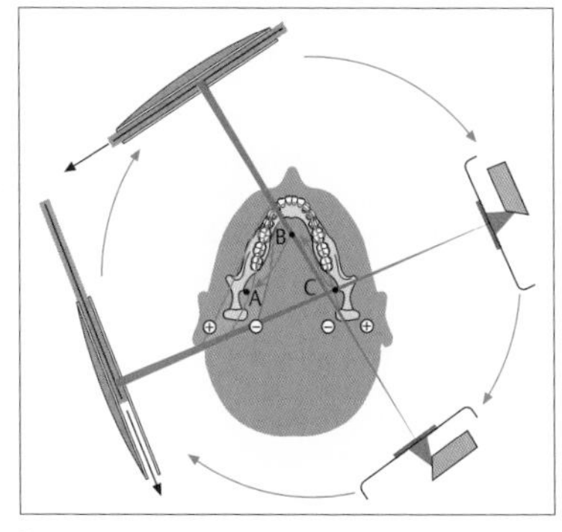

2 a

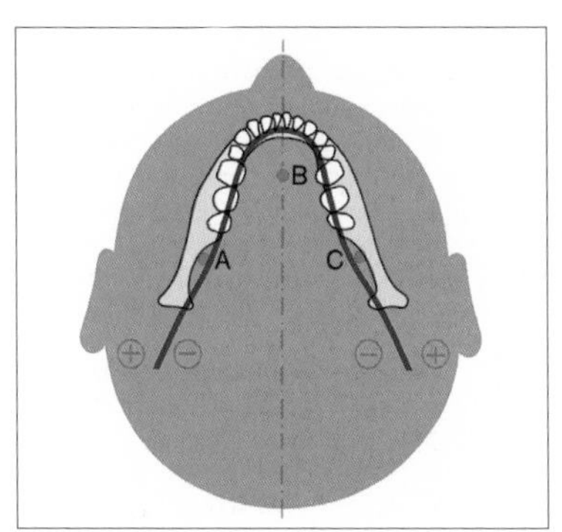

2 b

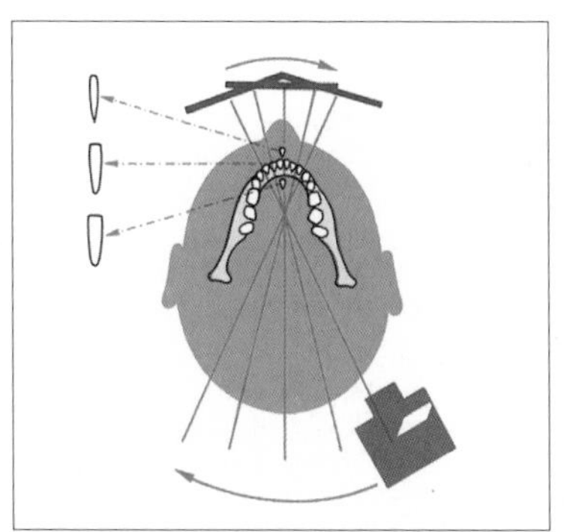

3 a

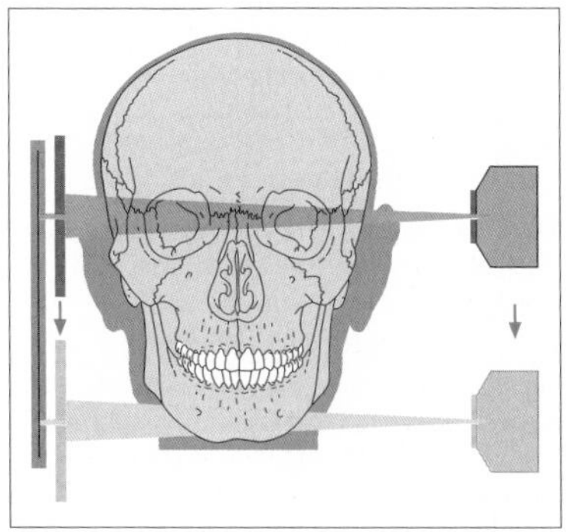

3 b

The “classic” 18-film intraoral radiograph examination of the teeth is relatively comfortable for the patient, and the overall radiation dose is generally acceptable; however, it is a time-consuming endeavor, and in some cases provides a less-than-optimum depiction of individual teeth. Nevertheless, it offers valuable information as a basis for treatment planning, is far superior to purely clinical observations, and often gives impetus for more extensive examination strategies. Finally, the 18-film “full series” exam provides a sense of security for both dentist and patient, and enhances confidence through communication. On the other hand, clear radiographic depiction of not only the teeth, but also the jaws, the temporomandibular joints, and the alveolar lobes of the maxillary sinuses will reduce the risk of an incomplete and possibly incorrect examination, which in the worst-case scenario could lead to malpractice. In this regard, the panoramic radiograph always leads to a broadening of horizons because it improves the dentist’s knowledge of radiographic anatomy and thus improves her/his skill in distinguishing between and among normal and pathologic conditions. This, in conjunction with a better understanding of the interrelationships of systemic medical problems and dental/oral problems can open new avenues for treatment planning.

The question of whether the treating dentist her/himself actually takes the radiographs or delegates this task to auxiliary personnel is really a question of responsibility for the radiographic quality that is achieved, and the radiation dose that this requires. If, for whatever reason, this assignment is delegated, the person who bears the primary responsibility must see to it that the auxiliary personnel are well-trained and have received legal certification. They must not only become expert in the production of high-quality radiographs, but must also be knowledgeable regarding the dental indications and the procedures for protecting patients and staff from excessive radiation exposure. Auxiliary dental personnel who are given the responsibility of taking radiographs must remain current in all continuing education standards in order to insure high radiographic quality and the lowest possible radiation dose for every patient. This is critical!

Fig. 4 Panoramic radiograph prepared using a bite plane. Using a bite plane, the maxillary and mandibular anterior teeth can be positioned vertically in an end-to-end bite, and be depicted clearly and sharply in the plane of focus. With this technique, however, it is important to carefully position the occlusal plane and the median-saggital plane in order to avoid subsequent errors of interpretation or the necessity for re-takes.

Fig. 5a Positioning the anterior segments in the bite plane. If it is possible to position the anterior maxillary and mandibular teeth in edge-to-edge arrangement parallel with and within the layer in focus, the result will be a clear and sharp radiographic depiction of the anterior teeth, and the proportions of these teeth will be portrayed in their correct relationships.

Fig. 5b Positioning in habitual occlusion. In patients where it is indicated to perform panoramic radiography in habitual occlusion, it is often really not possible to depict the anterior teeth or portions of these teeth sharply and with proper dimensions. The schematic diagram shows that the roots of the anterior teeth are behind the plane and are therefore depicted as blurred and widened.

Fig. 6a Positioning the occlusal plane. It is often recommended that the head/skull should be positioned so that from the lateral aspect the Frankfurt horizontal plane is horizontal (**red**). However, in many cases this leads to an unacceptable image, because the occlusal plane (**green**) occurs at a variable angle to the Frankfurt horizontal.

Fig. 6b Positioning the occlusal plane. The occlusal plane (**green**) should (with some exceptions) be positioned such that it is either horizontal (**black line**), for example with small children or periodontal patients, or rises slightly dorsally, in which case the Frankfurt horizontal (**red**) can be disregarded. For orientation, the Camper plane (**yellow**) can also be considered as it is identified coursing from the nasal spine (subnasale) to the tragion, and in almost all cases closely parallels the occlusal plane.

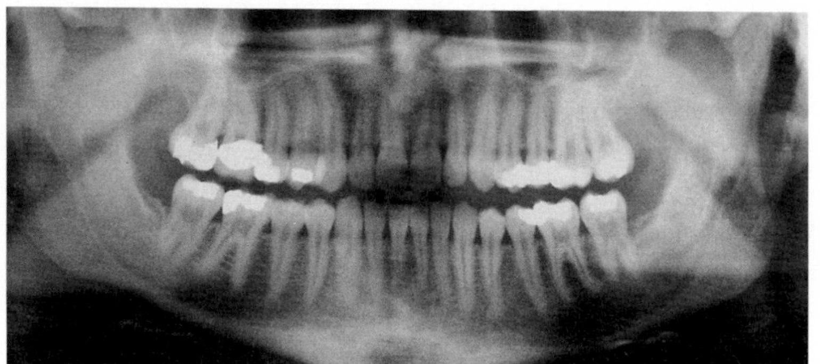

4

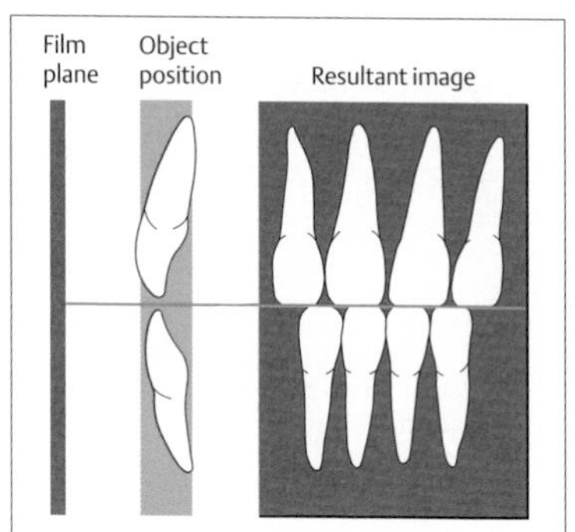
Film
plane
Object
position
Resultant image

5 a

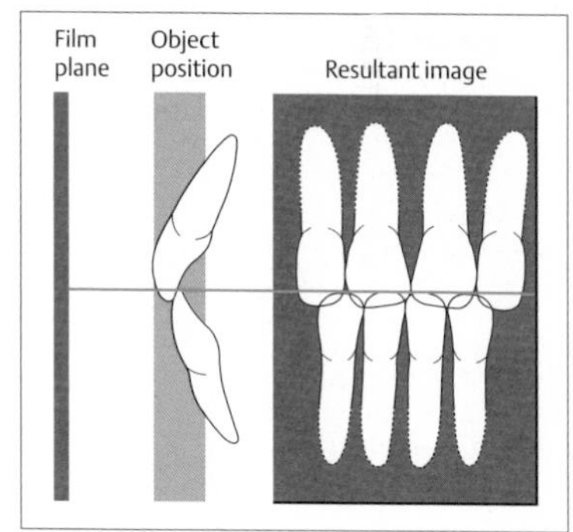
Film
plane
Object
position
Resultant image

5 b

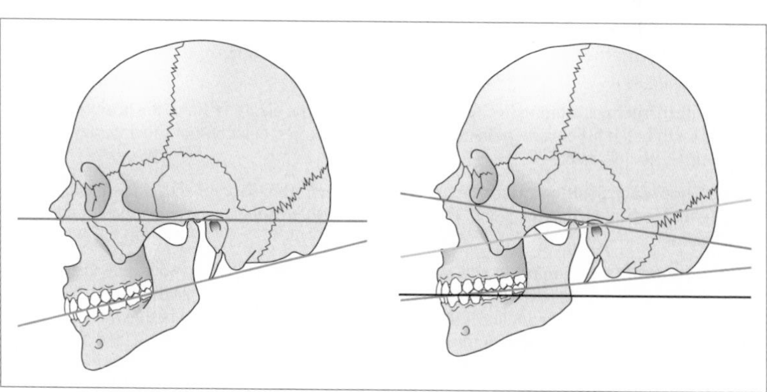

6 a

6 b

Modern panoramic imaging systems are available in various configurations with many different computer programs from which the dentist can select ones suitable for either conventional film images or digital images. The dentist can isolate a section of an image and digitally enhance it, thereby making it possible to monitor the course of treatment with a minimum of radiation exposure. Details can be enlarged and the brightness and contrast adjusted so that fewer additional exposures are needed. Intraoral radiographs are then necessary only for complementing the panoramic radiograph with individual projections for specific purposes. The most common example of this is the bite-wing radiograph for the detection of dental caries. Furthermore, because the panoramic radiograph is a two-dimensional image, it must sometimes be supplemented with additional intra- or extraoral radiographs in order to determine the exact position of an object in the third dimension. Knowledge of the myriad of radiographic diagnostic tools that are available, and use of low-dose techniques in utilizing them are essential parts in the foundation of a modern, high-quality dental practice. Since its introduction more than 50 years ago, the panoramic radiograph machine has evolved into a multifunctional panoramic tomographic imaging system with spiral attenuation. With its use, it is now possible to make high-quality transverse tomograms of the jaw in the dental office. The diagnostic value of various other programs, however, remains controversial.

Those dentists, who have the desire and ability to equip their practices with the full array of radiographic diagnostic possibilities, possess an enormous larder of radiographic diagnostic and examination possibilities that were unimaginable only a few years ago.

Fig. 7 Incorrect positioning in the anterior region. In this radiograph, the maxillary and mandibular anterior segments are positioned behind the plane of focus and therefore appear unsharp and broadened in the radiograph. The median saggital plane is obliquely positioned (note the asymmetric depiction of the zygomatic bone). The mandible is shifted toward the left. (See midline and the asymmetric depiction of the antagonistic arch segment.)

Fig. 8a Incorrect positioning in the anterior segment. The diagram shows the positioning of the anterior teeth behind the plane of focus. The result is a blurred depiction of the anterior teeth and their width is exaggerated.

Fig. 8b Improper positioning of the anterior segment. The diagram shows the positioning of the anterior teeth in front of the plane. The result is an unsharp appearance and apparent narrowing of the incisors.

Fig. 9 Incorrect positioning in the anterior segment. The maxillary and mandibular anterior segments were positioned in front of the plane of focus and the result is narrowing and blurring. In addition, the midline of the mandible is shifted to the left. Depending upon whether the skull is tilted backward or forward, the maxillary anterior anatomy may be widened or narrowed, and the mandibular anterior segment narrowed or widened in the image. Careful patient positioning is a decisive factor in determining the quality of the images of the anterior teeth and also the necessity for re-takes, which cause an unnecessary elevation of radiation exposure for the patient.

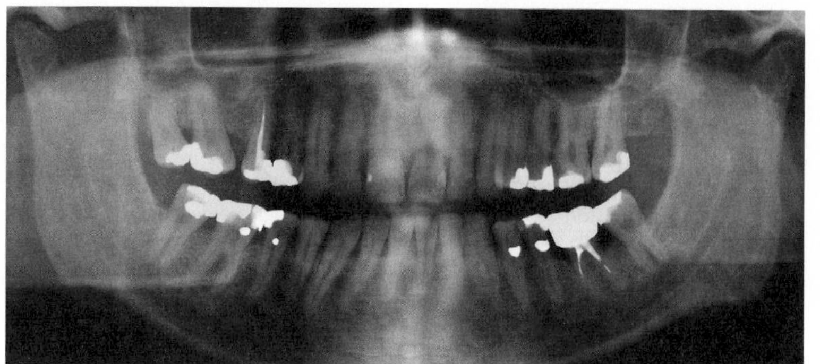

7

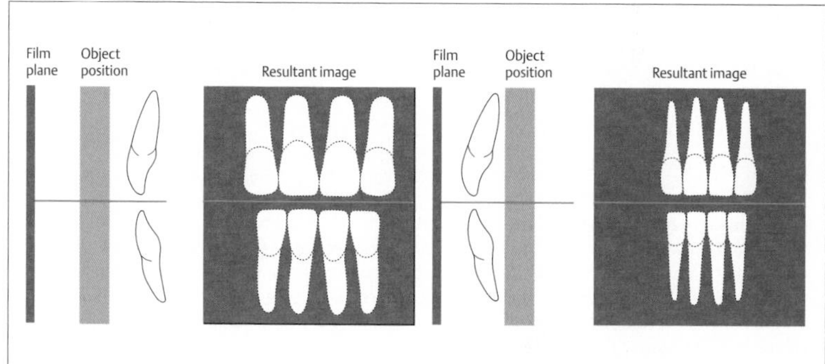
Film plane
Object position
Resultant image
Film plane
Object position
Resultant image

8 a

8 b

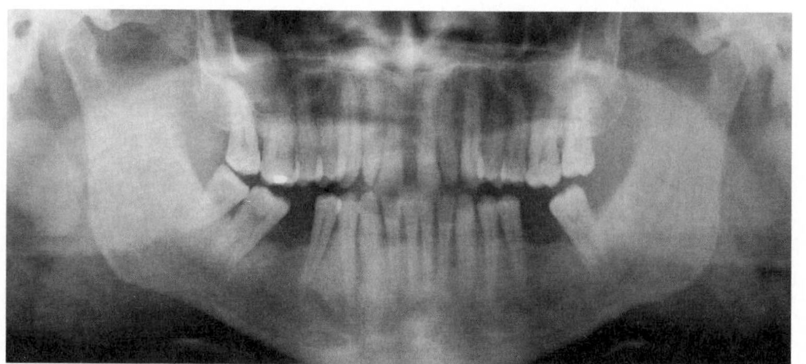

9

Panoramic radiographs (tomograms) have enriched and even revolutionized radiographic diagnostic possibilities in dental practice. In their implementation, important roles are played by the thickness of the target layer, the type of attenuation figure, and the magnification factor. The latter allows measurements to be calculated accurately. A distinction can be made between thick-layer imaging (zonography) and thin-layer imaging (tomography). Slice thickness is dependent upon the slice angle (see Fig. **1a**), which means it depends on the lengths of the paths traveled by the radiation source and the image receptor. These paths, in turn, are influenced by the attenuation figure, which is determined by technical considerations. A general premise is: the thinner the slice, the less the presence of an artifact at a given distance from the plane of focus will interfere with the interpretation of structures lying within the targeted layer, and the finer the resolution will be. However, a thinner slice does require greater exposure parameters, subjecting the patient to a higher dose of radiation. Demands for ever higher image quality carry not only a noticeably higher monetary price, but also necessitates special technical skills. Furthermore, the desired image quality is achieved not only through technical finesse but also, to a certain extent, through greater precision in positioning the targeted structures within the layer predetermined by the apparatus. Under these circumstances it is easy to understand that the preparation of qualitatively high-value radiographs demands, in addition to perfect technical knowledge and clinically consistent routine, above all perfect knowledge of craniofacial anatomy, which can only then be practically applied. The effective use of a high-performance panoramic unit is, in addition, extremely time-intensive, and this is frequently underestimated in the daily scheduling of a clinic or a private practice.

Fig 10 Improper positioning of the skull. With the head tipped back during exposure, the occlusal plane and the radiopacity from the palate and the floor of the nasal cavities appear as an inverted saucer. In such a case, the apices of the roots of the maxillary teeth will be more or less obscured by intervening bone. The roots of the maxillary anterior teeth will often appear extremely widened. In the mixed dentition stage, this type of incorrect positioning prevents observation of the permanent tooth buds in the maxilla (see Fig. **21**).

Fig. 11a Improper positioning of the skull. The diagram shows the skull tilted posteriorly, which often occurs inadvertently during correction of the cephalostat upward in an already correctly positioned patient. In comparison to a horizontal plane (**black**), the occlusal plane (**green**), and the Camper plane (**yellow**) sink dorsally, and the result is superimpositioning onto the maxilla of the palate and the floor of the nose. Especially in children in the early mixed dentition stage, this type of improper positioning leads to overshadowing of the permanent tooth buds in the maxilla, and prevents their evaluation.

Fig. 11b Improper positioning of the skull. The diagram shows the skull tipped forward, which is often caused by the lowering of the cephalostat in an already properly positioned patient. In comparison to the true horizontal (**black**), the occlusal plane (**green**) and the Camper plane (**yellow**) tip upward dorsally. The proximal surfaces of the maxillary posterior teeth overlap and the temporomandibular joints are usually not completely depicted. On the other hand, using this approach, the apical regions of the roots and the nasopalatine space can be well observed. In the early mixed dentition stage, maxillary tooth buds can be more clearly depicted.

Fig. 12 Improper positioning of the skull. In this panoramic radiograph, taken with the skull tipped forward, the occlusal plane appears saucer-shaped. With this positioning, the temporomandibular joints are frequently incompletely depicted. The mandibular ramus, and especially the proximal surfaces of premolars, are obscured by interfering shadows, while the nasopalatine region is depicted with no superimposed shadows except for that created by the tip of the nose.

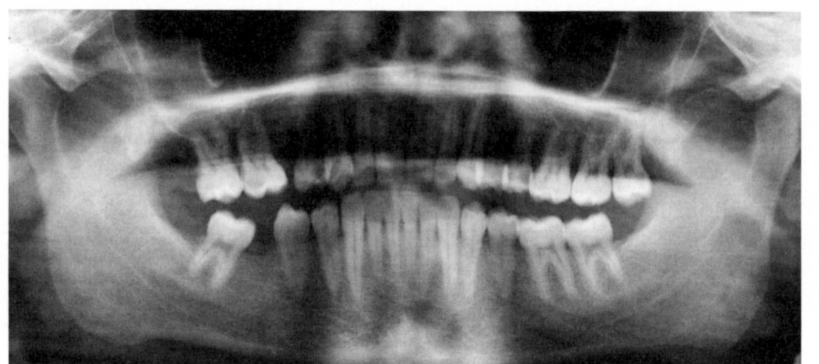

10

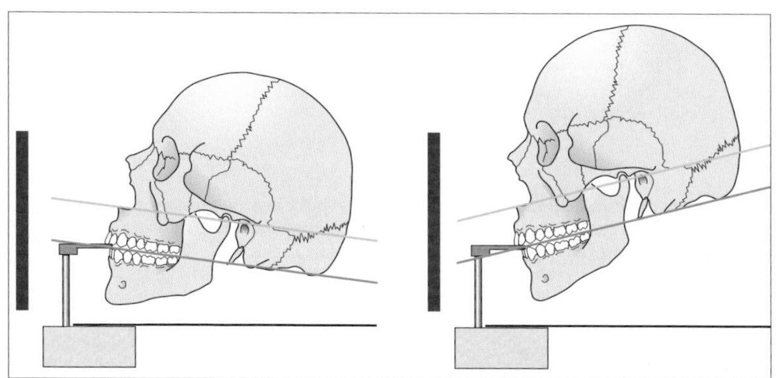

11 a 11 b

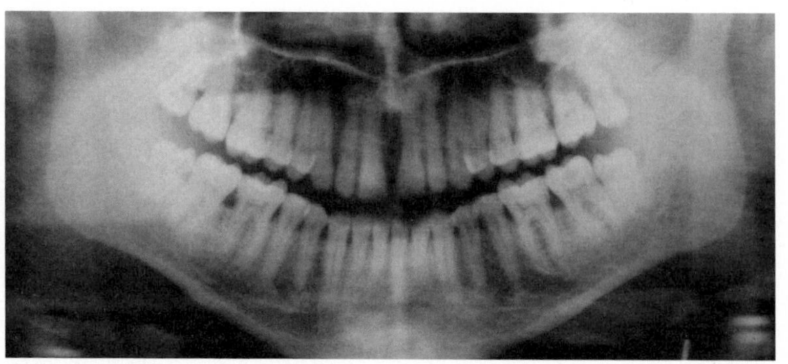

12

Panoramic radiographs represent zonographies (or thick-layer images), with layer thicknesses that change during the exposure, combined with a slot technique. For a clearer depiction of the anterior region, especially in elderly patients, the shadowing caused by the radiopaque cervical vertebrate must be reduced by lowering the speed of motion of the radiation head or by elevating the exposure setting during the procedure. Depending upon the manufacturer, layer thickness varies from about 9 mm in the anterior segments up to ca. 20 mm in the region of the TMJ. By employing this technique of "arch-form layer thickness determination," the jaws and the dental arches can be depicted two-dimensionally in a single image.

Within this predetermined (or minimally adjustable) layer thickness, the desired structures of the jaw must be properly positioned. This begins with a centric and controlled positioning of the patient within the panoramic unit. The varying anatomy of the jaws within the individual architecture of the facial skeleton is manifest as a variable angle between the Frankfort horizontal plane and the occlusal plane; this must be carefully considered in order to achieve optimum depiction of the teeth. Of additional importance is positioning of the median saggital plane for a symmetrical depiction of both sides at each jaw.

Fig. 13 Panoramic radiograph depicting periodontal bone loss. This picture clearly shows that advanced bone loss can be depicted in a panoramic radiograph that offers not only a clear overview of the entire situation, but also a *uniform* overall projection; contrariwise, the use of individual, intraoral periapical image receptors, even using the parallel technique, is associated with differing angles of central ray projection in the various segments of the dental arch. To obtain a perfect panoramic radiograph, it is important for the patient to press the tongue against the roof of the mouth, and to have the occlusal plane parallel to the horizontal but never tipped dorsally. For periodontal patients, complete depiction of the chin region and/or the TMJs is less critical. The observation/diagnosis of secondary alterations within the condyle-fossa relationships in conjunction with generalized periodontal bone loss can only be achieved with a panoramic image taken in habitual occlusion.

Fig. 14a Diagram of the technique. From the lateral aspect, the occlusal plane should be tipped only slightly dorsally, in order to avoid any superimposition (overlapping) in the interdental areas. Attention must also be given to the positioning of the Camper plane (nasoauricular plane, **yellow**).

Fig. 14b Diagram of the technique. As previously described, the symmetric horizontal and vertical positioning of the skull is of prime importance for perfect radiographic depiction and diagnostic interpretation. Here also, a critical consideration is the positioning of the median sagittal plane in the projection axis of the panoramic device. It is critically important to check the positioning from the dorsal aspect, in order to avoid an asymmetric depiction in the final result.

Fig. 15 Panoramic radiograph of periodontal bone loss. This image provides an additional example for the use of panoramic radiography to clearly reveal the extent of advanced and generalized periodontal diseases. Noteworthy in this radiograph is the shift of the mandibular midline toward the right and the resultant slightly asymmetric depiction of the opposing jaw, but in this image this does not compromise diagnostic clarity. If, however, distortion or lack of clarity in the anterior segments occurs due to superimposition of the cervical vertebrate, a targeted intraoral, periapical radiograph can be taken. This entire procedure lowers the overall radiation dose when one considers that the exposure dose with a panoramic radiograph does not exceed that of about four periapical exposures.

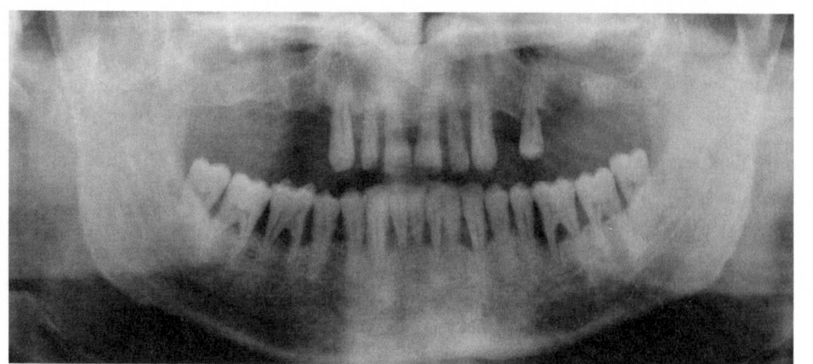

13

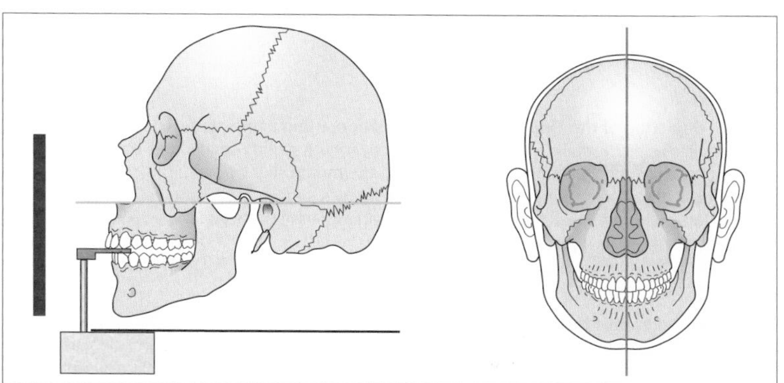

14 a

14 b

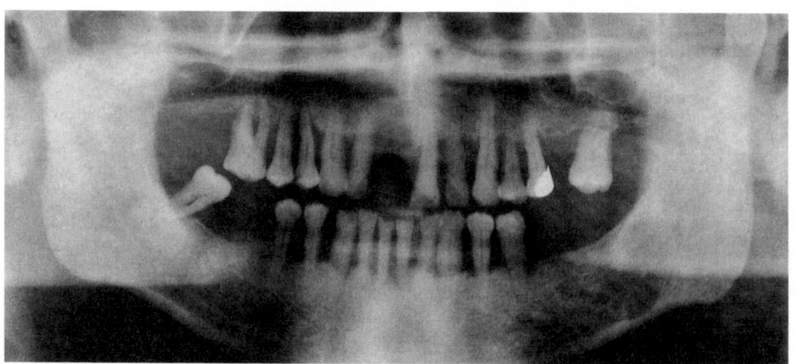

15

For various and diagnosis-specific indications, one can modify the standard positioning of the skull in the panoramic radiographic unit. A thorough understanding of the apparently simple but in reality quite complex patient positioning begins with the taking of panoramic radiographs in the "normal position," in adults with normal interocclusal relationships, and is then further developed with growing experience to include a thorough understanding of individual and indication-targeted special approaches.

The decision to take panoramic radiographs with other than standard/normal patient positioning can only be made by the dentist after a comprehensive initial clinical examination and the elucidation of clear indications for any necessary nonstandard projections.

Taking a standard panoramic radiograph in the normal position can be described as follows:

- The patient is informed about the function and movements of the radiographic unit in order to motivate the patient to the highest level of cooperation.
- The patient is requested to remove eyeglasses and jewelry, partial denture prostheses made of metal, any piercing jewelry or hairpins, and finally to open any metal zippers in the neck region.

Fig. 16 Depiction of the TMJs in the normal position, using a bite plane. The panoramic radiograph is taken using the standard projection. With the mouth slightly opened, the condyles exhibit a varying position during the opening motion. With the mouth slightly open, the condyles are projected free of any superimposed osseous structures, which permits observation of the morphology, the function, and sometimes even pathognomonic alterations of the heads of the condyles. Any radiographic analysis of the occlusion in conjunction with the TMJs is, however, only possible with projections taken in habitual occlusion. This image depicts signs of arthrosis (left) with osseous apposition and osteophytes, as well as limitation of the opening movement (right).

Fig. 17 Radiographic technique in habitual occlusion. This diagram shows the proper positioning in habitual occlusion, with slight dorsal tipping of the occlusal plane. When positioning the patient in the device, the clinician must observe the position of the Camper plane. If the projection angle is too steep, the joints will appear abnormally cranial, and with a down projection dorsally the joints will be projected laterally. It is better to position the anterior segment in front of rather than behind the projection plane. Because the entire TMJ in a panoramic radiograph is superimposed by the medial wall of the joint fossa, consisting of the styloid process and the border of the temporal tympanic bone, the TMJ cannot be clearly depicted; in practice it is only the positional relationship between the posterior edge of the articular tubercule and the anterior segment of the condyle (**4**) that provide information for the recognition of secondary arthropathies (see p. 235). Improper position of the condyle, either anteriorly or posteriorly, can then only be assumed with any certainty if the radiograph has been taken symmetrically. The ascertainment of symmetry can be performed via the position of the median saggital plane (**1**), the length of both halves of the mandible (**2**), and the shape and position of the superimposition caused by the opposing arch segments (**3**).

Fig. 18 Depiction of the TMJs in habitual occlusion. This is the same case as depicted above (Fig. **16**), to compare the second radiograph, which was taken in habitual occlusion. In this image one also sees that the left condyle exhibits arthrosis with bone apposition, which ends anteriorly in an osteophyte (the so-called *crow's beak*). Observation of this panoramic radiograph taken in habitual occlusion leads to suspicion of a disk lesion as the expression of the pathologic condition on the left side. The limited mouth opening on the right side can be interpreted as a "protective position," if the necessary clinical information is available. Clinically, it was possible to diagnose an acute arthritis leading to inhibition in jaw opening (see Fig. **16**).

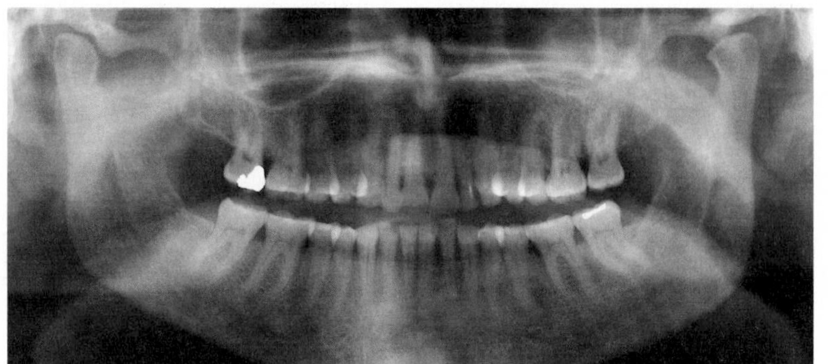

16

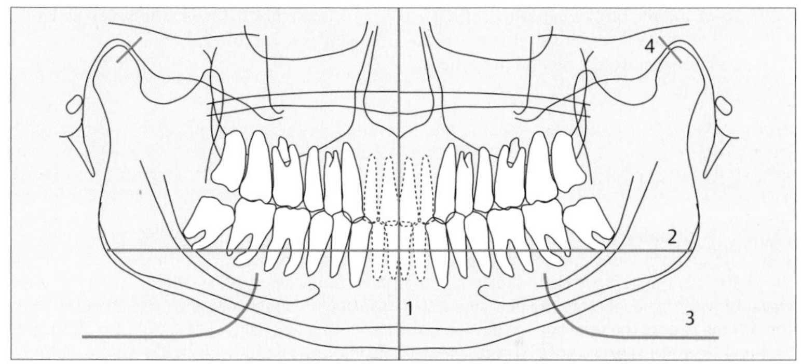

17

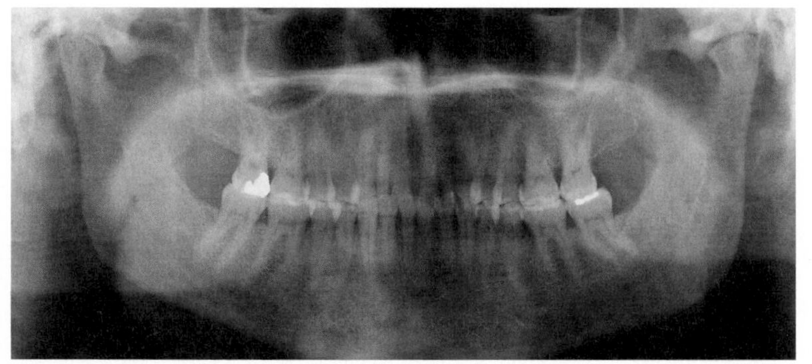

18

- Explain to the patient the functions of the control mirror and the bite block.
- Point out to the patient the markings on the floor upon which the patient must be positioned in order to be centered in the unit.
- Explain the correct body position ("sway-back," with loose, drooping shoulders).
- Have the patient demonstrate and practice the proper tongue position (see p. **17**).
- Explain to the patient not to breathe deeply during the exposure, but rather to breathe lightly and normally (see Fig. **33**).
- Make it absolutely clear to the patient that during the exposure neither the head nor the mandible in the bite plate must be moved (see Fig. **31**).
- Before positioning the patient in the apparatus, always first select the appropriate program and the proper exposure settings.
- Place the protective apron with the prescribed lead-equivalent around the patient, making certain that there are no gaps around the neck that could hinder the translation of the apparatus of the unit around the head.
- The patient is now positioned in the apparatus, with the neck stretched and a loose shoulder position. The patient must hold tightly to the handgrips.
- Establish the height of the bite block so that the patient's anterior teeth engage the groove in the bite block **without nodding or raising the head**, and with a horizontal orientation of both the occlusal plane and the Camper plane (spina nasalis-Tragion plane) (see Fig. **11 a**, **b**).
- The orientation of the Camper plane and therewith also the position of the occlusal plane are then corrected, *slightly* dorsally inclined. It must never, however, sink dorsally (see Fig. **14a**).

Fig. 19 Positioning in early childhood. Taking a panoramic radiograph of a child will require patient positioning that deviates somewhat from the normal position for adults. The occlusal plane and therewith also the Camper plane should be positioned somewhat more steeply, in order to permit clear vision of the location of the permanent tooth buds, i. e., to prevent superposition of the structures of the floor of the nose and the palatal roof. To insure a high quality radiograph, it is also important that the tongue position be correct, and this can only be achieved with children using appropriate patience! From the lateral viewpoint it must be kept in mind that the primordia of the permanent dentition lie high and behind the deciduous teeth. If the deciduous teeth are aligned in the focal plane, the permanent tooth buds, especially the anterior teeth, will appear enlarged and, depending upon distance from the focal plane, will appear more or less blurred and distorted. When taking a panoramic radiograph of a small child, it is prudent to position the vertical, lateral light guide at the level of the deciduous canines.

Fig. 20a Position of the tooth buds from the frontal view. The schematic illustrates that the permanent tooth buds in a 5-year-old child develop dorsal to the deciduous teeth.

Fig. 20b Location of the tooth buds from the lateral view. The schematic illustrates the position of the permanent tooth buds in relationship to the anterior teeth of the deciduous dentition.

Fig. 21 Positioning error in a patient traversing early mixed dentition age. This panoramic radiograph exhibits a typical patient positioning error, with a dorsally tipping occlusal plane, superposition of the palatal roof and the floor of the nasal sinus, apparent widening of the maxillary anterior teeth, a flat mandibular angle, and laterally projected TMJs. This type of patient positioning error with the head tipped backward frequently occurs if the cephalostat is positioned further upward after the patient is already positioned and without consideration for the position of the Camper plane. Images taken in this way frequently appear under-exposed because of the radiopacity of the superposed structures, despite proper selection of the exposure settings.

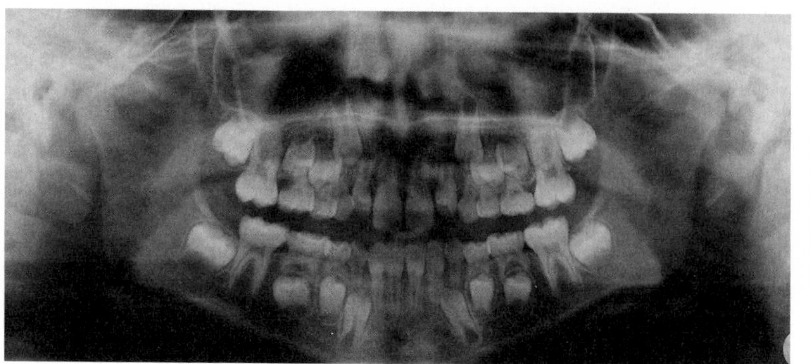

19

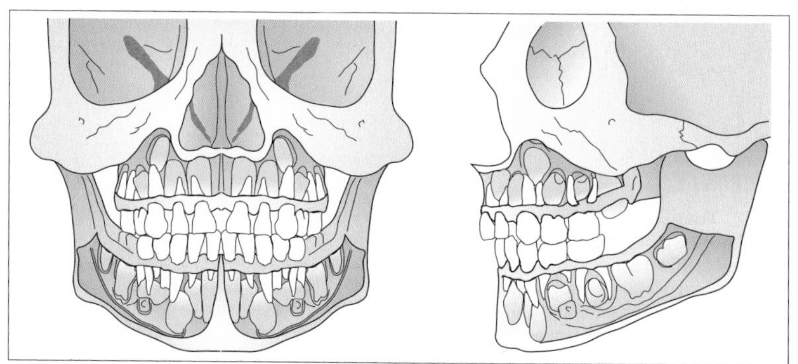

20 a 20 b

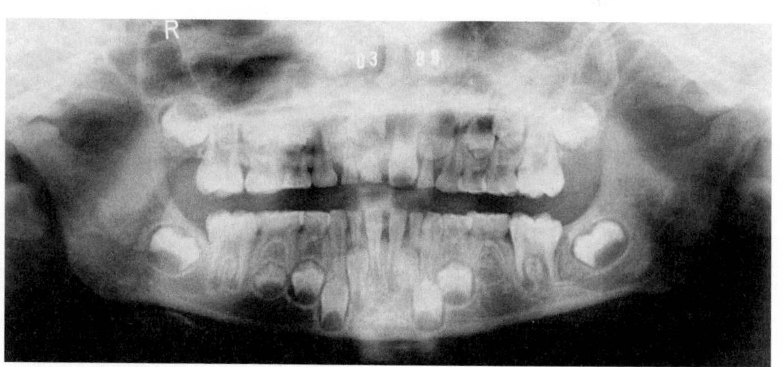

21

- From this moment on, the height of the bite plane should not be further adjusted (see Fig. **11a** and **b**, and the corresponding figure legends).
- Finally, check the positioning of the anterior dental segments using the lateral and vertical light guides, and orient it to the lateral incisors.
- Using the swing-out mirror, one checks the adjustment of the median saggital plane in the device, and then checks its position on the back of the head. **Note:** The application of the so-called "head holder" does not by any means guarantee that the median saggital plane on the back of the head is not tilted toward the side thus creating "technical asymmetries," which can obfuscate diagnostic observations (see Fig. **25**).
- After telling the patient "Please don't move, and breathe normally," the start switch is pressed.
- The patient should be observed during the entire exposure by auxiliary personnel who are appropriately protected from radiation.

Fig. 22 Improper tongue position during panoramic radiography. One observes in this radiograph that the roots of the maxillary teeth, the structures of the maxilla, and the boundaries of the nasal and maxillary sinuses are scarcely discernable because air, a "negative contrast substance," has effectively obliterated them. Radiation that passes through air-containing spaces is not dampened, rather it over-irradiates structures in the path of the central ray and effectively effaces such structures from the final result. This effect, which is known as the "**burn-out effect**" in radiographs of the teeth, can be avoided if the tongue is pressed firmly against the palate during the exposure; the tongue thus acts as a radiation-diminishing filter. Breathing deeply or holding the breath during the period of exposure causes an effacement of the structures of the angle of the mandible and the ascending ramus (see Fig. **33**).

Fig. 23a Radiograph technique using the tongue position as a filter. If the tongue is not pressed onto the palate (**pink**), but rather only onto the palatal surfaces of the maxillary anterior teeth (**blue**), there exists between the dorsum of the tongue and the palatal roof an air-containing space, which does not dampen radiation, leading to obliteration or effacement of maxillary structures.

Fig. 23b Radiographic technique for edentulous patients or those wearing complete dentures. In edentulous patients, the thin alveolar ridge of the maxilla, in contrast to the dense bone of the mandible, is usually over-irradiated and rendered invisible. In such cases, it is recommended to leave the complete denture in situ, and to employ the tongue as a filter in order to render the maxillary structures visible.

Fig. 24 Panoramic radiograph, tongue in proper position. The radiograph depicted above (Fig. **22**) was re-taken, but with the tongue in the proper position. This dampened the irradiation and permitted clear observation of all maxillary structures and the roots of the teeth. It has proven effective to have the patient practice achieving proper tongue position before placing the patient in the unit; this can prevent nondiagnostic results and also prevent unnecessary repetition of the radiographic exposure.

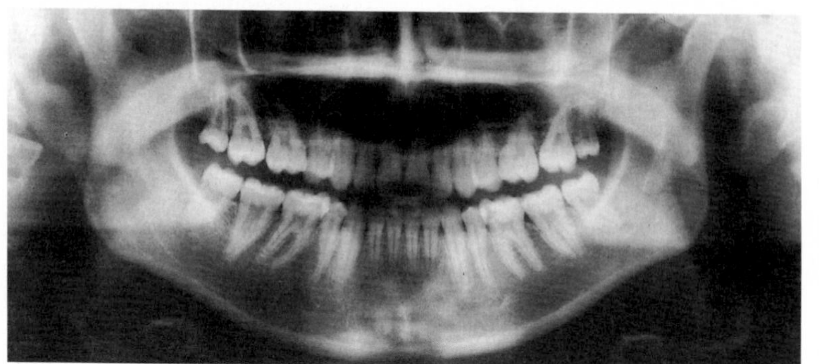

22

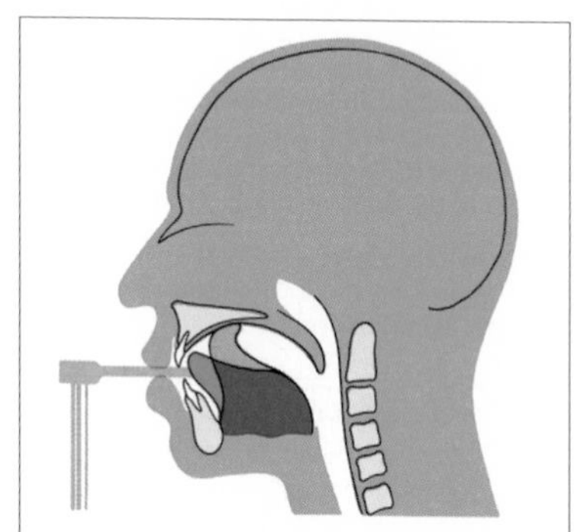

23 a

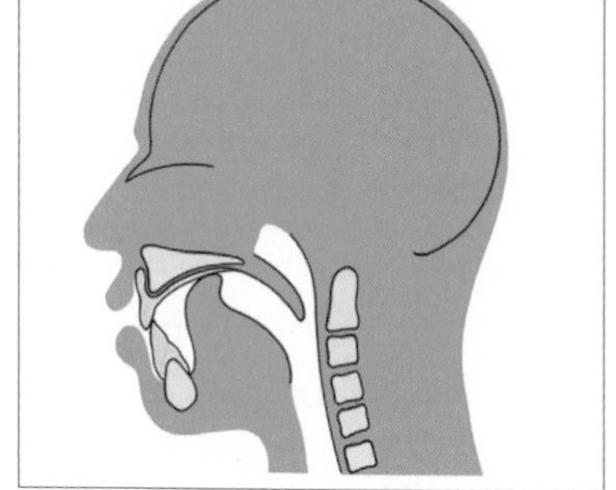

23 b

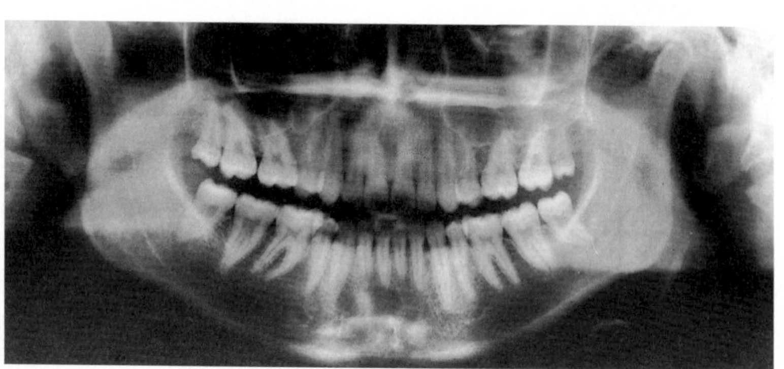

24

Fig. 25 Asymmetric positioning errors. This panoramic view resulted from asymmetric positioning with incomplete jaw closure, resulting in apparent enlargement of the right side ramus and zygomatic bone, which are far lingual in the focal plane. A visual left-to-right comparison reveals that the right side of the mandible appears elongated, and the posterior teeth of both mandible and maxilla on this side appear enlarged, and they overlap each other. The furcations of the right mandibular molars exhibit "enamel pearls" due to the overlapping.

Fig. 26a Improper positioning of the median saggital plane. The less than perpendicularly (**black**) positioned median saggital plane (**red**) leads to a varying overlapping effect of the opposing arch and to apparent widening of the far lingually positioned mandibular angle on the left side, with apparent enlargement.

Fig. 26b Improper positioning of the median saggital plane. The median saggital plane (**black**) appears to be properly positioned after checking the mirror, but without additional checking from the *dorsal* aspect it can deviate to one side or the other (**red**). Carefully checking the position of the median saggital plane cannot be neglected even if an effective head holder device is used. Otherwise, side-to-side comparisons will often exhibit asymmetric depiction of the vertebrate as well as apparent enlargement of the half of the facial skeleton depicted behind the plane of focus.

Fig. 27 Evaluation of achieved radiograph quality. In many cases, all of the details and criteria depicted here schematically cannot be found in a single panoramic radiograph; for this reason numerous aspects of radiographic quality are illustrated. In addition, experience has demonstrated that improper positioning in routine daily practice is only slowly realized and even seldom noticed early on; for these reasons, constant self-critique to maintain and elevate radiographic quality is necessary, and also to reduce radiation exposure. It is of course obvious that the evaluative possibilities depicted in this "case" will not be applicable to connatal asymmetries of the skull and the facial skeleton.

1a The connection line between the two points is drawn through the deepest point of the articular eminence, and provides in normal cases information about whether improper positioning with oblique position of the median saggital plane has occurred.

1b The line connecting the two red dots is drawn through the deepest part of the innominate line of the *Facies temporalis* of the zygomatic bone and the maxilla, and also provides information about the horizontal positioning of the skull and the position of the median saggital plane.

1c In normal cases, this line is perpendicular to 1a and 1b, and also demonstrates the vertical positioning of the median saggital plane.

2a Bilateral comparison of the width of the ascending mandibular ramus exhibits an asymmetric positioning of the entire skull, or nearly lateral displacement of the mandible.

2b A comparison of the distance between the midline of the mandible to the dorsal border of the ascending ramus also provides information about any asymmetric positioning of the skull or of the mandible, and will be obvious through apparent lateral displacement of the mandibular midline.

3a,b The centric or asymmetrical presentation of the radiolucency through the atlantooccipital articulation and the centric or laterally displaced radiopacity caused by the cervical vertebrate demonstrate that the median saggital plane was laterally positioned improperly in the dorsal aspect.

4 A bilateral comparison of the apparent teeth sizes in the maxilla with asymmetric positioning of the skull and the mandible is also an indication of improper patient positioning.

5 If a side-to-side comparison reveals different depictions of the overlap by the opposing arch, this is also evidence of an asymmetric and improper positioning of the skull and/or the mandible.

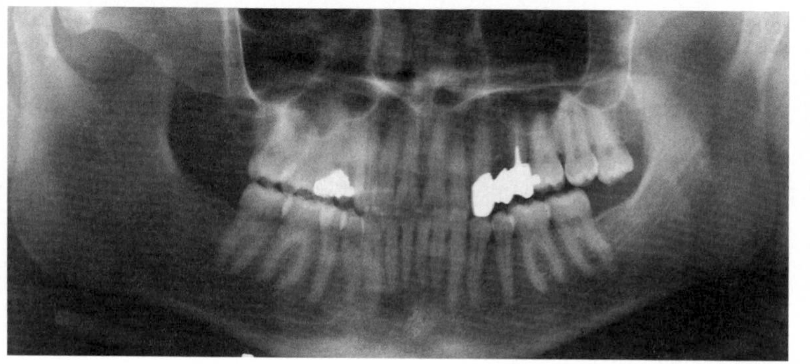
25

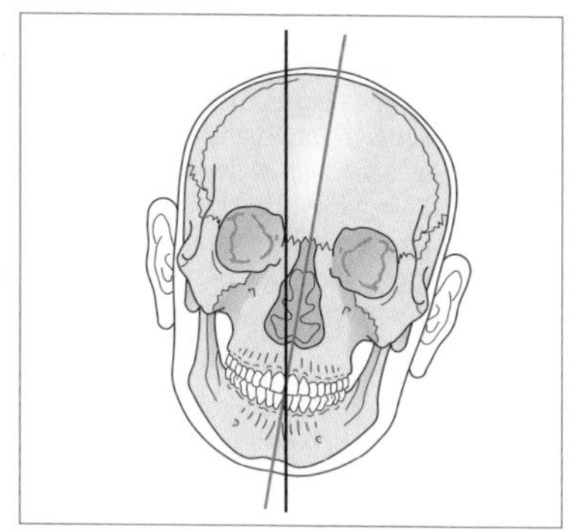
26 a

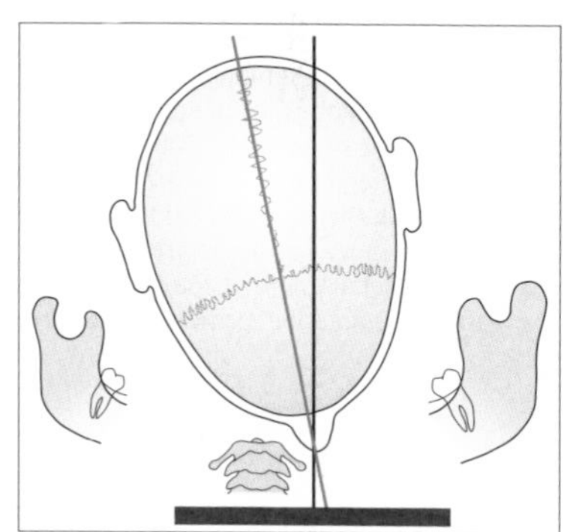
26 b

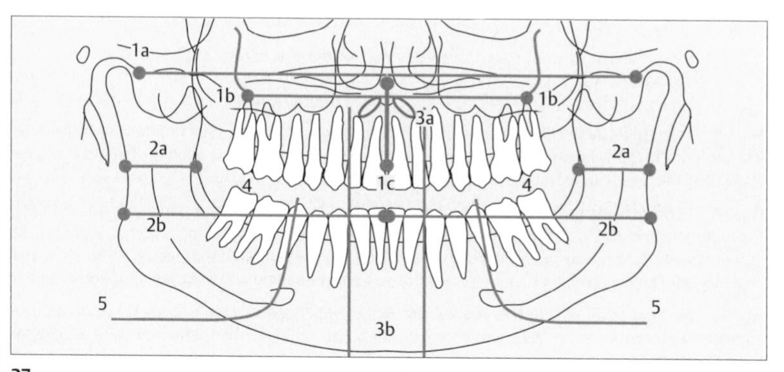

27

On the basis of standard panoramic radiography with the patient in the normal position, it is possible in some cases and with specific indications to modify the procedure described on p. **12**, in order to provide appropriate radiographic documentation with optimum quality for any particular clinical circumstance. Even in the face of extreme occlusal relationships within Class II it is important to note that in many patients who attempt to bring maxillary and mandibular anterior teeth into an edge-to-edge relationship by forcing the mandible forward, the head will be unintentionally tipped forward. This causes the occlusal plane (or the Camper plane) into a dorsally tipped position, which can lead to less than diagnostic pictures. On the other hand, patients exhibiting a Class III occlusion will attempt to retrude the mandible, which can cause the head to be unintentionally tipped forward, also resulting in nondiagnostic radiographs. If the main desire is to prepare a panoramic radiograph with accurate overall depiction including proper positioning of the occlusal plane, it may be necessary to sacrifice radiographic detail in either the maxillary or the mandibular anterior segment. If the main goal is to sharply depict the anterior teeth, it will be necessary to accept a less-than-ideal depiction of all other structures, or to subsequently employ other standard projection techniques to achieve a perfect depiction of the anterior segments. Special modifications to portray generalized periodontal bone loss or secondary alterations of the TMJ elicited by occlusal disturbances, and also even with small children, show the many possibilities offered by the panoramic radiographic device. **Quality assurance and quality control** serve in the clinic and private practice to preserve radiographic quality at a high level and with a low failure rate, coupled with low exposure dose for each patient; this can only occur in combination with continuous self-critique or quality-control mechanisms (see Fig. **27**). Nevertheless, with the preparation of panoramic radiographs, a failure rate of about 10% must be tolerated because here—in contrast to computed tomography scans (CT)—one does not have the advantage of an orienting tomogram (scout or pathfinder) nor the opportunity to select individual sections by marking upon the screen the exact positioning of the patient.

Fig. 28 Foreign body within the central ray. This radiograph reveals stark radiopacity in the anterior segment of both jaws elicited by jewelry (piercing) perforating the tongue (behind the focal plane) and the lower lip (in front of the plane, cf. Fig. **3a**).

Fig. 29 Foreign body within the central ray. The ear ring, which was not removed prior to taking the radiograph, is viewed on the right side as higher, enlarged and out of focus because the central ray coursed from below and upwards. In this case (luckily!) the completely impacted tooth 29, with a follicular cyst, in the maxillary tuberosity was not superimposed and was therefore also not missed.

Fig. 30 Foreign body within the central ray. Metal zippers on women's dresses, necklaces, and improperly positioned protective lead vest (folds near the neck), or the metal frames of eyeglasses will also cause disturbing superimposition effects, which often necessitate re-taking the radiograph, which brings with it additional radiation exposure.

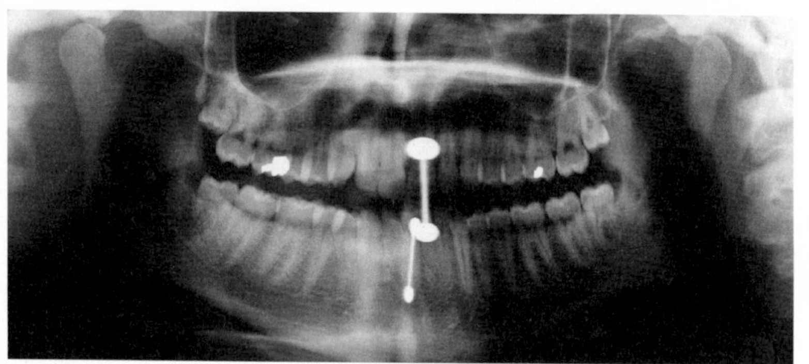

28

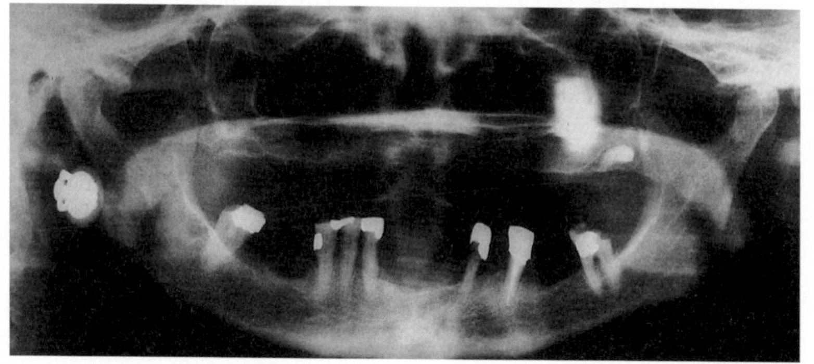

29

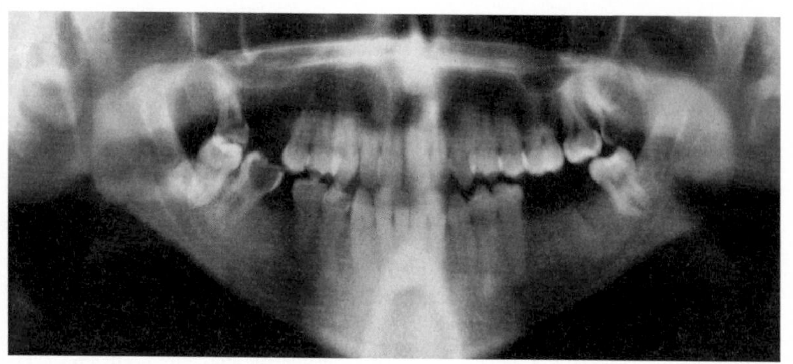

30

It is certainly true that as one gains experience the clinical technique of panoramic radiography becomes routine; however, it is also possible that "tolerances" may sneak in with time, and become manifest as radiographic failure in the sense of less-than-perfect or even nondiagnostic images. In order to achieve a high standard and to maintain that standard, an uncompromising and continuous self-critique is necessary. More than any equipment improvements or technical progress, it is the consequential performance of self-critique that brings and guarantees a reduction of radiation dose to that which is absolutely necessary to achieve the desired radiographic quality. The most important goal is to employ a low-radiation examination strategy, coupled with optimum clinical technique, to ensure minimum irradiation for each patient. Government and professional regulations demand periodic continuing education for personnel, and re-standardization of radiographic equipment. In addition, the authors of this book strongly suggest periodic evaluation of clinical techniques to ensure radiographic quality. In today's modern dental practice and using state-of-the-art equipment, it is possible to *store* ideal radiographic projections and also failure resulting from improper patient positioning in the computer for future reference, which can enhance the constancy of effective self-critique.

Furthermore, nondiagnostic images may also result from radiopaque foreign bodies outside the plane of focus, because these cannot be suppressed using the thick-layer panoramic radiography technique; thus, they become "projected onto" the structures of interest within the plane of focus (see p. **169**). In addition, movement of the head or even movement of the mandible, as well as an incorrect breathing technique (see Fig. **33**) during exposure will elicit artifacts and therefore a significant reduction of radiographic (diagnostic) quality.

Fig. 31 Asymmetric depiction. If the median saggital plane is not symmetrically positioned before the exposure, and also checked from the dorsal aspect, or if the skull moves horizontally during the exposure, a radiographically nondiagnostic image will be the result, and the radiograph will have to be re-taken.

Fig. 32 Movement during exposure. If the patient moves the mandible during exposure, the radiograph will depict what appears to be a transverse fracture of the mandible. Note here the depiction of tooth 48 and the "step" on the right side, and compare this with the depiction of the deep collum fracture (left). If the patient moves the entire head during the exposure, artifacts and distortions will be visible within the entire picture, effecting both jaws and all vertically adjacent structures.

Fig. 33 The influence of breathing on radiographic quality. Deep breathing before exposure and holding the breath during the exposure can lead to an extremely air-filled epipharynx which can distort or obscure the ascending mandibular rami, and affect a more or less complete radiographic obliteration of the osseous structures. Before starting the exposure, the patient must be instructed to continue breathing slowing and normally during the entire time the apparatus is in motion; this is critical to avoid unacceptable (nondiagnostic) radiographs.

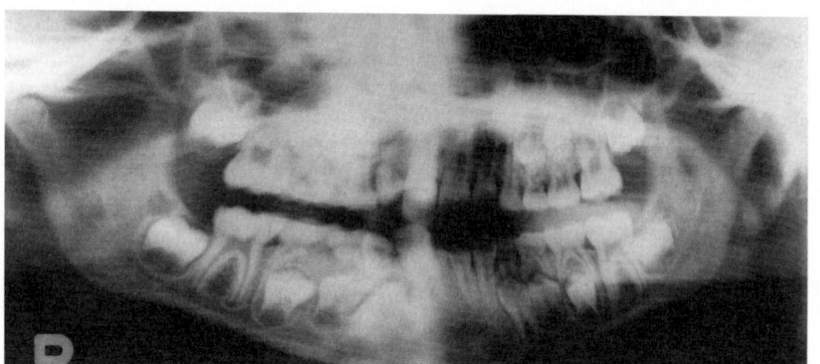

31

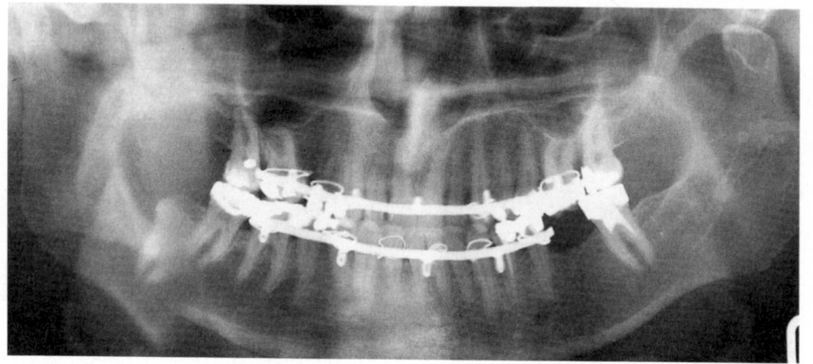

32

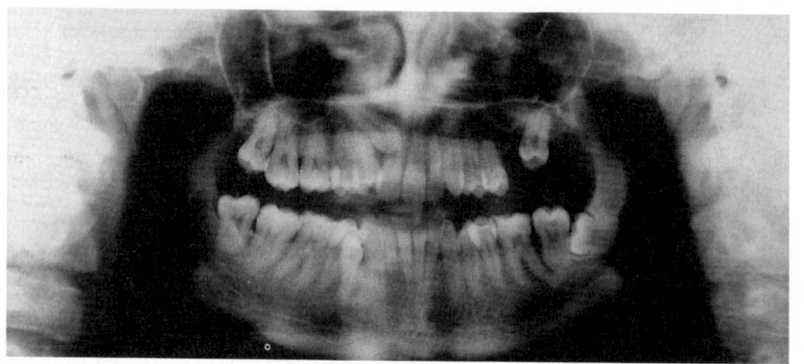

33

Numerous variations of the normal projection technique for panoramic radiography can be applied for indication-specific needs; these will often involve modifications of patient positioning. Modified programs make possible not only a targeted radiographic overview in the mixed dentition stage, but also low-radiation segment projections of jaw areas, which can be very useful for post-therapeutic check-up. Supplementary programs also make possible depiction of the TMJs in both frontal and lateral aspects, with multi-layering; these can, however, not be used for any functional evaluation in habitual occlusion, rather only for depiction of the morphology of the condular hard tissues and a purely radiographic (anatomic) diagnosis. Radiolucent tissue such as the articular disk can only be successfully examined using magnetic resonance imaging (MRI, see p. **237**). Panoramic radiographic depiction of the maxillary sinus is seldom necessary, and there remains controversy about the quality of panoramic radiographs for this purpose. For the oral surgeon, however, it is extremely important that the radiographic equipment include supplementary programs for transversal layered projections of the jaws, to permit before-and-after comparisons following osseous surgical interventions, including three-dimensional evaluation (see p. **27**). Such radiographic equipment can be used to precisely determine the position of impacted teeth vis-à-vis the mandibular canal and the maxillary sinuses, or the amount of bone available prior to placement of dental implants, as well as the orofacial expanse of intraosseous lesions.

The production of optimal transverse slice radiographs requires that the appropriate technical settings be made and that great care be taken in positioning the patient correctly. The greater the slice angle, i.e., the longer the path of the cone and the image receptor (IR) during exposure, the more free of superimposition (overlapping) will be the individual tissues in the selected sections (see Fig. **1b**).

Fig. 34 Segment projection with reduced radiation dose. The radiograph shown here was taken primarily to check the developing dentition, and was made using a reduced level of irradiation. It represents the numerous technical possibilities for low-dose segment projections such as, for example, unilateral or isolated TMJ depictions. Unilateral or anterior depictions are especially necessary and indicated diagnostically during or following treatment as control radiographs; simultaneously, such limited projections reduce the radiation load to the patient.

Fig. 35 Temporomandibular joint radiograph using linear zonography in the multi-layer procedure. Lateral multi-layer projections of the TMJ in habitual occlusion and with maximum mouth opening. Lacking in such isolated depictions of the TMJ, however, is the relationship of the joint itself to the patient's habitual occlusion, and this is an element of radiographic diagnosis that is particularly important and of clinical significance.

Fig. 36 Temporomandibular joint radiograph using linear zonography in the multi-layer procedure. Multi-layer depiction of the TMJ in the frontal plane. As these images illustrate, capturing an excellent depiction in the frontal plane is not always easy in practice. For example, in this case thorough interpretation of the anatomic situation is hindered by the fact that the lateral extremity of the condyle is not completely depicted.

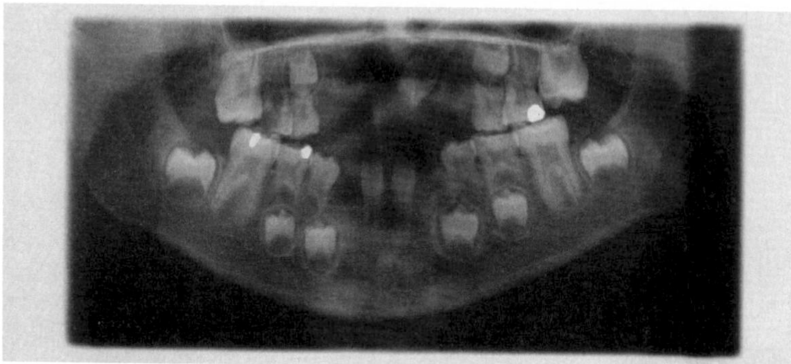

34

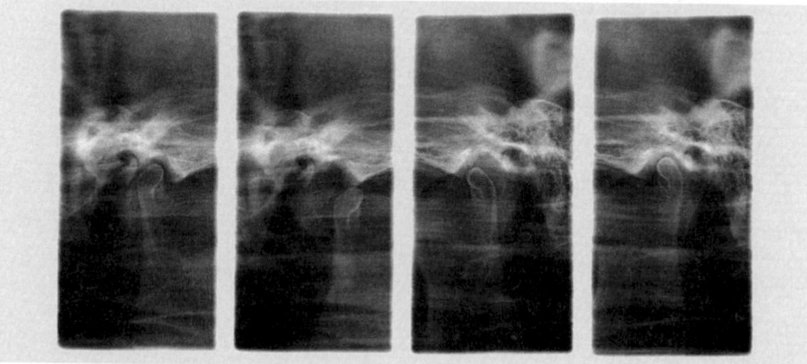

35

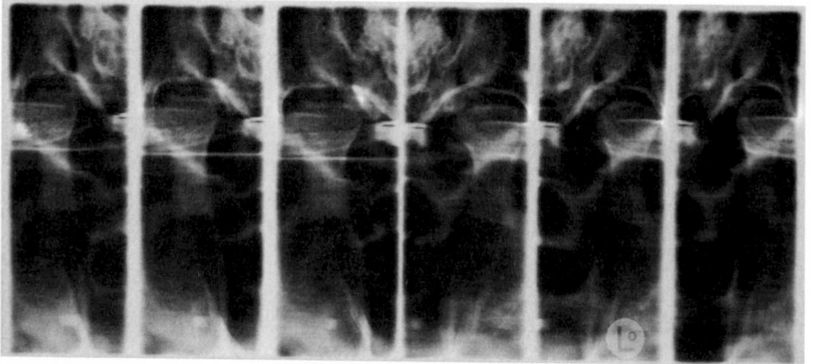

36

The tight pattern of movement in spiral tomography is clearly superior to the linear path used in most tomography machines in that it more effectively suppresses volumetric artifacts (see Fig. **1b**). An important consideration, however, is the unfortunately frequently observed overexposure, through which the relatively poor resolution of conventional tomography is only rendered poorer. In comparison to the DENT-programs of computer tomography or CBT (cone beam tomography), it is not possible to achieve enlargements in the ideal 1:1 relationship, whereby a less-than-perfect positioning of the desired structures of the maxilla or mandible in the predetermined plane represent an essential problem, namely that measurements corresponding to the actual relationships are frequently impossible to achieve.

In all of these technical procedures, the central problem is that the patient and the structures of interest must be precisely positioned in a predetermined plane, and this demands faultless knowledge of anatomy, as well as well-practiced clinical routine.

With regard to the quality of a panoramic radiograph optimally prepared via spiral tomography, innovative developments are unlikely to be forthcoming from new procedures deriving from conventional tomography. For today's practitioner the new, digital microcomputer tomography is not yet available; however, in the near future, this new approach and new technology will fundamentally change dental radiology (see Figs. **151**, **152**).

Fig. 37 Panoramic radiograph; spiral tomography (Scanora). As a means for basic data collection and preliminary treatment planning, a panoramic radiograph is taken. In the maxilla (**arrow**) one notes a poorly demarcated and apparently enlarged fully impacted tooth 23, also exhibiting a follicular cyst. The crown of the tooth is localized palatally and the root vestibularly (see p. **111**).

Fig. 38 Transverse multi-layering with spiral tomography in the maxilla. These transversal radiographs taken with spiral tomography clearly depict the palatal location of tooth 23, and the follicular cyst (**arrow**) located distal and vestibularly to tooth 22.

Fig. 39 Transversal multi-layer with spiral tomography in the mandible. In the same patient, the treatment plan included placement of a dental implant in the right mandible. The transverse projections (made with the Scanora apparatus) show on the left side (**arrow**) the position/location of the mandibular canal and the availability of bone at the level of tooth 46. On the right side one notes the mental foramen (**arrow**) distal to tooth 44.

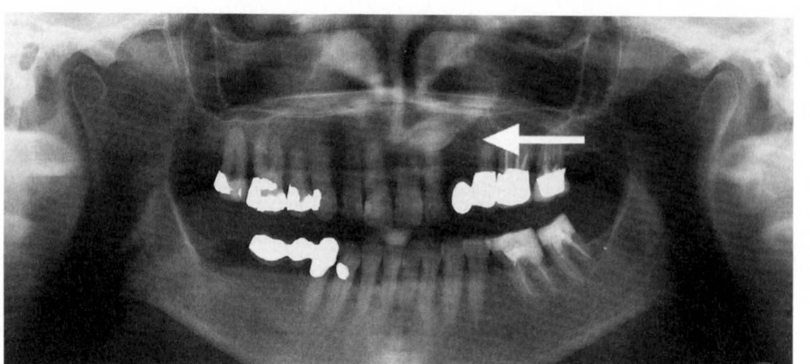

37

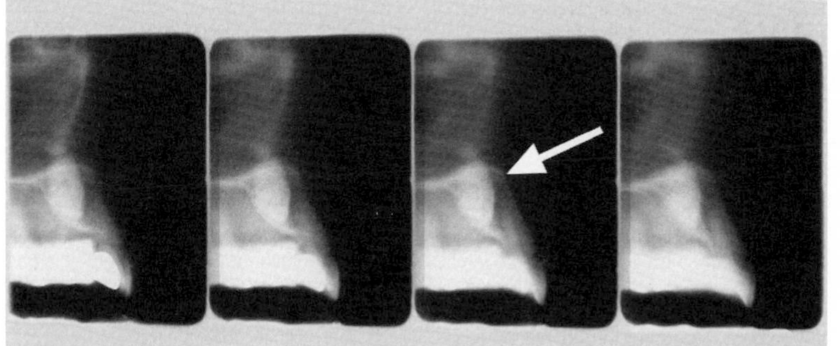

38

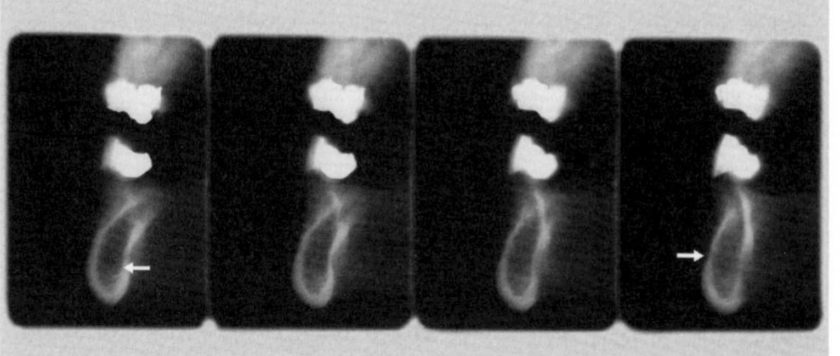

39

Radiographic anatomy

With conventional summation radiographs such as intraoral or skull projections, conventional thick-layer tomography (zonography) and panoramic radiographs, the normal tissues and structures that have been well defined in macroscopic (gross) anatomy fall within the central ray to be superimposed upon each other. The actual three-dimensional situation is reduced to a two-dimensional picture (exception: thin-layer tomography). The observation and interpretation of such two-dimensional depictions must therefore follow a strict protocol, which provides the fundamental basis for each and every radiographic interpretation. Furthermore, a solid basic knowledge of irradiation effects and of normal anatomy are absolutely necessary in order to assess the spatial orientation that is dependent upon the selected projection angle. Even *minor* alterations in the direction of the central ray projection will result in depictions of the desired spaces and structures in quite varying perspective, and this means that the positioning of the patient, the direction of the central ray, and the position of the image receptor are of extreme importance. The positioning of the patient plays a very important role, especially with panoramic radiographs, when one considers the quite individual architecture of the facial skeleton; proper and appropriate positioning of each individual patient must be carefully considered in order to ensure adequate radiographic quality.

It is therefore clear that optimization of radiographic technique actually creates the basis for interpretability of panoramic radiographs, because in the *pano* the structures in the three-dimensional context are not only projected as superimposed upon each other, but there is also dependence upon their spatial removal from the plane of focus, which may render them blurred or even obliterated. On the other hand, hollow spaces at a distance from the focal plane, or radiopaque structures, may be located in the plane of focus and thus negatively influence the structures of primary interest. With its varying layer thicknesses adapted to the jaw anatomy, the panoramic radiograph is not true tomography in the sense of a thin-layer projection with a layer thickness of maximally 4 mm, but rather a zonography or thick-layer projection in which structures that reside outside of the plane of focus are also depicted, and this can disturb the interpretability of desired structures. The anatomy provided by a panoramic radiograph (and naturally, of course, also radiographic pathology) therefore follows the individual and predictable characteristics of radiographic picture production and can, despite even intensive efforts, not provide measurement values approaching 1:1 ratios to the true clinical (anatomic) relationships.

Fig. 40–42

1 Orbit
2 Atlantooccipital articulation
3 Cheek, with nasolabial fold
4 Infraorbital canal
5 Compact basal bone of the opposing jaw
6 Nasal septum, with maxillary nasal ridge
7 Inferior nasal concha
8 Lacrimal fovea
9 Maxillary sinus (borders)
10 Nasopalatine canal, with nasal orifices and incisive foramen
11 Anterior nasal spine
12 Horizontal osseous palatal lamina
13 Laterobasal border of the nasal cavity; the palatal roof is between 12 and 13
14 Dorsum of the tongue
15 Palatal velum
16 Pterygopalatal fossa
17 Body of the zygomatic bone, with innominate line
18 Zygomatic arch

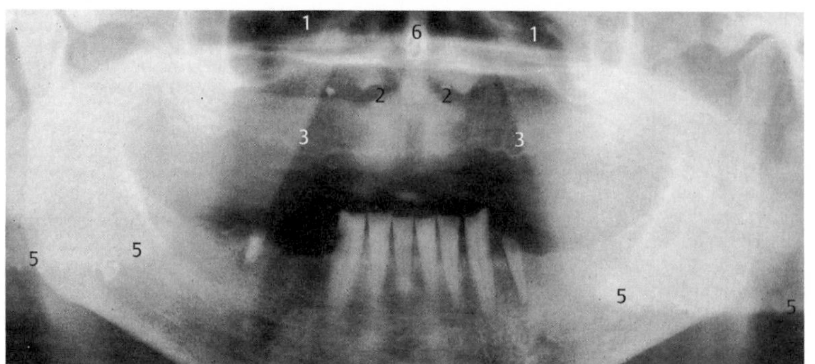
1
6
1
2
2
3
3
5
5
5
5

40

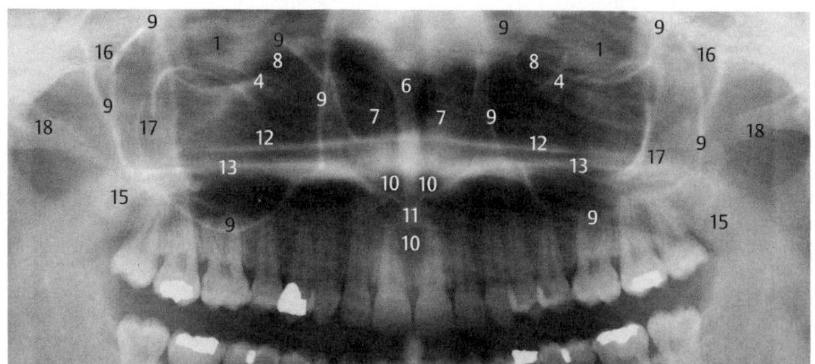
9
16
1
9
8
4
6
9
9
8
1
4
16
9
18
17
12
7
7
9
12
9
18
13
13
17
15
10
10
11
9
9
15
10

41

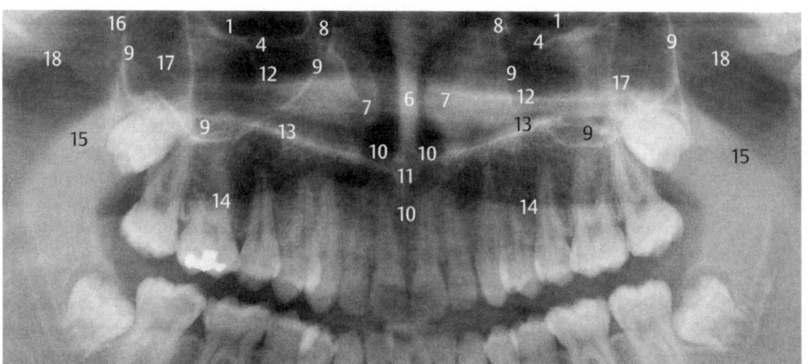
16
1
8
8
1
4
4
18
9
17
12
9
9
18
17
7
6
7
12
15
9
13
13
9
15
10
10
11
14
10
14

42

Roentgen rays elicit characteristic effects in radiographs, which are referred to by radiologists as "summation effects" and also as "tangential effects."

Summation effects occur when the central ray along its traverse of the tissues penetrates various objects and superimposes such objects upon each other and portrays the third dimension in a two-dimensional radiograph. If the central ray, on its pathway toward the desired and targeted object encounters an air-containing space, the ray will not be weakened by any substance and when it encounters (without any dampening) some portion of the object of interest it may over-irradiate the desired structures, or obliterate them entirely in the radiograph. But if, during its trip to the desired object, the central ray encounters soft tissues, osseous structures, or other radiopaque objects, the ray is weakened or diminished by such material and therefore encounters the object of interest with less radiation intensity. As a result, this causes a more or less circumscribed shadowing, which can render more difficult any effective interpretation of the desired structures, or render this entirely impossible.

In the first case, the structures of interest lose clarity because of over-irradiation. This type of summation effect has been referred to as a "**subtraction effect**." In the latter case, the structures of interest lose clarity due to the summation of the radiopaque objects, and one refers to this type of summation effect as the "**addition effect**."

These effects, which are unavoidable when attempting to portray three dimensions in a two-dimensional picture can only be minimized by careful and well-considered manipulations of the radiographic technique (see p. **169**).

Typical examples of the summation effects in panoramic radiographs include:

1. **Subtraction effects** caused by air-containing spaces
   a. For example, if the dorsum of the tongue is not pressed against the palate when taking a panoramic radiograph, an air-containing space will exist between the tongue dorsum and the palatal roof. This permits uninhibited penetration of the central ray onto the maxillary anterior region, resulting in a subtraction effect that diminishes or even obliterates the possibility of accurate and diagnostic interpretation of these structures (see p. **17**).
   b. The air-containing epipharynx will elicit a sharply demarcated zone of radiolucency in the ascending mandibular ramus with resultant radiographic obliteration of osseous structures (i.e., a subtraction effect), if the patient has been improperly advised to breathe deeply before the radiographic exposure and to hold his breath. This potential problem can be avoided simply by informing the patient that he/she should breathe slowly and normally during the entire exposure time (see Fig. **33**).

Fig. 43–45

1 Orbit
2 Cervical vertebrate, with tooth axis
3 Basal compact bone of the opposing jaw
4 Nasal septum
5 Inferior nasal concha
6 Maxillary sinus (borders)
7 Anterior nasal spine
8 Horizontal osseous palatal lamina
9 Laterobasal border of the nasal cavity
10 Palatal velum
11 Pterygopalatal fossa
12 Body of the zygomatic bone, with innominate line
13 Zygomatic arch
14 Basal compact bone
15 Mylohyoid line
16 Mandibular canal
17 Mental foramen
18 Digastric fovea or mental fovea, depending upon the positioning of the mandibular anterior segment in the plane of focus
19 External ear, with auditory opening
20 Mandibular articular process (condyle)
21 Muscular process of the mandible
22 Styloid osseous temporalis process
23 Hyoid bone
24 Base of the tongue

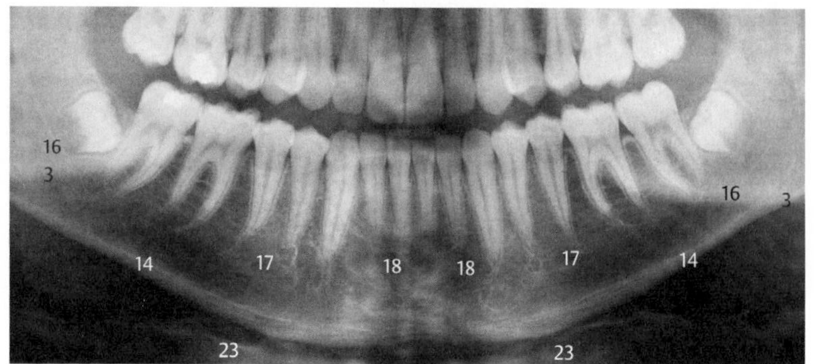
16
3
16
3
14
17
18
18
17
14
23
23

43

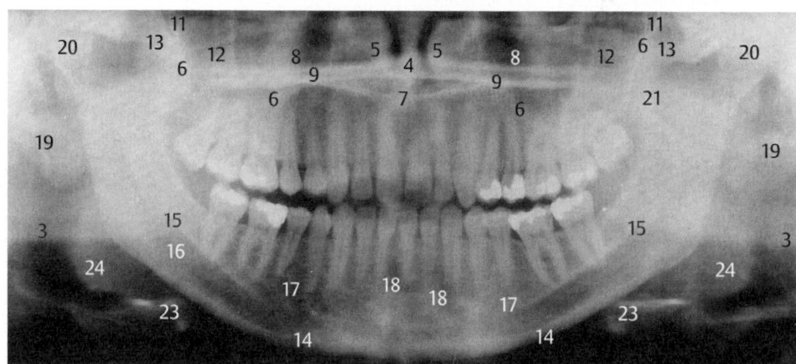
11
11
20
13
12
8
5
4
5
8
12
6
13
20
6
9
9
6
7
6
21
19
19
15
15
3
3
16
24
24
17
18
18
17
23
23
14
14

44

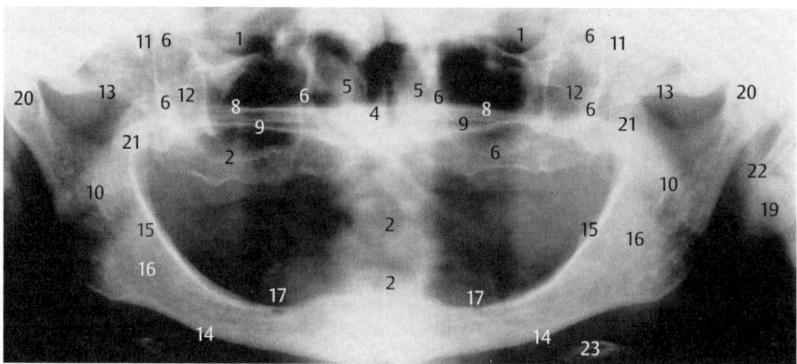
11
6
1
1
6
11
20
13
6
12
8
6
5
4
5
6
8
12
6
13
20
9
9
21
21
2
6
22
10
10
19
2
15
15
16
16
2
17
17
14
14
23

45

   c. The air-containing region of the external auditory meatus may be projected onto the mandibular condyle. This can cause a circumscribed subtraction effect resembling osteolysis and leading to an incorrect diagnosis (see Fig. **48**).
2. **Addition effects** caused by summation (overlapping) of radiopaque structures and objects
   a. A typical addition effect is caused by superimposition of the mandibular anterior region by the vertebrate. In the case of children and adolescents, this superimposition is less disturbing because the hydroxyapatite content of the vertebrate is still quite low. With increasing age, increasing content of hydroxyapatite, and not least following loss of the mandibular anterior teeth, the addition effect increasingly disturbs radiographic observation and interpretation, and cannot be completely eliminated by technical manipulations such as increasing the kV number or slowing the speed of rotation in the area of the vertebrae (see Fig. **45**).
   b. The targeting of the central ray and the pathway traversed by the radiograph head as it rotates around the patient's head are system-specific and nonadjustable; the consequence for the final radiograph is the appearance of vague shadowing because those parts of the jaws closest to the image receptor are superimposed by segments of both sides of the mandible, which are further from the image receptor. In many cases and especially in asymmetrically positioned patients, this can lead to addition effects that will disturb or inhibit observation and interpretation of structures of the ascending ramus of the mandible (see Fig. **44**).
   c. Radiopaque normal and pathologic structures and also foreign bodies outside the plane of focus can exert addition effects in the radiograph that will inhibit interpretation or even lead to incorrect diagnostic conclusions. The nasal wing (especially in dark-skinned races), sialoliths, phleboliths, and calcified lymph nodes, as well as earrings and necklaces, hairpins, eyeglasses, piercing jewelry, etc., may mask structures and impair interpretation and therefore must, as far as possible, be removed before positioning the patient in the device. Only in this way can the necessity for re-takes and excessive irradiation of the patient be avoided (see p. **21**).

Fig. 46–48

1 Maxillary sinus (borders)
2 Shadowing due to the horizontal lamina of palatine bone and the laterobasal border of the nasal cavity
3 Muscular (coronoid) process superimposed with the pterygoid process of the sphenoid bone, the maxillary tuberosity, and the connective tissues of the soft palate
4 Body of the zygomatic bone, with innominate line
5 Innominate line (demarcation line in the wall of the temporal surface of zygomatic bone)
6 Zygomatic arch
7 Zygomaticotemporal suture
8 Glenoid fossa
9 Articular eminence
10 Soft tissue of the external ear
11 Auditory meatus, with the auditory canal appearing as a radiolucency
12 Articular process, with mandibular condyle
13 Styloid process of temporal bone
14 Radiolucency caused by the air-containing epipharynx
15 Soft palate
16 Dorsum of the tongue
17 Mandibular foramen
18 Mandibular canal
19 Anterior tubercle of the atlas
20 Dens axis (epistropheus)
21 Transverse foramen, axis
22 External oblique line (continuation of the anterior margin caudally and laterally)
23 Temporal crest
24 Maxillary tuberosity
25 Pterygopalatine fossa

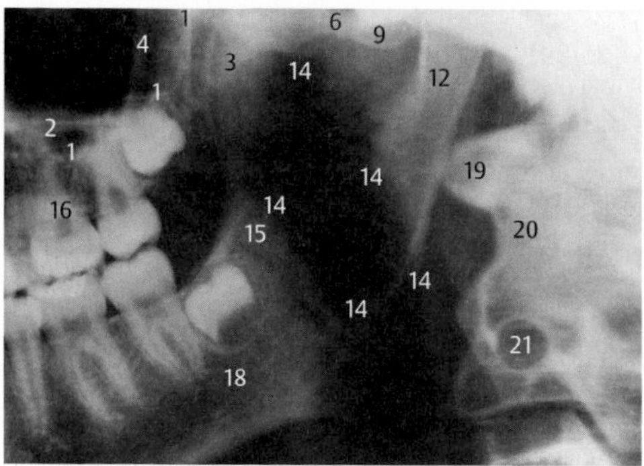
1
6
9
4
3
14
12
1
2
1
19
14
16
14
15
20
14
14
21
18

46

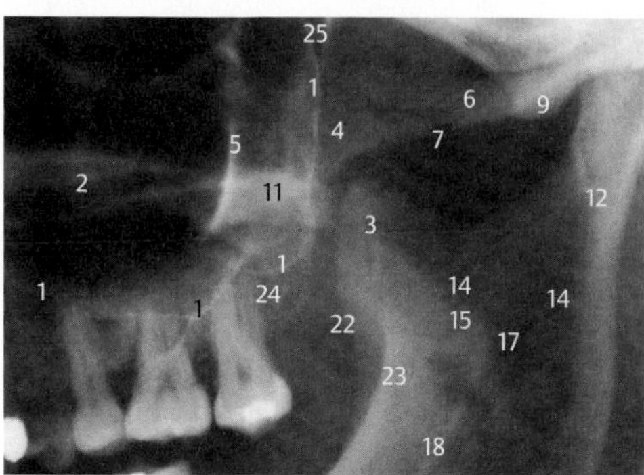
25
1
6
9
4
7
5
2
11
12
3
1
1
24
14
14
1
22
15
17
23
18

47

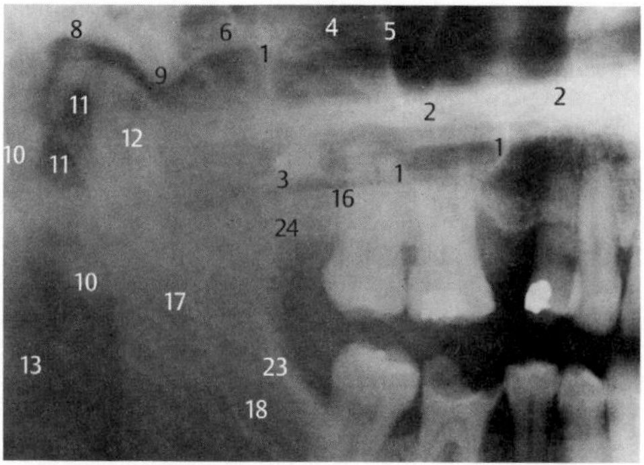
8
6
4
5
1
9
2
11
2
12
1
10
11
1
3
16
24
10
17
13
23
18

48

The **tangential effect** is another characteristic effect of roentgen rays. If structures are at a 90° angle to the central ray, they will only be visible in the radiograph if they are of sufficient thickness or density, when using normal exposure settings. Thin osseous lamella will only be clearly depicted if they are parallel to the central ray. In terms of curved surfaces or spherical objects, only those portions that are struck tangentially by the central ray will be observed in the radiograph because this region, in contrast to other objects, is parallel to the path of the central ray. For example, only the lateral border of a round rod will be depicted, and a dense sphere will be portrayed only as a circle. Depending upon the thickness and the density of the structure, such objects within the clearly demarcated area will appear more or less evenly opaque.

Typical practical examples for the consequences of the tangential effect include:

1. Structures with flat surfaces
   a. In addition to the above-mentioned example of the bony lamella, the depiction of cancellous bone is a further example. All portions of the cancellous bone that are transverse to the central ray will be depicted in the image only as general shadowing, so that in reality only a portion of the actual cancellous bone will be visible in the radiograph.
2. Structures with curved surfaces
   a. One sees only the basal portion of the compact bone of the mandible, because this is traversed tangentially by the central ray (see Fig. **50**).
   b. The curved and dorsally indented surface of the temporal surface of the zygomatic bone courses axially, and appears in the panoramic radiograph as the dorsal border of the body of the zygomatic bone within the dominating radiolucency of the maxillary sinus because it is encountered tangentially by the central ray (see Fig. **47**).

Fig. 49–51

1 External oblique line (continuation of the anterior margin caudally and laterally)
2 Mandibular crest with retromolar triangle
3 Mandibular foramen
4 Mandibular canal
5 Mental foramen
6 Angular process on the masseteric tuberosity
7 Angle of the mandible
8 Basal compact bone
9 Hyoid bone, with greater horn of the hyoid bone
10 Cervical vertebra exhibiting clearly the dense osseous plates on each vertebra
11 Maxillary sinus (borders)
12 Dorsum of the tongue
13 Condyle (medial pole)
14 Condyle (lateral pole)
15 Muscular process (coronoid process) in superimposition with the pterygoid process, the maxillary tuberosity, and the connective tissues of the soft palate
16 Neck of the condyloid process of the mandible
17 Soft palate
18 Radiopacity caused by the roof of the palate and the floor of the nasal sinus
19 Epipharynx
20 Long, ossified styloid process, with its jointed connection
21 Radiopacity cause by the compact bone of the contralateral jaw

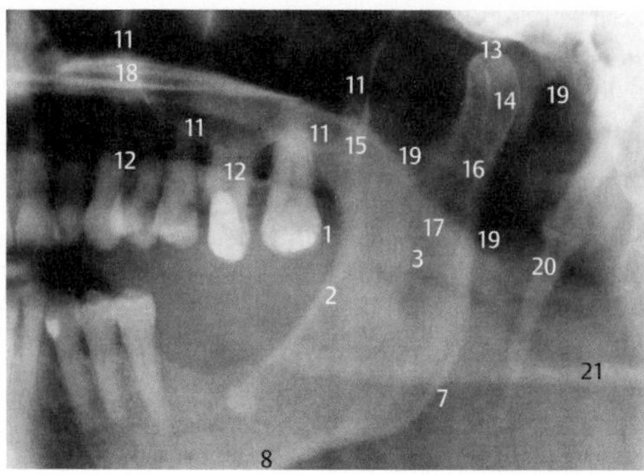
11
18
11
11
11
11
15
19
13
14
19
16
12
12
1
17
19
3
20
2
21
7
8

49

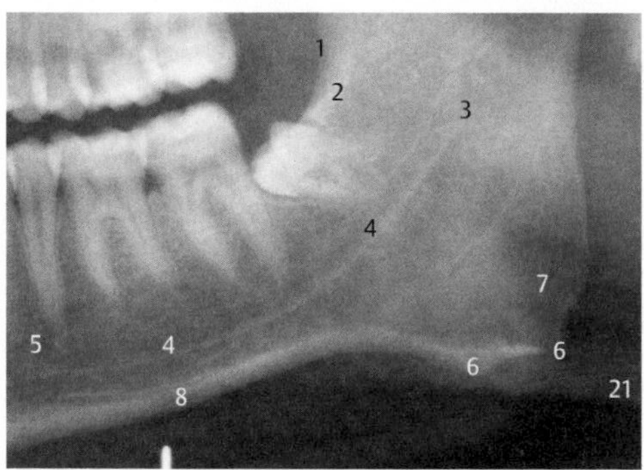
1
2
3
4
7
5
4
6
6
8
21

50

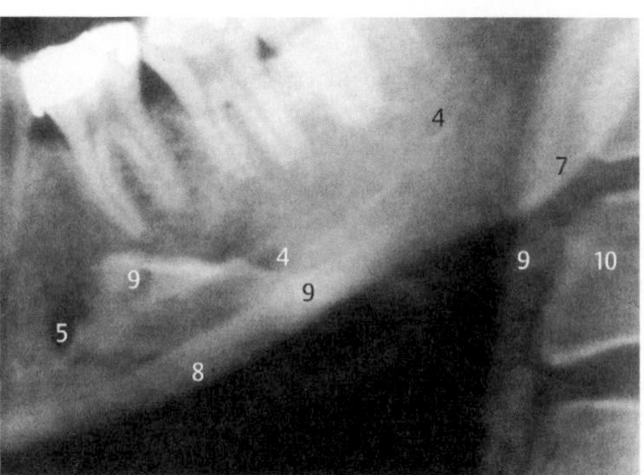
4
7
4
9
9
9
10
5
8

51

For the accurate depiction of anatomic and pathologic structures, exposure settings of course play an important role, and these settings must be selected based upon the indication and with regard to the thickness and density of the desired structures.

With the exception of the extremely variable eruption times of third molars, complete eruption of the permanent dentition occurs in females at about age 17 and in males about age 18. The following developmental phases have been differentiated:

- Infantile phase: up to 3 years.
- Juvenile phase: from 3–11 years.
- Pubertal phase: from 11–18 years.
- Adult phase.

This classification can be expanded and rendered more complete by subdividing the juvenile phase into an early childhood phase (up to 6 years) and school age with a pre-pubertal phase (8–11 years).

Clear and significant growth spurts occur usually between 3 and 8, and 11 and 18 years. These periods of rapid growth are hormonally elicited and generally begin following the pre-juvenile age in girls, about 1–2 years earlier than in boys; furthermore, it is important to note that the development of condyles in males may continue into the 23rd year of life due to the adaptive changes in the mandible. Therefore, in this chapter, illustrations of jaw growth and maturation will be illustrated using radiographs of females.

In terms of radiographic diagnosis, it is important to note in this context that *dental* developmental age is not necessarily correlated with skeletal age. With regard to forensic identification, the determination of the age of a young person is therefore not always possible with precision, especially in individuals of color.

During the course of advancing ventral and caudal development of the mandible under the influence of dorsal and cranial growth pressures, the retruded position of the mandible that is typical of early childhood normally progresses to a more typical adult facial appearance with a prominent chin region, i.e., the angle between the Frankfort horizontal plane and the nasopogonion line becomes larger during the course of development of the dentition.

Fig. 52 Schematic depiction of development and eruption of the primary dentition.

Fig. 53 Panoramic radiograph of a 6-year-old female. The mandibular central incisors and the first permanent molars have erupted, and their root formation is almost complete. The ascending ramus and the articular processes with the condyles, as well as the tuberosity regions, remain in the growth phase, and at this stage do not exhibit sufficient space for the development of the third molars.

Fig. 54 Panoramic radiograph of a 9-year-old female. All of the permanent incisors have erupted, but their apical foramina, especially in the maxilla, have not yet assumed the normal diameter, indicating incomplete maturation at this point. Note that tooth 12 is rotated about its axis. Note in the bifurcation of the first permanent molars a radiographic addition effect caused by superimposition of the root trunks; this appearance is not due to *enamel pearls*.

Eruption of the maxillary deciduous teeth occurs according to the following schedule
(eruption of the mandibular deciduous teeth is more or less analogous):

Central incisors	6–8 months
Lateral incisors	8–12 months
Canines	15–20 months
First molars	12–16 months
Second molars	20–40 months

6 months

1 year

2 ½ years

4 years

52

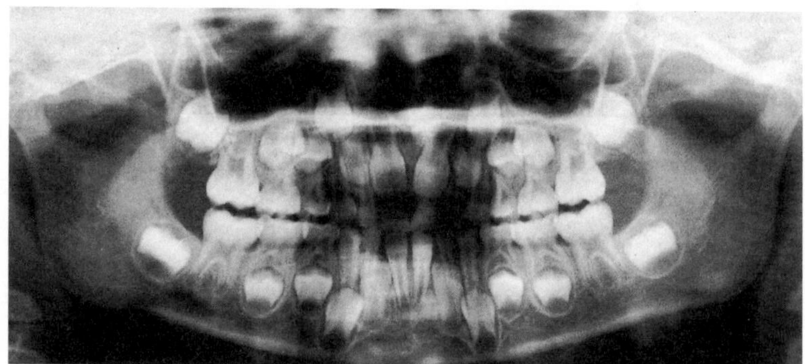

53

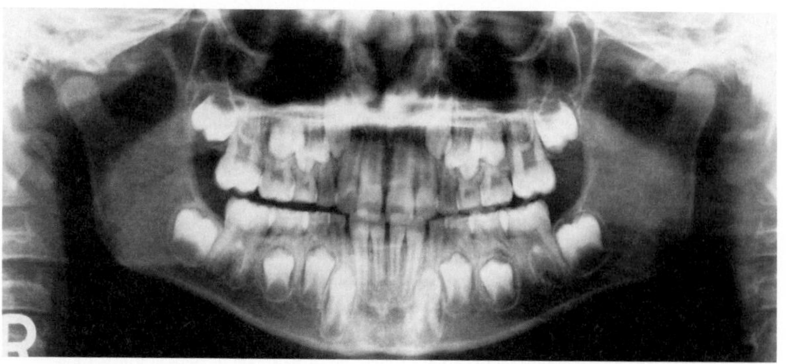

54

The relationship between the Frankfort horizontal plane and the occlusal plane changes correspondingly as the final form of the facial skeleton develops,and exhibits in adults angular relationships with a relatively broad range of variation; for this reason, routine use of the Frankfort horizontal as a reference plane during the preparation of panoramic radiographs can lead to improper patient positioning. These types of positioning errors can only be avoided through prior examination by the dentist, and clear instructions to the auxiliary personnel actually taking the radiographs.
It is therefore very important, especially with small children, that the **radiographic technique** using the panoramic device be extremely carefully performed, in order to avoid unnecessary radiation exposure that would be the consequence of any necessity to re-take the radiograph.
With small children, it is important to make sure that during positioning in the bite holder with protrusion of the mandible that the patient does not lift the entire head, because that would cause the tooth buds of the maxillary permanent teeth to appear overlapped by the structures of the floor of the nose and the palatal vault, rendering them impossible to examine thoroughly. From the lateral view, positioning of the skull can, at this age, be oriented to the Frankfort horizontal, because the occlusal plane of the deciduous dentition is still parallel to that plane.
Whenever possible, the dorsum of the tongue should be firmly pressed against the roof of the mouth, in order to avoid overexposure of the developing buds of the permanent anterior teeth. The tooth buds of the maxillary anterior region are also better depicted if the occlusal plane is not parallel to the Frankfort horizontal, but rather positioned slightly steeper ventrally. Nevertheless, using a normal-size panoramic image receptor it is to be expected that the buds of the maxillary premolars will be projected as superimposed (overlapped) upon each other. For any special depiction of the maxillary anterior region, a radiographic program with a limited field of irradiation is indicated. Again, especially with small children, the positioning of the back of the head in the device should be checked from the dorsal aspect and corrected as necessary before exposure. Deviations of the median saggital plane from the perpendicular axis of the unit will otherwise lead to asymmetric radiographs, which can lead to an *incorrect* diagnosis of facial asymmetry.

Fig. 55 Schematic diagram of development and eruption of the permanent dentition.

Fig. 56 Panoramic radiograph of a 15-year-old female. Root formation of the erupted teeth is complete. In this patient, teeth 35 and 45 have developed into taurodonts with a coronoapically expanded pulp chamber. During the pubertal growth spurt, dorsally and cranially directed growth of the maxilla and the mandible created space for the buds of the wisdom teeth (third molars), and their root development has begun. The neck and condyle of the mandible are not yet fully developed.

Fig. 57 Panoramic radiograph of a 20-year-old female. Development of the dentition is complete. The apical foramina and the root canals exhibit normal diameter of adult age. The third molars are completely erupted, but exhibit a long axis that is oriented slightly dorsally.

Eruption of the maxillary permanent teeth occurs according to the following schedule (eruption of the mandibular teeth is more or less analogous):

Central incisors	6–8 years
Lateral incisors	8–12 years
Canines	10–14 years
First premolars	9–12 years
Second premolars	10–13 years
First molars	6–7 years
Second molars	10–13 years
Third molars	16–30 years

6 years

9 years

10 years

11 years

12 years

55

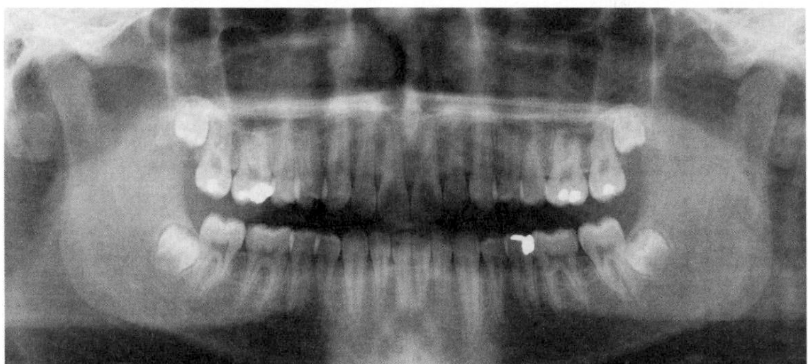

56

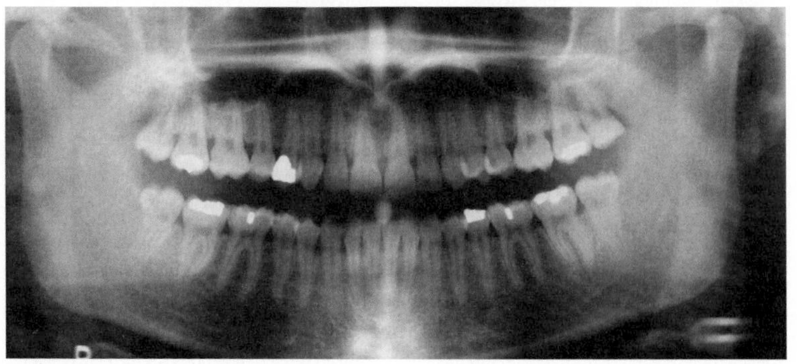

57

For all dentists who elect to use a panoramic radiograph for basic data collection during the initial examination of a patient, individual intraoral dental radiographs are relegated to a supplementary role to answer special, specific questions that demand exceptional radiograph quality. A complete 18-film intraoral radiographic survey in patients of all ages should—today—only be performed if the practice does not have panoramic radiographic equipment. There exists considerable risk for both the patient and the dentist if the radiographic examination is incomplete, i.e., if pathologic conditions go undetected. This is especially true concerning incomplete initial examinations performed using individual intraoral radiographs (of all types).

From the standpoint of direction of the central ray, intraoral dental radiographs can be differentiated into the following types of special films:

a. **Apical projection** with the central ray directed through the region of the tooth apex, for optimum depiction of apical or periapical lesions.
b. **Periodontal projection** with the central ray directed through the upper third of the tooth root for radiographic examination of periodontal lesions.
c. **Coronal projection (bitewings)** with the central ray directed at the height of the tooth crown; this is particularly indicated for caries detection.
d. **Occlusal projection** with axial (mandible) or half-axial (maxilla) central ray projection for depicting the jaws in the third dimension.

The lowest level of distortion and the highest level of image clarity will always be found in the region of the central ray projection. The *clinical indication* actually sets the priority for selection of the individual types of intraoral radiographs, and the radiographic quality of other structures is of secondary importance. The image receptor should be as perpendicular as possible to the central ray and as parallel as possible to the tooth long axis in order to guarantee optimum radiographic interpretability.

Fig. 58 Intraoral radiographic survey in the mixed dentition. This figure shows a 10-film series using 2 x 3 cm films in the mixed dentition stage, taken using a film holder for the right-angle technique. Depending upon the age and size of the child, a radiographic survey may also be possible using only six films (for anterior regions and posterior segments), or with use of 3 x 4 cm film format. With digital radiography, a mixed dentition survey will be similar, but using similar sizes of phosphor-coated imaging plates or a digital sensor. The use of an image receptor holder (IRH) and a targeting device is highly recommended.

Fig. 59 Intraoral radiographic survey for adolescents or adults. This figure depicts the "classic" 14-film series using 3 x 4 cm film in a young adult patient, performed using the right-angle technique in an IRH holder as the targeting device. If, in a patient of this age, the third molar is not captured on the molar radiograph, a different projection angle must be attempted. The radiographic survey depicted here can also be performed digitally using imaging plates or sensors of similar sizes. If it is necessary to use a small sensor, the posterior teeth must be radiographed in vertical format, and this will require an extra 1–2 exposures per quadrant. It is recommended that an image receptor holder be used as the targeting device.

Fig. 60 Periodontal survey. In comparison to a normal, apically targeted radiographic survey, individual intraoral projections or even entire surveys for periodontitis patients should be targeted more toward the alveolar ridge margin, so that the central ray directly impacts the primary area of interest, the alveolar bone crest. This guarantees a sharp and undistorted view of osseous periodontal lesions. Such periodontal (marginal) projections, taken to supplement a panoramic radiograph, need not necessarily display the root apex; therefore, during placement and adjustment of the selected IRH, one need concentrate only on the alveolar ridge. The periodontal survey shown here, with a total of 14 films, can be viewed as a variation of a normal radiographic survey in completely dentulous adults. The use of bite-wing radiographs in the posterior areas can reduce radiation exposure significantly (see pp. **54–57**).

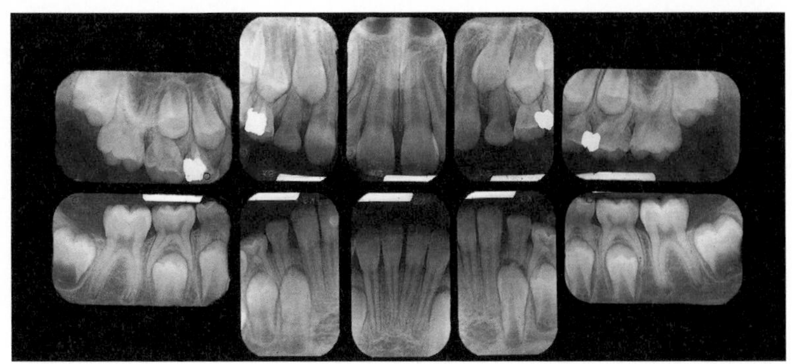

58

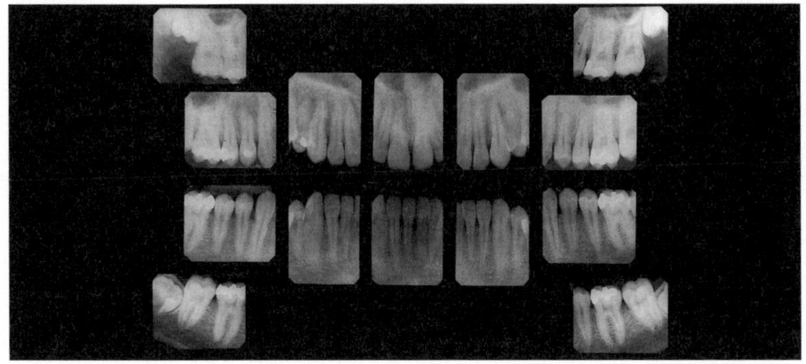

59

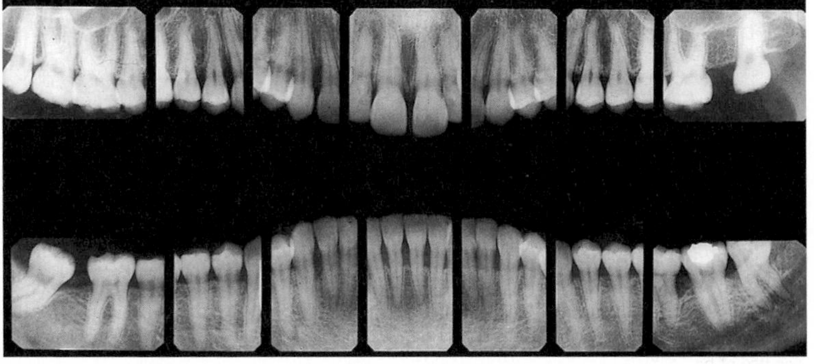

60

Fig. 61 a Vertical central ray projection angle adjustment for the intraoral bisecting angle technique. In all instances where it is not possible for anatomic reasons to place the image receptor parallel to the tooth long axis, the plane of the IRH (**2**) assumes a vertical angle of varying degree to the tooth long axis (**1**). It is therefore not easy to target the central ray onto the tooth so that the tooth is depicted in its true length. A tooth will only be depicted in its correct length if the central ray (**4**) can be projected through the apex perpendicular to the bisected angle (**3**). Otherwise the tooth will be depicted as too short (**5**) or too long (**6**). In any case, the root will appear more or less widened depending upon the relationship of the distance of the apex from the image receptor.

Fig. 61 b Intraoral right-angle technique. Proper targeting of the tooth of interest will be considerably simplified through use of a device that both holds the image receptor (IR) and permits precise targeting of the central ray (**4**) and which defines definitively that the central ray will be at a right angle (**3**) to the plane of the selected IR (**2**). Using the naked eye to position the IR parallel to the tooth long axis (**1**) will guarantee correct depiction of the tooth in proper size and spatial relationships. If the intraoral anatomic relationships make it impossible to position the image receptor over the apex and parallel to the entire tooth, the position of the receptor holding device can be slightly altered more toward the bisecting angle technique.

Fig. 62a Indication-based use of the intraoral radiographic technique. For proper depiction of a mandibular molar, the central ray (**4**) is directed perpendicular to the tooth long axis (**1**) and the plane of the IR (**2**). Given these circumstances, the tooth will be depicted in its true size, and without distortion. On the other hand, if the tooth is targeted steeply cranially (from below; **5**), it will appear much shorter in the final image. But if the intent is to evaluate the location of the root apex vis-à-vis the mandibular canal, it will be necessary to combine the steeper projection (**5**) with a modified receptor position (**2a**). The important concept is that the projection of the central ray will be dictated in each individual case by the clinical indication for taking the radiograph. This must be clearly conveyed to the person taking the radiographs.

Fig. 62b Horizontal angle adjustment for intraoral radiographs. In general, teeth are radiographed orthoradially in the horizontal angle (i.e., perpendicular to the chord of a section of the dental arch). The figure illustrates the "orthoradial" shadow of a vertical bar with a square cross-section on the image receptor (**7**). If the same metal bar is targeted laterally (i.e., eccentrically; **8**), it is depicted on the image receptor as both distorted and in some areas blurred.

Fig. 63a Orthoradial projections for individual teeth or groups of teeth. The illustration shows the proper direction of the central ray and the proper positioning of the IR in the horizontal angle for the ideal orthoradial projection. The IR should be positioned at a right angle to the central ray and must therefore be positioned where there is adequate space, i.e., as near as possible to the middle of the palatal vault and not necessarily near to the teeth. This is also true for the mandible, where the IR should be placed toward the tongue and in such a position that no pain is elicited at the floor of the mouth.

Fig. 63b Excentric positioning for intraoral radiographs. For special diagnostic questions such as depiction of complicated root canal relationships and localization of impacted teeth or root fragments, one may employ excentric central ray targeting, which is described as mesial-excentric (**9**) or distal-excentric (**10**) projections depending upon their deviation from a normal projection. Such radiographs are usually taken as supplements to standard orthoradial projections. The position of the IR will therefore not be identical to that used to take the original radiograph. The most important consideration is the proper targeting of the central ray.

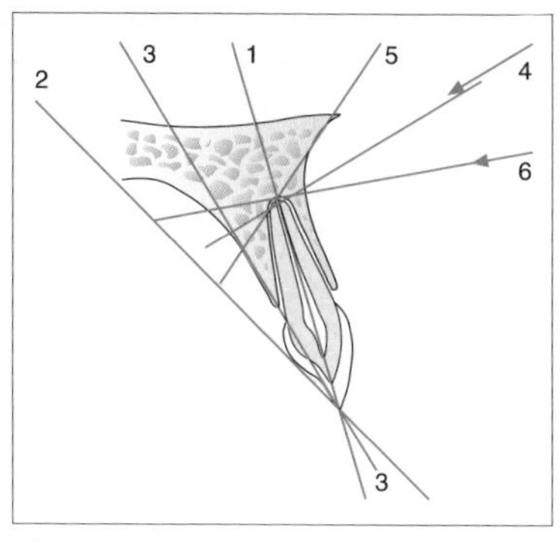

61 a

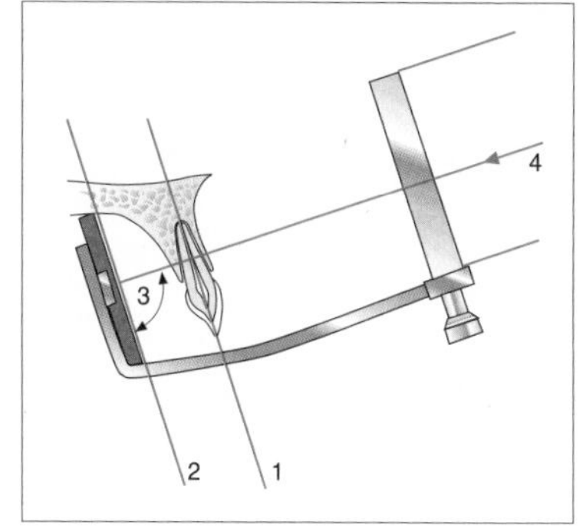

61 b

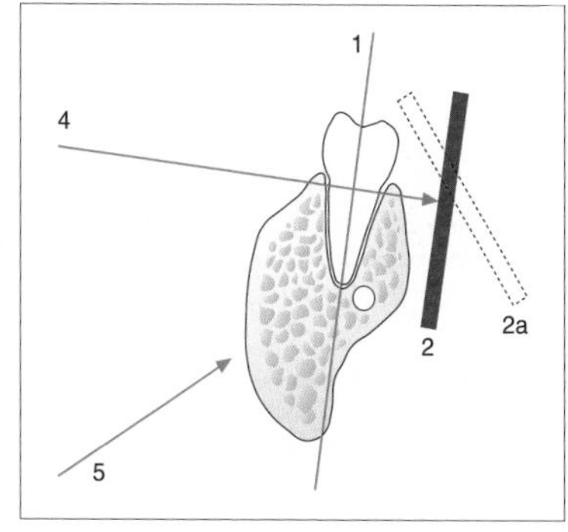

62 a

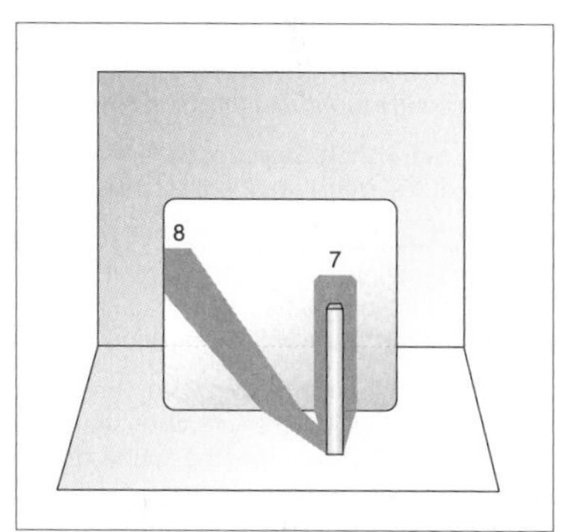

62 b

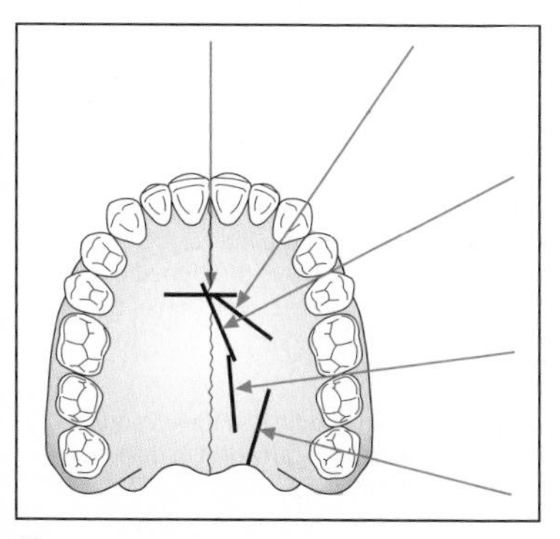

63 a

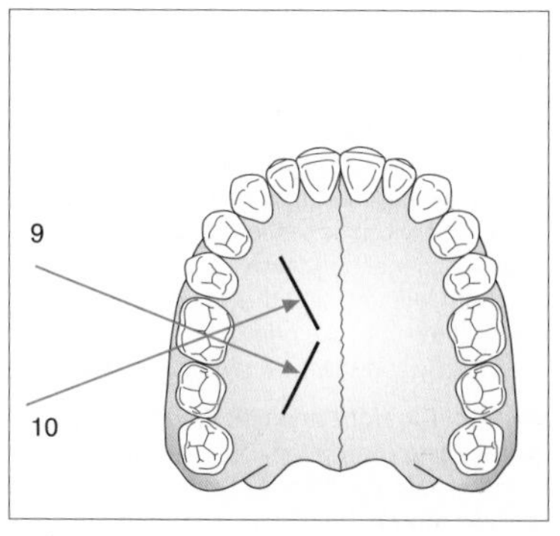

63 b

Fig. 64a Skull photograph, labial view of anterior region. Visible are the cementum surfaces of the tooth necks, the median suture, nasal crest of the maxilla, the anterior nasal spine, and the incisive foramen dorsal to the piriform aperture.

Fig. 64b Periapical radiograph of the maxillary anterior region. The lateral incisors are usually not completely depicted. The tip of the nose overlaps the tooth roots. The cervical areas exhibit the typical burn-out effect (see also Fig. **106a, b**).

Fig. 64c Proper position for taking a radiograph of the maxillary anterior region. The occlusal plane of the maxillary teeth is horizontal, with the mouth slightly open. The central ray is focused laterally symmetrically. The position of the IR device as described by Pasler (1982): The IR is positioned in the palatal vault without touching the teeth.

Fig. 65a Skull photograph, maxillary canine region. This view shows tooth 13 with an orthoradial projection. The mesial and/or distal osseous septa are often not optimally visible.

Fig. 65b Periapical radiograph of the region of the maxillary canine. This image was taken with the central ray targeted slightly too mesially, but provides an excellent view of the apical relationships. Note the typical trabecular bone structure of the maxilla, the anterior lobe of the maxillary sinus and the soft tissue of the wing of the nose (alar nasal cartilage).

Fig. 65c Proper position for taking the maxillary canine radiograph. This frontal view shows that the horizontal angle of the central ray should be clearly from the side in order to avoid superimposition of the first premolar over the canine. Using a mechanical holder to establish the right-angle technique, the IR can be placed free and deeply within the palatal vault, which greatly simplifies proper targeting of both vertical and horizontal angles.

Fig. 66a Skull photograph of the distal osseous interdental septum of the maxillary canine for a periodontal radiograph. The photograph demonstrates the necessity for accurate targeting in order to depict the interdental septum distal to the canine in an intraoral periodontal (periapical) radiograph free of overlapping. The horizontal angle must be perpendicular to an imaginary line connecting teeth 13–15.

Fig. 66b Skull photograph showing projection targeting to depict the mesial interdental septum of the maxillary canine. The photograph shows that a different projection angle will be necessary in an intraoral periodontal (periapical) radiograph to clearly depict the osseous septum mesial to the maxillary canine without any overlap. The horizontal angle must be perpendicular to an imaginary line connecting teeth 13 and 12. The IR held in the right-angle holder is positioned parallel to the tooth long axis and this can be checked visually before exposure. Perfect depiction of the apical region does not take priority, except in cases of severe periodontal bone destruction, and usually need not be considered when setting up to take this targeted radiograph.

Fig. 66c The right-angle IR holder as described by Pasler. The IRH is indicated for intraoral radiographs using conventional IRH packets, or digital sensors. It simplifies the targeting of desired structures because the central ray-to-receptor plane relationship is clearly defined and fixed. When employed properly, the device is patient-friendly and easy-to-use by the clinician; however, the technique must be learned and thoroughly practiced.

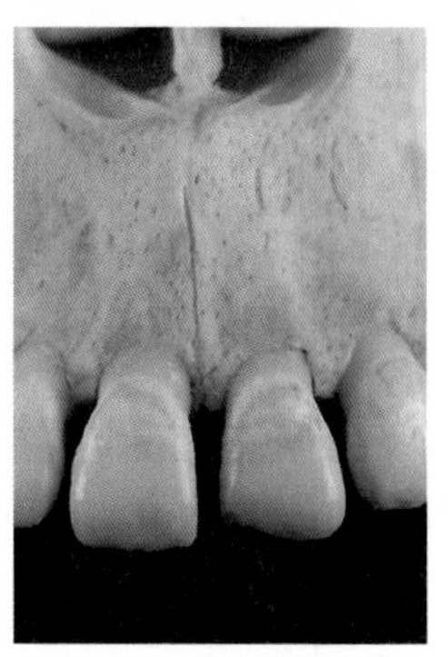
64 a

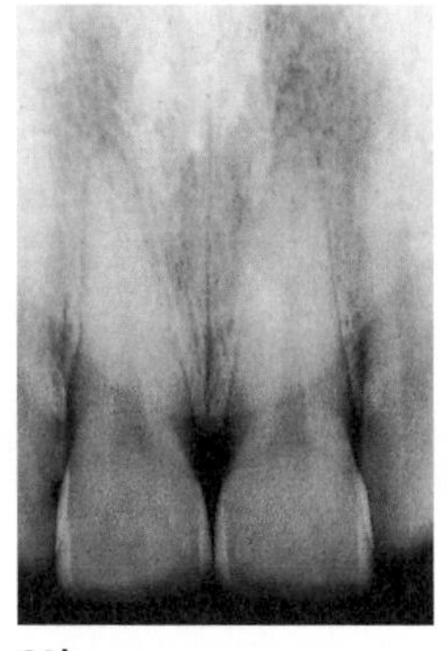
64 b

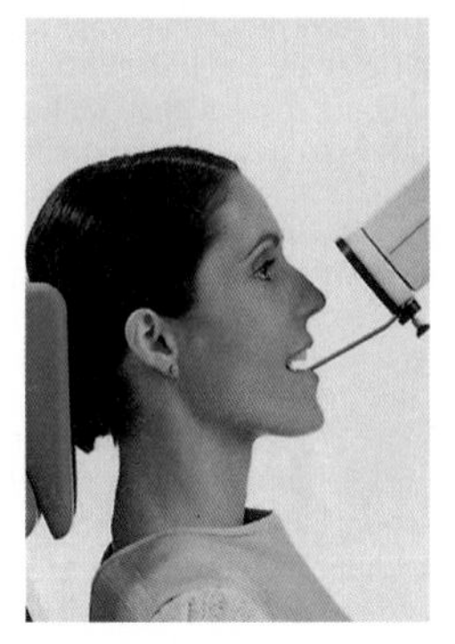
64 c

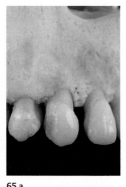

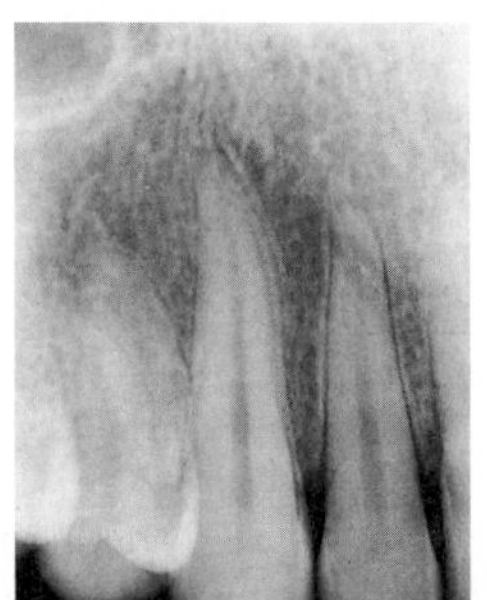

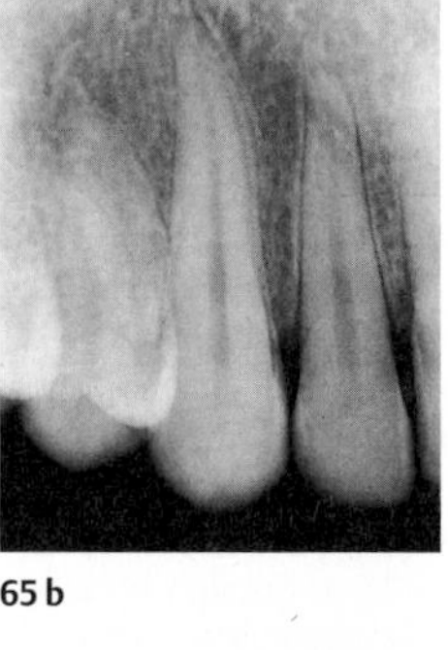

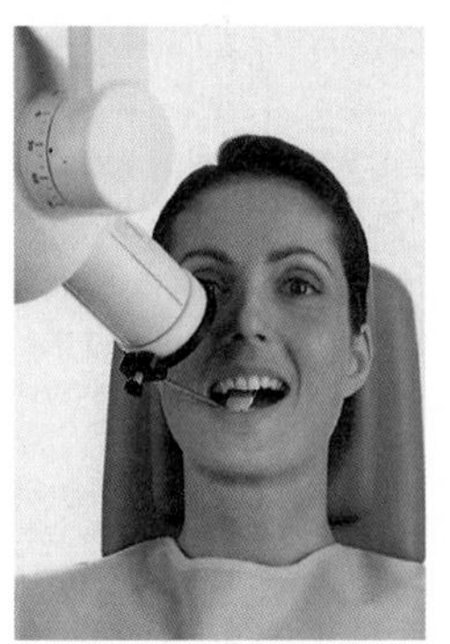

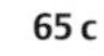

65 a

65 b

65 c

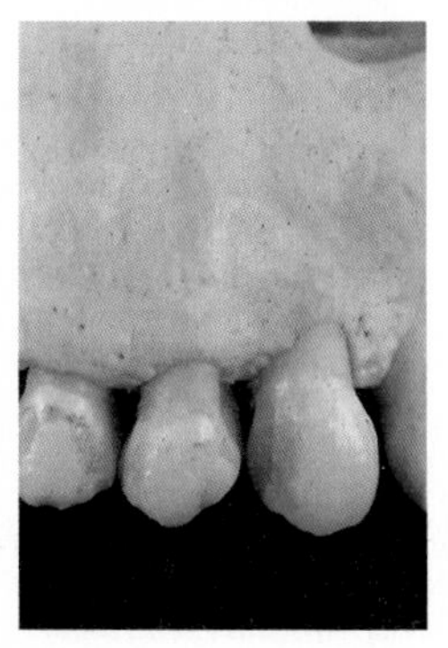
66 a

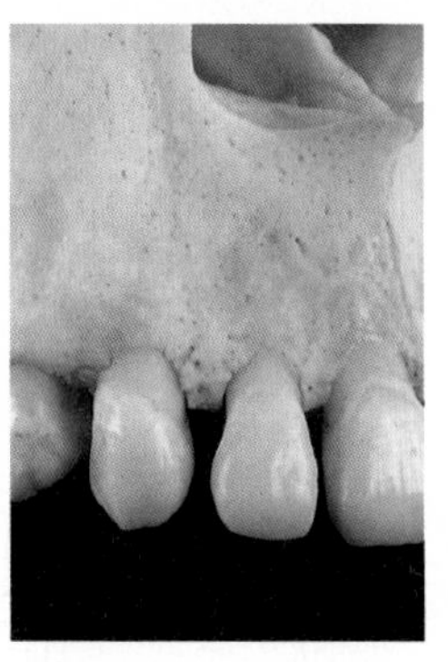
66 b

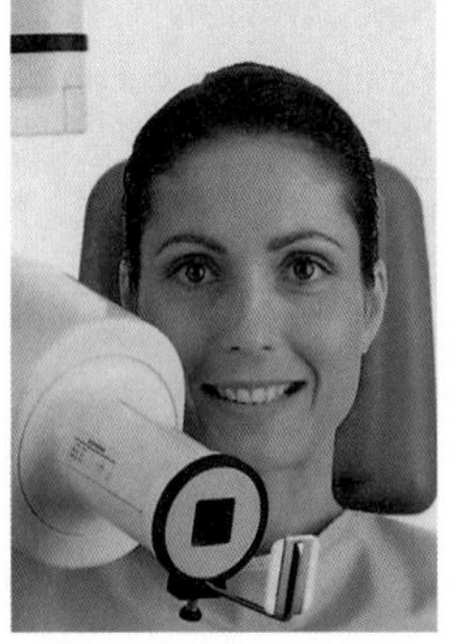
66 c

The concepts and principles described in this chapter are applicable to both digital and traditional/conventional radiography. Our primary goal is to present the radiographic techniques for various individual teeth or groups of teeth as performed according to defined indications, using roentgen film or digital sensor technology. Intraoral, periapical radiographs taken to supplement the panoramic film should be considered as "targeted radiographs" that fulfill the highest quality standards in order to guarantee optimum interpretation. Fulfilling such stringent demands will be considerably simplified by the use of image receptor (IR) holders that reliably secure central ray projection. The dentist or the auxiliary personnel taking the radiographs can concentrate on proper targeting of the desired structures because the image receptor holder device insures the proper relationship between the projection surface and the central ray. It is important to point out, however, that becoming completely familiar with any type of targeting device requires time, and the use of such devices must be thoroughly learned and continually practiced. The right-angle holder (see Fig. **66c**) designed by the author in 1982 is indicated for use with both conventional film packets and digital sensors.

Fig. 67a Skull photograph, maxillary premolar region. The photograph presents an orthoradial view of the maxillary premolars. Very frequently, the central ray is not targeted perpendicular to the middle of an imaginary line connecting the maxillary premolars (see Fig. **63a**), but rather more steeply and mesial-excentric (see Fig. **62b**).

Fig. 67b Radiograph of the maxillary premolar region. This radiograph was taken using a 3 x 4-cm size IR in landscape format. With smaller sensors and an appropriate targeting device (IRH), images such as this can also be taken in portrait format.

Fig. 68a Clinical technique for maxillary premolar radiographs. This frontal photograph clearly shows that the central ray will strike both maxillary premolars orthoradially, and at a relatively flat angle from the lateral aspect.

Fig. 68b Incorrect positioning for taking a radiograph of the maxillary molars, with an excessively steep central ray projection. This photograph shows the most common technical error when taking intraoral radiographs of the maxillary molars. The excessively steep vertical angle results in superimposition and overlapping of the zygomatic bone over the molars, especially the second molar (addition effect).

Fig. 68c Correct clinical positioning for radiographs of maxillary molars. This photograph shows that with use of the right-angle technique IRH holder, the central ray is targeted beneath the zygomatic arch, directly onto the molars, thus preventing superimposition of the zygomatic bone upon the molar roots.

Fig. 69a Radiograph of maxillary molars. This radiograph depicts the molar group of the maxilla taken using a somewhat vertical projection angle; the zygomatic process of the maxilla can be seen at the upper edge of the picture. With the use of an IHR, the central ray was targeted relatively flatly beneath the zygomatic arch.

Fig. 69b Radiograph of the maxillary molars with a steep vertical projection angle. This radiograph resulted from an incorrect projection in which the central ray was targeted slightly from the mesial and very steeply from above onto the molar region. The zygomatic bone is superimposed upon the roots of the first and second molars (addition effect) so that the roots cannot be adequately observed and interpreted. With this type of incorrect projection, periodontal osseous lesions will also be distorted and no longer adequately diagnosed.

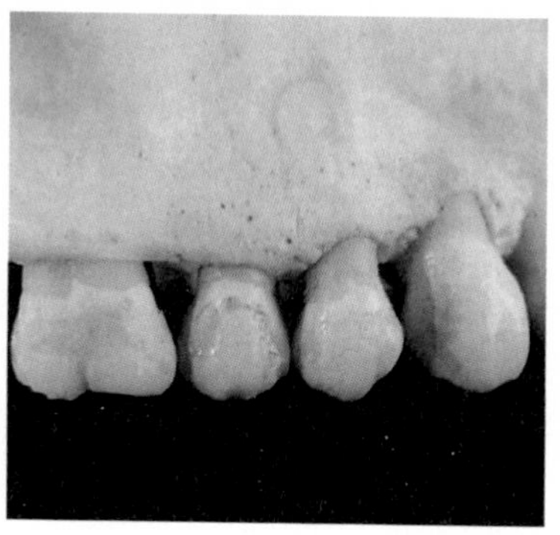

67 a

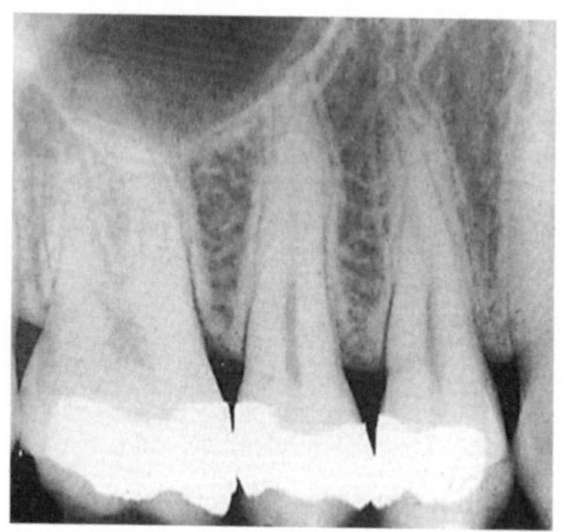

67 b

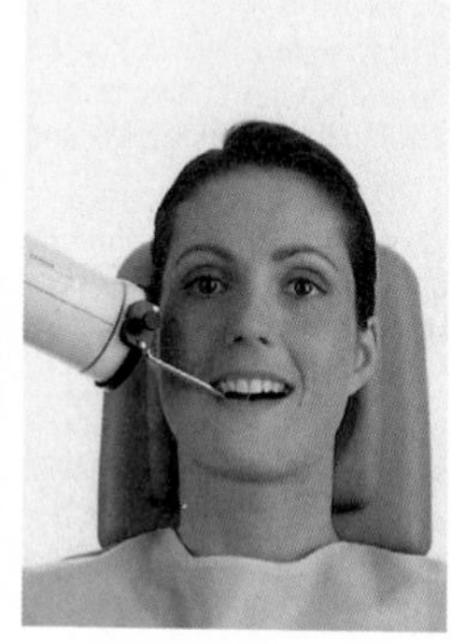

68 a

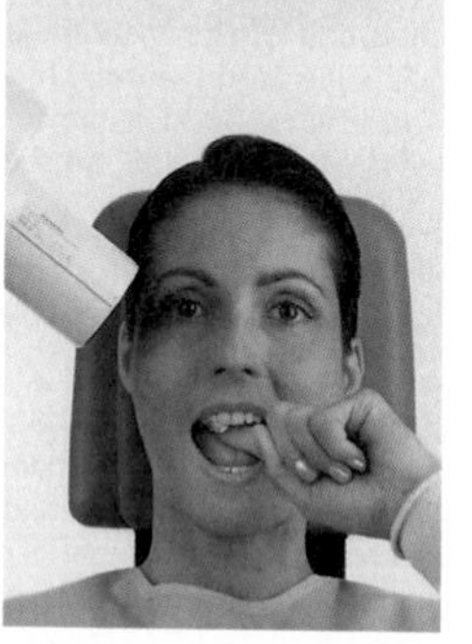

68 b

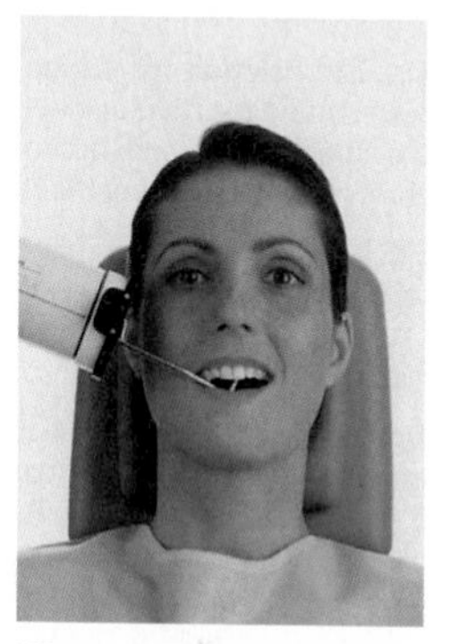

68 c

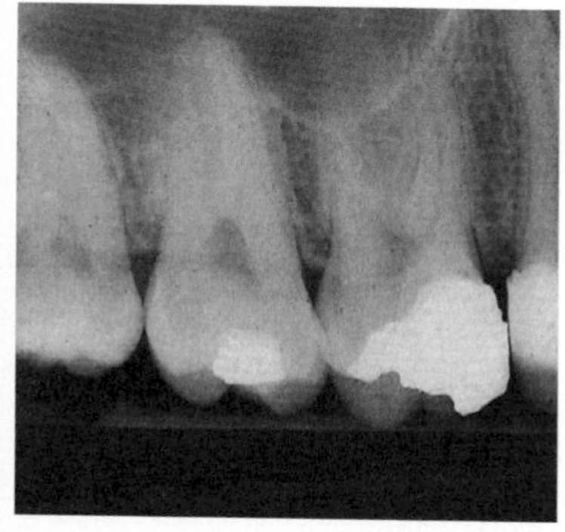

69 a

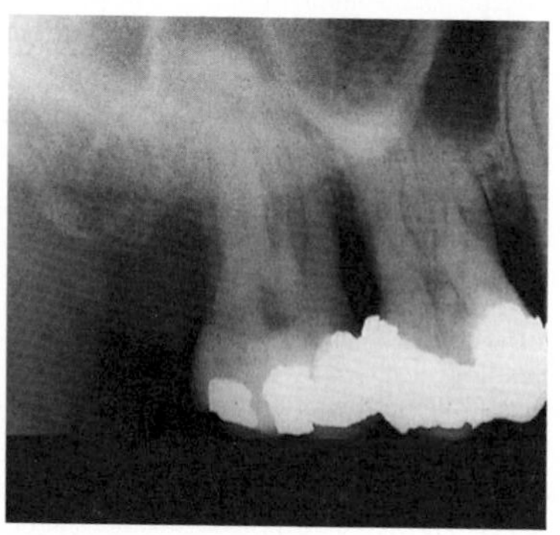

69 b

Fig. 70 a Skull photograph, mandibular anterior region. The photograph reveals slight horizontal bone loss around the lateral incisors and extensive labial osseous dehiscence on the central incisors. It is important to note that the two-dimensional intraoral radiograph cannot reveal the failing labial alveolar bone (dehiscence) because of the radiopacity of the superimposed tooth roots; it is for this reason that the periodontal relationships exhibited by such radiographs do not always correspond to the expectations of the clinician based upon clinical data gathering.

Fig. 70 b Radiograph of the mandibular anterior region. Apically projected radiographs often reveal the labial course of the alveolar ridge as overexposed because it is freely projected without superimposition of any other structures. On the other hand, the lingual course of the alveolar ridge is more clearly depicted because it is brought into prominence by the summation effect of the overlying alveolar bone.

Fig. 70 c Position for taking a radiograph of the mandibular anterior region. The IR can be placed using the right-angle technique holder further toward the tongue and parallel to long axes of the anterior teeth, and must not be forced into a position immediately behind the anterior teeth and against the resistance of the stretched floor of the mouth, which can cause pain.

Fig. 71 a Skull photograph, region of the mandibular canine. The photograph shows a properly targeted mandibular canine that will not be overlapped in the image by either the first premolar or the lateral incisor. It is not always possible to depict both the mesial and the distal interdental osseous septa free of overlapping.

Fig. 71 b Radiograph of the mandibular canine region. The osseous structure of the mandible and especially the body of the mandible is far more reticulated than the bone of the maxilla. The labial course of the alveolar ridge is directly impacted by the central ray and therefore overexposed. The periodontal ligament space appears to be narrower in the apical region than in the coronal area; this is due to increasing superimposition of the alveolar bone. In general, the periodontal ligament space will appear wider if the central ray strikes the root surface tangentially.

Fig. 71 c Clinical positioning for a radiograph of the mandibular canine. An IRH permits correct targeting of the mesial or the distal interdental septum of the mandibular canine. The IR packet can be placed posteriorly toward the tongue and parallel to the tooth long axis.

Fig. 72 a Skull photograph showing the projection direction to depict the mesial interdental septum of the mandibular canine. The septum will be optimally depicted in a periapical radiograph if the central ray is projected perpendicular to an imaginary line connecting teeth 43 and 42.

Fig. 72 b Skull photograph revealing the distal interdental osseous septum of the mandibular canine, for a periodontal radiograph. With regard to the horizontal angle, the central ray must be targeted perpendicularly to an imaginary line connecting teeth 44 and 43 in order to perfectly depict the distal interdental osseous septum of the mandibular canine. If the canine is malpositioned in the arch, it is likely that difficulty will be encountered in properly placing the IR near to the arch without **bending** the film. Narrow image receptors can be positioned further from the tooth and toward the tongue through use of a right-angle IR device.

Fig. 72 c Clinical positioning for depiction of the distal interdental osseous septum of the mandibular canine. Using the right-angle IRH, the image receptor can be placed far posteriorly in the tongue space. The rigid connection between the radiograph cone and the IRH simplifies targeting the central ray onto the desired structure.

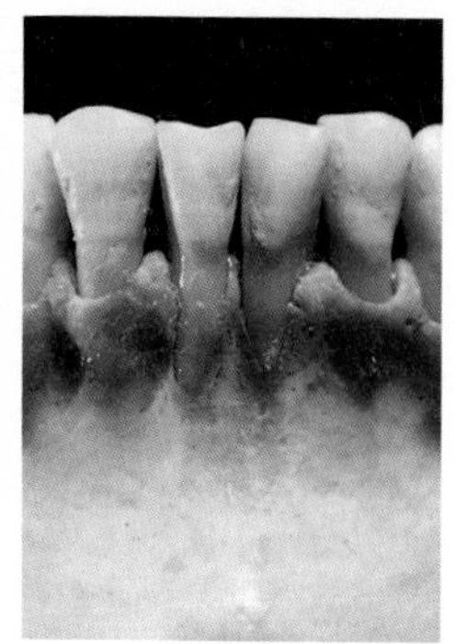

70 a

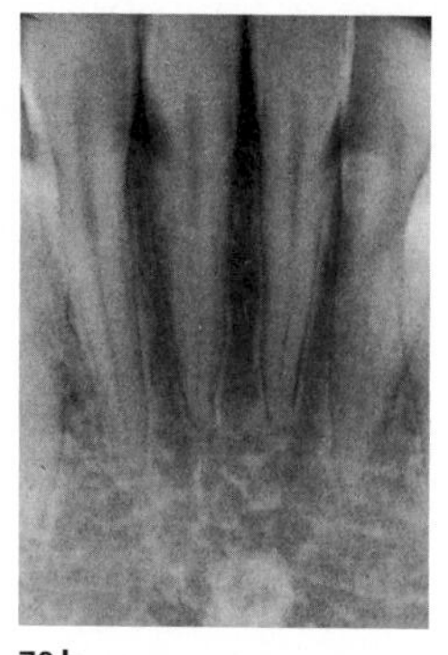

70 b

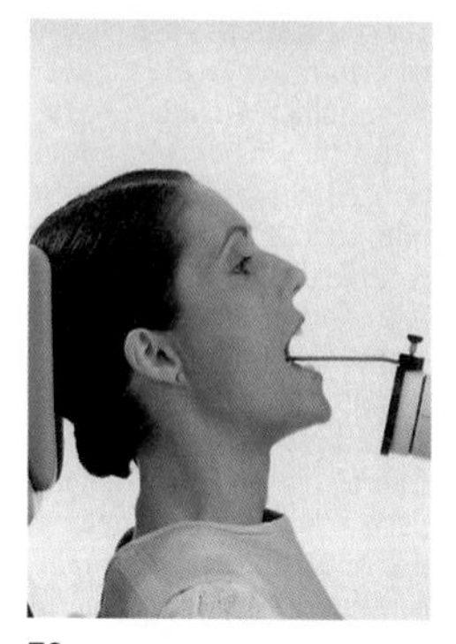

70 c

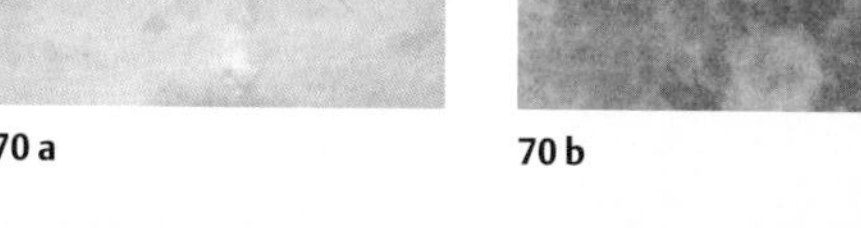

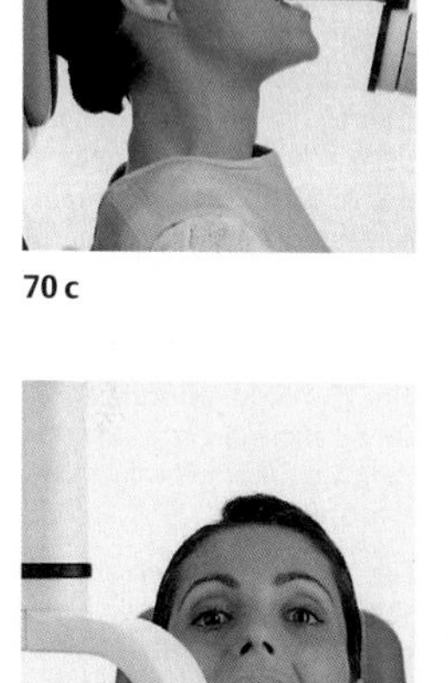

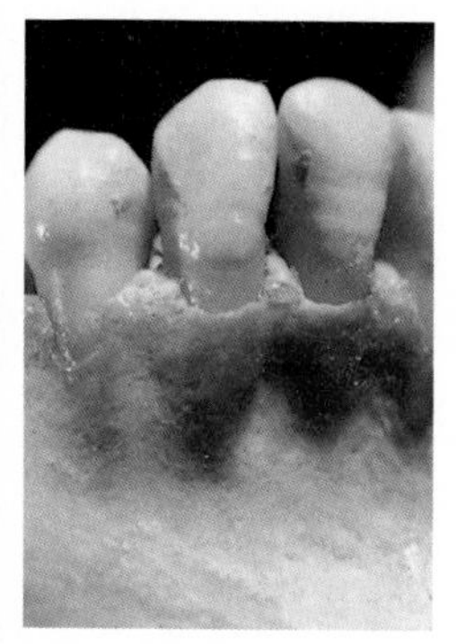

71 a

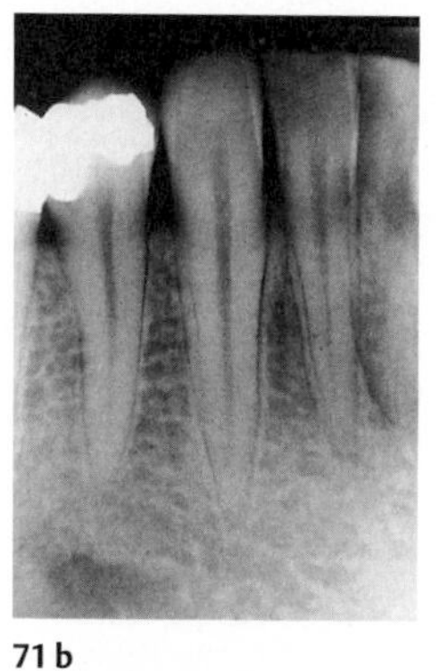

71 b

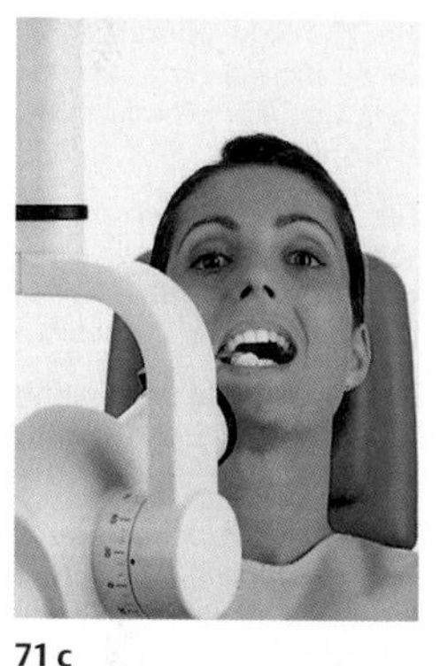

71 c

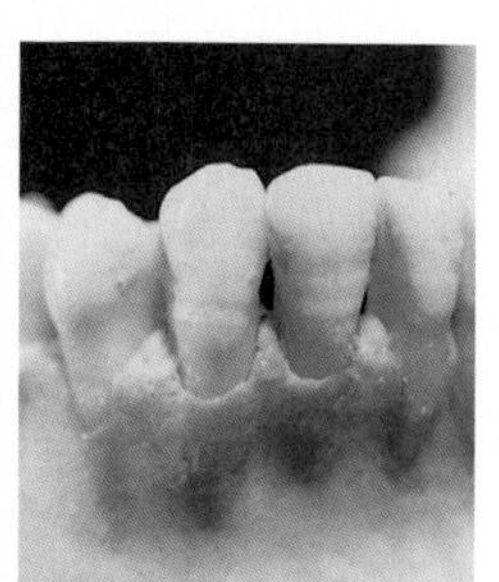

72a

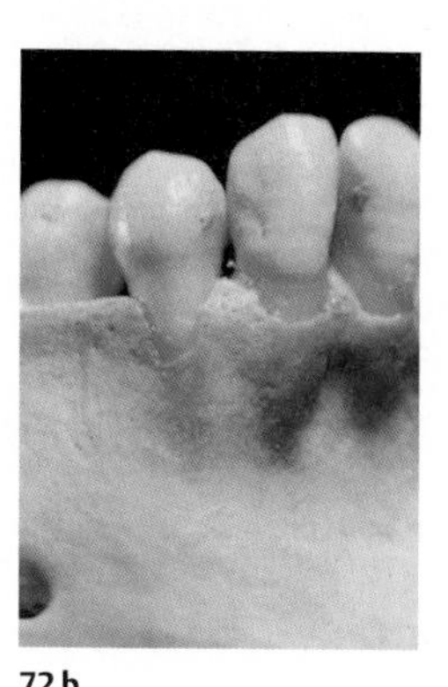

72 b

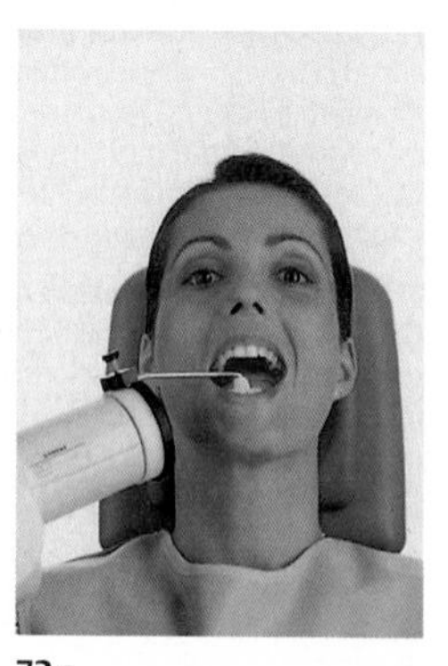

72 c

The illustrations we have used thus far to portray intraoral radiographic techniques may seem to some readers to be "antiquated" because they have been produced using traditional radiographic films. It is important to note that the basic rules for intraoral radiographic techniques are the same, whether using conventional radiography or the newer digital radiography. The only basic difference is film processing.

Regardless of the technique employed for intraoral radiography, the most important aspects will remain proper positioning of the image receptor and proper targeting of the central ray in order to depict the desired structures properly, thus permitting correct radiographic interpretations. The clinical technique used to achieve these goals will be determined to a great degree by the anatomy of the oral cavity and its spatial relationships. Some theoreticians have smiled and often considered the bisecting angle technique to be dead; however, even now in the digital age it remains the only method that is applicable in almost every situation to produce radiographs of high diagnostic quality. Still today, the isometry rule first published by Cieszynski (1907) remains the fundamental basis for the preparation of diagnostically satisfactory intraoral radiographs.

Fig. 73a Skull photograph, mandibular premolar region. If the central ray is targeted in its horizontal angle directly between the two premolars and perpendicular to an imaginary line connecting the two, the result will be an orthoradial depiction without overlapping if the proper vertical angle is also used.

Fig. 73b Radiograph of the mandibular premolar region. The coarsely trabeculated osseous structure of the mandible is particularly evident in this region of the body of the mandible; in elderly patients, fatty marrow islands or signs of cancellous bone are often observed. The mandibular premolars can also be depicted in portrait format, using a narrow image receptor.

Fig. 74a Clinical positioning for the mandibular premolar region. Especially with narrow image receptors, a targeting device is of great advantage. Using this device, the IR can be placed further toward the tongue space, and parallel to the long axes of the teeth.

Fig. 74b Incorrect clinical positioning for depiction of the mandibular molars. In an effort to completely depict the apical portions of the mandibular molar roots, the central ray is often projected too steeply from below. This results in an apparent shortening of the roots of the teeth and the coronoapical dimension of the body of the mandible is reduced; in addition, the crowns of the teeth will appear enlarged.

Fig. 74c Proper clinical positioning for a radiograph of the mandibular molars. The inexperienced clinician will often attempt to force the IR packet into the stretched floor of the mouth near to the teeth, eliciting a response from the mylohyoid muscle at its point of attachment. If the patient is asked to close the mouth slightly during positioning of the IR, the muscle will relax, and it can be placed without pain further toward the tongue and removed from the sensitive muscle attachments, into the desired position. A right-angle IRH can be used to advantage.

Fig. 75a Radiograph of the mandibular molar region. If the IR is placed at a right angle to the central ray and parallel to the tooth long axis, one will always achieve undistorted radiographs thanks to the favorable spatial relationships. The mandibular molar region has always been the subject of numerous publications concerning questions of quality in the preparation of intraoral dental radiographs.

Fig. 75b Nondiagnostic radiograph of a mandibular molar, resulting from excessively steep vertical angle of projection. If the central ray is projected to steeply from below, the body of the mandible will be depicted as coronoapically compressed and the surfaces of the mylohyoid line and the oblique line will be superimposed, thus rendering the radiograph nondiagnostic in many instances.

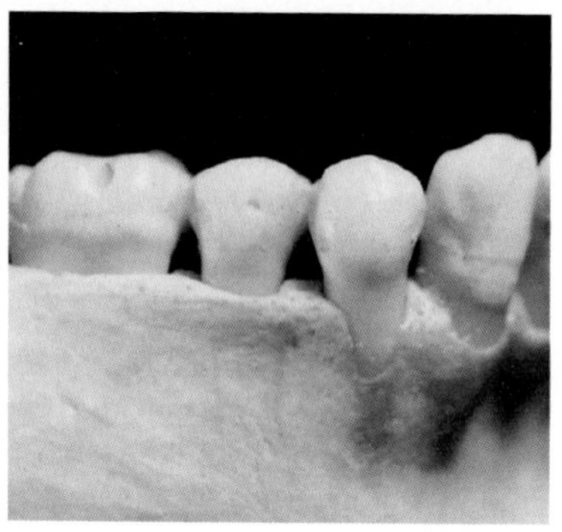
73 a

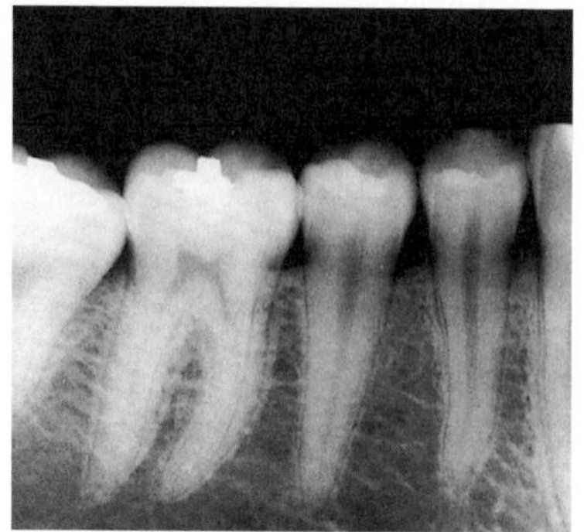
73 b

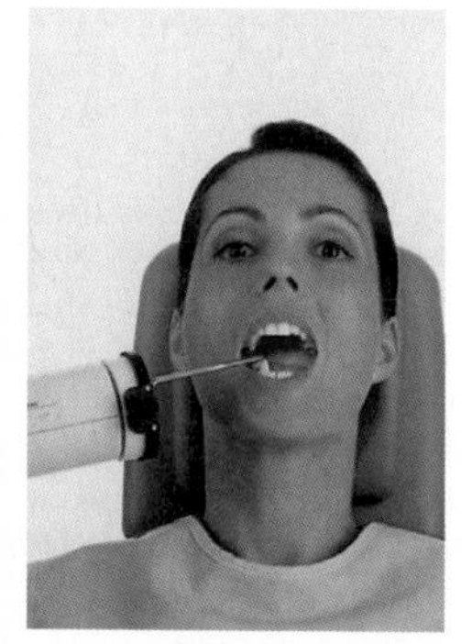
74 a

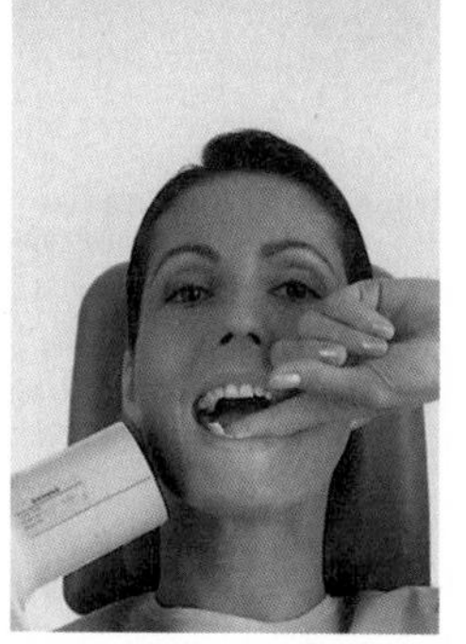
74 b

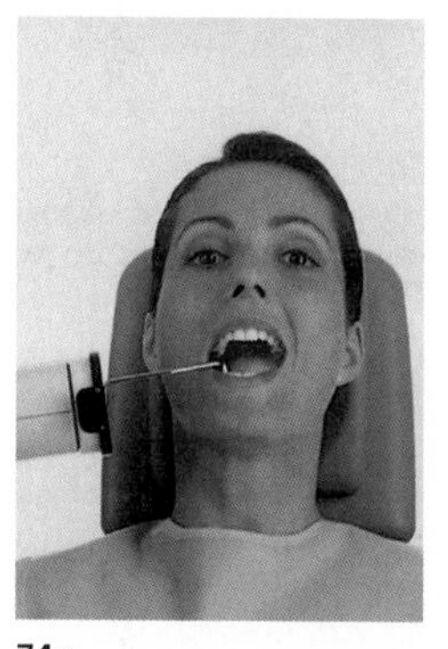
74 c

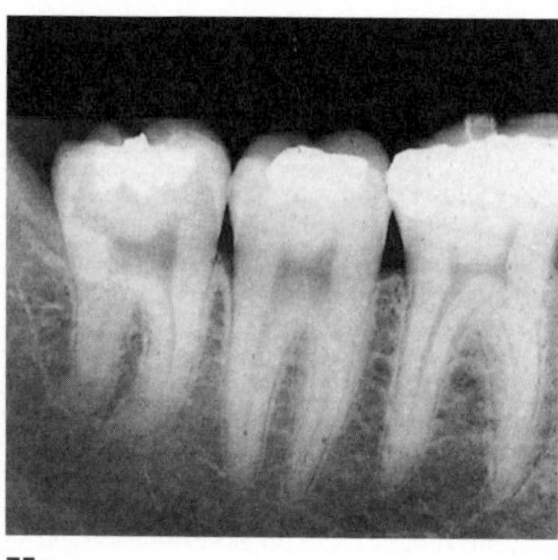
75 a

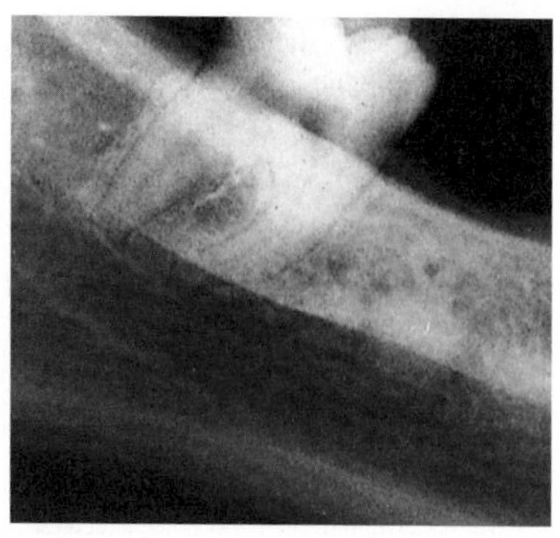
75 b

From the original text of the isometry rule (Cieszyński 1907): "The projected image will correspond to the actual size if the central ray is targeted vertically upon the middle plane; i.e., the central ray must be projected perpendicular to the line bisecting the angle between the tooth long axis and the film packet. Establishing the focus, i.e., the direction of the central ray, is performed in the following manner: One visualizes the long axis of the tooth, which represents one leg of the necessary angle; the second leg of the angle is determined by the position of the film. Next a plane dividing the angle between the tooth's long axis and the film is visualized. This angle-bisecting plane corresponds to the so-called 'middle plane'. A line perpendicular to this middle plane and passing through the apex of the root gives the correct direction for a central ray that will produce an image of the tooth with the same length as the actual tooth."

Fig. 76a Radiograph of a partially impacted maxillary third molar. This radiograph was taken with the central ray aimed steeply from above and dorsally, with ventral placement of the IR. Note the consequently overlapped projection of the maxillary molars.

Fig. 76b Radiograph of a fully impacted mandibular third molar. The central ray was not targeted steeply from below (as is often attempted), but rather coursed dorsally and somewhat above and forward onto the IR. Note the depiction of the ascending ramus of the mandible.

Fig. 77a Clinical positioning for a radiograph of the maxillary third molar. Proper central ray projection from the lateral view in order to achieve a diagnostic radiograph of a completely impacted maxillary third molar, from dorsal (above) toward ventral (below).

Fig. 77b Depicting wisdom teeth using the commercially available "Emmenix" IRH. For an intraoral depiction of third molars, the right-angle technique is usually inadequate because the cheek inhibits proper positioning of the IRH. The Emmenix IRH permits positioning of the IR with the mouth closed. If it becomes necessary to use intraoral radiography instead of a panoramic view, the clinician must remember and apply the principles of the bisecting-angle technique.

Fig. 77c Clinical positioning for a maxillary third molar radiograph. The photograph shows the proper central ray direction for an intraoral radiograph using the bisecting-angle technique.

Fig. 78a Clinical positioning for a mandibular third molar radiograph. The effort to depict a mandibular third molar is often accompanied by an error, namely targeting the tooth steeply from below with IR placement correspondingly far distally. This procedure is uncomfortable for the patient and also has risks for the clinician. It is easier and safer to place the IR *not* in a far distal location and to target the central ray from above and anteriorly in order to project the tooth optimally.

Fig. 78b Correct and incorrect projection for mandibular third molar radiograph. The appropriate technique will project the mandibular third molar from "distal excentric" onto the IR (**1**), and **not** "orthoradially" (**2**) onto a far distally positioned image receptor.

Fig. 78c Clinical positioning for a mandibular third molar radiograph. This frontal view shows the proper aiming of the central ray, which targets the desired object (third molar) to anterior and inferior onto the projection surface of the image receptor.

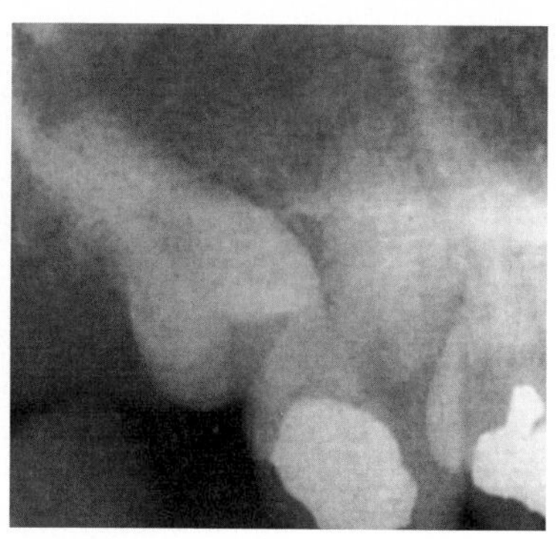

76 a

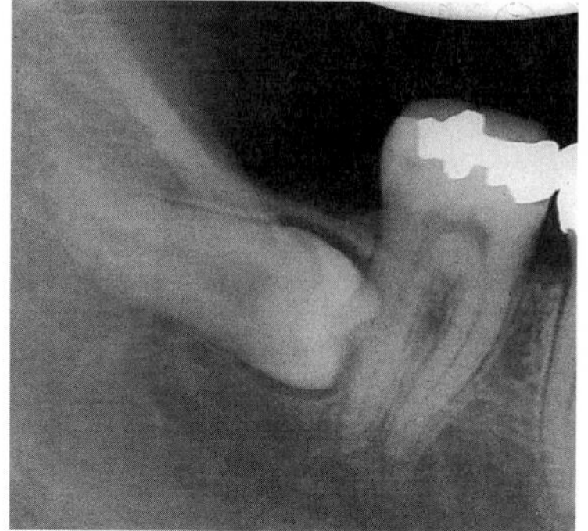

76 b

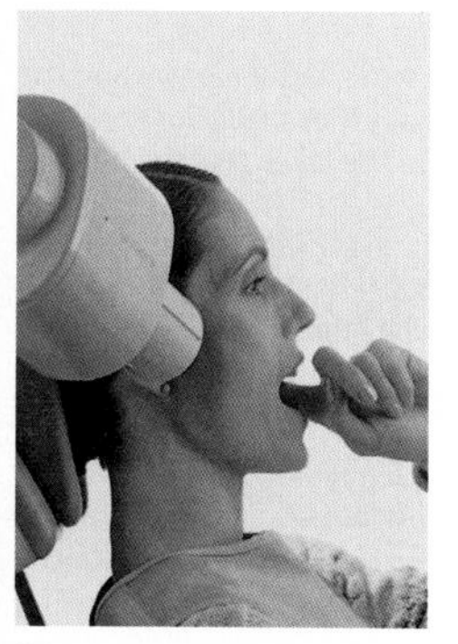

77 a

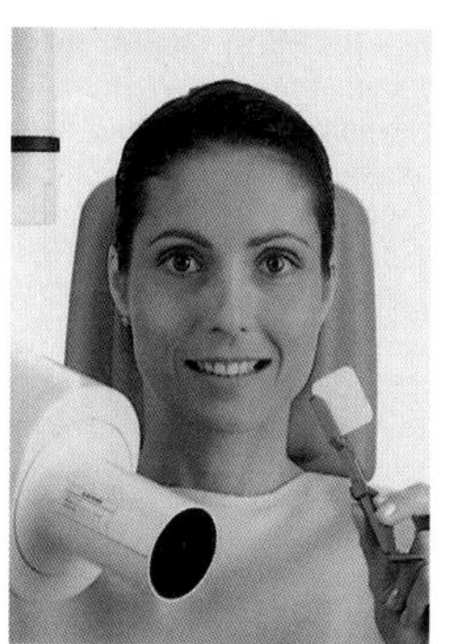

77 b

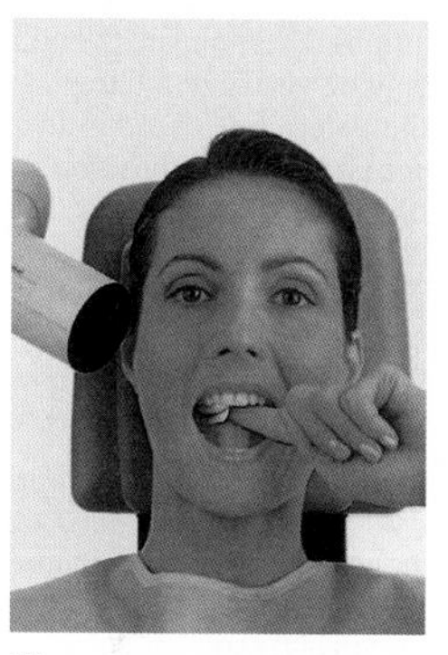

77 c

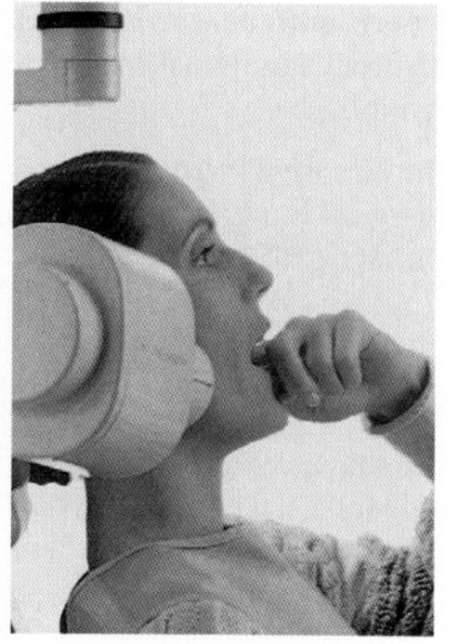

78 a

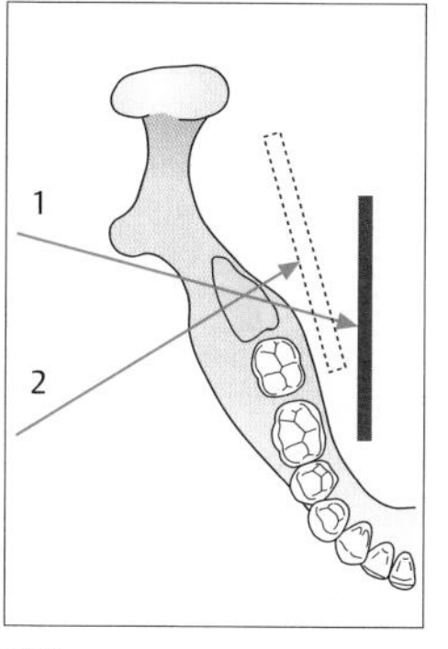

78 b

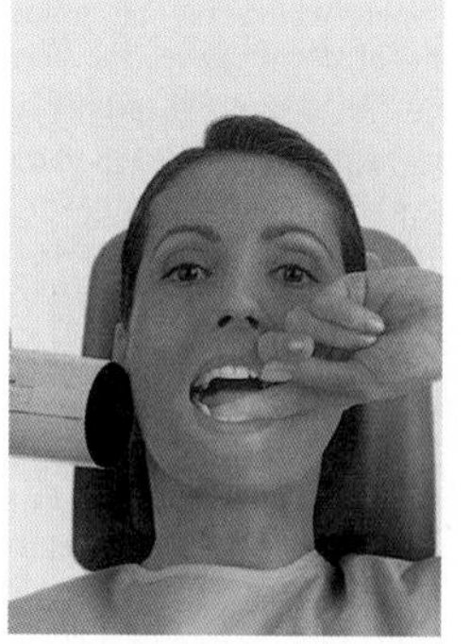

78 c

Bitewing radiographs have been used in dental practice for many decades. The central ray is targeted interocclusally with the mouth closed. These radiographs can be used to answer many questions concerning health and/or disease in the posterior regions of mandible and maxilla. Most frequently, however, bitewing images (Raper 1925) are used for the early detection/diagnosis of proximal carious lesions, because the roentgen rays target the proximal surfaces tangentially and loss of hard substance can be noted early as a radiolucency (or subtraction effect) in dental enamel. On the other hand, cervical caries on buccal or lingual surfaces expands transversely to the central ray, and will therefore often be diagnosed by careful clinical examination *earlier* than in the radiograph. Carious lesions developing in the occlusal fissures will only be visible in a bitewing radiograph after the defect has become deep and expansive, because the superposition (addition effect) of the intact enamel of the tooth crown masks the occlusal substance loss (especially in molars) for a long period of time during development of the lesion.

The masking of initial caries by intact hard structure of the tooth crown and the soft tissues of the cheek, in combination with low exposure setting, lead to a situation in which the size of a carious lesion is often underestimated radiographically. Periapical radiographs are almost totally *useless* for early diagnosis of dental caries, because of the unfavorable direction of the central ray.

Today, the bitewing radiograph remains the method of choice for the early diagnosis of proximal carious lesions. Despite the tremendous progress in caries prevention in recent decades, early detection of carious lesions remains one of the most important radiological diagnostic measures for the maintenance of dental health. Failure in this arena leads frequently to continuing loss of tooth hard structure in the posterior segments, and this inevitably leads to much more expensive treatment later on.

When taking bitewing radiographs using the various holders that are available for positioning the IR, care must be taken that the film not be pressed laterally against the lingual surfaces of the teeth, because upon mouth closure the distal upper end of the IR will be pushed downward by the maxilla.

Fig. 79 Bitewing radiographs, mixed dentition stage. These bitewing radiographs of a 7-year-old child, somewhat enlarged in this illustration, depict a carefully performed and proper radiographic technique. It is important not only that the IR (e.g., in an IRH) and the central ray are properly aligned, but also that the exposure settings are selected correctly. With overexposure, radiolucencies resembling caries will frequently appear, especially on the mesial surfaces of maxillary second deciduous molars; this artifact results from the shape of the crown of deciduous molars (see Fig. **262b**).

Fig. 80a Clinical positioning for bitewings in small children. Into the mixed dentition age, it is generally advantageous to focus the central ray in its vertical angle almost horizontal and *never* too steeply from above. The horizontal angle of the central ray is slightly from the mesial so that it traverses the second deciduous molars perpendicular to the IR as much as possible.

Fig. 80b Diagram of the bitewing technique. In adults, and when the IR is used in landscape format, the central ray is directed ca. 5° from above and slightly from the mesial through the first permanent molars. If narrower image receptors are used in portrait format (*vertical bitewings*), the premolars and the molars must be separately targeted.

Fig. 80c Technique for bitewings in adults. This profile photograph shows that in adults the central ray is targeted slightly from the mesial and interocclusally onto the image receptor.

Fig. 81 Bitewing radiographs using the long bitewing films from Kodak. Given ideal tooth position in the jaws, and with an extremely carefully performed bitewing technique, it is often possible in adults to completely depict the posterior arch segments using only two exposures. Excessively faint radiographs made with very low exposure doses are not indicated for early caries diagnosis because of the superimposition (overlapping) with intact segments of enamel. Note the radiolucency distally on the cervical area of tooth 37, which is due to the subtraction effect of the transparent dental sac, a burn-out effect.

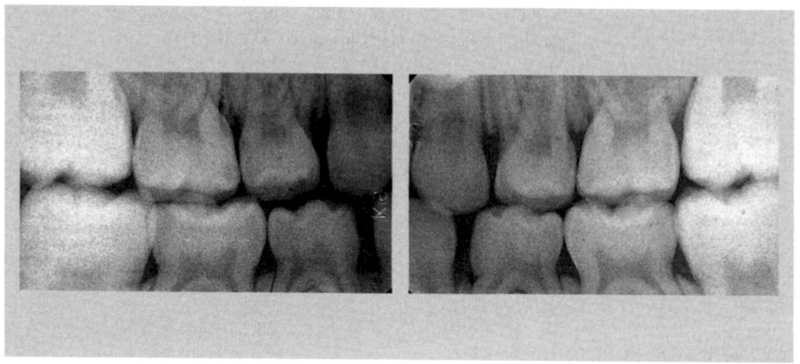

79

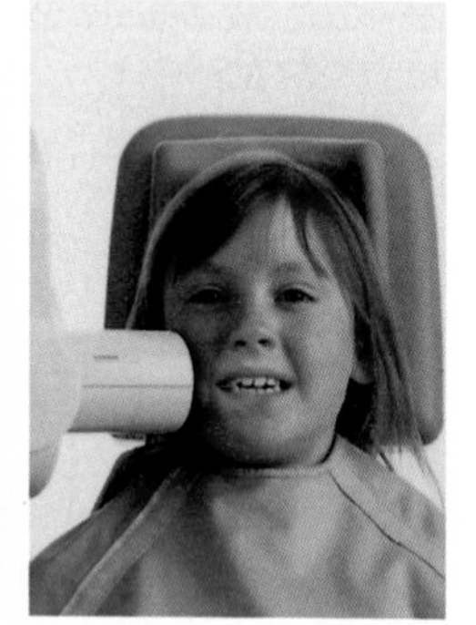

80 a

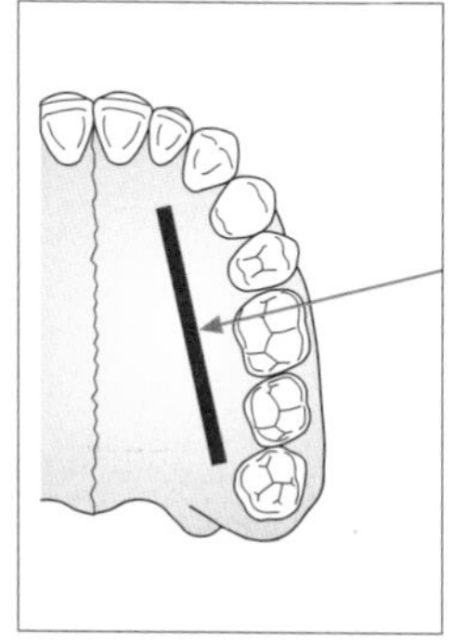

80 b

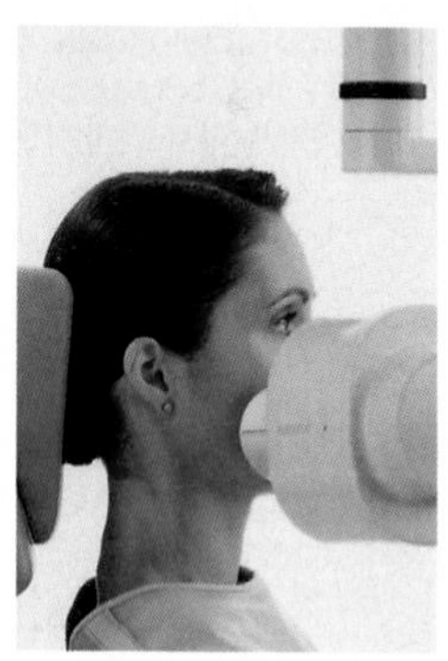

80 c

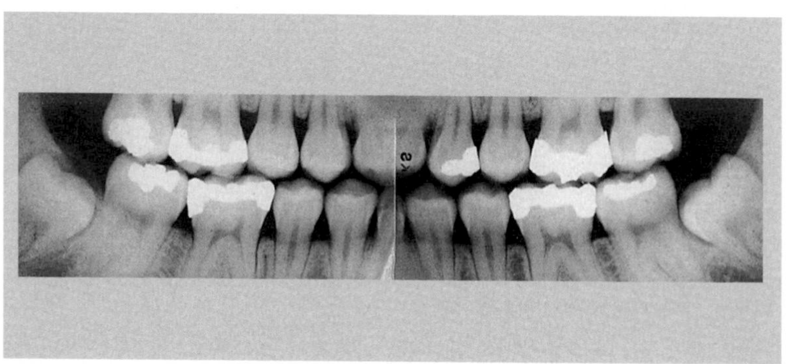

81

The result will be loss of diagnostic information in the maxillary molar region and/or in the mandibular premolar region. Additional loss of diagnostic information in the radiograph will occur if the jaws are not completely closed together. Finally, difficulties of interpretation will result if the horizontally directed central ray is not targeted enough from the mesial aspect and tangentially onto the proximal tooth surfaces, resulting in overlapping (see Fig. **101a**).

Bitewing radiographs can also be used to advantage for examination of the alveolar ridge in adults. Depending upon the size of the image receptor that is used, the marginal osseous structures of the maxilla and mandible can be depicted with a single or eventually two exposures per side; this leads not only to the creation of a diagnostically effective periodontal survey, but also considerably reduces the radiation exposure for the patient.

Bitewing radiographs can provide the following diagnostic information:

- Early recognition of proximal caries.
- Secondary caries beneath restorations and crowns.
- Proximal marginal integrity of restorations and crowns. (**Note:** With high exposure settings, the root near the restoration margin will be overexposed, leading to the diagnostic impression of an overhanging crown margin.)
- Calculus accumulation in the proximal regions.
- Condition of the alveolar ridge in the early stages of periodontal lesions.
- Malocclusions resulting from tooth positional anomalies, missing teeth, or missing antagonists.

Depiction of peri-implant osseous structure at the implant shoulder (neck).

Fig. 82 IR placement in adults:

Left: Possible applications in landscape format using film or sensor size 2.5 x 5.5 cm (**orange**) and the film or sensor format of ca. 3 x 4 cm (**green**).

Right: Possible applications in portrait format (*vertical bitewing*) using film or sensor of ca. 2 x 3 cm (**violet**) and 3 x 4 cm (**orange**).

Fig. 83 Radiographs taken with various image receptors. Conventional radiographic film packets as well as digital sensors in the 3 x 4 cm format can be used in both young people and adults for caries diagnosis. In comparison to the long bitewing film from Kodak, the diagnostic information is somewhat limited in length, but improved in height if the arches are closed completely together. For bitewing radiographs in children, special small films or small sensors are used in landscape format.

Fig. 84 Radiographs taken using various image receptor formats:

Left: For diagnosis and evaluation of advanced cases of periodontitis, image receptors (film or sensor) of various sizes can be used in portrait format (*vertical bitewings*).

Right: Experimental testing of an IR of size 3.5 x 5 cm clearly revealed that this size and format would be ideal for virtually all diagnostic questions in the posterior segments. This format could also be used to advantage as an occlusal film in cases of tooth injury in children.

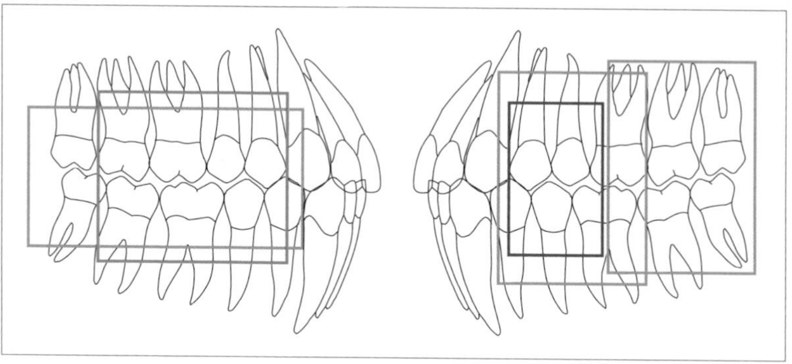

82

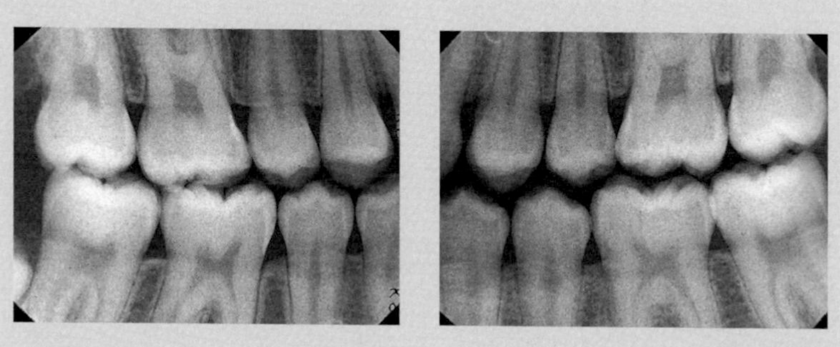

83

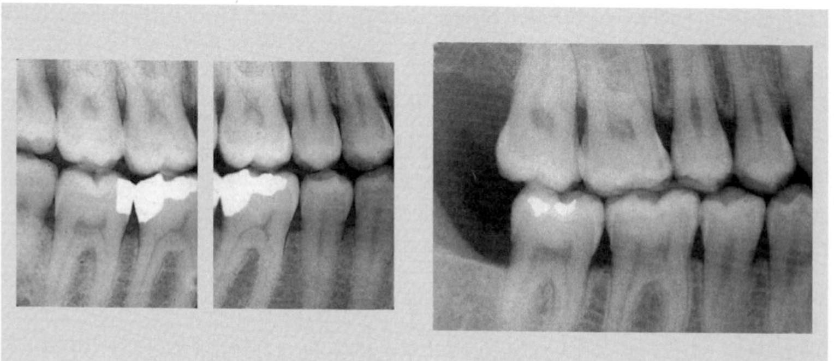

84

Intra- and extraoral use of occlusal radiographs: Not only the well-known and traditional occlusal films in 7.5 x 5.5-cm format, but also digital sensors of larger format can be used to answer numerous intra- and extraoral diagnostic questions, especially in small children and individuals in the early mixed dentition stage. Unfortunately, the broad array of diagnostic possibilities offered by occlusal radiographs is only seldom taken advantage of, even though their use in dental practice is relatively simple. One reason is that digital image receptors of appropriate sizes are not yet commercially available. For the proper indication and with technically perfect performance, the occlusal radiograph can often provide the diagnostically important third dimension, which cannot be achieved with periapical radiographs, or with standard panoramic views. The occlusal radiograph is particularly well indicated as an overview radiograph, above all in small children in the anterior region (e.g., following accident or injury); especially with fearful small children, the use of a right-angle holder offers advantages for pain-free positioning of the IR packet. The properly taken occlusal radiograph can also be helpful in daily practice for the solution of localization problems, e.g., a palatally impacted canine (see Fig. **169b**). For this procedure, adjacent teeth must be used as reference objects and be targeted along the tooth long axis by the central ray. If the central ray is projected obliquely, for example to depict a palatally impacted tooth in the maxilla, the desired object will be distorted and not depicted in its actual position, and this can lead to incorrect diagnosis and errors during subsequent therapeutic procedures. With appropriate positioning and technical procedures, a high-quality occlusal radiograph can be an excellent means to depict sialoliths within Wharton's duct of the submandibular gland, or in the sublingual gland.

Fig. 85a Skull photograph, anatomic position for taking a maxillary overview occlusal radiograph. This photograph reveals how steeply the central ray must be focused in order to achieve the best possible and most inclusive overview of the maxilla. When aiming the central ray it is important to note whether the subnasale is behind or in front of a vertical line through nasion (see p. **94** for skeletal points), which is to say, whether the maxillary portion of the face is receding or protruding. A concave facial profile can, depending on its severity, make it difficult to render a complete depiction of the maxilla.

Fig. 85b Overview occlusal radiograph of the maxilla. The central ray must be targeted as steeply as possible and must follow the median-saggital plane in order to achieve a symmetrical view of the maxilla; this is critically important for the bilateral comparative interpretation and diagnosis.

Fig. 86a Clinical photograph showing proper aiming of the central ray for an overview occlusal radiograph of the maxilla. The patient's head is straight up and the central ray enters perpendicularly through the region of the maxillary first molars.

Fig. 86b Clinical photograph showing the central ray projection for an overview occlusal radiograph of the mandible. The patient's head is tipped far backward and the central ray is targeted perpendicularly through the region of the mandibular molars onto the projection surface of the IR. The patient's head position will significantly influence the radiographic quality.

Fig. 87a Skull photograph shows the anatomic situation for central ray targeting for an overview occlusal radiograph of the mandible. The photograph shows the mandible and the IR packet from the point-of-view of the central ray.

Fig. 87b Overview occlusal radiograph of the mandible. Because the teeth are depicted axially, this radiograph is useful for localization of retained, impacted, or supernumerary teeth (exception: third molars). For the visualization of expansive lesions that extend beyond normal anatomic boundaries in the mandible, the exposure settings will have to be varied according to the thickness and density of the object in question.

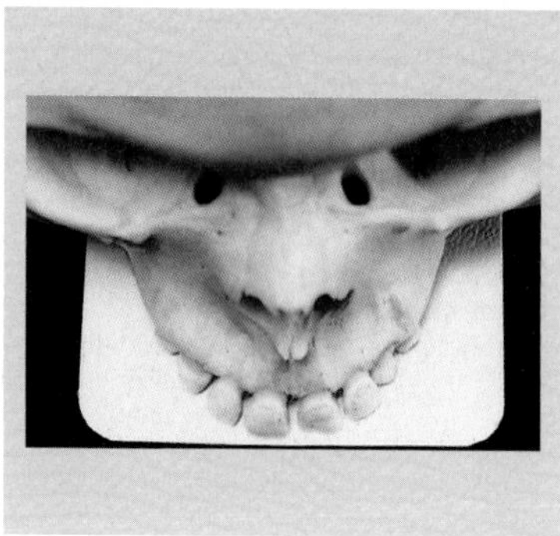

85 a

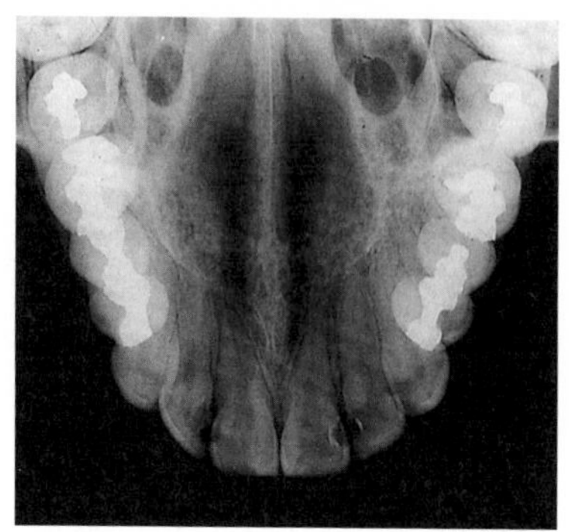

85 b

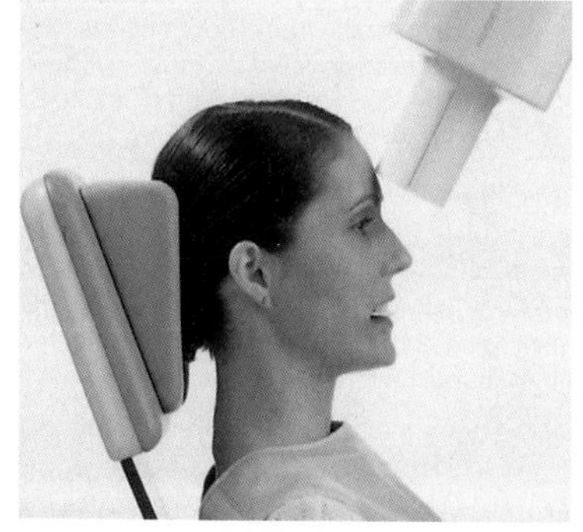

86 a

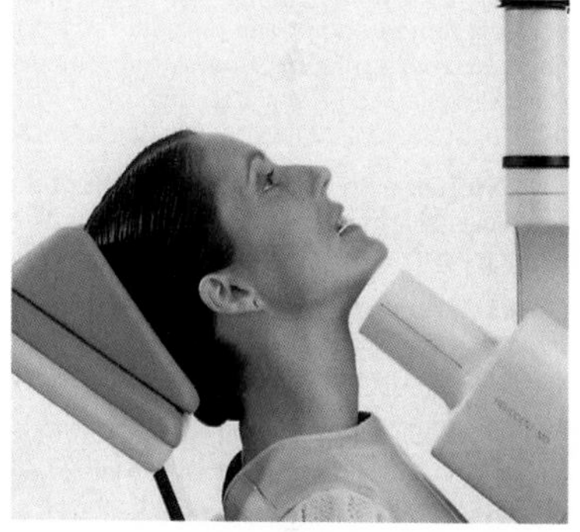

86 b

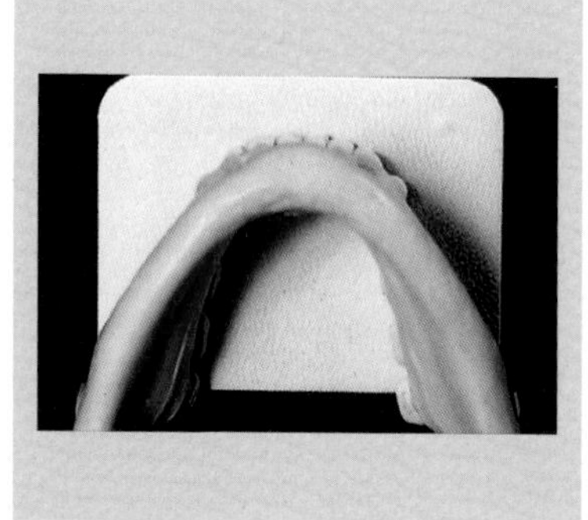

87 a

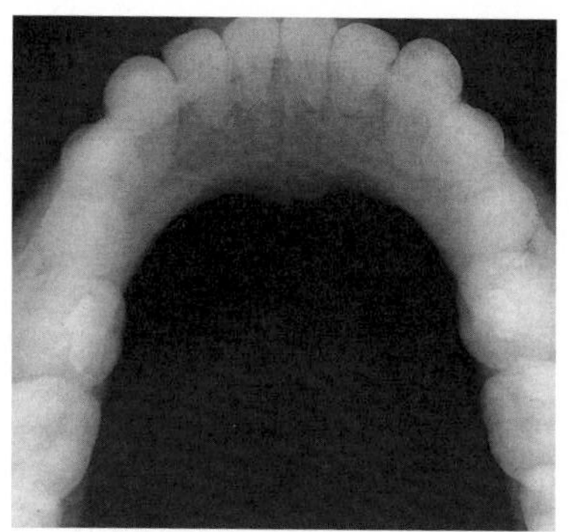

87 b

With spatially expanding pathologic processes such as odontogenic and nonodontogenic cysts, tumors, or tumor-like lesions, the occlusal radiograph can clearly depict the pathologic structures and any lesions that expand or extend beyond anatomic boundaries in the mandible, providing the third dimension; however, this will only occur if the operator has appropriately adjusted the exposure settings for the thickness and density of the desired structures of interest, and appropriately adjusted the central ray. Also in the maxilla, a properly positioned and exposed occlusal radiograph can provide important information concerning normal structures and pathologic alterations; however, the clinician must be aware that the radiograph is the result of oblique projections and must therefore be correspondingly interpreted.

Fig. 88a Skull photograph showing the direction of the central ray, from above, for a half-arch occlusal radiograph of the maxilla. The central ray is targeted laterally from above and medially downward to clearly depict one side of the maxilla. High and vestibularly located structures will however, be projected palatally, so that use of this radiographic technique for localization of impacted teeth high above the root tips of adjacent teeth will not always provide optimum views.

Fig. 88b Half-arch occlusal radiograph of the maxilla. In this case, the impacted canine was located palatally at the height of the root tips of teeth 12 and 11. Note the resorption of the cusp of the impacted canine.

Fig. 88c Diagram showing the central ray direction for a half-arch occlusal radiograph of the maxilla. The entrance point for the central ray is in the region of the infraorbital foramen. The red line indicates the traverse of the roentgen rays through the maxilla and roof of the palate.

Fig. 89a Clinical positioning for a half-arch occlusal radiograph of the maxilla. The photograph shows horizontal positioning of the IR packet and indicates the direction of the central ray.

Fig. 89b Clinical positioning for a half-arch occlusal radiograph of the mandible. With consideration for the axis of the cross-section of the mandible in the posterior segments, the central ray must be projected from below and laterally upwards and lingually in order to ensure depiction of structures exhibiting pathologic alterations of bone, or sialoliths in Wharton's duct or within the sublingual duct. When using this half-arch technique for the mandible, the patient's head must be tilted very far backward in order to be able to properly position the cone of the equipment.

Fig. 90a Skull photograph showing the direction of the central ray for a half-arch occlusal radiograph of the mandible. The photograph shows that the central ray must be targeted according to the axis of the jaw cross-section in order to freely project the mandibular molars along their long axes, or to depict sialoliths.

Fig. 90b Half-arch occlusal radiograph of the mandible. The radiograph depicts the posterior tooth segment of the right half of the mandible, with an axial projection of tooth 46. Depending on whether the goal is to depict the teeth, pathologic alterations of the bone of the mandible or sialoliths, the exposure settings must be adjusted for the thickness and density of the desired structures.

Fig. 90c Schematic showing proper positioning of the IR for a half-arch occlusal radiograph of the mandible. Depicted is the position of an occlusal film, size 7.5 x 5.5 cm. It is obviously considerably more difficult to achieve a good result using a sensor of ca. 3 x 4 cm in size. Nevertheless, with proper positioning of the image receptor and careful targeting of the central ray it is possible in emergency situations to appropriately depict a section of the dental arch.

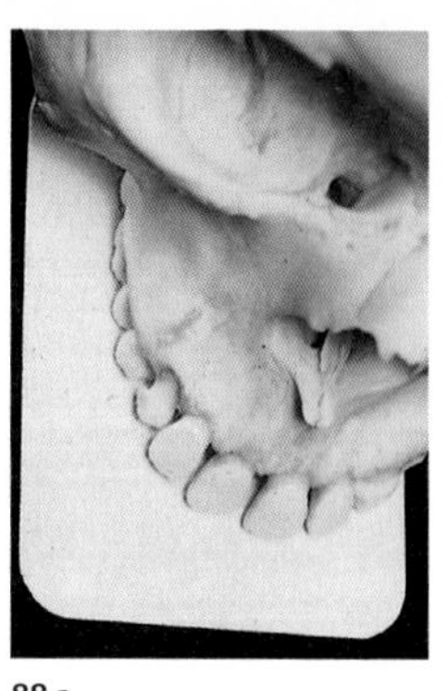
88 a

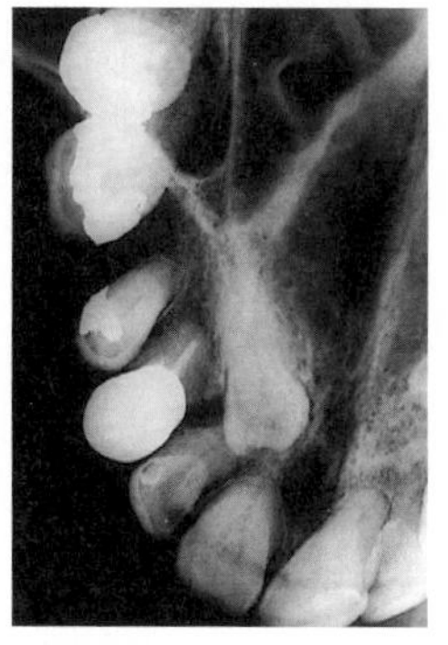
88 b

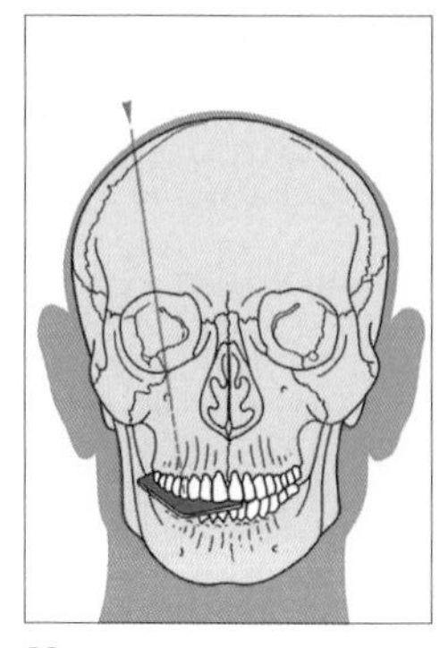
88 c

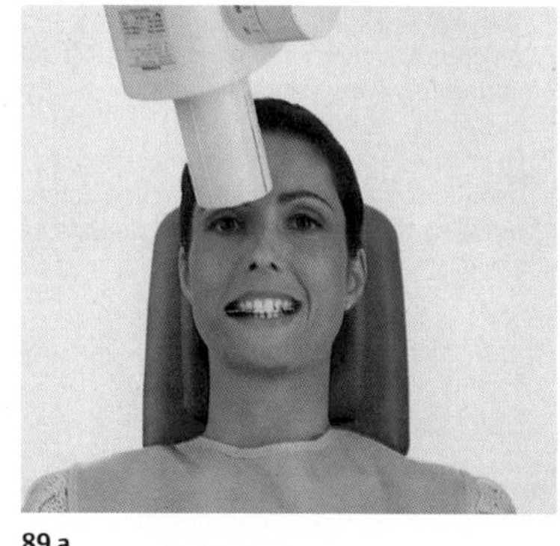
89 a

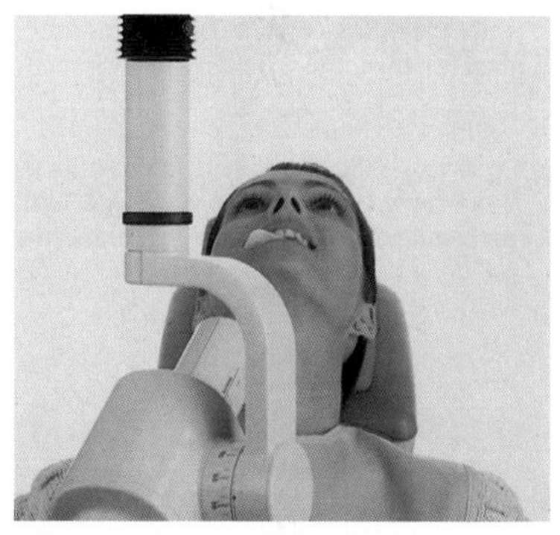
89 b

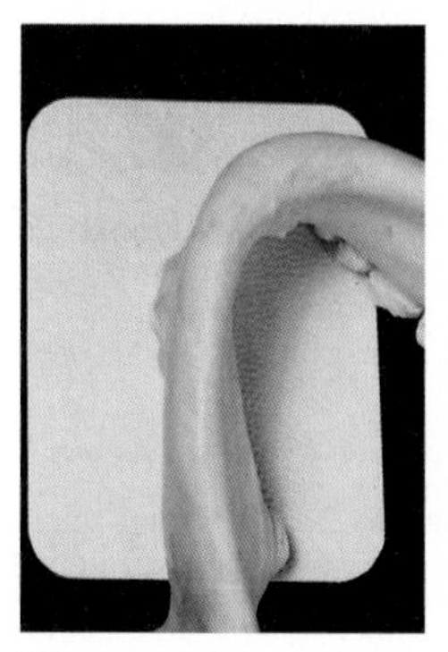
90 a

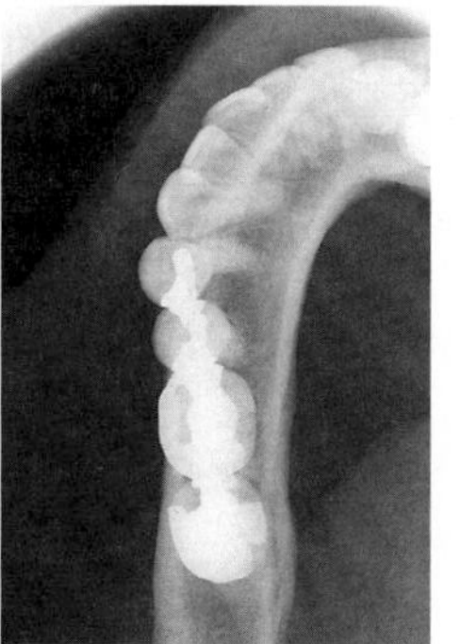
90 b

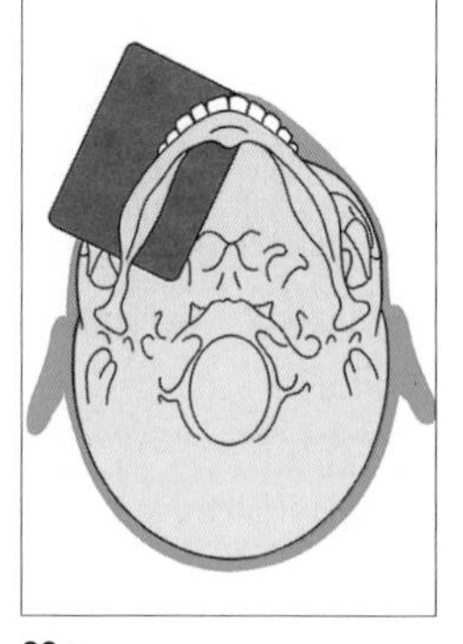
90 c

Presented here is a summary of what can be accomplished using **intraoral** occlusal radiographs; these can be performed with conventional occlusal film packets and to a more limited degree also using large digital sensors.

Maxilla:

1. Overview occlusal radiographs using a steep, median-saggital central ray projection that symmetrically captures the region of the maxillary first molars and the entire maxilla.
2. Partial (smaller) occlusal radiographs employing a flat, median-sagittally directed ray for depiction of the maxillary anterior region.
3. Half-arch occlusal radiographs employing a steep lateromedial central ray projection with the entrance point near the infraorbital foramen.

Mandible:

1. Overview radiograph with the patient's head tipped steeply backward and with perpendicular median-saggital central ray projection onto the image receptor at the level of the first mandibular molars.
2. Partial (smaller) radiograph with a flat, median-saggital central ray projection to depict the anterior region of the mandible or the genial apophysis.
3. Half-arch occlusal radiograph with lateromedial central ray projection along the axis of the mandibular cross-section in the molar region, and entrance point of the central ray at the deepest point of the compact bone of the body of the mandible in the molar region. Use of appropriate variations in exposure settings for depiction of expansive or expanding lesions and, with special central ray targeting, depiction of the position of mandibular wisdom teeth in the third dimension.

Occlusal radiographs in small children:

1. Overview radiograph of the maxillary and mandibular anterior segments for examination following dental injuries caused by accidents.
2. Overview radiograph of the maxillary and mandibular anterior regions to supplement bitewing radiographs in a radiographic survey of small children.

Fig. 91 a Improper head position for an overview occlusal radiograph of the maxilla. With the head position and the central ray projection depicted here, it will not be possible to achieve a satisfactory overview radiograph. In this configuration, one will achieve only a depiction of the anterior region of the maxilla.

Fig. 91 b Incorrect head position for taking an overview occlusal radiograph of the mandible. The photograph shows that the patient's head is **not** tipped backward to permit right-angle positioning of the central ray to the image receptor. This positioning *would* permit adequate depiction of the mental spine.

Fig. 92 a Clinical positioning for an occlusal radiograph of the maxillary anterior segment in a small child. The photograph shows proper positioning for examination of the maxillary anterior region; often necessary because of childhood accidents. With a resistant or fearful child, the IR packet must not come into contact with the sensitive palatal tissues. Use a right-angled image receptor holder!

Fig. 92 b Clinical positioning of a small child for depiction of the anterior region of the mandible with the occlusal technique. The photograph shows head position and radiation source direction for depicting the anterior segment of the mandible.

Fig. 93 Occlusal radiographs of maxilla and mandibular anterior segments in a small child. Such occlusal radiographs of the anterior regions can be coupled with the smallest available image receptors for posterior bitewings, resulting in a satisfactory radiograph survey of small children.

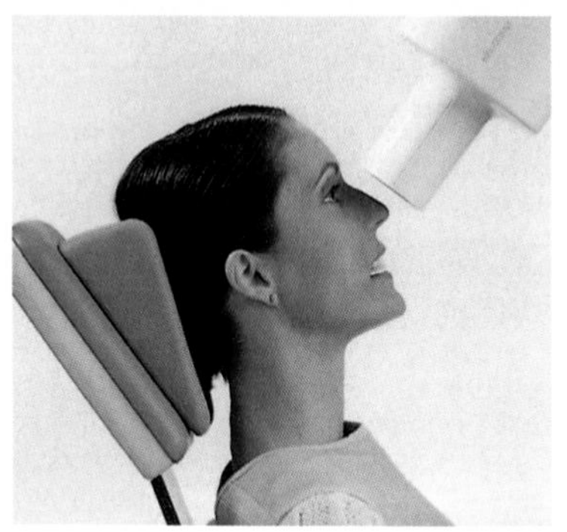
91 a

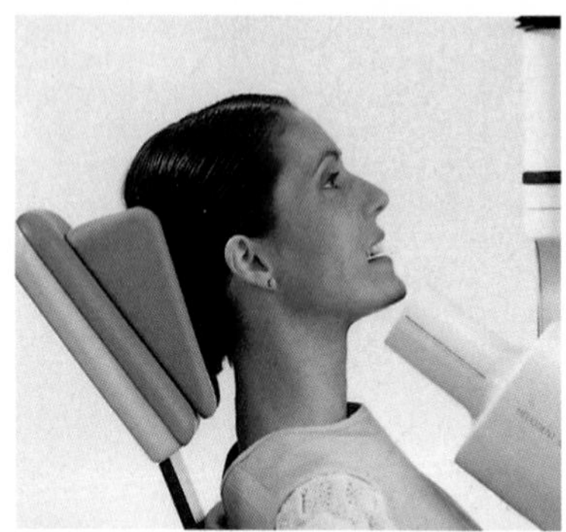
91 b

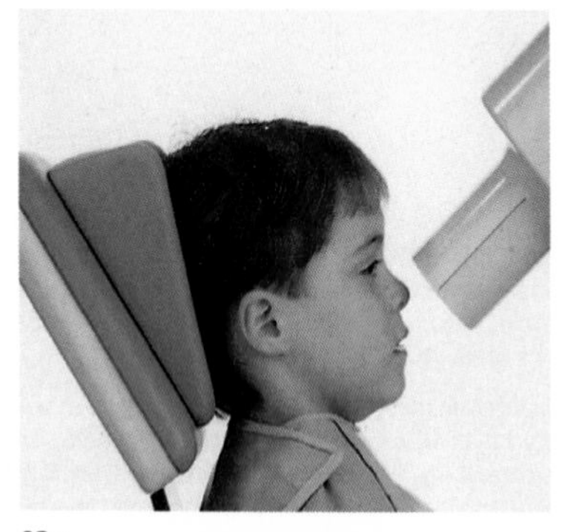
92 a

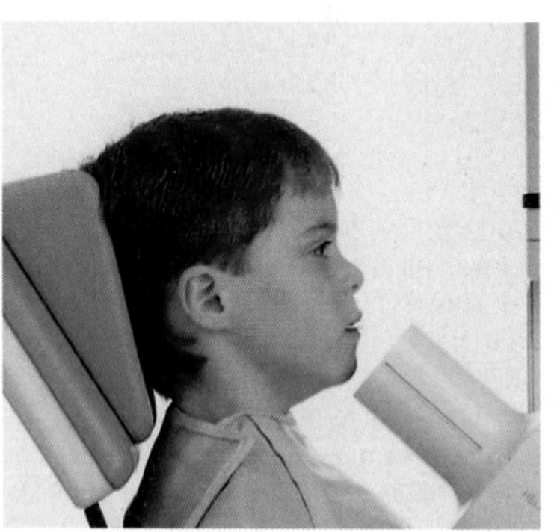
92 b

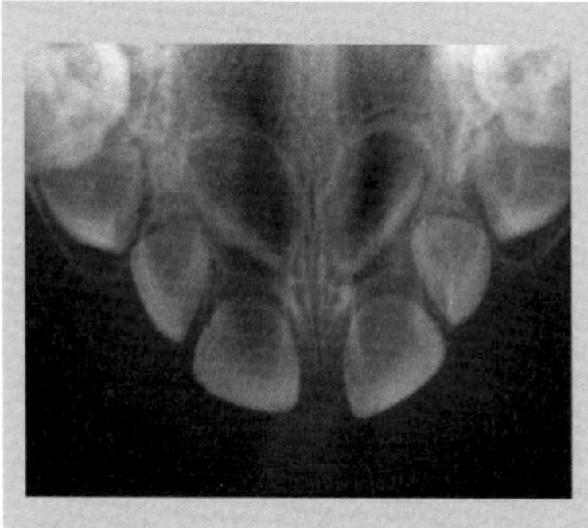
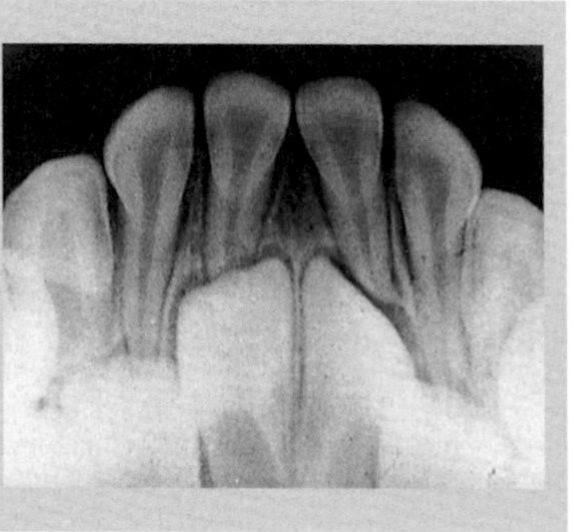
93

Occlusal films (also digital image receptors) may also be used infrequently **extraorally** to address special diagnostic questions. They serve to supplement a panoramic radiograph, and can be taken with a "free hand" projection or with use of an appropriate IRH. Extraoral use of an occlusal image receptor is indicated above all in the chin region, where it can be used following trauma to verify fracture lines or dislocation of bone fragments when the panoramic view does not bring clarity because of the overlapping of the cervical vertebrate.

Occlusal image receptors can also be used for lateral projections of the maxilla to depict the precise location of an ectopic anterior tooth, if the dental practice does not have access to a panoramic unit with a cephalostat to take a lateral skull projection.

Fig. 94a Clinical positioning for depiction of the mandibular third molar in its third dimension. The patient's head is tipped back and also tipped laterally toward the healthy side. The central ray is projected anteriorly and upward through the third molar onto the IR packet, which can only be inserted up to the anterior border of the ascending ramus of the mandible.

Fig. 94 b and c Half-arch extraoral occlusal radiograph revealing the third dimension of a mandibular third molar. Both images reveal the third molars in positional relationship to the mandibular second molars, because of the axial orientation of the central ray. When targeting the central ray, it is necessary to ascertain the access direction of the second molars. This type of radiograph can also be taken using digital sensors of about 3 x 4 cm in size.

Fig. 95a Clinical positioning for taking a radiograph of the chin. The patient's head is positioned so that the IR packet is horizontal with the mouth slightly open. The central ray is targeted so that the chin is projected onto the IR, free of overlap by the anterior teeth.

Fig. 95b Radiograph of the chin, taken using an extraoral occlusal IR packet. Especially in elderly patients, the panoramic radiograph may provide unsatisfactory depiction of the chin region because of overlapping by the cervical vertebrate; this technique provides a view of the chin with no superimposed structures. It is especially indicated in cases of chin fracture.

Fig. 96a Extraoral lateral radiographic technique of the anterior region of the maxilla. The photograph shows the position of the occlusal IR packet. If the packet is placed somewhat more cranially, the nasal bone can also be depicted for diagnosis of facial osseous fractures.

Fig. 96b Diagram of the lateral maxillary anterior region radiograph. The illustration shows the position of the IR packet, which should be pressed onto the zygomatic arch and **not** contact the cheek anteriorly. The red line indicates the lateral central ray projection which passes anterior to the nasal spine in order to impact the IR at a right angle.

Fig. 96c Lateral radiograph of the anterior region of the maxilla. Taken following an accident, this radiograph reveals splinters of glass in the upper lip (**arrows**).

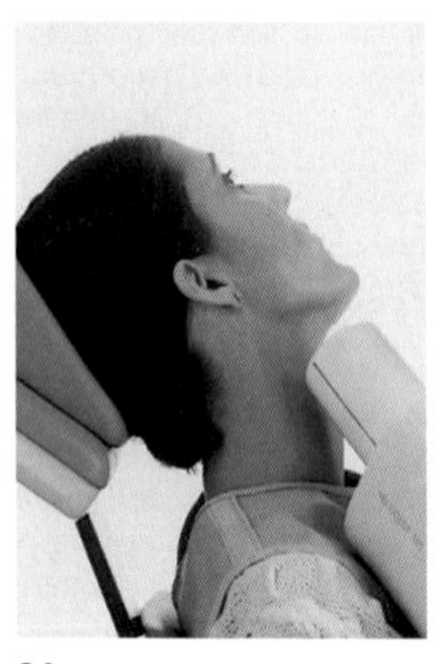
94 a

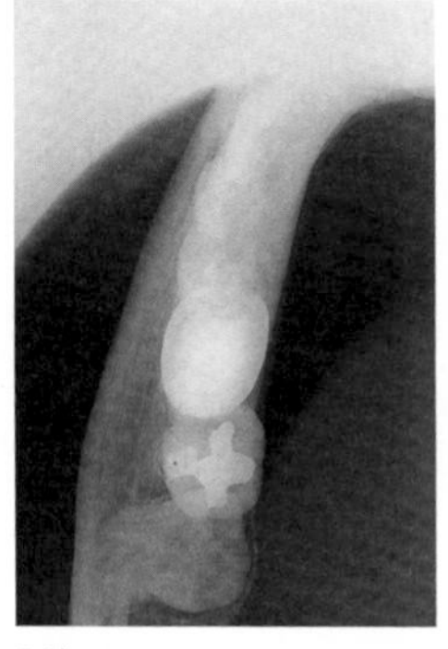
94 b

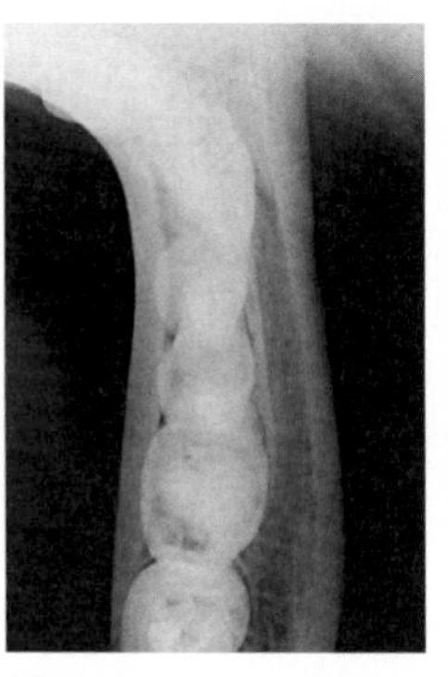
94 c

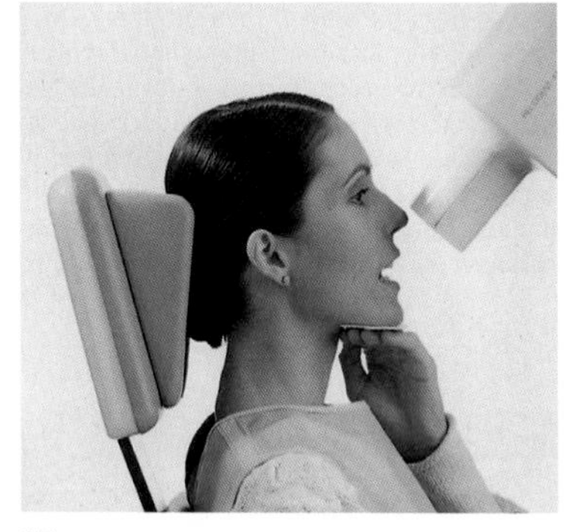
95 a

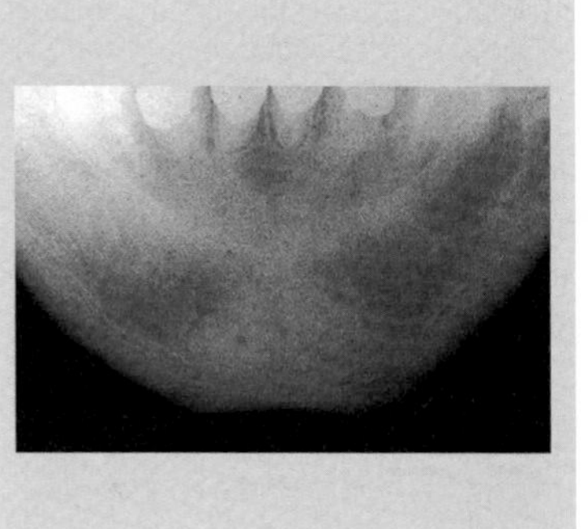
95 b

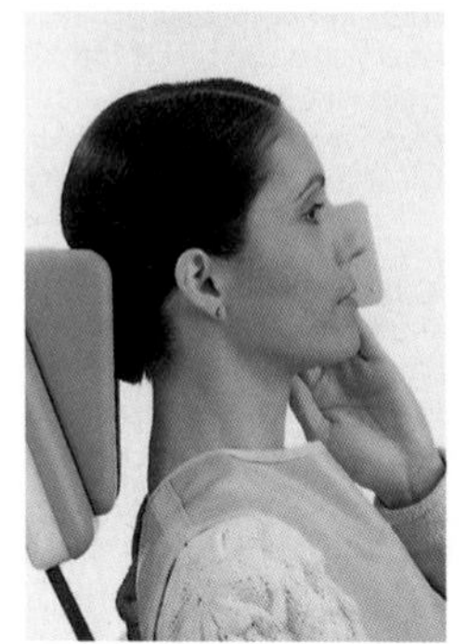
96 a

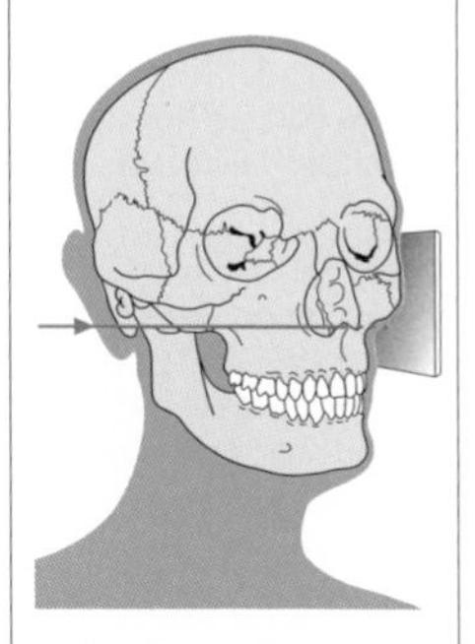
96 b

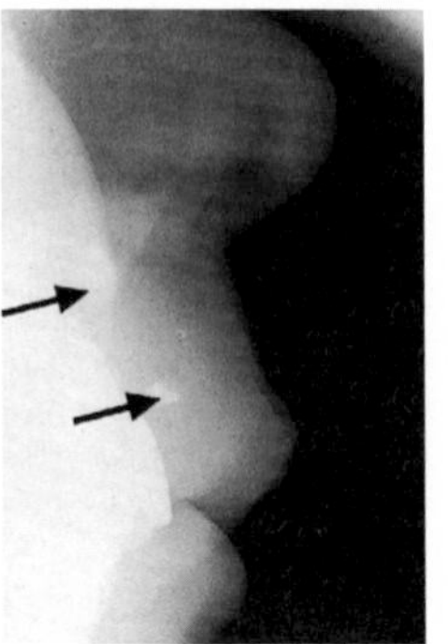
96 c

For the intraoral radiograph necessary in a routine dental practice today several image receptor systems are commercially available, which permit either conventional or digital processing of the primary image. The quality of the final image that appears on the radiographic film or on the screen of a PC is, aside from certain limited correction possibilities, dependent on the quality of the initial or primary image, which itself is determined by the quality of the clinical exposure technique employed. In the final analysis it is the radiographic technique that is responsible for the quality and also for the *interpretability* of every radiograph; the developing or processing systems play a much less important role. Technical errors lead in many cases to the necessity to re-take the radiograph, and this unnecessarily increases the radiation exposure for the patient. In summary, the following factors will *negatively influence* the technical quality of intraoral radiographs:

- Proper indication for any given radiograph, with consideration for the radiographic-diagnostic question.
- Careful and complete preparation of the patient, the necessary instruments, and materials.
- Proper and as far as possible pain-free placement of the selected image receptor.
- Proper targeting of the central ray in both vertical and horizontal angles, and use of an appropriate IRH.
- The **clinical time** necessary for taking the radiographs!

In this chapter we will use typical results to show the effects of technical errors on radiographic quality. In addition to the correct application of the basic indication for any radiograph, preparation of the patient plays a not insignificant role. *This can be time-intensive.* A patient who is thoroughly informed is more likely to be motivated to participate in achieving success with the radiographic procedure. All radiopaque foreign bodies and also removable metal-based partial dentures must be removed from the path of the central ray. Once exposed, the intraoral films should be arranged in the proper format so that they can be immediately labeled; digitally derived images should be checked in the PC and properly arranged. It is much more comfortable for the patient if the exposure data are set *before* positioning the image receptor.

Fig. 97 Technical errors. a An excessively steep projection angle results in a radiograph wherein the teeth appear shortened; the proportions are also incorrect. **b** A projection angle that is too flat results in a radiograph wherein the tooth roots appear elongated, often even beyond the edge of the radiograph. **c** If the central ray is targeted obliquely from above and steeply from the mesial aspect, the maxillary premolars will exhibit overlapping and, as depicted here, the laterobasal wall of the nasal cavity will be visible in the image.

Fig. 98 Technical errors. a Excessively flat targeting of the central ray with obvious apparent lengthening of the tooth root. **b** This film was bent near the floor of the mouth, leading to distortions of the teeth due to the oblique projection. In this particular case, the patient held the film with his finger! **c** Central ray projection too steeply from below the chin led to complete loss of visualization of the mandibular anterior incisor crowns and clear depiction of the basal compact bone of the anterior mandible.

Fig. 99 Technical errors. a Excessively steep projection in a molar periapical radiograph in the maxilla. The zygomatic bone overlaps the endodontically treated tooth 17 (with secondary caries). **b** A metal partial denture was not removed before exposure, and completely obscures the tooth roots.

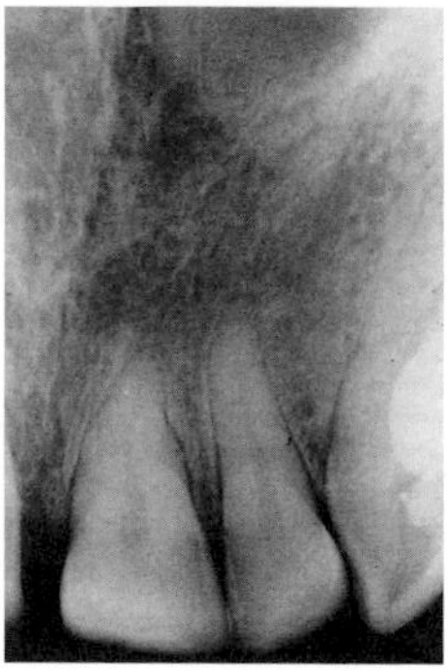

97 a

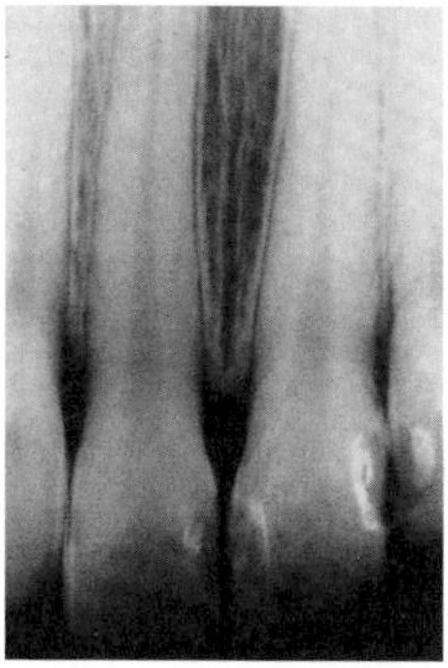

97 b

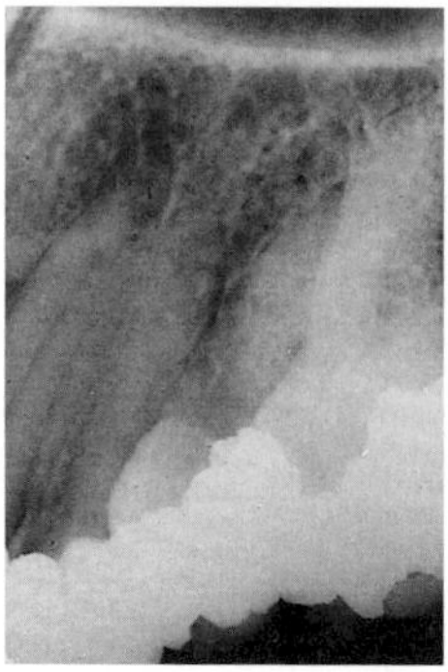

97 c

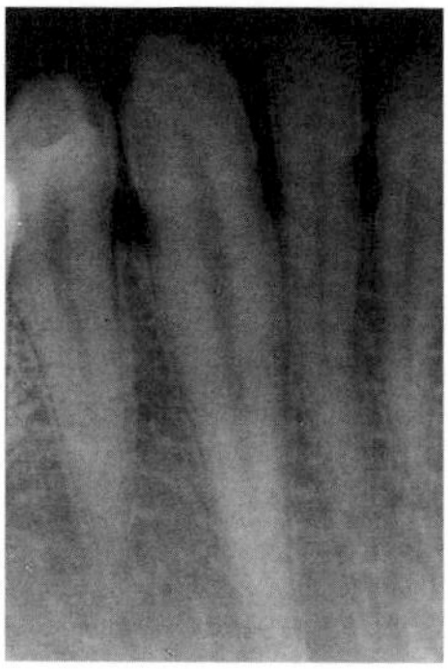

98 a

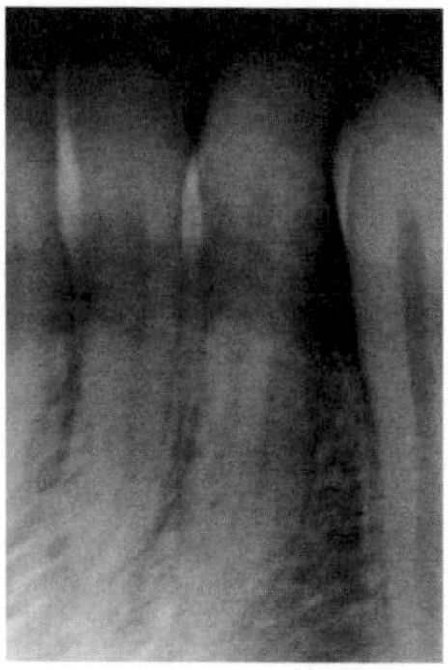

98 b

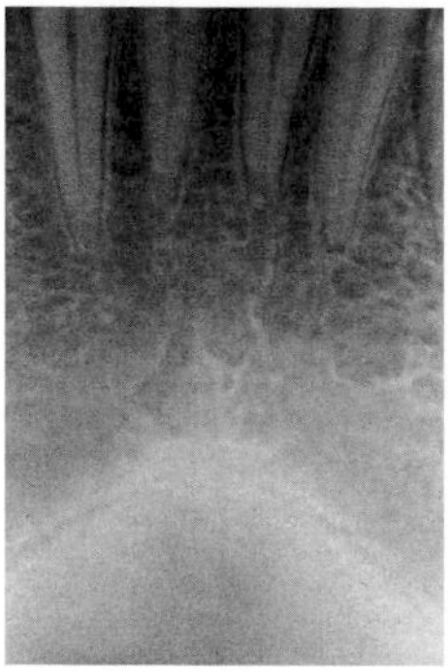

98 c

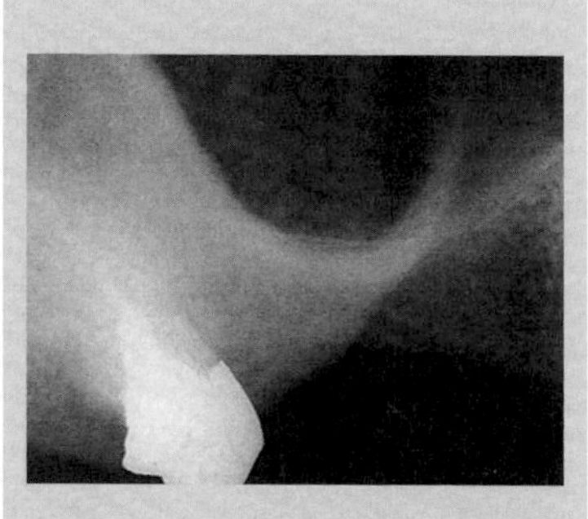

99 a

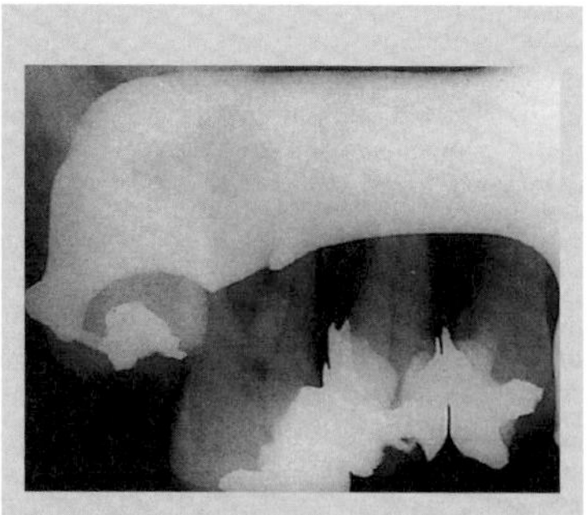

99 b

Conventional radiographic film packets or storage phosphor image receptors should **never** be “prebent” and, like digital sensors, should always be placed as parallel as possible to the long axis of the tooth. Whenever possible, an appropriate holding and targeting device should be used for secure and comfortable positioning of the image receptor. The central ray must be targeted in its vertical as well as its horizontal angle such that the desired object is depicted at its actual length and in proper proportions, as well as free of overlapping by other anatomic structures.

The question of *time* in a dental practice can always play an important role. If radiographs are taken in a hectic or hurried environment, the failure rate and therefore the number of necessary re-takes will virtually always increase.

Fig. 100 Technical error. a The body of the mandible has been targeted too steeply from the caudal aspect. Adjacent to the basal compact bone, the surface of the mylohyoid line dominates the radiograph. This surface is formed from the compact lamella lingual to the mylohyoid line. **b** Artifact caused by the diaphragm of the radiograph head. The incorrect horizontal angle of the central ray effectively missed the object and the IR.

Fig. 101 Technical error. a Because the central ray was not targeted perpendicularly to the plane of the IR, but rather distal excentric, severe overlapping of the proximal crown surfaces occurred. Early detection of proximal caries cannot be achieved with such projections. **b** It appears that the bitewing IR was placed obliquely and that the patient did not completely close the jaws; the image is blurred because of movement by the patient, an indication of a pain response.

Fig. 102 Technical error. a The central ray was targeted asymmetrically (instead of median-saggitally), which effectively inhibits the diagnostically important left-to-right comparison in the maxilla. This was an “overview” radiograph with the IR in portrait rather than landscape occlusal IR format. **b** Flat and asymmetric targeting of the central ray (see cone cut on the upper right IR edge), and the portrait-format positioning of the occlusal IR inhibits any examination of the distal segments of the mandible. Note the amalgam particle lingual to tooth 47.

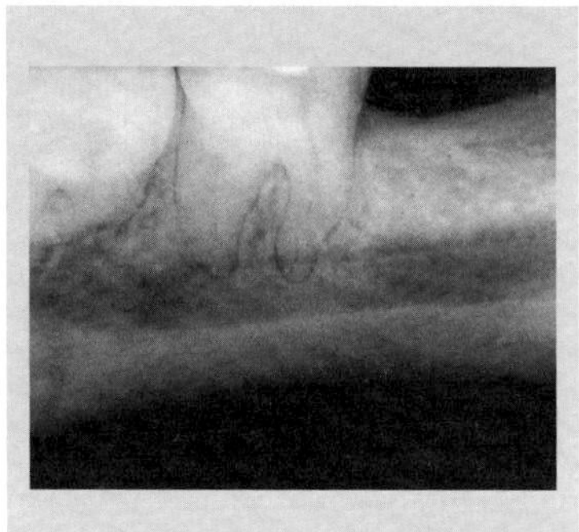

100 a

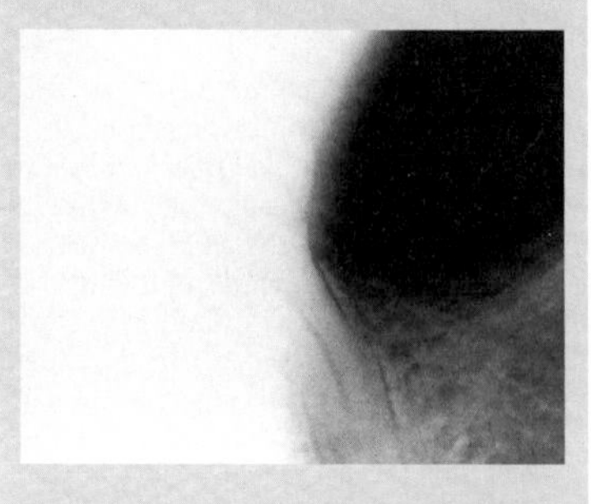

100 b

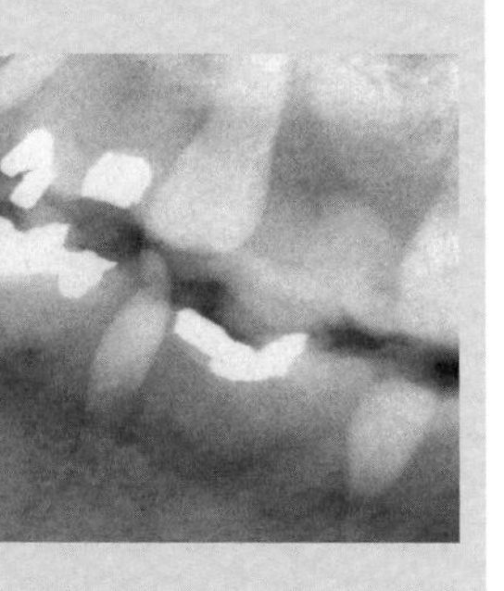

101 a

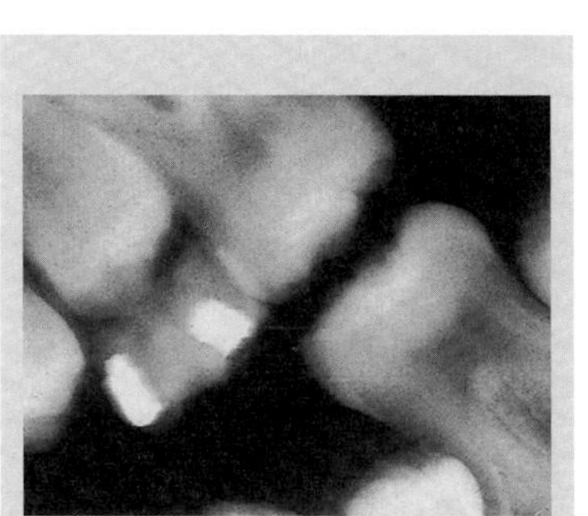

101 b

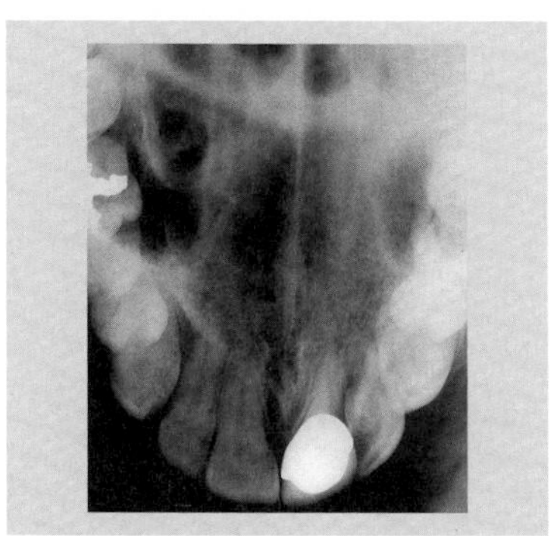

102 a

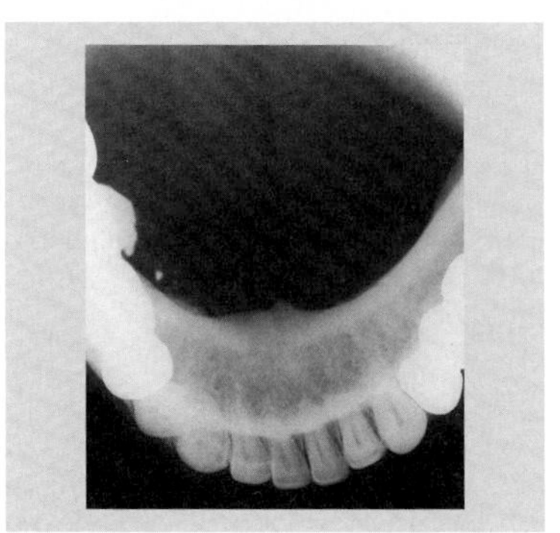

102 b

Introduction: All conventionally or digitally prepared intraoral dental radiographs follow the same rules of radiographic anatomy that apply to the technique for two-dimensional radiographs without contrast medium.

Here also, the **summation effect** and the **tangential effect** play important roles in the radiographic depiction of the anatomic realities and the borders of structures in the third dimension of space. The size and image sharpness of the desired objects are dependent upon the relationships of focus-object and object-image receptor. By purely optical laws, a 1:1 measurable depiction of the object is impossible. The relationship of the depicted structures to one another will change in three-dimensional space according to the selected projection angle of the central ray. The projected radiographic transposition of the diagnostic question is therefore of considerable significance for the interpretive and therefore diagnostic value of the radiograph.

Thick and dense structures, e.g., tooth roots, cause thinner structures (e.g., alveolar walls) to effectively disappear because of additive overlapping (**addition effect** = enhancement of overlapping), while the superposition of a tooth by air- or soft tissue-containing objects leads to a subtractive overlapping (**subtraction effect** = radiolucency) because of their lower radiation absorption. Relatively thick structures such as compact bone positioned transversely to the central ray will be depicted as a more or less dense structural shadowing, while thinner osseous lamella become visually accentuated if they are parallel to the central ray. With curved surfaces or with a spherical object, only those portions of the object that are parallel to the roentgen rays will be clearly depicted, or those struck tangentially by the roentgen rays (**tangential effect**).

Fig. 103a Macerated skull of a newborn. Symphysis of the mandible with mental ossicula and tooth buds of the primary dentition.

Fig. 103b Bitewing radiograph of a 4-year-old girl. Radiograph of the deciduous tooth crowns. In this projection, the Carabelli tuberculum (palatal of tooth 64) creates a radiographic addition effect in the tooth crown. The apparent radiolucency mesial to the Carabelli cusp is frequently misdiagnosed as proximal caries. The visual clarity of this phenomenon is dependent upon projection angle and exposure time and dose.

Fig. 104a Structures in the mixed dentition. Permanent teeth 34 and 35 exhibit fully developed tooth crowns in this 7-year-old girl. The apex of the root of tooth 36 is not yet completely developed.

Fig. 104b Structures in the mixed dentition. Nine-year-old boy following early extraction of teeth 74 and 75. Root development has already begun on the premolar (tooth 35). The apex of the root of tooth 36 is well formed but the root canals remain broadly open.

Fig. 105a Disturbed eruption in the mixed dentition. Asymmetric root resorption. It is likely that the mesial root of the resorbing deciduous tooth 75 will remain as a "root fragment following extraction" in the alveolus.

Fig. 105b Disturbed eruption in the mixed dentition. The endodontically treated (pulpal amputation) and now nonvital tooth 85 is inhibiting the eruption of permanent tooth 45. The consequences of such disturbances of tooth eruption may include positional anomalies of the permanent teeth.

Legends:

1 Symphysis of the mandible, with mental ossicula
2 Normal eruption, with initial resorption of the deciduous tooth roots
3 Root development not yet complete
4 Apical foramen and wide-open root canals
5 Initial root development
6 Asymmetric root resorption on tooth 75
7 Apical periodontitis on tooth 85, inhibiting the normal path of eruption

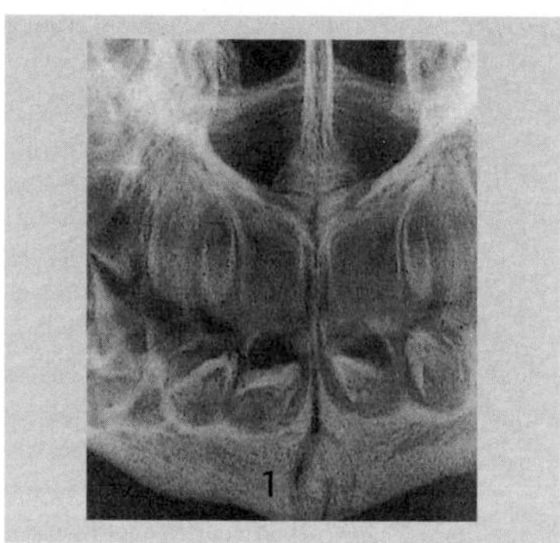

103 a

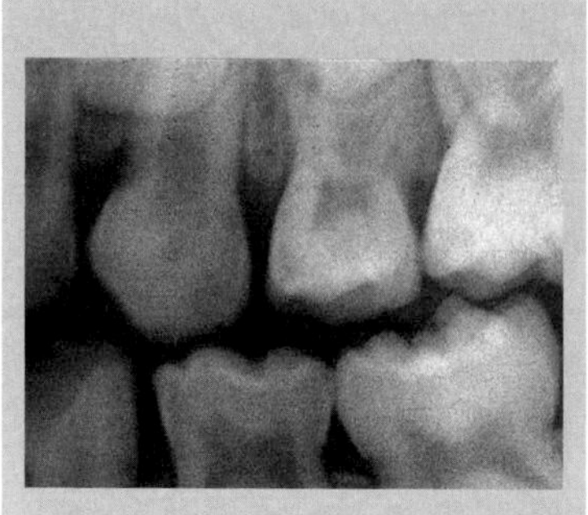

103 b

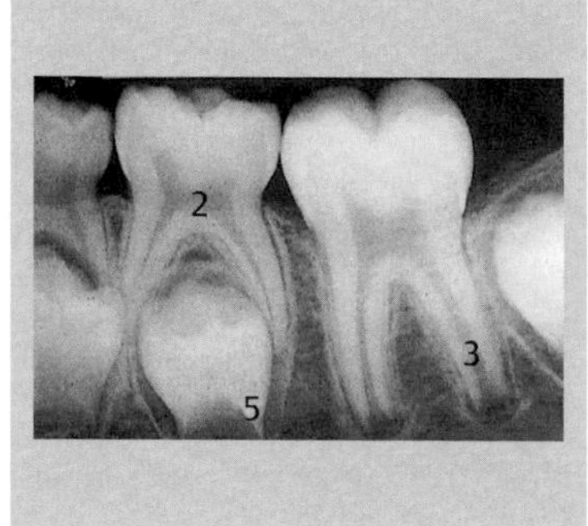

104 a

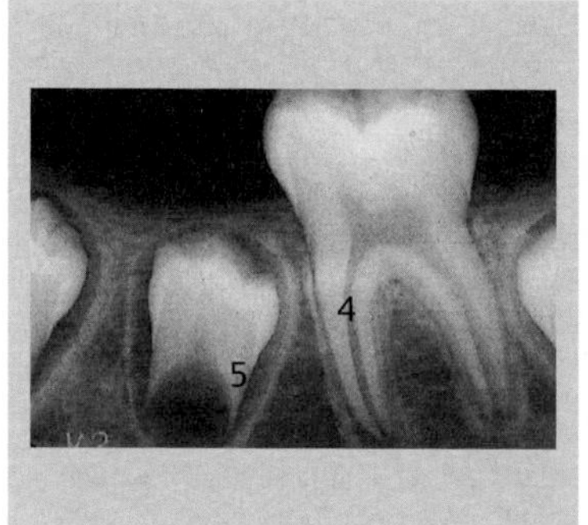

104 b

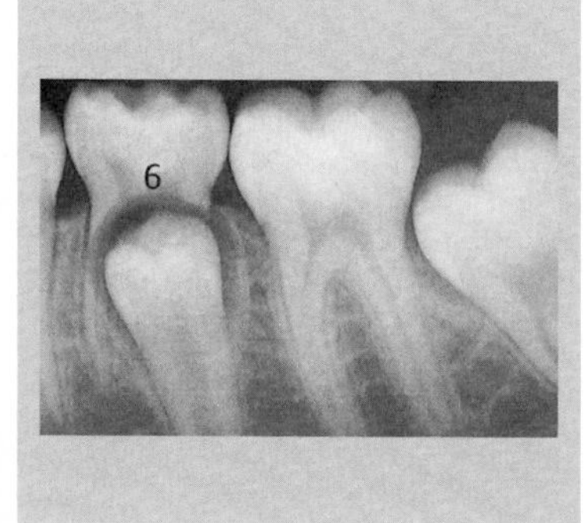

105 a

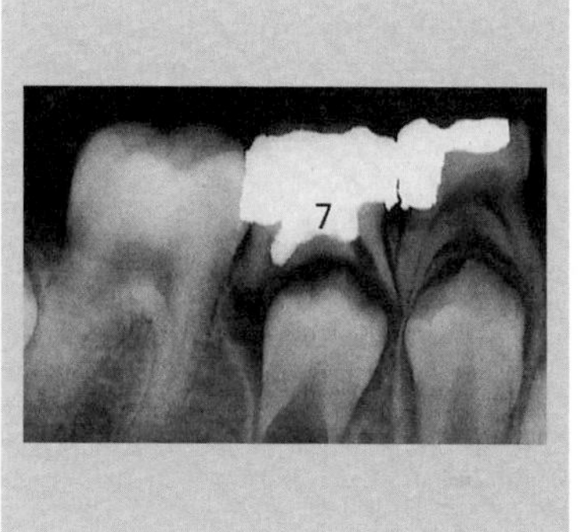

105 b

The primary dentition: At the end of the infantile period of growth and development, usually all deciduous teeth have erupted and the development of the tooth buds for the permanent dentition has begun. If the Carabelli cusp of the maxillary first deciduous molar is especially pronounced, and if there is any radiographic overexposure, the image may exhibit what appears to be dental caries on the mesial surface; even the experienced clinician may be fooled!

The permanent dentition—maxillary anterior region: The cervical dentin, which is covered by neither bone of the alveolar ridge nor the enamel cap, appears as a radiolucent band because of the burn-out effect. This effect may also be observed in the crown of rotated lateral incisors. The slight depression of the incisal foramen is usually not visible because of lack of radiographic contrast.

Maxillary canine region: All too often, the central ray is targeted too far from the mesial aspect when attempting a radiograph of the canine. This leads to ideal depiction of the lateral incisor, but the canine is often superimposed by the palatal root and palatal portion of the crown of the first premolar.

Maxillary premolar region: The maxillary first premolar exhibits two roots in most cases. The roots are often thin, and connected by a cementum bridge. The mesial aspect of the cementoenamel junction is often concave in shape, which can lead to caries-like radiolucency (burn-out effect) in the crown, especially if the teeth are rotated in the arch.

Fig. 106a Anterior tooth exhibiting overlapping effects. Intact tooth 21 exhibits summation effects. Apically, the thickness of the alveolar bone increases, which is why the periodontal ligament space appears narrowed in the apical region.

Fig. 106b Maxillary anterior segment. The palatal dental cingula (tubercula dentalia) intensify the radiopacity through the tooth crown. Note the obvious burn-out effect at the cervical area.

Fig. 106c Canine region of the maxilla. Radiolucency caused by the anterior lobe of the maxillary sinus. The radiopaque structure is the wing of the nose.

Fig. 107a Canine region of the maxilla. In the floor of the nose one notes the entrance to the nasopalatine (incisive) canal. That and a portion of the incisive foramen overlie the root of tooth 11.

Fig. 107b Nasopalatal structures. Note the nasopalatal canal system and the incisive foramen.

Fig. 107c Summation effects caused by soft tissues. The nasal orifices and the nasal soft tissues produce both addition and subtraction effects that superimpose the osseous structures.

Fig. 108a Premolar region of the maxilla. Three-rooted tooth 24 is a variation from the norm.

Fig. 108b Premolar and molar regions of the maxilla. The radiopaque line of demarcation of the maxillary sinus is not the floor of the sinus. That is found between the palatal and vestibular apices of the roots of tooth 26.

Legends:

1 Enamel cap enhanced by the tangential effect
2 Cervical region between the enamel cap and the alveolar crest; burn-out effects
3 Periodontal ligament space and lamina dura
4 Root canal
5 Vestibular crest of the alveolar bone
6 Palatal crest of the alveolar bone
7 Soft tissues of the nose
8 Entrance into the nose
9 Median suture, incisive foramen, nasopalatal (incisive) canal
10 Foramen of the nasal nasopalatal canal
11 Piriform aperture
12 Laterobasal border of the nasal cavity
13 Palatal root, tooth 14
14 Palatal cusp, tooth 14
15 Vestibular cusp, tooth 14
16 Anterior lobe of the maxillary sinus
17 Maxillary nasal crest with anterior nasal spine
18 Laterobasal border of the maxillary sinus
19 Floor of the maxillary sinus
20 Three-rooted tooth 24

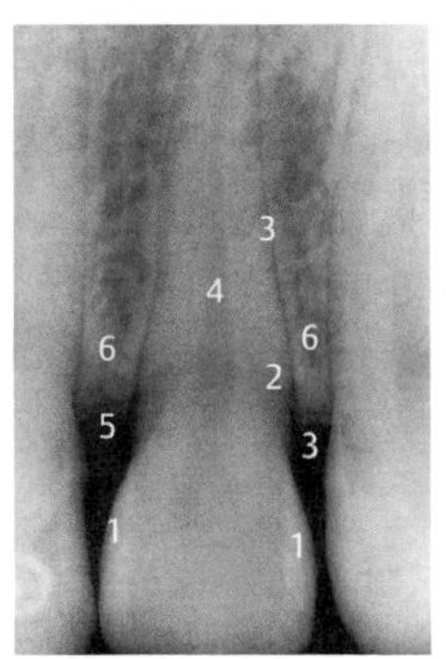

106 a

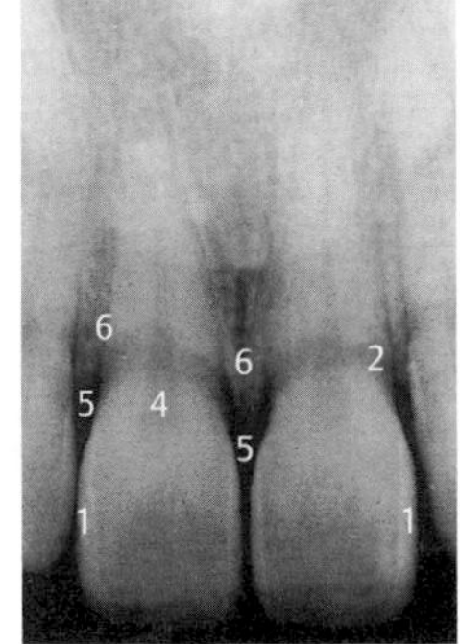

106 b

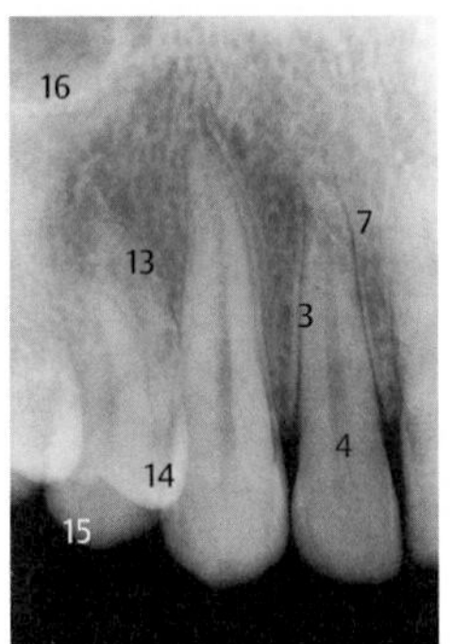

106 c

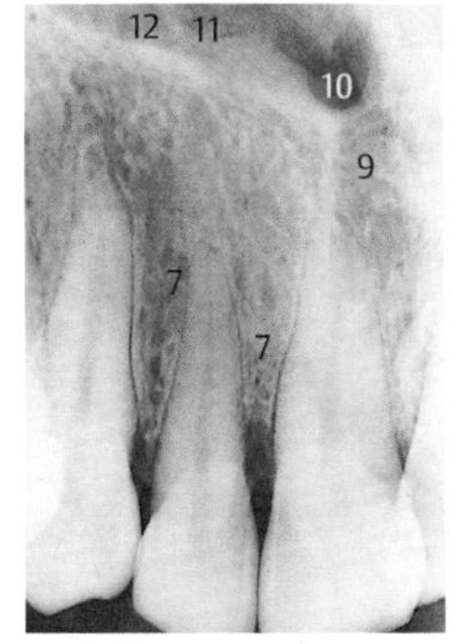

107 a

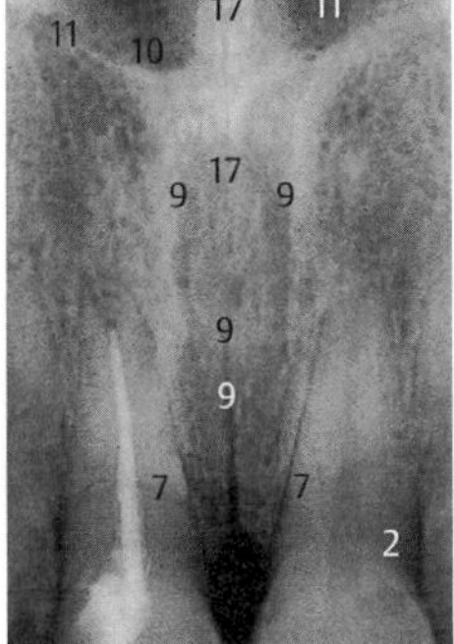

107 b

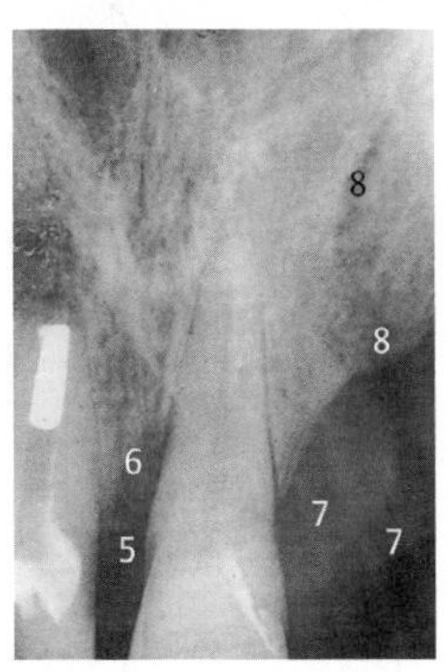

107 c

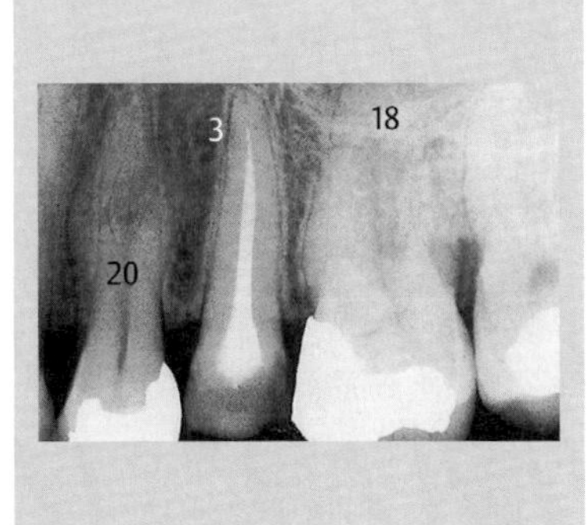

108 a

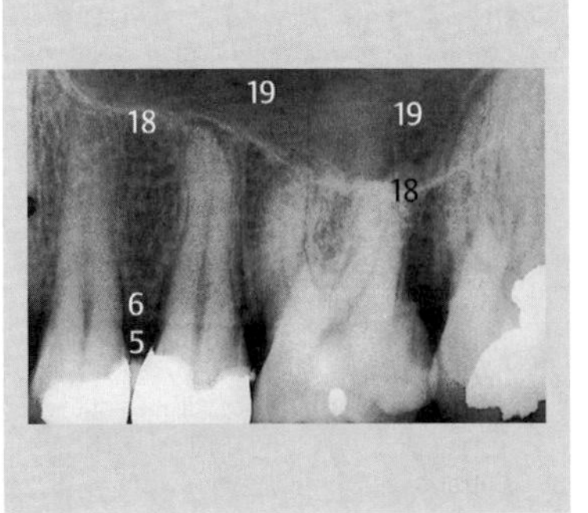

108 b

The premolar region of the maxilla is frequently radiographed using portrait format. Frequently one observes a radiopaque septum above the second premolar; this septum separates the anterior lobe of the sinus from the alveolar lobe.

Maxillary molar region: If the central ray is targeted too steeply from above, the zygomatic bone will be visible in the radiograph. The floor of the maxillary sinus is located between the buccal and the palatal roots of the first permanent molar.

Maxillary sinus and tuberosity region: The two maxillary sinuses are often quite asymmetric vis-à-vis each other. Radiographs often reveal radiopaque septa projected over the second premolars and the second molars; these septa divide the sinus into an anterior, alveolar, and posterior lobe. The relationship of the floor of the sinus to the individual tooth roots is usually close; sinusitis may simulate pulpitis. Especially after tooth extractions, the maxillary sinus may extend almost to the alveolar ridge.

Fig. 109a Premolar region of the maxilla. Following early loss of the molar, the sinus may extend almost to the alveolar ridge. Note the burn-out effect on tooth 14, and compare this with the true secondary caries mesially and distally on tooth 15.

Fig. 109b Premolar region of the maxilla. The medial portion of the sinus is "traversed" by the laterobasal border of the nasal cavity. Note secondary caries distally on tooth 24.

Fig. 109c Premolar region of the maxilla. The central ray was targeted much too steeply from above in the premolar regions, and the radiograph revealed a delicate septum in the sinus that separates the anterior from the alveolar lobe.

Fig. 110a Premolar and molar region of the maxilla. The zygomaticomaxillary suture is sometimes viewed as an irregular, fracture-like radiolucency in the sinus. The apparently closed anterior lobe of the sinus simulates an apical cyst. However, it is possible to trace the entire lamina dura around the apex of vital tooth 25.

Fig. 110b Tuberosity region. This radiograph of the tuberosity region depicts the floor of the sinus between the apices of tooth 27, the coronoid process, and the pyramidal process of the palatal bone.

Fig. 111a Tuberosity region. The maxillary zygomatic process and the zygomatic bone overlap and obscure the root apices of tooth 26. The hamulus of the medial lamina of the pterygoid process is freely projected, as is the coronoid process of the mandibular ramus.

Fig. 111b Tuberosity region. The maxillary sinus is depicted here with its posterior lobe traversed by a bony septum. Following early extraction of molars, the maxillary sinus may approach the alveolar ridge and the posterior border of the maxillary tuberosity.

Legends:

1 Laterobasal boundary of the nasal cavity
2 Floor of the nasal sinus
3 Laterobasal border of the maxillary sinus
4 Floor of the maxillary sinus
5 Intrasinus septum
6 Anterior lobe of the maxillary sinus
7 Alveolar lobe of the maxillary sinus
8 Zygomatic lobe of the maxillary sinus
9 Zygomatic process of the maxilla
10 Body of the zygomatic bone
11 Zygomatic arch
12 Alveolar ridge
13 Lateral lamina of the pterygoid process
14 Hamulus of the medial lamina of the pterygoid process
15 Pyramidal process of the palatal bone
16 Maxillary tuberosity
17 Zygomaticomaxillary suture
18 Coronoid (muscular) process of the mandibular ramus
19 Root tips of the maxillary first premolars. The longer root is the palatal root
20 Burn-out effect
21 Secondary caries

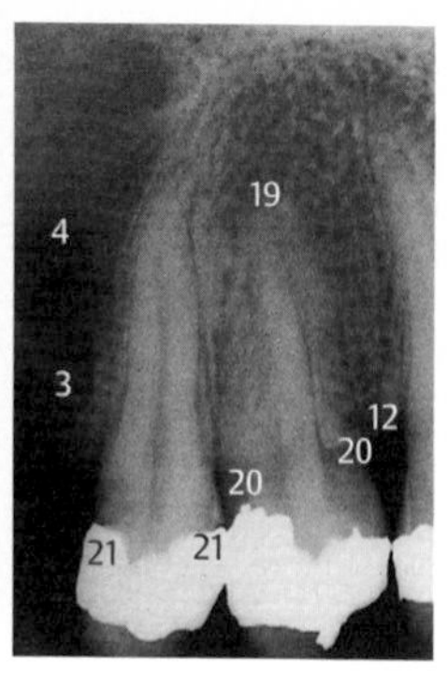

109 a

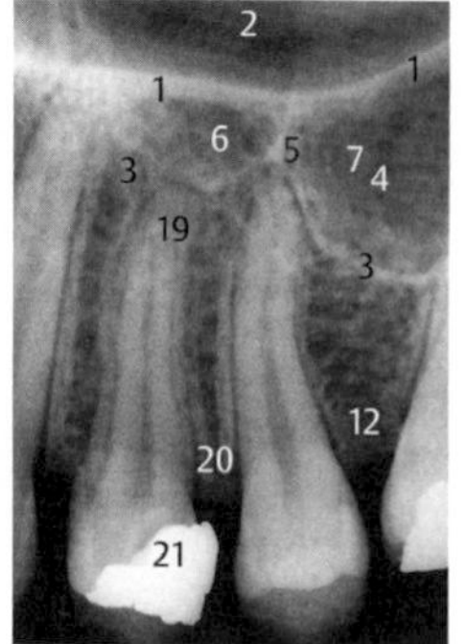

109 b

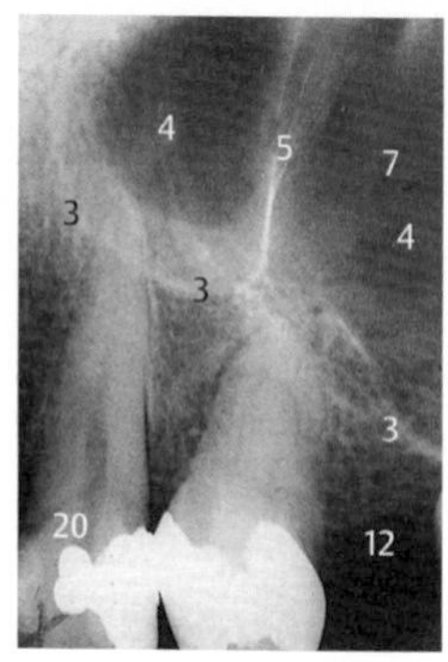

109 c

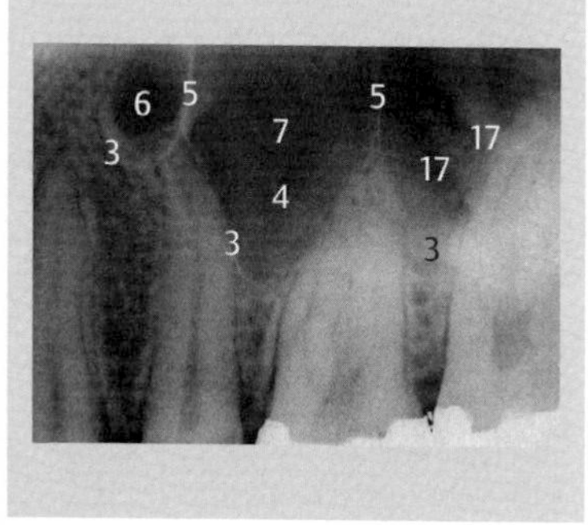

110 a

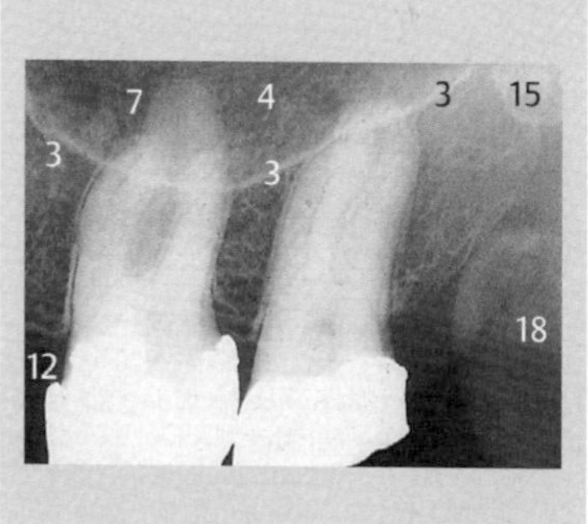

110 b

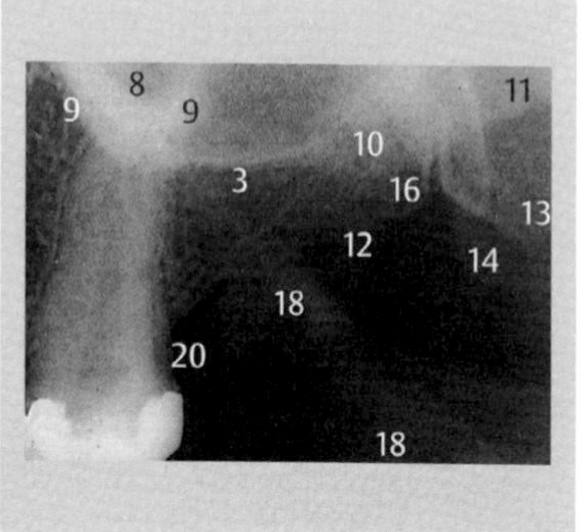

111 a

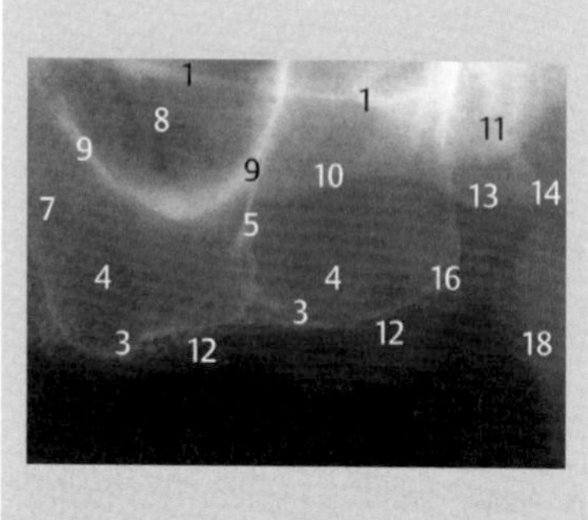

111 b

Mandibular anterior region: The vestibular portions of the alveolar ridge are projected beyond the lingual portions. The mental fovea corresponds to a vestibular depression in the area of the anterior tooth roots and can produce a well-demarcated radiolucency.

Mandibular canine region: The canine is not always a single-rooted tooth. The variations can only be visualized by use of excentric central ray projection. The appearance of several periodontal ligament spaces is evidence of a depression in the root's cross-section.

Mandibular premolar region: The alveolar process exhibits a broadly reticulated trabeculum. The porous mandibular canal and the mental foramen located between the two premolars are therefore often difficult to visualize in the radiograph. The mental foramen may be projected directly over the root apex of a premolar, thus giving the impression of an apical lesion.

Fig. 112a Anterior region of the mandible. The film shows that the central ray entered obliquely and that the labial portion of the alveolar crest is projected above the lingual aspect of the alveolar crest. Note the width of the periodontal ligament space; the crestal bone (interseptal tip) is narrow at the cemento-enamel-junction (CEJ) but becomes ever wider apically. The lamina dura is thickest at the apex of the root, which gives the impression that the periodontal ligament space has become progressively narrower.

Fig. 112b Anterior region of the mandible. Note the vertically coursing vascular canals in this case of chronic periodontitis.

Fig. 112c Summation effects in the mandibular anterior region. Note the round and rather sharply demarcated radiolucent area in the midplane of the alveolar ridge (dark area, #6) caused by a deep mental fovea.

Fig. 113a Anterior region of the mandible. The central ray was targeted steeply upward; the film clearly shows the mental spine on the lower border of the compact bone, and also an additional radiopacity caused by overlapping with the chin prominence.

Fig. 113b Canine region of the mandible. Teeth 33, 34, and 35 exhibit numerous periodontal ligament spaces, corresponding to their root cross-sections. On teeth 33 and 34, obvious burn-out effect is observed.

Fig. 113c Canine region of the mandible. The film depicts a two-rooted mandibular canine and distal burn-out effect. Also on teeth 42 and 41, several periodontal ligament spaces can be discerned.

Fig. 114a Premolar region of the mandible. As a result of the focal sclerosing osteomyelitis emanating from the nonvital tooth 34, the mental foramen and the mandibular canal are clearly depicted.

Fig. 114b Premolar region of the mandible. The mental foramen creates a radiolucency near the apex region of tooth 45 due to the subtraction effect.

Fig. 114c Premolar region of the mandible. This radiograph permits a direct comparison between the normal anatomic conditions around the apex of vital tooth 33, with subtraction effect from the mental foramen, and the pathologic alteration on nonvital tooth 34. One can trace the apical lamina dura on both teeth.

Legends:

1 Vestibular interdental bony septum tip
2 Lingual bony interseptal tip
3 Mental spine
4 Vertically coursing vascular canal
5 Vascular canal in cross-section
6 Mental fovea
7 Burn-out effect
8 Radiopacity due to the chin prominence
9 Basal compact bone of the mandible
10 Periodontal ligament space irregularities due to variations in the cross-sectional profile (depressions)
11 Trabecular bone of the alveolus in the depression of the root cross-section
12 Slender root tip massively superimposed by trabecular bone
13 Alveolar crest
14 Root fragment
15 Mandibular canal
16 Mental foramen
17 Incomplete root canal filling with chronic apical periodontitis

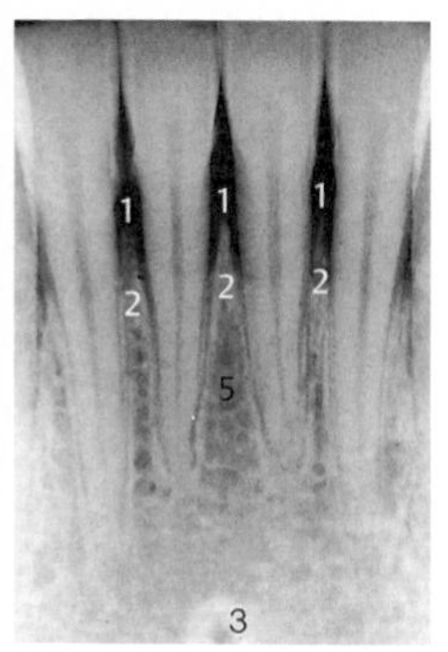

112 a

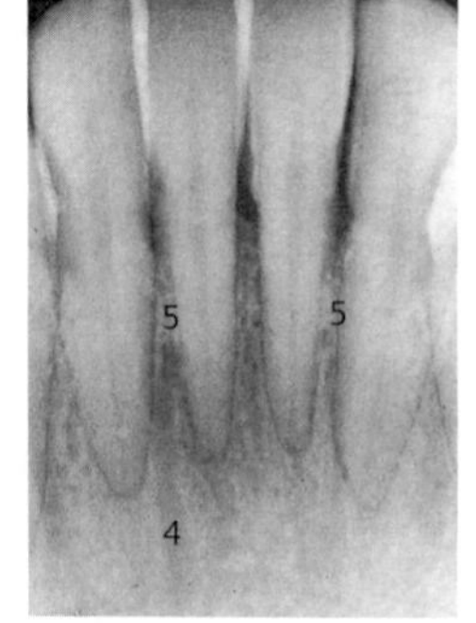

112 b

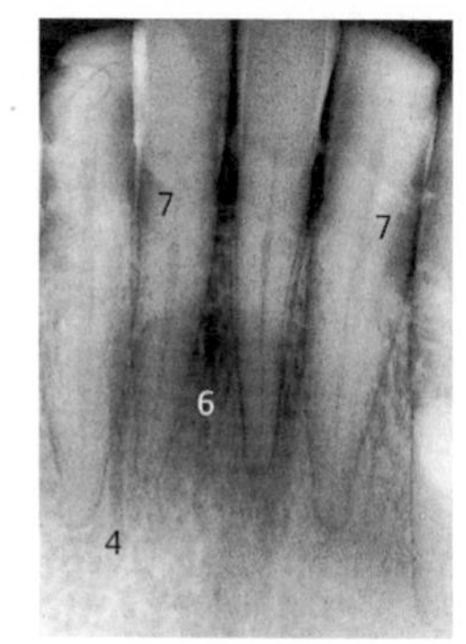

112 c

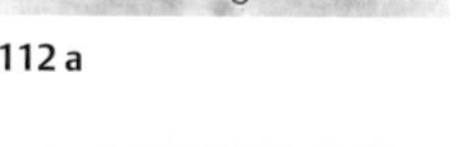

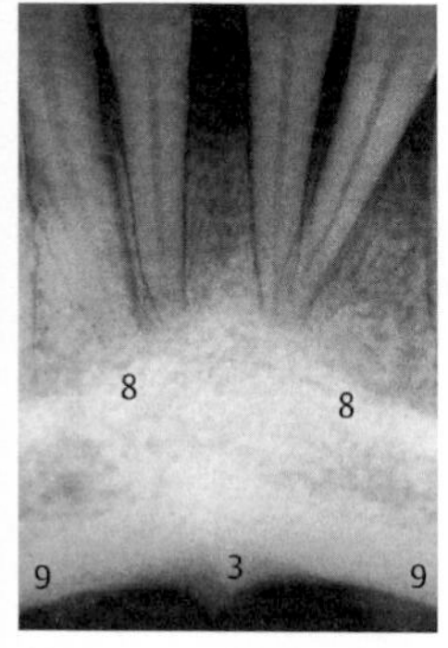

113 a

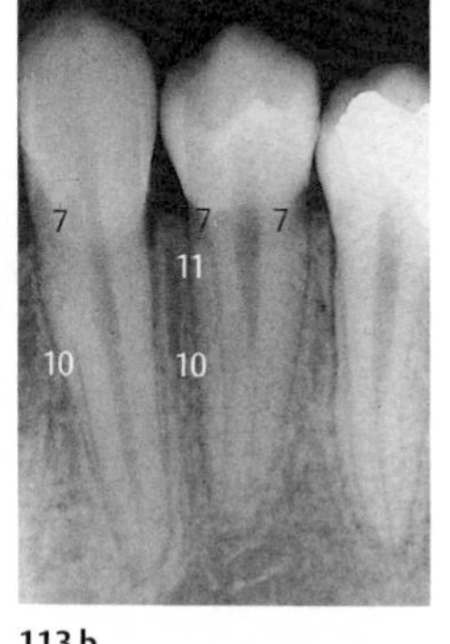

113 b

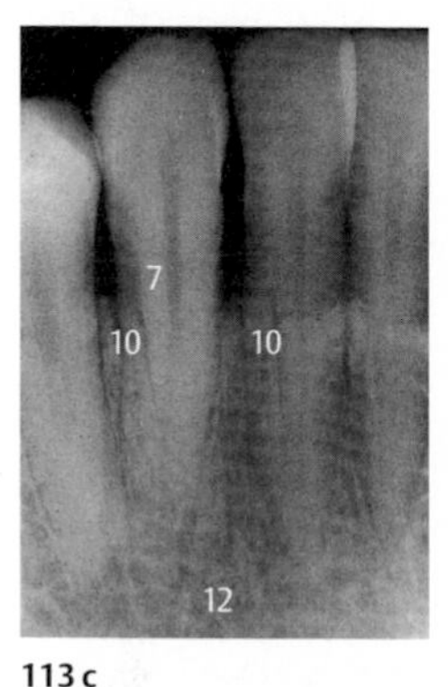

113 c

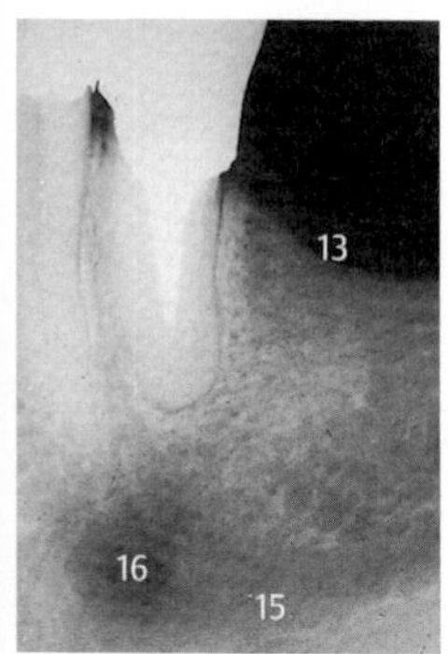

114 a

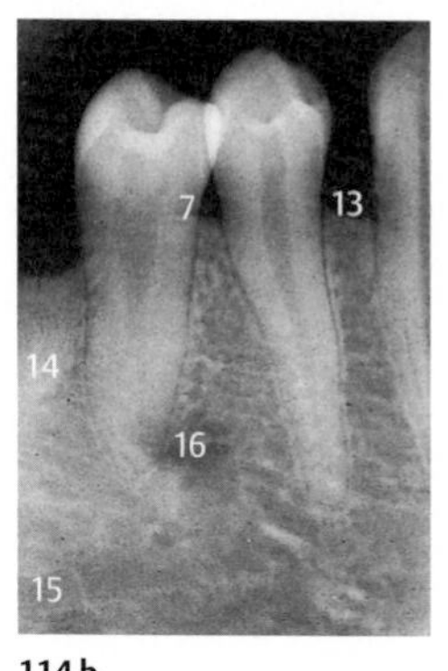

114 b

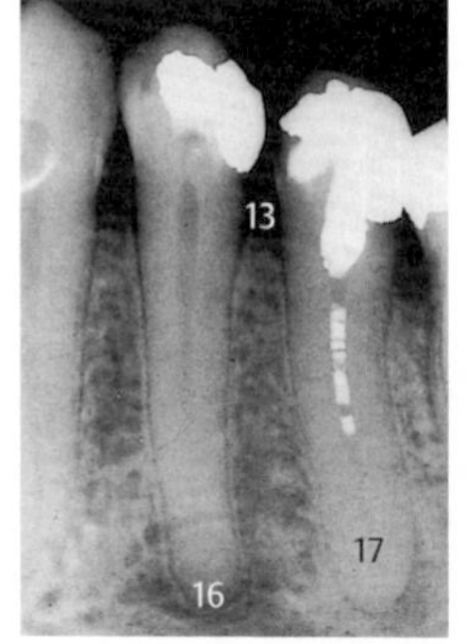

114 c

Premolars having short roots and a coronal pulp chamber that is extended coronoapically are not infrequently encountered; these are referred to as **taurodont**. The first premolar may have two and in extremely rare cases even three roots, while the second mandibular premolar is almost always single-rooted with a single root canal.

Mandibular molar region: The distal root of the first molar is typically roundish in shape, while the mesial root is usually flat, exhibiting a distal concavity and two root canals. The second molar often exhibits fusion of the roots. The mylohyoid line is frequently observed at the upper border of a trabecula-poor zone, and the radiolucency is additionally affected by the depression of the submandibular fovea. Usually only the thicker floor of the mandibular canal can be visualized in the region of the second molars because of its porous walls. The full course of the mandibular canal can often be only discerned with a background of chronic sclerosing osteomyelitis. In the retromolar area, the anterior border of the ramus is depicted as the lateral external oblique line ventral to the molar. Medial to the coronoid process, the internal oblique line begins lingual to the body of the mandible. Distal to the molars is the retromolar triangle with the medial and lateral crura.

Fig. 115a Premolar region of the mandible. The radiograph depicts the typical osseous structure of the alveolar process and the typical trabecular pattern within the body of the mandible. Within the trabecula-poor zone of the body of the mandible, the mental foramen is often difficult to discern.

Fig. 115b Premolar region of the mandible. Tooth 34 and tooth 35 exhibit short roots and a coronal pulp chamber that is elongated. The term for this sort of tooth is taurodont.

Fig. 116a Premolar and molar regions of the mandible. In this radiograph, the mental foramen is superimposed partially over the root apex of tooth 44. It is almost impossible to discern the mandibular canal, because of the porosity of its walls and especially its roof, which is overlapped by the radiolucency of the submandibular fovea.

Fig. 116b Molar region of the mandible. Horizontal periodontal bone loss, and spurs of supragingival calculus in the interdental spaces. The spongy bone of the alveolar process exhibits a reactive sclerosing ostitis.

Fig. 117a Molar region of the mandible. Course of the floor of the mandibular canal within the radiolucency caused by the submandibular fovea (below the mylohyoid line).

Fig. 117b Molar region of the mandible. Adjacent to the apical radiopacity of nonvital tooth 47, one can discern the roof of the mandibular canal. In the retromolar area, one notes the course of the external oblique line and the internal oblique line, continuations of the temporal crest.

Legends:

1 Typical trabecular structure in the alveolar process of the mandible
2 Radiolucency (subtraction effect) caused by the submandibular fovea
3 Typical trabecular structure of the body of the mandible
4 Mental foramen
5 Taurodont
6 Mandibular canal
7 Internal oblique line (continuation of the temporal crest of the right mandible)
8 External oblique line (anterior margin of the right mandible)
9 Mylohyoid line
10 Retromolar triangle, with medial and lateral crura
11 Island of bone marrow following tooth extraction
12 Basal compact bone of the mandible
13 Interdental calculus

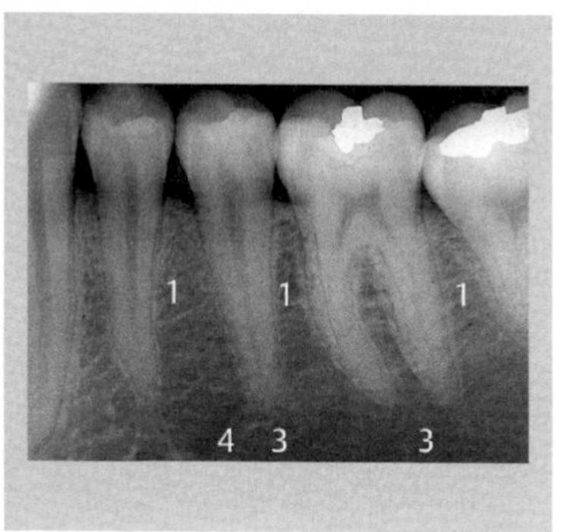

115 a

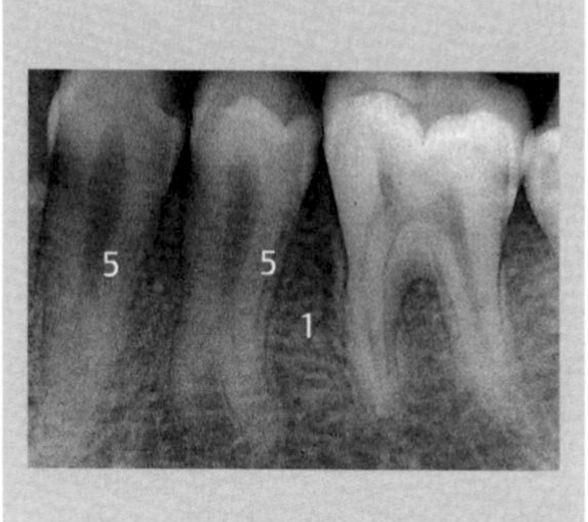

115 b

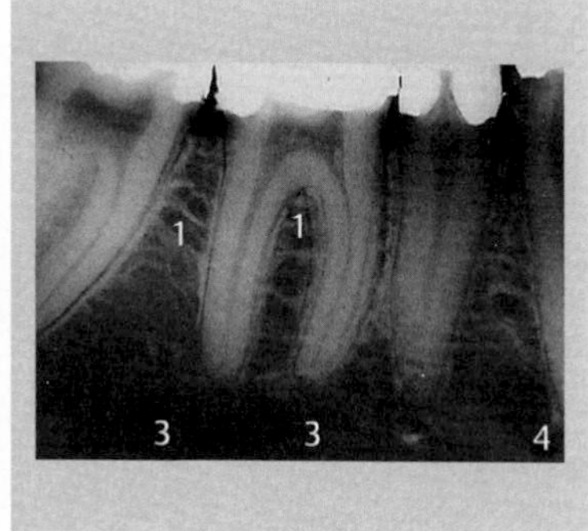

116 a

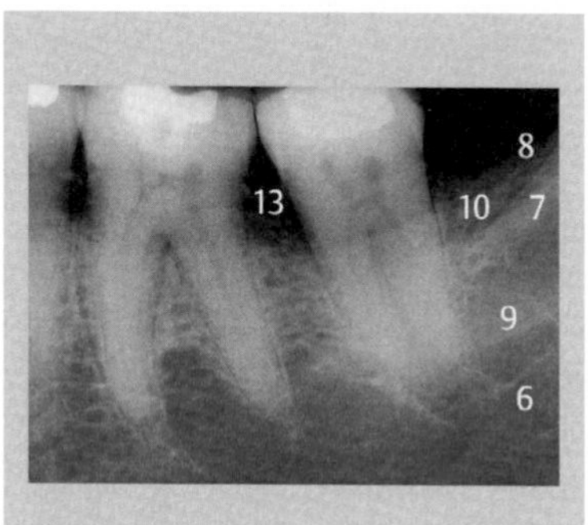

116 b

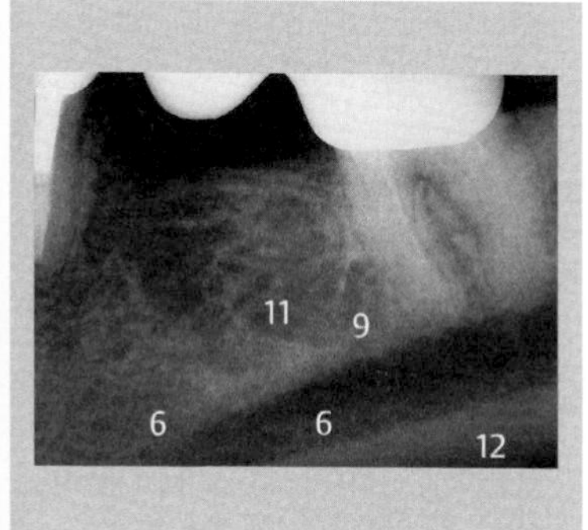

117 a

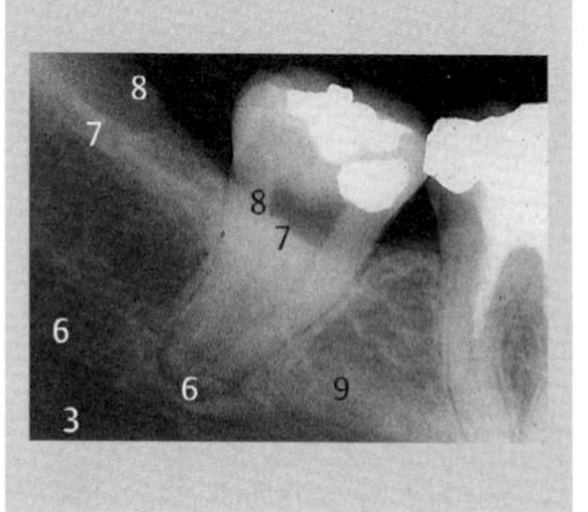

117 b

Maxillary occlusal radiographs: Except for axial computed tomography (CT), only occlusal radiographs offer the possibility to examine the jaws in the diagnostically important third dimension (see also p. 58). On the other hand, the anatomic relationships of the facial skeleton and maxilla prohibit a truly axial central ray, so only an oblique projection can be achieved, with attendant distortion of structures. For example, teeth that are impacted high in the maxilla cannot be reliably localized. Figures **118a** and **119** depict occlusal radiographs of a fully dentulous and an edentulous patient, respectively.

Mandibular occlusal radiographs: Overview radiographs of the mandible can be taken with axial central ray projection. If this is performed precisely, localization of impacted teeth, foreign bodies, or also pathologic structures can be revealed with a high level of precision. The anatomy of the mandible, however, precludes adequate depiction of the retromolar regions in an occlusal radiograph.

Image optimization: With the exception of occlusal radiographs, virtually all intraoral radiographs should always be taken using an appropriate image receptor holder (IRH) in order to optimize the quality of the resulting image (see also p. **61**).

Fig. 118a Occlusal radiograph of the maxilla in a fully dentulous patient. Even a cursory inspection of the depicted anterior segment of the maxilla shows how the oblique projection of the central ray appears to lengthen the anatomic structures dorsally. Nevertheless, this type of maxillary overview radiograph does provide a para-axial depiction of the maxilla, and provides a view of the third dimension to complement intraoral projections and a panoramic radiograph.

Fig. 118 b Diagram of the technique for taking an occlusal overview radiograph of the maxilla. This procedure cannot be performed with digital sensors that were available as of the date of publication of this book.

Fig. 119 Maxillary occlusal radiograph of an edentulous patient. This radiograph depicts the anatomic structures of the maxilla without superimposition of the teeth.

Fig. 120a Mandibular occlusal radiograph of an edentulous patient. The alveolar process and the body of the mandible can be recognized by the radiographic depictions of the compact bony walls. It is clear to see how the dental arch in the molar regions extends beyond the arch of the jaw medially. Tooth 48 was completely impacted!
An occlusal radiograph of a fully dentulous mandible is not presented here because of the almost total overlapping by the teeth.

Fig. 120b Diagram of proper technique to take a mandibular occlusal radiograph. At the date of this publication, digital sensors were not commercially available for this technique.

Legends:

1 Nasal septum (cartilage)
2 Anterior nasal spine
3 Median suture
4 Maxillary nasal crest with the osseous nasal septum
5 Incisive foramen
6 Incisive canal, nasal apertures
7 Borders of the nasal cavity
8 Nasal conchae (superimposition)
9 Frontal bone
10 Maxillary sinus (borders)
11 Nasolacrimal canal
12 Canine fossa and infraorbital margin
13 Groove for the palatal artery
14 Alveolar process of the maxilla
15 Chin
16 Alveolar process, course of the vestibular and lingual compact bone
17 Body of the mandible, course of the vestibular and lingual compact bone
18 Mental spine
19 Mental foramen
20 Mandibular canal
21 Insertion of the genioglossus muscle, superimposed by the alveolar process
22 Impacted tooth 48

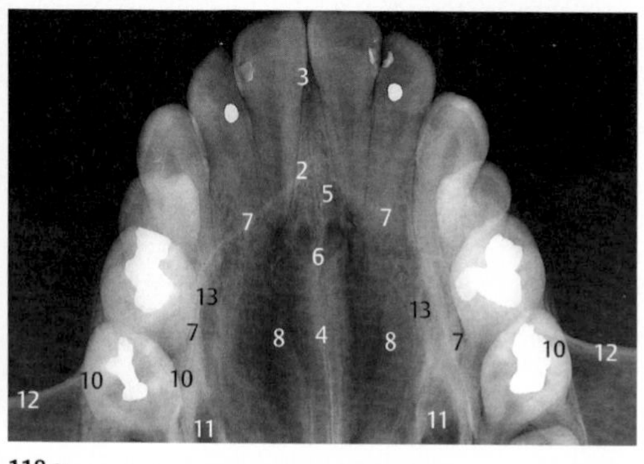

118 a

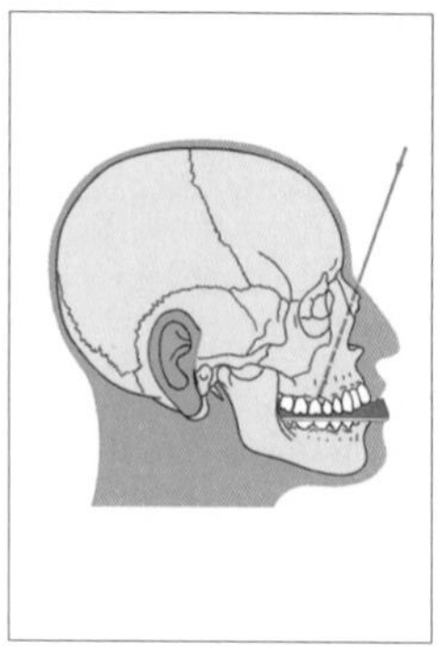

118 b

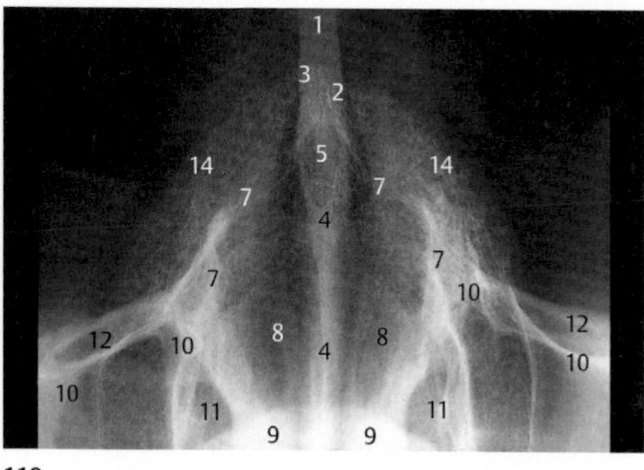

119

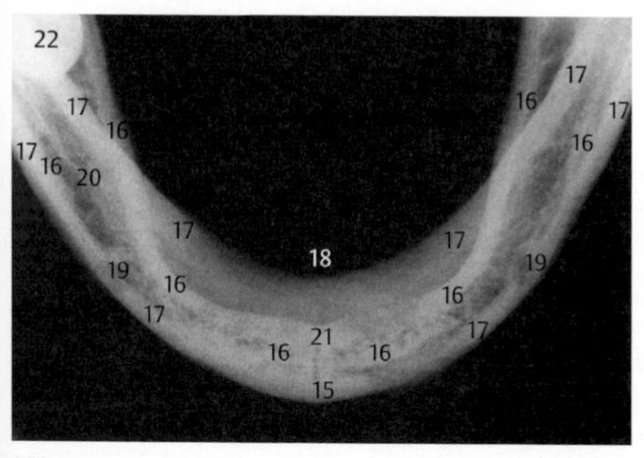

120 a

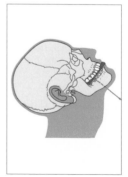

120 b

The term "native" radiographs connotes a two-dimensional radiograph that reproduces a three-dimensional space without the use of a contrast medium.
Advantages of this procedure include without doubt the lower radiation exposure in comparison to computed tomography (CT), and the comparatively low cost. With appropriate scanners, the images can be digitized.
The disadvantages become obvious because of the numerous cranial structures that would lend various summation effects, leading to superimpositioning of structures, and therefore rendering impossible a clear depiction of the third dimension of the desired structures.
Clearly very few dentists have either the need or the desire to purchase and possess large pieces of radiographic equipment (which would, after all, be seldom used). Therefore, dentists are sometimes dependent upon collaboration with radiologists; however, the dentist should have a full understanding of large-format skull radiographs and must possess the necessary fundamental knowledge of cranial anatomy.

Conventional skull overview radiographs depict the skull completely in the three planes of projection: the frontal plane, the median saggital plane, and axially in the plane of the Frankfort horizontal. Therefore, these "standard radiographs" are designated as follows, together with the selected central ray targeting:

1. Posteroanterior skull projection, overview.
2. Lateral skull projection, overview.
3. Axial skull projection, overview.

Within this system of standard projections, the following radiographs are also integrated: Partial skull radiographs such as the half-axial radiograph of the mid-face (Waters projection), the posteroanterior overview of the mandible (reverse Towne's projection), the cephalometric radiograph of the facial skeleton, half-arch radiographs of the mandible, and special conventional views of the temporomandibular joints (TMJs) (Schüller).

Indications for the first standard projection: This is used above all for documentation of skull and facial skeletal asymmetries.

Fig. 121a Diagram of proper head positioning. Note the position of the frontal bone (forehead), supported by a foam rubber wedge. Note also proper targeting of the central ray.

Fig. 121b Positioning the patient. In this lateral view, the superior border of the petrosal bone meets the middle of the orbit. The protective apron covers the patient's back. The field of irradiation is kept to the necessary minimum using various collimators.

Legend for Figure 122:

1 Saggital suture
2 Coronal suture
3 Lambdoid suture
4 Parietal bone
5 Diploic canal
6 Anterior cranial fossa, lateral wall
7 Minor ala of the sphenoid bone
8 Frontal sinus
9 Crista galli
10 Orbit
11 Superior orbital fissure
12 Innominate line, fundus of the major ala of the sphenoid bone
13 Petrous part of the temporal bone, upper edge of the petrous pyramid
14 Sphenoidal sinus in superimposition with the ethmoid labyrinth and the nasal septum
15 Lamina orbitalis
16 Round foramen of the sphenoid bone
17 Frontal process of the zygomatic bone
18 Mastoid process
19 Mandibular condyle
20 Coronoid process of the mandible
21 Zygomaticoalveolar crest
22 Zygomatic bone
23 Maxillary sinus, borders
24 Nasal cavity with conchae and nasal septum
25 Base of the skull
26 Styloid process
27 Transverse process
28 Angle of the mandible
29 Mandibular canal
30 Median maxillary suture

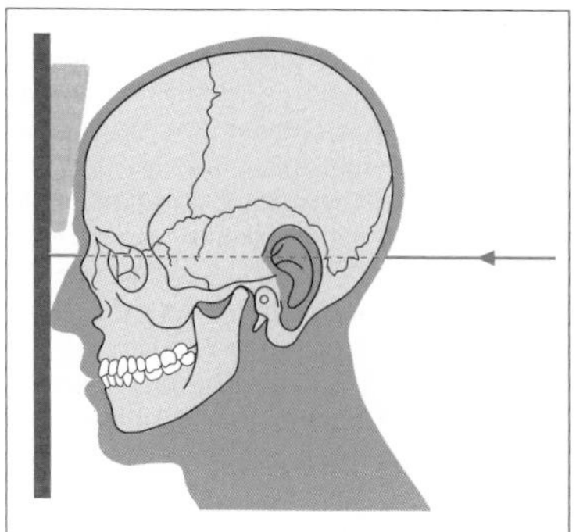

121 a

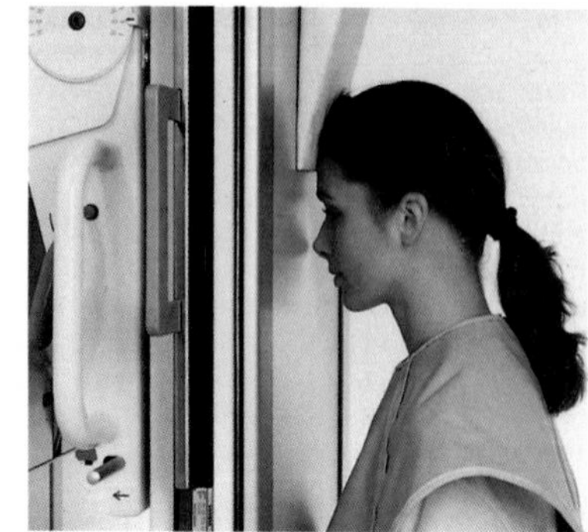

121 b

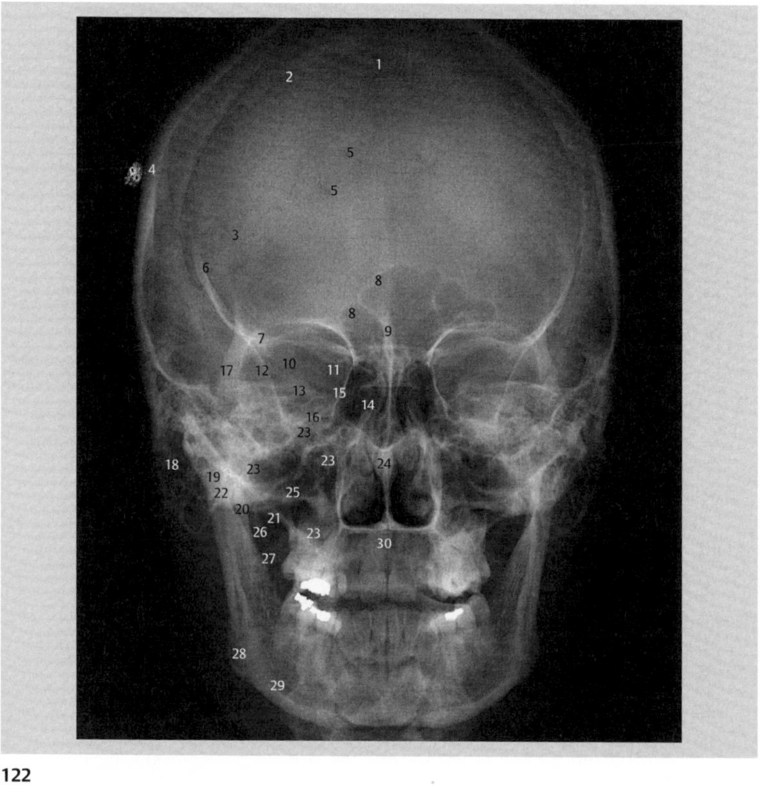

122

The lateral overview radiograph of the skull may depict symmetrically positioned structures such as the frontal process of the zygomatic bone or the angle of the mandible superimposed upon each other in the third dimension. Structures near the plane of focus will appear enlarged. These parallactic central ray displacements are reduced when the object-source distance is enlarged; this is possible with a cephalometric radiograph, devices with which a distance of 1.5 m or greater from the image receptor is possible. In contrast, special equipment for skull radiographs works with a focus-film distance of 1 m. Air-containing regions such as the nasal cavity with the adjacent sinuses and the epipharynx permit undiminished passage of the roentgen rays, and the hard tissues are accurately depicted.

Indications for the second standard radiograph: This radiograph retains even today its frequent use as the initial image for orientation, especially in post-traumatic cases. However, it is being replaced more and more by CT. In addition, this technique is used as an overview in orthodontics and for examination of patient facial profile in prosthodontics.

Fig. 123a Diagram of positioning. The median saggital plane must be parallel to the plane of the film cassette. The central ray (red line) enters at the level of the pituitary gland.

Fig. 123b Positioning the patient. The lateral skull radiograph is performed exclusively with the **right side** of the face against the cassette. The central ray enters just above the middle of the zygomatic bone.

Legend for Fig. 124:

1 Parietal bone
2 Diploic canal
3 Coronal suture
4 Groove for the medial meningeal artery
5 Lambdoid suture
6 Pineal body, with calcifications
7 Internal occipital protuberance
8 External occipital protuberance
9 Occipital squama
10 Internal occipital crest
11 Mastoid sinuses
12 Petrous part of the temporal bone (petrosal bone)
13 Occipital condyle
14 External auditory meatus
15 Internal auditory meatus
16 Atlas
17 Anterior tubercle of atlas
18 Dentoid process of axis
19 Styloid process
20 Temporomandibular joint
21 Clivus and basilar portion
22 Dorsum sellae, posterior clinoid process
23 Sella turcica
24 Anterior clinoid process
25 Sphenoidal sinus
26 Floor of the medial cranial fossa
27 Major and minor alae of the sphenoid bone
28 Anterior cranial fossa
29 Frontal sinus
30 Crista galli with the cribriform lamina
31 Nasal bone
32 Ethmoid labyrinth
33 Optic canal
34 Orbit
35a Frontal process of the zygomatic bone (distant from radiation source)
35b Frontal process of the zygomatic bone (near radiation source)
36 Fossa of lacrimal sac
37a Zygomatic process of the maxilla with the zygomatic lobe of the maxillary sinus (distant from plane of focus)
37b As 37a (near plane of focus)
38 Zygomatic arch
39 Inferior nasal concha
40 Maxillary sinus (borders)
41 Pterygopalatine fossa
42 Pterygoid process with laminae
43 Hamulus, medial lamina of the pterygoid process
44 Nasal cavity, floor
45 Bony palate
46 Anterior nasal spine
47 Posterior nasal spine
48 Coronoid process of the mandible
49 Condylar process of the mandible
50 Mandibular canal
51 Soft tissue shadow of the tongue
52 Radiolucency of the epipharynx
53a Compact bone of the mandible (distant from radiation source)
53b As 53a (near radiation source)
54 Chin
55 Lateral nasal cartilage
56 Alar nasal cartilage

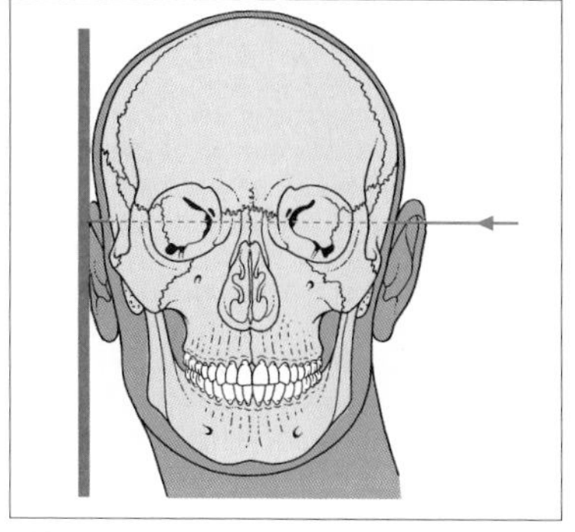

123 a

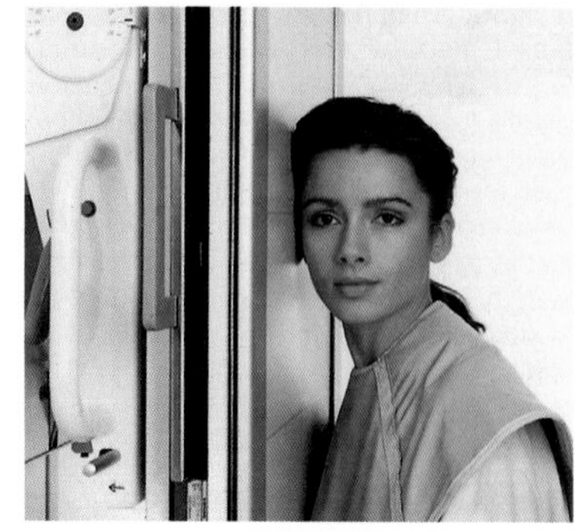

123 b

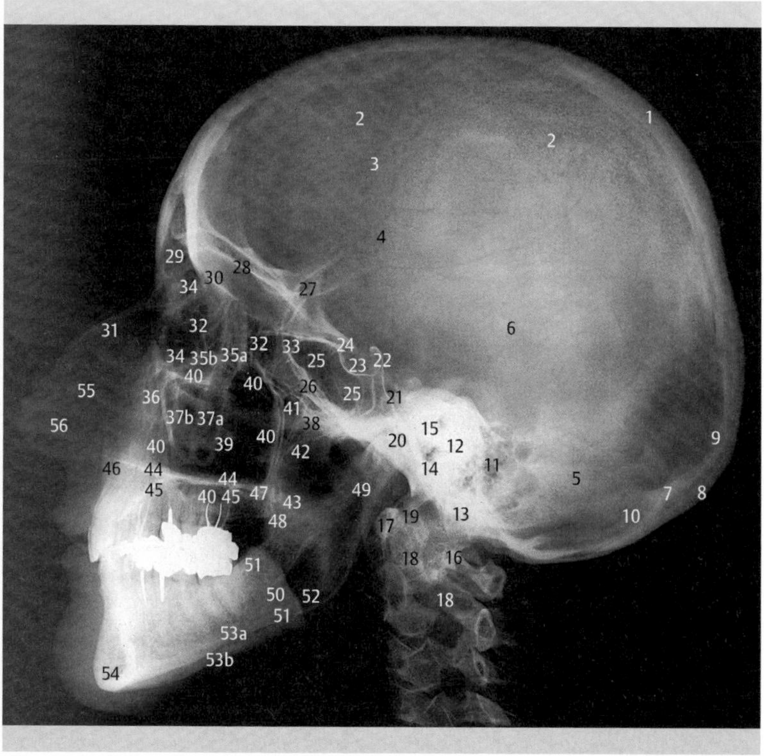

124

If the skull is precisely symmetrically positioned, the axial overview skull film permits left-to-right comparison of structures. For this reason, it is the radiograph of first choice for numerous indications. In dentistry, it can be used for localization of extremely ectopically impacted maxillary third molars that appear in the panoramic radiograph only in cross-section. Asymmetries of the condyles and deviations of the condyle axes can also be documented. In trauma cases, it can be used during initial examination for the detection of depressed fractures of the zygomatic bone, and to demonstrate blood within the sinuses; in ENT (ears, nose and throat) diagnosis, this projection is part of the conventional paranasal sinus survey (which includes frontal, ethmoid, maxillary sinuses). The Grashey–Schinz variation of this technique involves an excentric central ray projection from the submental in the direction of the frontal bone, with reduced exposure settings, leading to free projection of the zygomatic arch in isolation. Proper use and application of this radiographic technique will be attended by difficulty in elderly individuals with limited mobility of the cervical vertebrate.

Indications for the axial overview cranial radiograph: Because of the relatively low radiation dose required and the low cost of production, this technique is well indicated as an initial radiograph to check the condylar axes, or as a supplement to a panoramic radiograph for localization of extremely laterally impacted maxillary third molars. It is often also selected as the first radiograph for diagnosis and examination following zygomatic bone depressed fractures.

Fig. 125a Diagram of positioning. The top of the head is positioned on the cassette wall such that the Frankfort horizontal is parallel to the image receptor.

Fig. 125b Positioning the patient. With the head tipped severely backwards, the central ray can be projected submentovertically through the middle of the zygomatic arch and perpendicular to the image receptor (1). Central ray direction for the Grashey–Schinz variation (2) to achieve better presentation of the zygomatic arches.

Legend for Fig. 126:

1 Maxillary teeth
2 Mandibular teeth
3 Impacted tooth 48
4 Basal compact bone of the mandible
5 Anterior nasal spine
6 Osseous nasal septum
7 Nasolacrimal canal
8 Nasal conchae with ethmoid labyrinth
9 Palatal bone, dorsal border
10 Maxillary sinus, borders
11 Nasal cavity, lateral wall
12 Infraorbital margin
13 Canine fossa
14 Sphenoidal sinus
15 Pterygoid process, lateral lamina
16 Pterygoid process, medial lamina
17 Posterior nasal spine
18 Zygomatic bone
19 Zygomatic arch
20 Temporal fossa
21 Coronoid (muscular) process of the mandible
22 Lingula
23 Mandibular condyle
24 Angle of the mandible
25 Coronal suture
26 Foramen ovale
27 Spinous foramen
28 Middle lacerate foramen
29 Carotid canal
30 Dorsum sellae
31 Anterior tubercle of atlas
32 Transverse foramen of atlas
33 Odontoid bone (dentoid process of axis)
34 Great occipital foramen (foramen magnum)
35 Occipital condyle
36 Mastoid sinuses
37 Occipital bone
38 Cervical vertebrae

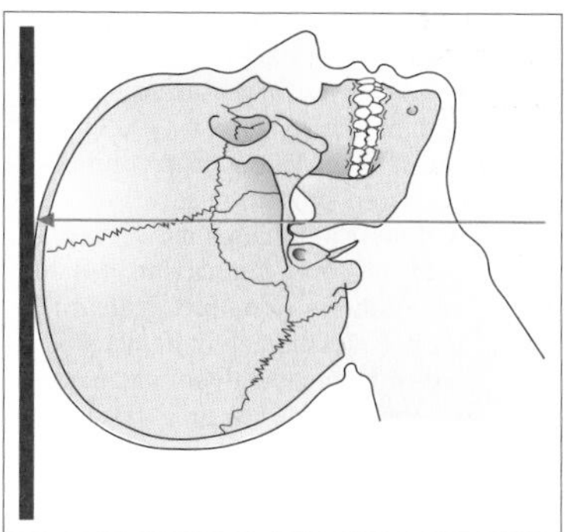

125 a

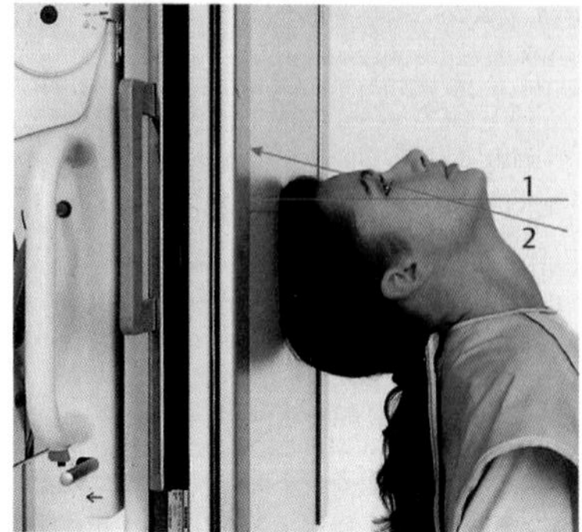

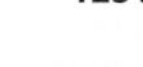

125 b

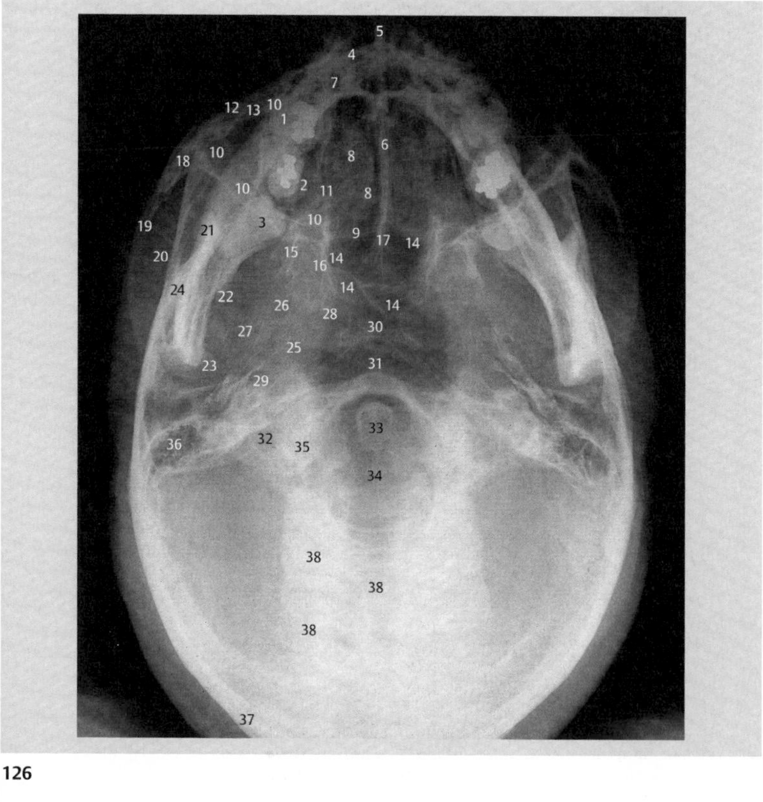

126

The Waters skull radiograph is not an overview, but rather a partial radiograph of the skull. It encompasses the orbits, the maxillary sinuses, and the zygomatic bone with the zygomatic arch. It is used by dental surgeons as supplemental information referred to as "maxillary half-axial," and is always taken with maximum mouth opening. The central ray is targeted horizontally, enters the skull about 10 cm above the external occipital protuberance, and exits the skull at the anterior nasal spine. If the patient has difficulty tipping the head extremely far back, the entry point of the central ray must be moved upward until the petrosal bone is below the sinus; this will ensure free and clear depiction of the maxillary sinus. With proper positioning of the patient and targeting of the central ray, the sphenoid sinus appears on the hard palate above the posterior nasal spine. Only with precisely symmetrical positioning will the radiograph permit the critically important bilateral diagnostic comparisons. Because of the oblique projection of the maxilla, this radiograph should not be used for localization of impacted teeth or foreign bodies.

Indications for the Waters projection of the skull: The Waters projection serves above all for conventional examination of the maxillary sinuses with bilateral comparison, although the posterior lobe in a completely dentulous patient cannot be completely depicted. As a component of the conventional paranasal sinus survey, the Waters view provides simultaneous depiction of the paranasal sinuses if there is suspicion of pansinusitis. In trauma cases, the Waters view is used for examination of depressed fracture of the zygomatic bone.

The Waters view is not indicated for localization of impacted teeth or foreign bodies in the maxilla because of the oblique projection of the structures.

Fig. 127a Diagram of positioning. With maximum mouth opening ensured by a bite cork, the petrosal bone (**violet**) must be positioned lower than the floor of the sinus (**pink**) in order to clearly depict the maxillary sinuses.

Fig. 127b Positioning the patient. The photograph shows the correct position of the patient against the cassette wall. The petrosal bone and the structures of the base of the skull will be depicted in the radiograph beneath the maxillary sinuses.

Legend for Fig. 128:

1 Saggital suture
2 Frontal sinus, with septa
3 Cirsta galli with falciform process of cerebrum
4 Cribriform lamina of ethmoid bone
5 Nasal bone
6 Orbit
7 Innominate line (of the major ala)
8 Minor ala of the sphenoid bone
9 Median cranial fossa (borders)
10 Optical canal
11 Superior orbital fissure
12 Infraorbital canal
13 Foramen rotundum (round foramen of sphenoid bone)
14 Ethmoid labyrinth
15 Osseous nasal septum
16 Nasal conchae
17 Maxillary sinus
18 Zygomatic bone
19 Frontal process of the zygomatic bone
20 Frontal zygomatic suture
21 Zygomatic arch
22 Zygomaticoalveolar crest
23 Condylar process of the mandible
24 Coronoid process of the mandible
25 Mastoid sinuses
26 Petrosal portion of the temporal bone
27 Anterior nasal spine
28 Posterior nasal spine
29 Sphenoidal spine
30 Basilar apophysis
31 Dorsum of the tongue
32 Lateral mass of atlas
33 Odontoid bone (dentoid process of axis)

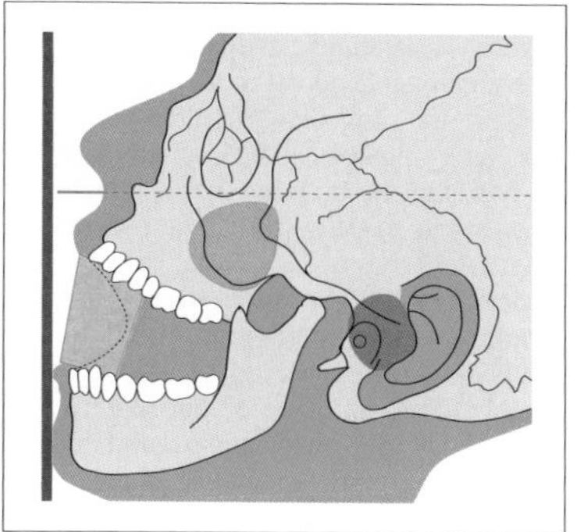

127 a

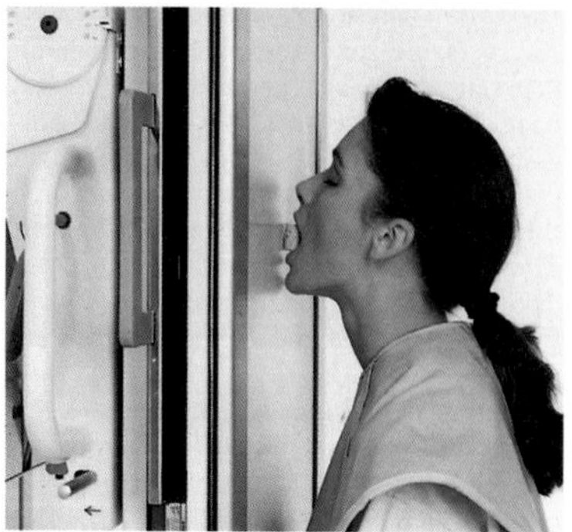

127 b

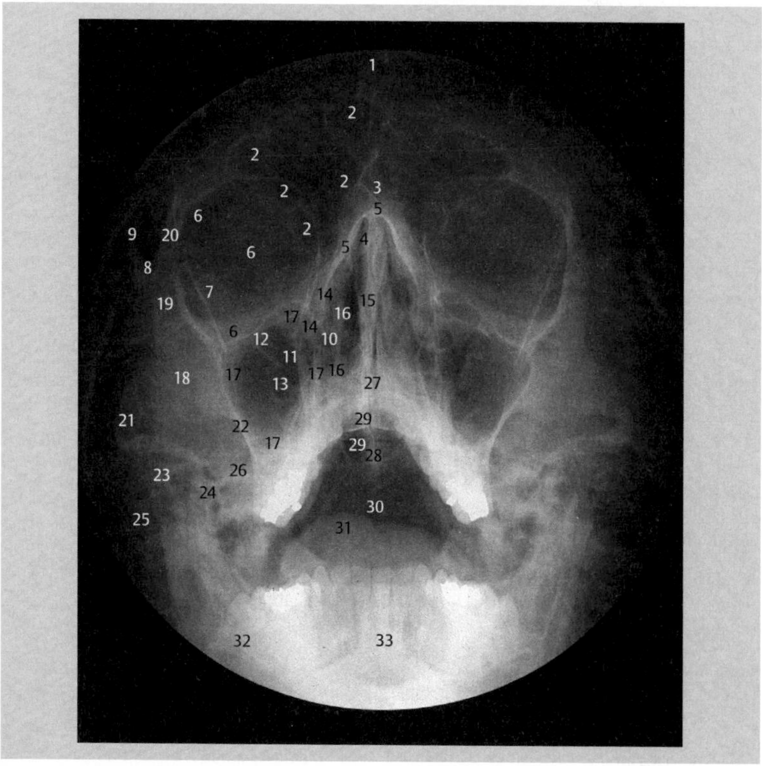

128

The posteroanterior mandibular overview is a very versatile conventional skull radiograph that can usually also be taken using the cephalometric attachment on panoramic radiograph equipment. It is a partial radiograph of the skull in which the mandible and especially the angle of the mandible, the neck of the condyloid process and the condyle can be clearly depicted without superimposition of other structures. With the patient's forehead pressed against the cassette wall and with maximum mouth opening, the central ray is directed so that is passes below the back of the head (occiput) and exits the skull on the bridge of the nose. A perfectly symmetrical central ray direction is a prerequisite for optimum and interpretable radiographic quality.
Using normal exposure settings, the neck of the condyle and the condyle itself will be overexposed, and the use of appropriate lateral filters is therefore recommended.
In addition, this technique is excellent to supplement a panoramic radiograph when, before surgery, it is necessary to definitively localize in the third dimension the position of completely impacted maxillary and mandibular third molars. Only the more radiation-intensive and more costly CT procedure provides better results.
Indications for the posteroanterior mandibular overview radiograph: This technique can be used to supplement a panoramic radiograph for localization of horizontally impacted maxillary and mandibular third molars. Trauma to the mandible, for example fractures at the angle of the mandible or fracture of the condyles, often cannot be definitively verified in a panoramic radiograph because the bone fragments are often superimposed upon each other.

Fig. 129a Diagram of positioning. With a bite block to insure maximum mouth opening, the skull should be positioned with the forehead pressed against the cassette wall so that the condyles are projected above the maxillary sinuses and below the petrosal bone.

Fig. 129b Positioning the patient. The photograph shows the patient leaning against the cassette wall with her forehead, to receive a horizontally aimed central ray. Special care must be taken to ensure symmetrical positioning of the skull.

Legend for Fig. 130:

1 Frontal crest
2 Squamous portion of temporal bone
3 Petrosal portion of temporal bone
4 Arcuate eminence
5 Mastoid process of the temporal bone
6 Sphenoid sinus in superimposition with portions of the frontal sinus
7 Crista galli
8 Sphenoid plane
9 Atlantooccipital articulation
10 Transverse process of atlantis
11 Pterygoid process of the sphenoid bone
12 Articular eminence
13 Zygomatic arch
14 Zygomatic bone
15 Orbit, inferior margin
16 Maxillary sinus
17 Nasal cavity
18 Inferior nasal concha
19 Osseous nasal septum
20 Odontoid bone (dentoid process of axis)
21 Atlantoaxial articulation
22 Anterior nasal spine
23 Condyloid process of the mandible
24 Articular surface of the condyle
25 Angle of the mandible
26 Coronoid process of the mandible
27 Mandibular canal
28 Mental foramen
29 Body of third cervical vertebra

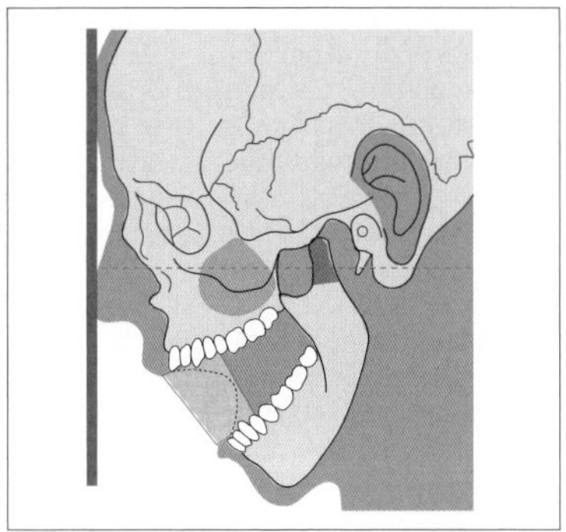

129 a

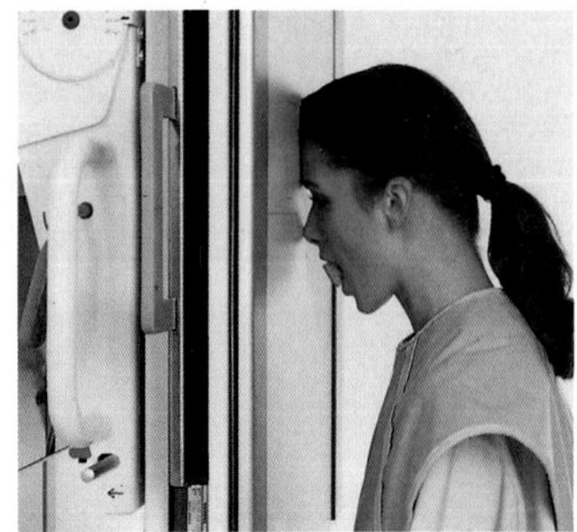

129 b

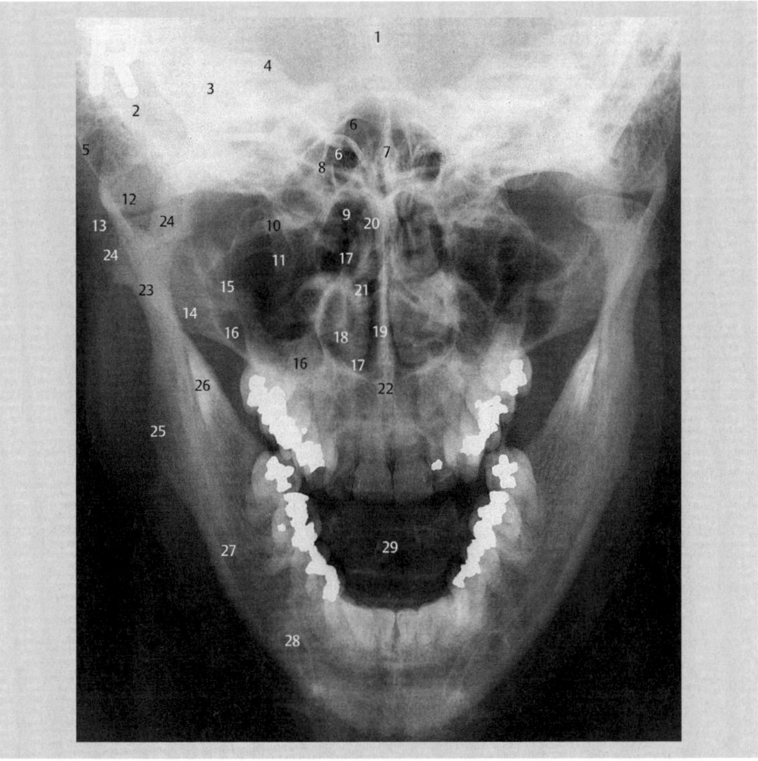

130

The mandibular half-arch radiograph can be taken with skull radiography equipment or with a conventional dental radiographic unit. However, a high level of experience and a firm grasp of 3-dimensional spatial relationships are necessary in order to properly depict the desired regions. Taking this projection with the cephalometric attachment device in the panoramic unit is possible, but difficult, because the necessary light gauge is lacking. When using the standard dental radiographic unit, the patient, film cassette, and radiograph head must be positioned free-hand. If this technique can be mastered, radiographic results can be achieved in various regions of the jaws that are considerably superior to those that can be achieved with intraoral radiographs. Worthy of consideration, however, is that because the film format (standard: 13 x 18 cm) is considerably larger than standard intraoral film packets, arrangements must be made for conventional film processing and eventually also for digitizing the radiographs.

With proper selection of exposure settings, the ramus of the mandible, the retromolar region, and above all the course of the mandibular canal can frequently be depicted more clearly than in a panoramic radiograph. If appropriate equipment is available, a conventional film cassette can be used to take orientation radiographs even with a patient under general anesthesia.

Indications for the mandibular half-arch radiograph: If the dental practice does not have a panoramic unit, this technique can be used with a low radiation dose to provide much more comprehensive views of entire sections of the jaws in comparison to individual intraoral radiographs. This radiograph can have a special significance for the clear depiction of the angle of the mandible, the ramus, and the mandibular canal, all of which are often not satisfactorily depicted in a panoramic radiograph.

Fig. 131 a Positioning using a standard dental radiographic unit. Note especially that the film cassette must not be pressed with excessive force onto the mandible, in order to avoid image distortions.

Fig. 131 b Positioning using a standard dental radiographic unit. Proper targeting of the central ray for depiction of the left half of the mandible (see Fig. **132a**).

Fig. 132 a Skull photograph reveals the target of the central ray. Projection angle, e.g., for depicting the body and angle of the mandible on the left side (see Fig. **131a**, **b**).

Fig. 132 b Radiograph of the ascending mandibular ramus. The angle of the mandible and its ramus must be targeted more steeply from the caudal aspect.

Fig. 133 a Radiographic anatomy in a mandibular half-arch radiograph. This radiograph resulted from the central ray projection angle depicted in Fig. **132a** and **b**. See legend.

Fig. 133 b Depiction of the mandibular anterior region. The anterior region of the mandible can be depicted if the central ray is targeted between the cervical vertebrate and the mandibular angle on the opposite side, targeting the canine.

Legend for Fig. 133a:

1 Condyle
2 Articular eminence
3 Zygomatic arch
4 Zygomaticoalveolar suture
5 Pterygoid process of the sphenoid bone
6 Zygomatic bone
7 Maxillary sinus
8 Maxillary tuberosity
9 Coronoid process of the mandible
10 Semilunar notch
11 Mandibular foramen
12 Mandibular canal
13 Mental foramen
14 Temporal crest
15 Hyoid bone
16 Angle of the mandible

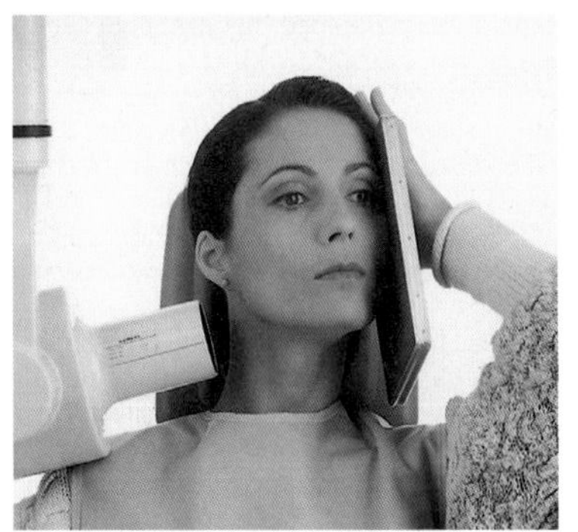
131 a

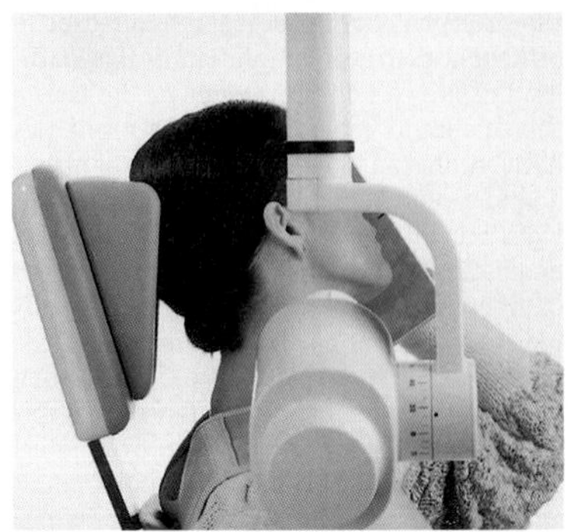
131 b

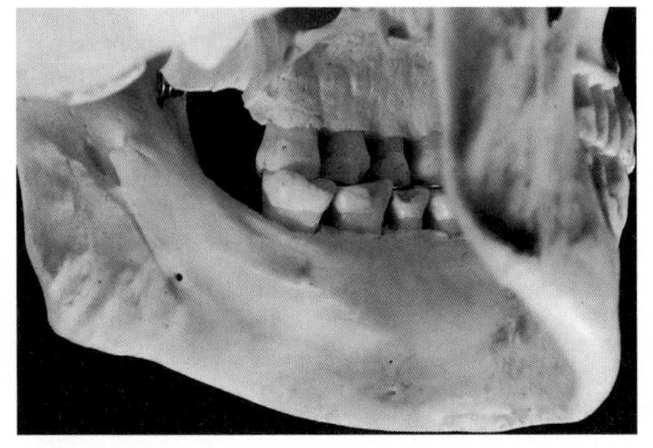
132 a

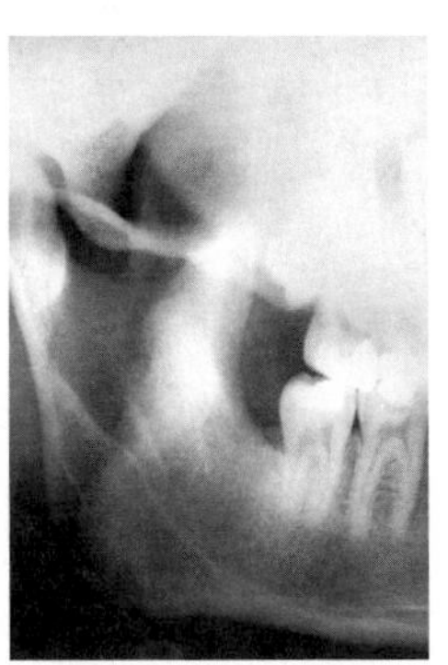
132 b

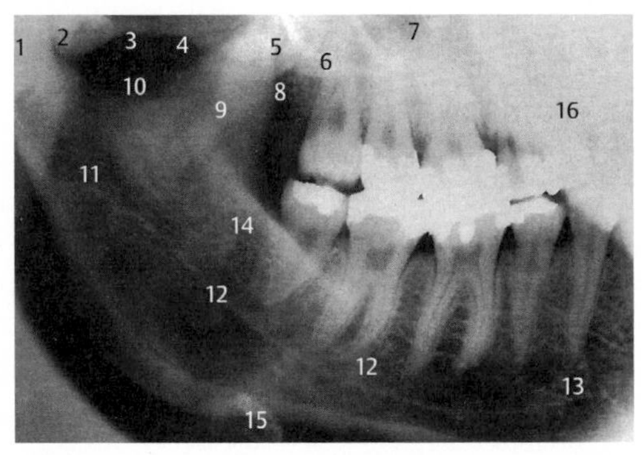

133 a

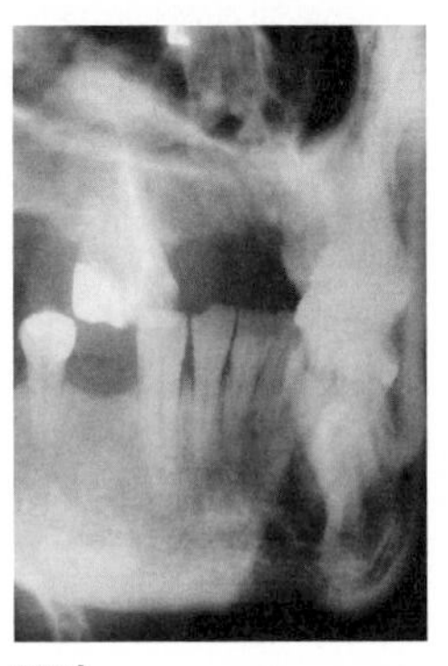
133 b

Lateral cephalometric radiographs are used in orthodontics to examine and clarify dysgnathias. Despite certain shortcomings, the lateral cephalometric radiograph and its analysis have become an integral component of orthodontic examinations. The "lateral ceph" provides accurate measurements of skeletal and dentoalveolar relationships within the myriad of different types of dysgnathias, and permits precise classification. In order to select the most effective therapy, a proper differential diagnosis is of extreme importance; it is this diagnosis that must be extracted from interpretation of the accurately measured values and relationships. The now-classic measurements are derived from linear connections and angular determinations emanating from skeletal and soft tissue fixed points. Measured values from a given patient can then be compared to population norms, and the evaluations will lead to a comprehensive and accurate differential diagnosis.

With regard to the cephalometric technique itself, the radiograph may be taken from the right side or the left side; there are several schools of thought in this regard. Nevertheless, generally in radiology the IR is taken with the right side touching the picture cassette and the central ray penetrating from the patient's left side. The Frankfort horizontal should be positioned horizontally. Radiographs that are taken with varying focus-object distances cannot be compared to each other. Space limitations here preclude a detailed discussion and description of the complex analysis of lateral cephalometric radiographs. This can be reviewed in appropriate clinical/scientific textbooks and professional journals.

For depiction of soft tissue structures, appropriately shaped and graduated aluminum filters can be employed. A clearly visible depiction of the soft tissue profile can be achieved by coating the median saggital plane of the face with a barium-containing paste.

A focused Potter–Bucky grid can increase the radiographic quality, but also requires a higher radiation dose; for this reason, today the slot-technique is preferred (see Fig. **3b**).

Indications for the lateral cephalometric radiograph: This lateral view of the skull is used primarily in the important differential diagnosis encompassing cephalometric analysis, while the posteroanterior radiograph is used more frequently for documentation of skeletal asymmetries.

The lateral cephalometric projection can be used to advantage as a supplement to the panoramic view for the localization of impacted teeth in the region of the maxillary sinuses.

Fig. 134 Principle of the lateral cephalometric radiograph. The patient is positioned with the right side of the face against the cassette. Using arbitrarily selected "measurement points" this diagram shows the interdependence of the enlargement factor with varying focus-film distances. Note that measurement precision *increases* with focal distance, but is also dependent upon the placement of the measurement points on the radiograph itself.

Fig. 135a Lateral cephalometric radiograph. With the right side of the patient's face positioned against the image receptor, the Frankfort horizontal is adjusted to the horizontal. Teeth are closed together in habitual intercuspation.

Fig. 135b Posteroanterior cephalometric radiograph. Using a p.-a. targeted central ray, skeletal asymmetries of the skull can be ascertained.

Legend for Fig. 135a:

Skeletal measurement points:

1 Nasion
2 Anterior nasal spine
3 Posterior nasal spine
4 A-point
5 B-point
6 Pogonion
7 Chin
8 Gonion
9 Basion
10 TMJ
11 Condyle
12 Porion
13 Orbit
14 Sella, midpoint

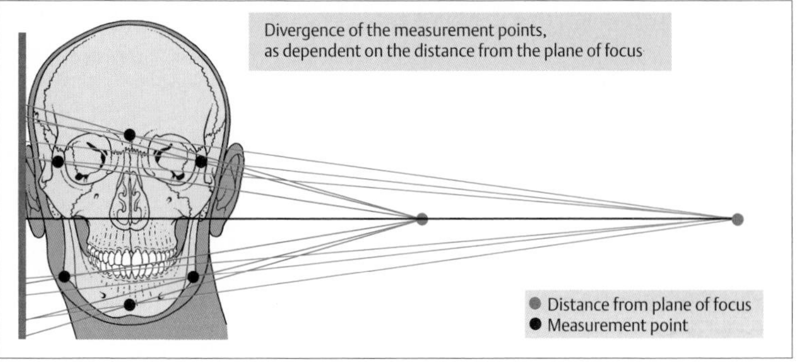

134

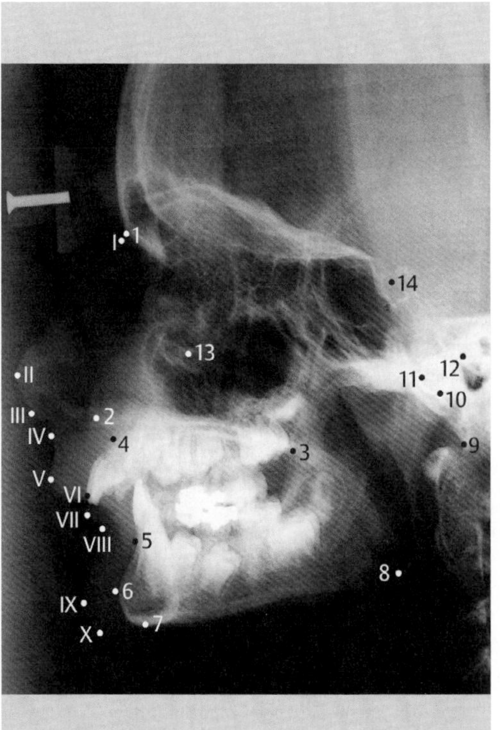

135 a

Soft tissue measurement points:

I	Skin, bridge of the nose
II	Tip of the nose
III	Subnasale
IV	Subspinale
V	Upper lip
VI	Stomion
VII	Lower lip
VIII	Submentale
IX	Skin pogonion
X	Skin gnathion

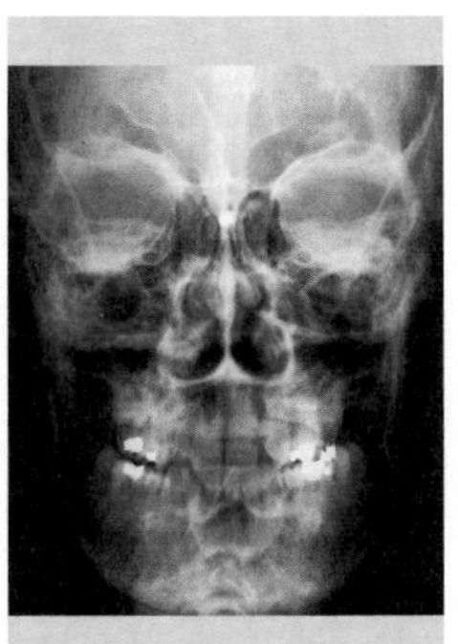

135 b

"Classic" TMJ radiographs, as modified by Schüller, lead one to the incorrect assumption that such films represent a lateral profile view of the TMJ; this is reflected in some of the older literature where one encounters the term "joint space." The oblique projections, with dorsal and cranial targeting of the central ray, necessary for depicting the joints without overlapping, provides a picture of the components of the joint two-dimensionally in an oblique view, so that the "upper" part of the condyle in actuality is the lateral pole of the condyle and the part near to the joint space of the "fossa" actually corresponds to the lateral portion of that structure as it transitions to its attachments on the zygomatic arch. These spatially variable anatomic relationships, resulting also from individual joint architecture are often interpretable only by those with broad experience, and really only provide gross diagnostic conclusions about condyle position or pathologic alterations. The condition of the articular disk, which is so important in secondary arthropathy, cannot be depicted because of its radiotransparency; it can only be discerned by its potential effects. If initial traumatic lesions of the articular disk, or degenerative alterations of the condyle, have occurred, other examination methods must be employed, e.g., CT or magnetic resonance imaging (MRI).

For reasons of film quality and protection from radiation overdose, partial skull radiographs must be performed using an appropriate collimator.

Indications for conventional TMJ radiographs: A radiograph taken with the teeth in habitual intercuspation (occlusion) depicts the structures of the TMJ in a transcranial, oblique-lateral projection, which as a result of the individual anatomic situation can only be interpreted with great care. If, however, no other method is available for examining the TMJ, this method can still provide useful information with optimum technical performance and adequate experience on the part of the evaluator; nevertheless, the interpretations must be limited only to functional disturbances and gross alterations of the hard tissues and the TMJ relationships.

Fig. 136a TMJ radiography, Schüller modification. The diagram shows the proper positioning of the skull vis-à-vis the cassette wall. Red = central ray.

Fig. 136b TMJ radiography, Schüller modification. Positioning of the patient against the cassette wall. The median saggital plane is perpendicular to the film cassette, at an angle of about 10°.

Fig. 137a TMJ, mouth closed. The Frankfort horizontal is positioned horizontally. The jaws are closed with the teeth in habitual intercuspation.

Fig. 137b TMJ, mouth open. When the mouth is opened, the Frankfort horizontal must not be elevated. Only the mandible moves, and the position is secured with a mouth prop.

Fig. 138a, b TMJ projections, mouth closed and open. If a patient complains of TMJ discomfort, the examination must always include radiographs of *both* TMJs! Depicted here is the right TMJ only (space limitations) with the mouth closed and open. Note that both images were positioned identically. (Note the shape of the external auditory meatus and the position of the zygomatic arch.)

Legend for Fig. 138:

1 Condyle, lateral pole
2 Condyle, medial pole
3 Condylar process of the mandible
4 Glenoid fossa, lateral portion
5 Articular eminence, lateral portion
6 Zygomatic arch
7 Sella turcica
8 Sphenoid sinus
9 Posterior clinoid process
10 Clivus
11 Petrosal part (distant from the cassette)
12 Petrosal part (adjacent to the cassette)
13 Upper pyramidal border (adjacent to the cassette)
14 External auditory meatus
15 Mastoid sinuses
16 Tympanic bone

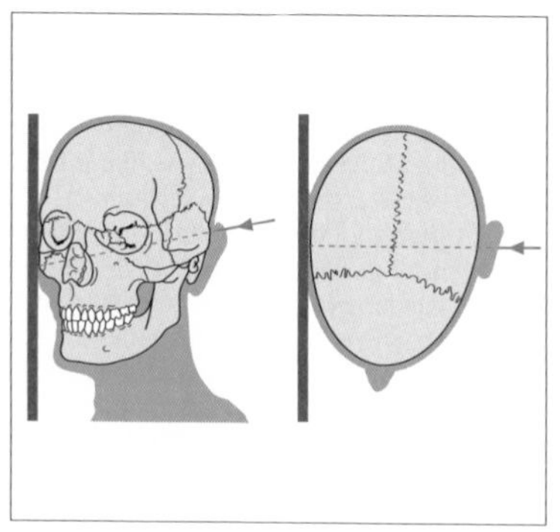

136 a

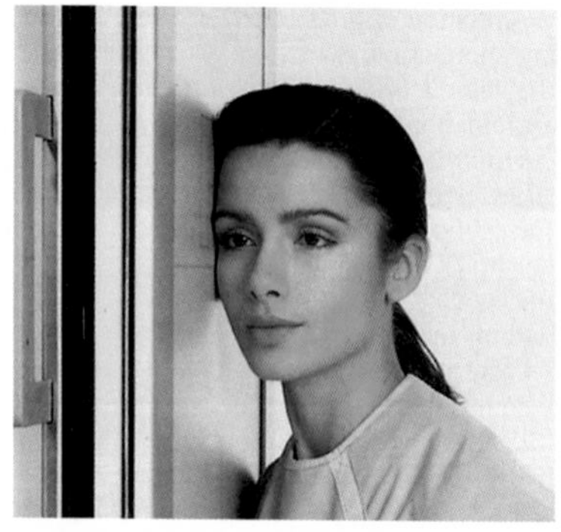

136 b

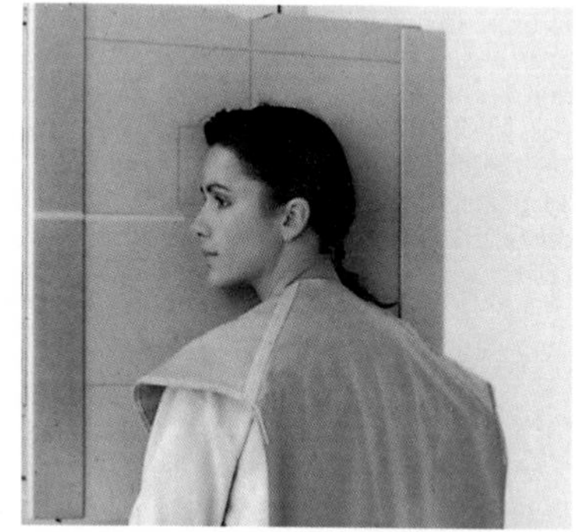

137 a

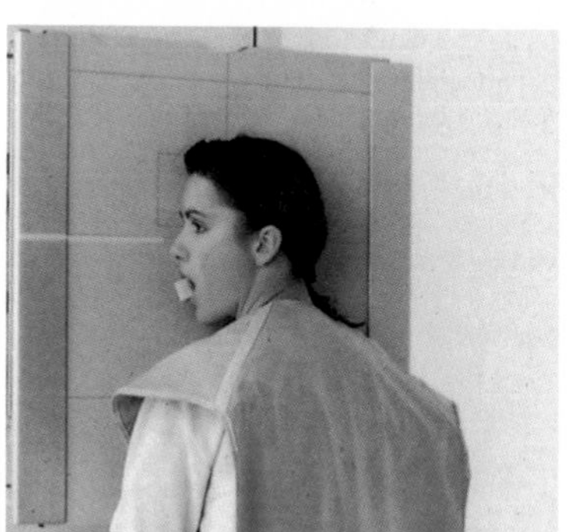

137 b

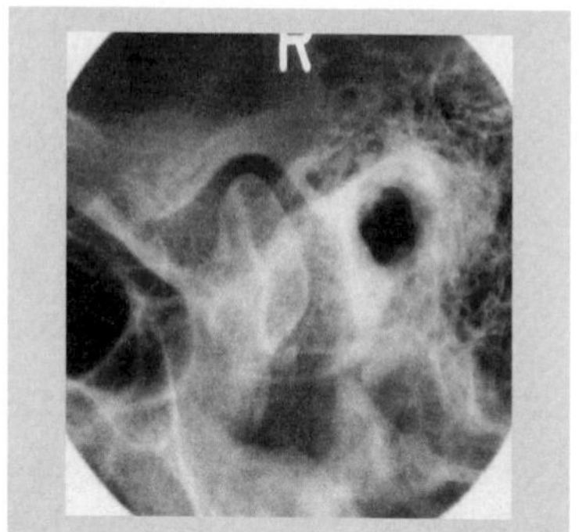

138 a

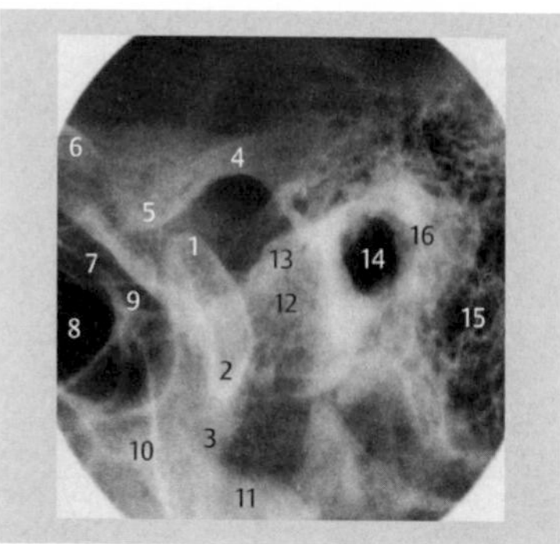

138 b

With computed tomography (CT), the disturbing summation effects are avoided, because the volume of the portion of the body under examination is cut into "slices" by a fanning out of the collimated roentgen rays. These slices can be considered as a grid-like layer consisting of volume elements (voxel) whose height is determined by the selected layer thickness. The anatomic structures located within these voxels dampen the incident roentgen rays according to the thickness and atomic number of the elements in the tissues. Its density is measured in Hounsfield units (HU). The attenuation coefficients encountered by rays passing through the volume elements are summated by detectors so that they can be transformed into electrical signals, multiplied and amplified, and converted into image elements. The values (linear or tangential integrals) emanating from a single direction are referred to as projections. For high image quality, numerous projections and the most measured values per projection must be achieved. The absorption values measured within a volume element are reconstructed using a high capacity computer and analog-digital converter into pixels, which together produce the image matrix.

In contrast to conventional film tomograms, computed tomograms reproduce only those anatomic and pathologic details that lie within the selected and computed slice (layer). But also here there are technical limitations because the thinner slices that are most desirable for optimization of interpretation themselves increase noise that reduces quality and furthermore requires higher mA values, thus increasing radiation exposure for the patient. On the other hand, thicker slices increase the undesirable volume artifacts. The solution to this apparent enigma is to combine the advantage of low image static with the artifact-reduction of the thinner layers by combining in a single image two or three desired slices; this is accomplished using a high capacity computer.

In order to improve the quality of digital image reconstruction, the highest possible number of projections from as many angles as possible are required, which can provide over 10^6 measurement values per rotation. An inadequate number of measurement points reduces the quality of resolution, and for this reason cones have been constructed that change the angle of irradiation during the rotation; the attenuation profiles from the various angle adjustments are measured and processed separately into data sets.

Figs. 139–141 Topogram (scout/pathfinder) and axial computed tomography of the mandible, with indicated radiographic anatomy.

Legend:

1 Mandibular rami
2 Angle of the mandible
3 Mandibular foramen, with lingula
4 Mandibular canal, lengthwise
5 Mandibular canal, transverse
6 Mental foramen
7 Mental spine
8 Mandibular torus
9 Styloid process
10 Hyoid bone, minor horn
11 Atlas, posterior tubercle
12 Axis, vertebral foramen
13 Axis, transverse foramen
14 Axis, vertebral body
15 Axis, spinus process
16 Body of vertebra III
17 Pharynx, oral portion
18 Submandibular gland
19 Parotid gland
20 Musculature of the floor of the mouth: genioglossus, hyoglossus, and mylohyoid
21 Masseter muscle
22 Sternocleidomastoid muscle
23 Medial pterygoid muscle
24 Muscles of the neck (semispinal muscle of head, inferior oblique muscle of head, splenius muscle of head)
25 Chin muscle (mentalis)

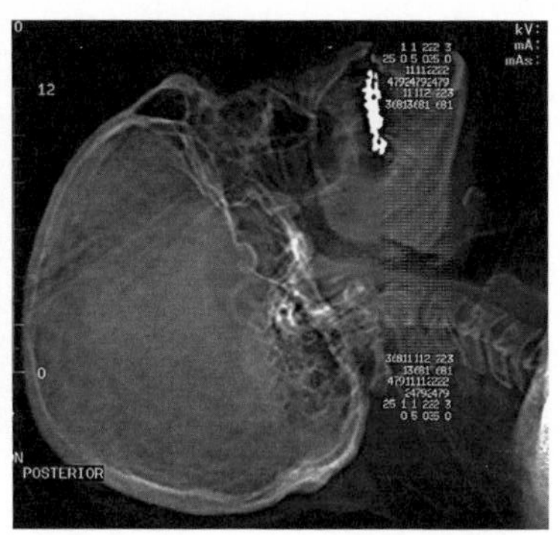

kV:
mA:
mAs:
12
0
POSTERIOR

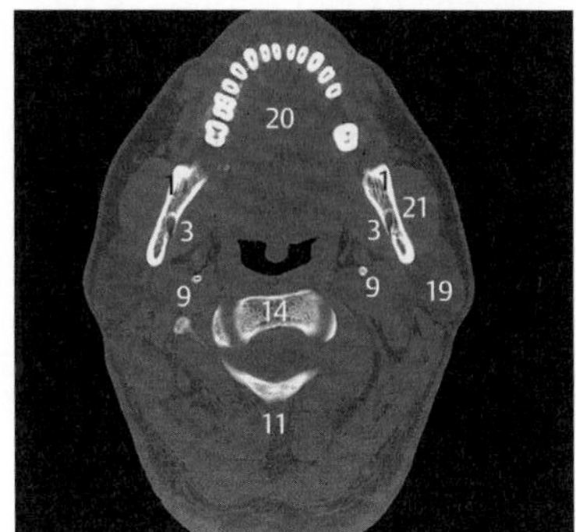

20
1
1
21
3
3
9
9
19
14
11

139

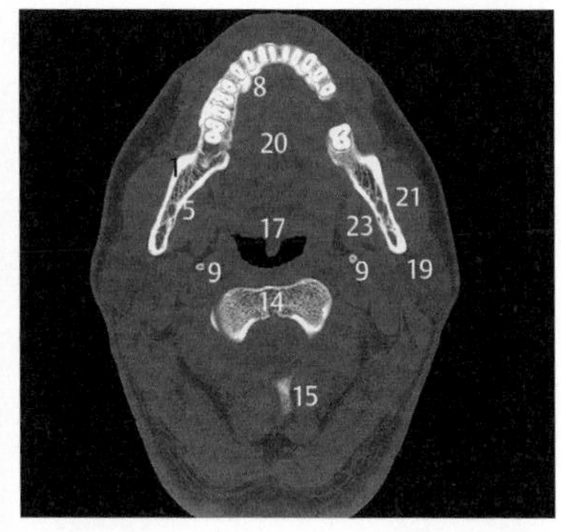

8
20
1
21
5
17
23
9
9
19
14
15

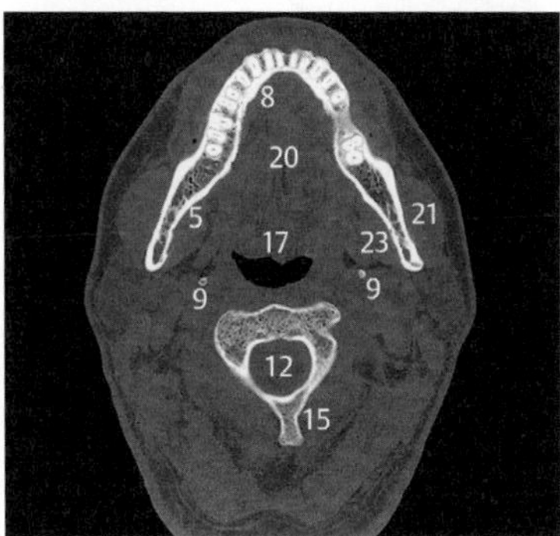

8
20
5
21
17
23
9
9
12
15

140

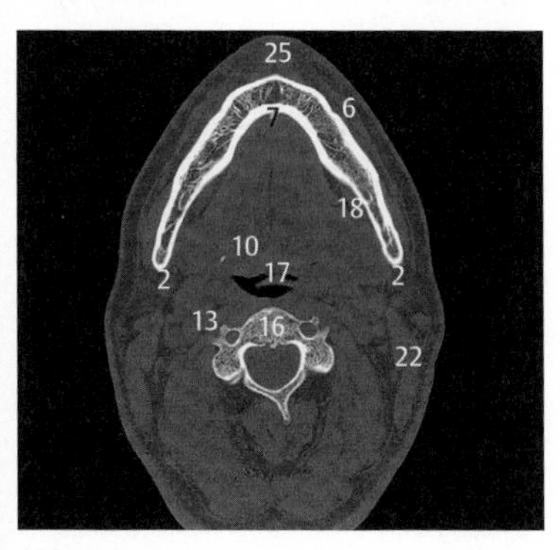

25
6
7
18
10
2
17
2
13
16
22

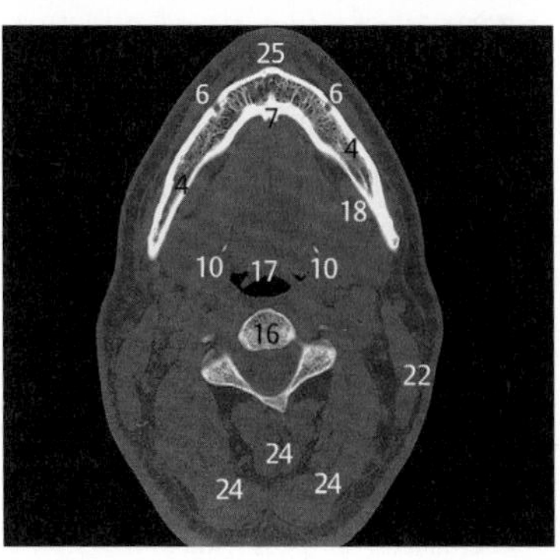

25
6
6
7
4
4
18
10
17
10
16
22
24
24
24

141

The concept of "pitch," as used in spiral tomography, is a function of the slice thickness in millimeters and the rate at which the table is advanced. It is expressed in "layers per rotation" (mm/360° rotation). Pitch 1 means that with a movement speed of one slice thickness per rotation scanning will be continuous. Depending upon the slice thickness selected, the result will be a shorter or a longer scan volume per rotation. By increasing the rotation speed and simultaneously exposing several layers, the exposure time will be reduced as well as the radiation dose, taking greater advantage of the capabilities of the roentgen tubes and improved axial image resolution. Generally speaking, with increasing pitch the slice thickness increases continuously, while the applied radiation dose is reduced. Elevated volume-scan-speed is used to improve axial resolution, which also optimizes the image quality of three-dimensional (3D) reconstructions. Multilayer spiral CT with sub-millimeter collimation makes it possible to achieve very high quality depictions, especially of skull and joints. From the same data set it is possible to extract high- and low-contrast images without additional irradiation, which was heretofore only possible with the use of bone or soft tissue window settings.

To achieve an image reconstruction in only a few seconds, the computer procedure of filtered back-projection coupled with a correction program is usually employed. The algorithm, based upon the Fourier transformations and integral functions, is simply referred to as filtering or folding. Errors can be caused by variable sensitivities of the attenuation profile detectors and by variations in the effect of radiation absorption on the longer wavelength regions of the radiation bundle. These errors can be compensated for by the correction function of the control program.

In order to fulfill contemporary patient demands for a both functional and esthetically satisfying replacement of missing teeth, enossal dental implants were developed, which created a new discipline within periodontology and oral surgery. This necessitated new techniques for radiographic assessment in order to adequately evaluate, *during the treatment planning phase*, the shape of the alveolar ridges, the positional/spatial relationships of adjacent anatomic structures, as well as the quantity and the quality of the bone destined to receive an implant. Initial efforts led to the development of appropriate and indicated programs and processors to create transverse sections using conventional tomography. Thereafter occurred the final breakthrough with the introduction of CT, which offered the possibility of multi-planar reconstructions of secondary panoramic views and depiction of slices, and finally transverse sections of the jaw with integrated measurement scales.

Fig. 142–144 Topogram and axial computed tomographies of the maxilla, with radiographic anatomy.

Legend:

1 Artifacts caused by metal dental restorations
2 Mandibular ramus
3 Mandibular foramen
4 Articular (condular) process
5 Coronoid process
6 Alveolar portion of the maxilla
7 Incisive canal
8 Anterior nasal spine
9 Maxillary tuberosity
10 Pterygoid process, with lateral and medial laminae
11 Hamulus of the medial lamina
12 Styloid process
13 Mastoid process
14 Maxillary sinus
15 Odontoid bone (dentoid process of axis)
16 Axis, spinus process
17 Axis, anterior tuberculum
18 Axis, posterior tuberculum
19 Atlas, lateral mass
20 Transverse foramen
21 Parotid gland
22 Lateral pterygoid muscle
23 Medial pterygoid muscle
24 Masseter muscle
25 Long muscle of head, long muscle of neck
26 Palatal vault

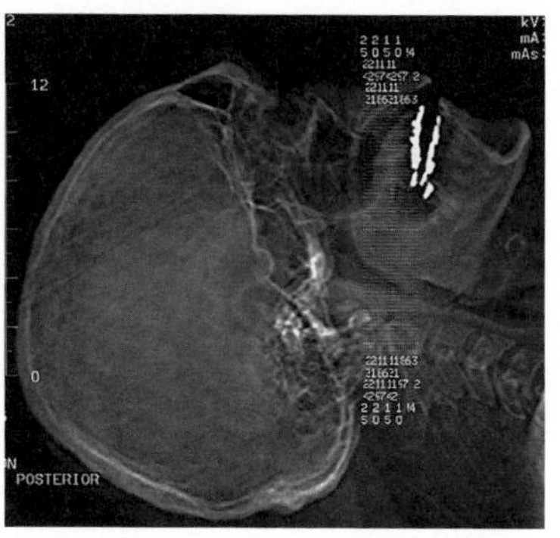
12
0
POSTERIOR

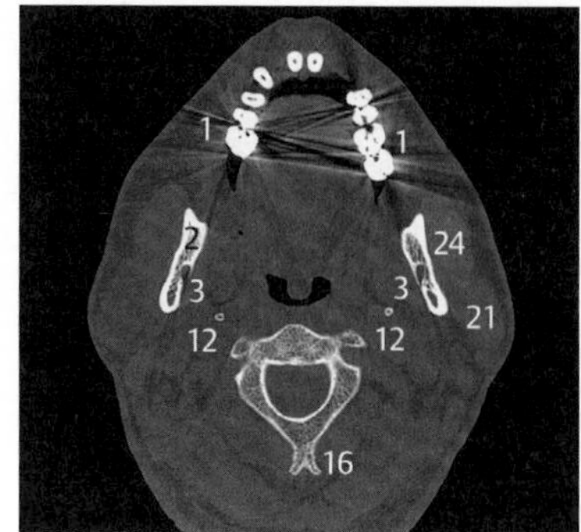
1
1
2
24
3
3
21
12
12
16

142

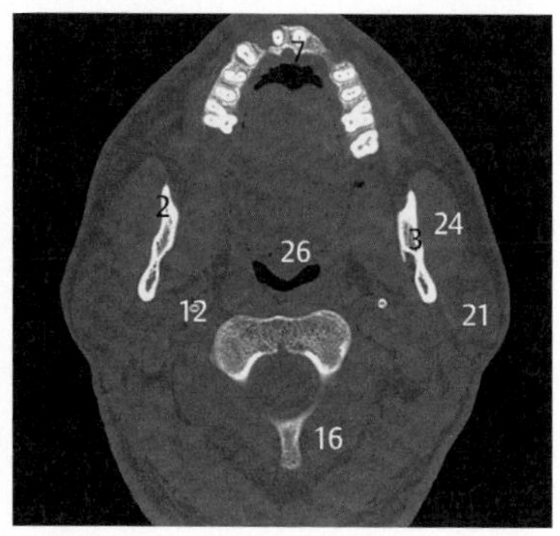
7
2
24
3
26
12
21
16

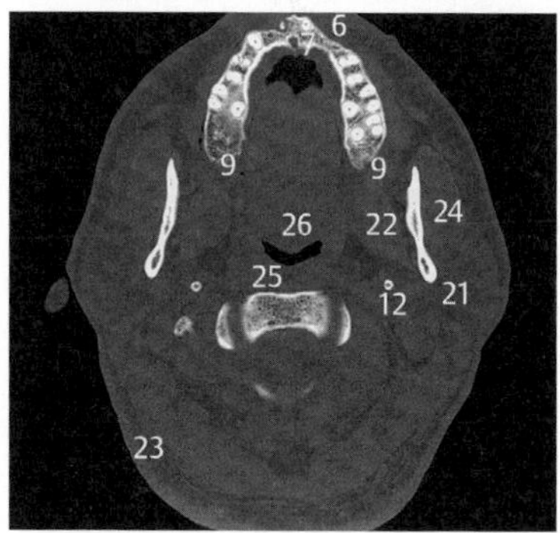
6
7
9
9
26
22
24
25
12
21
23

143

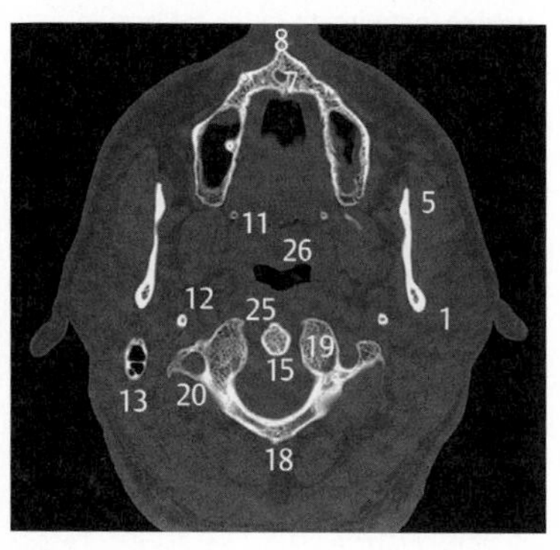
8
7
5
11
26
12
25
1
19
15
13
20
18

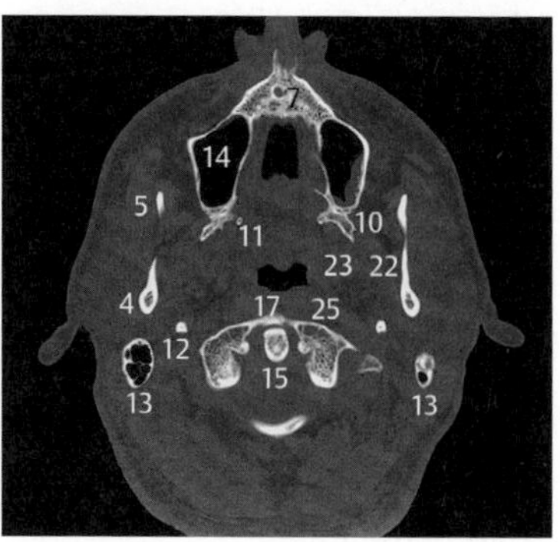
7
14
5
10
11
23
22
4
17
25
12
15
13
13

144

This procedure, known as dental-CT (Imhof 1992) permits a metric analysis of transverse sections of the jaw in three dimensions. After creating and processing the data set, the information is provided to the practitioner on film or per electronic data transfer. Critically important for this procedure is the correct adjustment of the primary slices that are programmed into the topogram (scout or pathfinder program) with graduations. For both completely dentulous and partially dentulous patients, it is recommended that the slice be adjusted parallel to the alveolar ridge so that the axes of the teeth are as perpendicular as possible to the central ray. Therefore, in order to avoid distortions that would lead to errors during metric analysis of secondary slices, the planes of the slices should not be oriented with the floor of the maxillary sinus nor with the inferior border of the mandible. The diagnostically important distance measurements in the region of impacted third molars should be undertaken in secondary slices only when the primary layers are adjusted parallel to the course of the mandibular canal. As is also the case with conventional panoramic radiographs, the mandibular canal from the mental foramen back to about the second molar is often not sharply demarcated due to the porosity of the canal walls and especially the canal roof in transverse sections of the mandible. The canal is easier to identify in cases where sclerosis of the surrounding cancellous bone has occurred.

Multiplanar Reconstructions

The tomogram of a desired cross-section retrieved directly from the data set is referred to as a primary multiplanar tomogram. Only slices that are reconstructed by data computations are referred to as secondary multiplanar tomograms. Computed tomography can also be used to depict and examine the facial skeleton in views other than the axial. Direct (primary) tomograms can also be created in other planes, if the problem of patient positioning in the gantry can be solved. The result fulfills the highest demands for image sharpness (resolution), while reconstructed secondary tomograms can only be generated with reduced image quality although without additional irradiation. An image with an appropriately large data volume will provide realistic views of all possible osseous and soft tissue structures. For any particular depiction or measurement, zones of interest can be marked with reconstruction lines, points, or measurement fields. For observation of tiny details, "zooming" optical enlargement of segments of the image can be made, to mention only one of many possibilities using digital technology. Images below the resolution capabilities of the system, such as the periodontal ligament space, usually cannot be adequately depicted.

Fig. 145–147 Topogram and modified coronar computed tomography of the TMJ region, with radiographic anatomy.

Legend:

1 Basal portion (clivus) of the occipital bone
2 Pharyngeal tubercule
3 External auditory meatus
4 Internal auditory meatus
5 Petrosal part of the temporal bone
6 Spine of the sphenoid bone
7 Mandibular (glenoid) fossa
8 Articular eminence (articular tubercule)
9 Temporal squama (squamous portion of the temporal bone)
10 Zygomatic arch, temporal root
11 Medial cranial fossa
12 Condylar (articular) process of the mandible
13 Neck of condyloid process of mandible
14 Mandibular lingula
15 Mandibular foramen
16 Mandibular canal
17 Head of the mandibular condyle
18 Mastoid sinuses (anterior portion)
19 Semilunar notch
20 Sphenoidal sinus
21 Body of the sphenoid bone
22 Hamulus of the medial lamina of the pterygoid process
23 Lateral lamina
24 Epipharynx

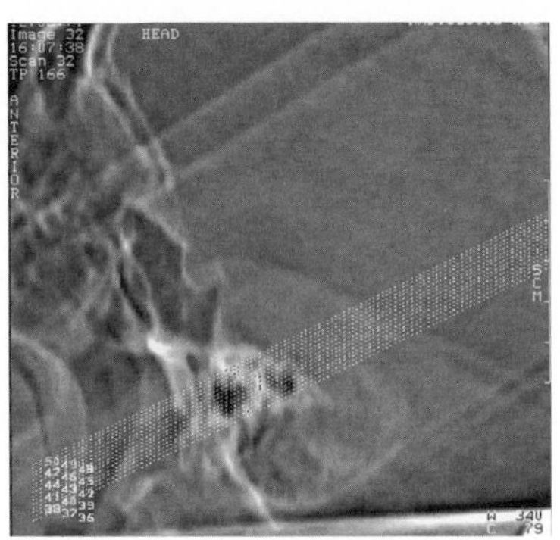

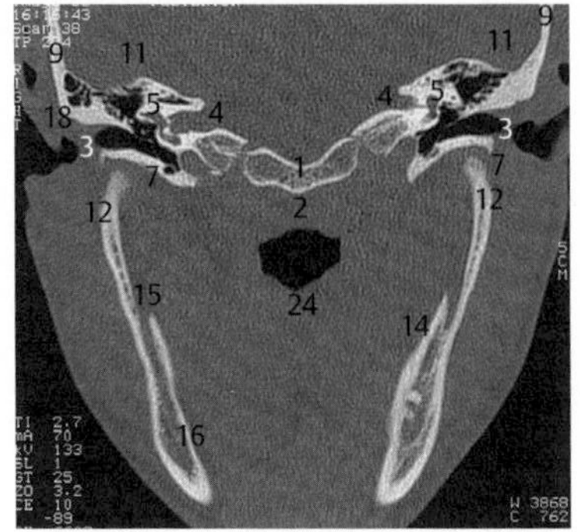
9
11
5
4
18
3
7
12
1
2
24
15
14
16

145

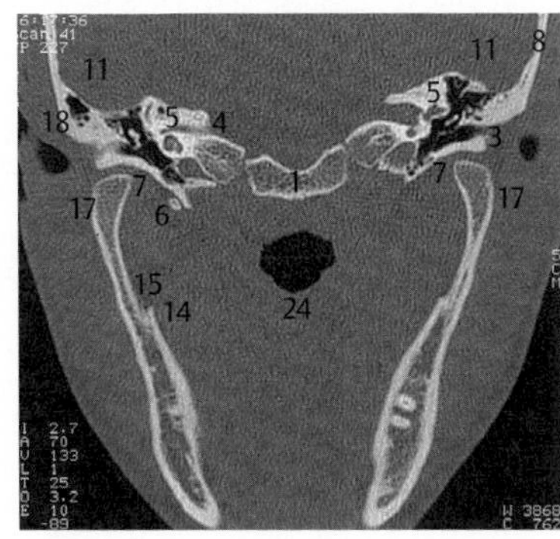
11
8
18
5
4
3
7
17
6
1
15
14
24

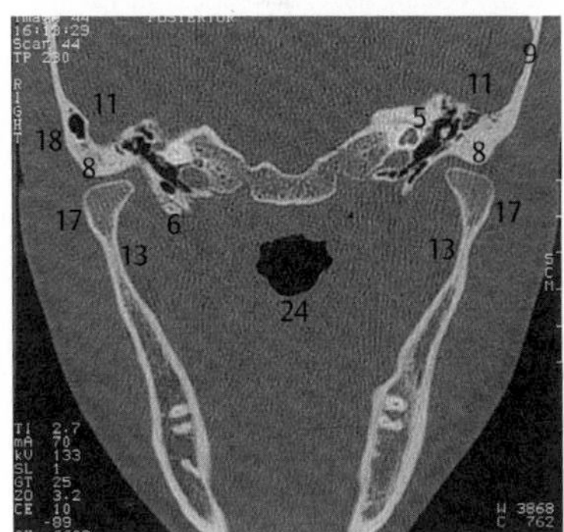
9
11
18
5
8
17
6
13
24

146

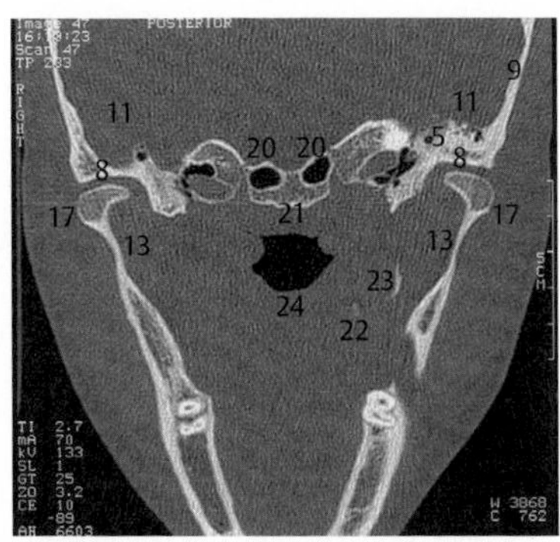
9
11
5
20
8
17
21
13
23
24
22

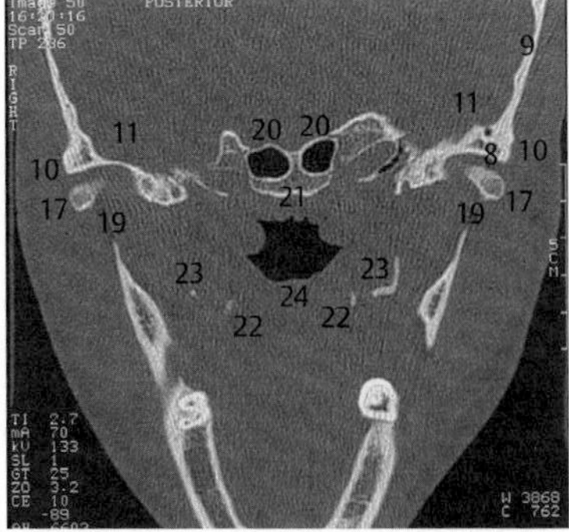
9
11
20
10
8
17
21
19
23
24
22

147

In the radiographic image, anatomic structures are depicted in various levels of gray. In the case of computed tomography, approximately 4000 levels of gray can be measured. Because the color-sensitivity of the human eye does not correlate with the scale of levels of gray, it has not yet been possible to develop a desirable and comprehensive color-coding system.

Tissue density is measured in Hounsfield units (HU), with a scale ranging from –1000 to +3000 HU; in this system, water has the value of 0 and air has a value of –1000 HU. Bone density, which is of particular interest to dental implantologists, is presented according to the classification of Misch (1990) with 500–1300 HU for compact bone and 100–240 HU for trabecular/cancellous bone, while soft tissue such as musculature is ca. 40 HU, with an image voltage of 120–150 kV.

The image quality of the secondary tomograms is dependent on care and precision during production of the primary tomogram; this is determined to a great extent by proper positioning of the patient and the adjustment of the measurement field in the topogram. Establishing and maintaining the position of the mandible is, especially in elderly and edentulous patients, whenever possible best secured using a pre-fabricated, radiation-transparent bite plate, in order to prevent spontaneous movements of the mandible during the exposure, for example due to muscles spasms. However, this is becoming less and less necessary with the use of spiral tomography, volume data acquisition, and higher examination speed. Metal restorations and metal reconstructions (e.g., bridge work) of all types elicit disturbing artifacts (see Fig. **142**), but this can be avoided by positioning the field of measurement inferior to the tooth crowns in the affected jaw.

Indications for CT in dentistry: The CT makes possible multiplanar radiographic examinations, and can depict every body volume three-dimensionally by means of directly taken or indirectly reconstructed (so-called secondary) tomograms. Axial tomograms of the facial skeleton can portray the third dimension to supplement conventional two-dimensional intraoral radiographs or the panoramic view; using the data set, indirect (secondary) reconstructions can be made in virtually any desired plane.

Fig. 148a Modified coronal CT, temporomandibular joint: Mouth closed, teeth in habitual intercuspation (occlusion).

Fig. 148b Axial CT, temporomandibular joint. Mouth closed, habitual intercuspation. Slice at the height of the condyles. Note the bifid condyle, right.

Fig. 149a Multiplanar reconstruction of sections of the maxilla. Topogram with markings for the maxilla. (Dental Package, Picker.)

Fig. 149b Multiplanar reconstruction of a transverse section through the maxilla. Marking of three slices for selection of a "panoramic view" of the maxilla, and position of the jaw cross-section with continuous numbering.

Fig. 150 Multiplanar reconstruction of a cross-section of the maxilla. Panoramic view from the middle marking, with scale indicated. The secondary tomographs of the maxillary transverse slices depict horizontally the position of the panoramic view and vertically that of the axial layers so that a precise localization in a 1:1 relationship is possible. Note the chronic apical periodontitis with an infected radicular cyst on tooth 11, and the depiction of the incisive canal (layers 22–25).

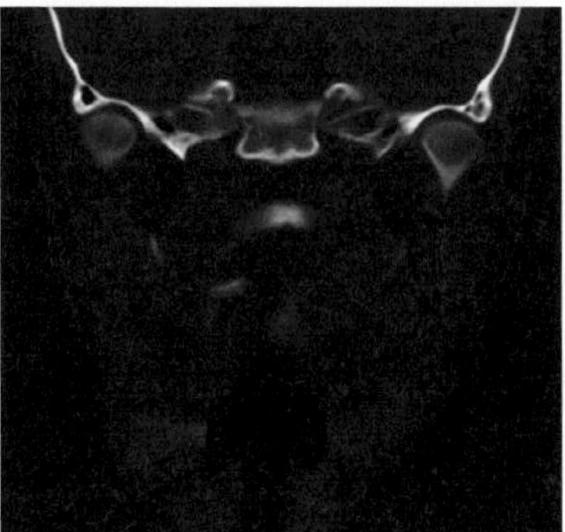

148 a

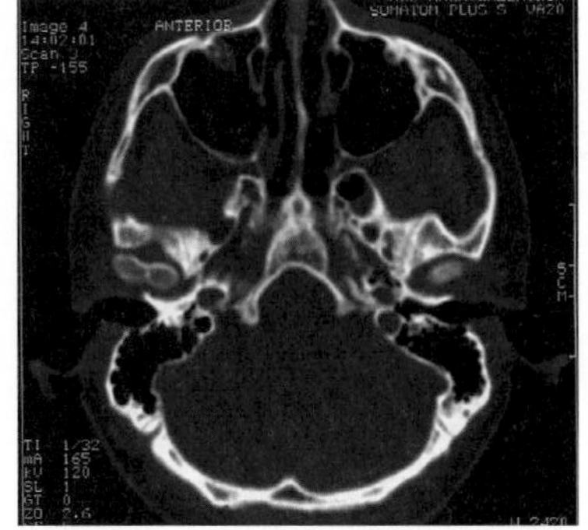

148 b

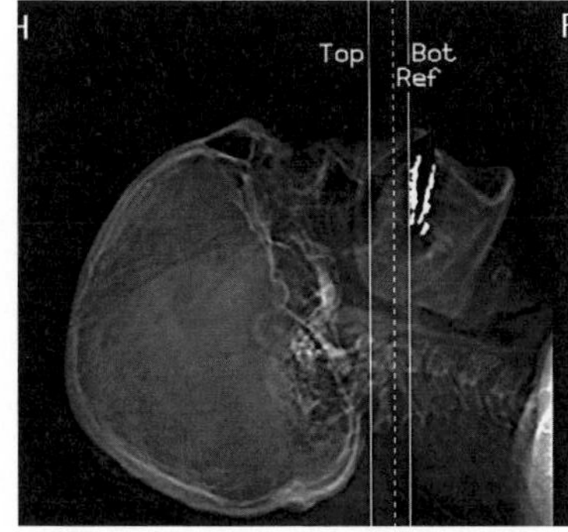

149 a

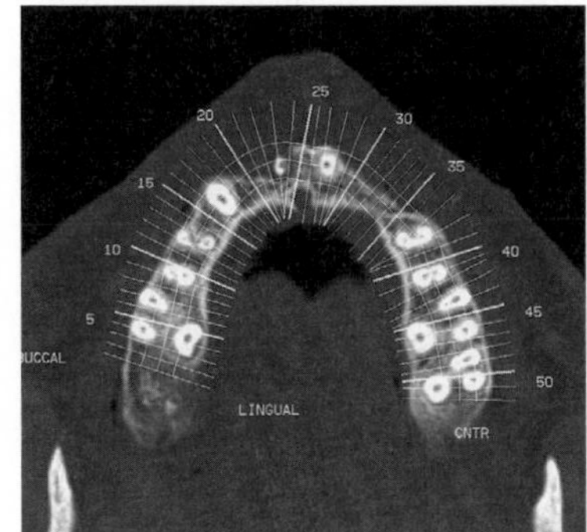

149 b

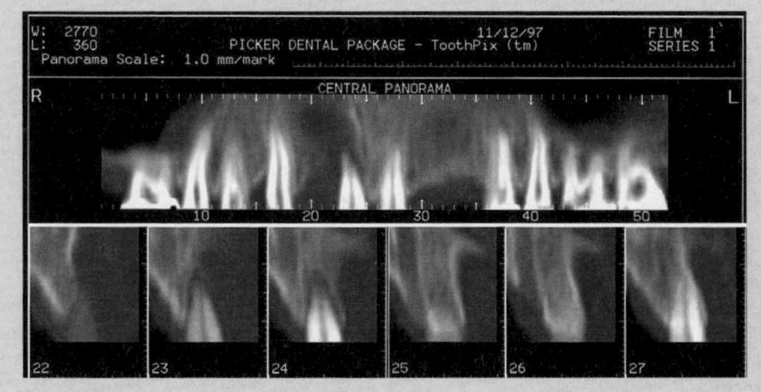

150

For oral surgeons and dental implantologists, important structures such as the mandibular canal, incisive canal, or the maxillary sinuses in their spatial relationships to the surrounding structures can be examined in images that also depict the third dimension. A periodontal surgeon can, in special cases, be oriented with regard to the expanse and shape of bony pockets. The newest possibility for image creation also significantly expands the observation and examination of primary and secondary TMJ disorders. Precise localization and the expanse of osseous or soft tissue lesions can be significantly clearly depicted, free of any masking overlaps. These new possibilities, which can be of significant value to the dentist in his/her daily practice, demand knowledge of radiographic anatomy in order to improve communication between the dentist and the general radiologist. This can be especially useful and important for limiting radiation exposure.

Radiographic operation planning in dental implant surgery: Optimum planning of any procedure increases the chances for success of the operation because it can reduce surgical risks and shorten the length of the clinical procedure. The techniques developed using CT technology for the three-dimensional and metrically accurate depiction of cross-sections of the jaws are far superior to conventional methods of examination, despite the necessity to collaborate with a general radiologist in most cases. The raw data accumulated from the axial primary tomograph are transformed with a workstation and read into the dental practice computer via a special program. A spiral CT provides optimum data sets. The panoramic views and jaw cross-sections reconstructed from the axial slices make it possible to measure distances and diameters and to determine angles as well as the thickness of osseous structure expressed in Hounsfield units. By placing implant outlines directly upon the computer screen, the planned surgical procedure can be simulated and checked using various programs and 1:1 size relationships.

Volume Tomography: 3-D Surface Reconstructions

A noteworthy and in some ways remarkable capability is digital three-dimensional volume tomography (3D-Accuitomo, Morita). Out of a circumscribed, cylindrical volume, the accumulated measurement values can be used for reconstructions of extraordinary quality in any desired plane, and the structural details are rendered visible on the computer screen.

A factor of ever-increasing significance to implantologists will be the continuing refinement of navigation techniques which simplify implantation methods.

Fig. 151 a Volume tomography (3D Accuitomo [Morita]). Above: Axial section through the left side of the mandible at the mid-root level. **Left:** Vertical section through the premolar-molar region at the level of the tooth long axis. The mental foramen is clearly visible. **Right:** Cross-section of the mandible through the mental foramen.

Fig. 151 b Volume tomography (3D Accuitomo). Above: Axial section through the left side of the maxilla at the mid-root level. Left: Vertical section through the premolar-molar region along the level of the tooth long axis. The clarity of the image will vary according to the course of the dental arch. Right: Cross-sectional image of the maxilla through the interdental osseous septum between the buccal roots of tooth 26.

Fig. 152 a–c Volume tomography (3D Accuitomo). Three images of cross-sections through the mandible, cusps, enamel cap, and crown of tooth 48; note also the mandibular canal.

Fig. 153 a 3D surface reconstruction. Three-dimensional surface reconstruction of the base of the skull at the level of the condyles. Note the dysplastic right condyle.

Fig. 153 b 3D surface reconstruction. Lateral three-dimensional surface reconstruction of the skull at the level of the affected TMJ on the right side.

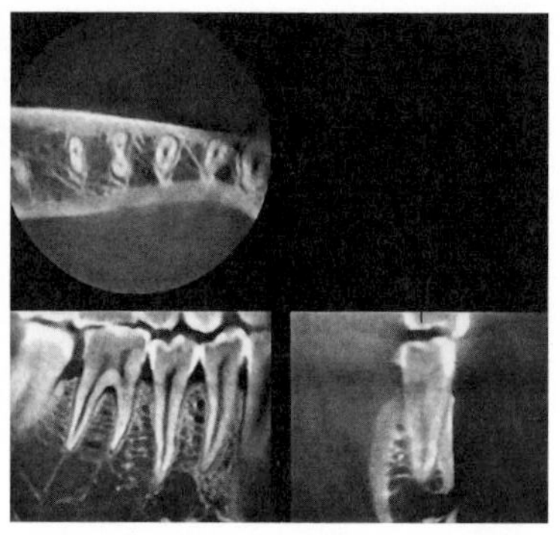

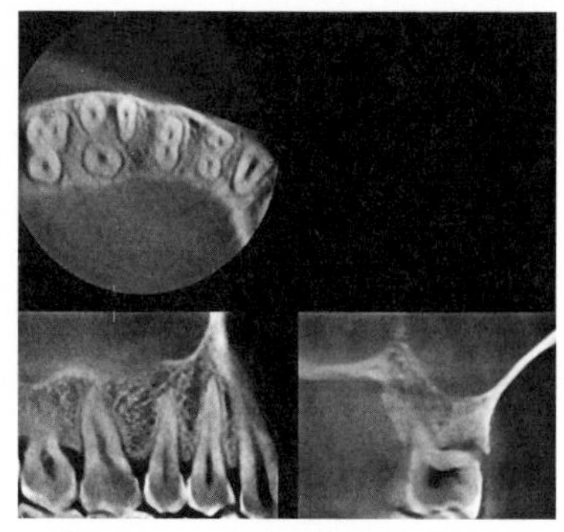

151 a

151 b

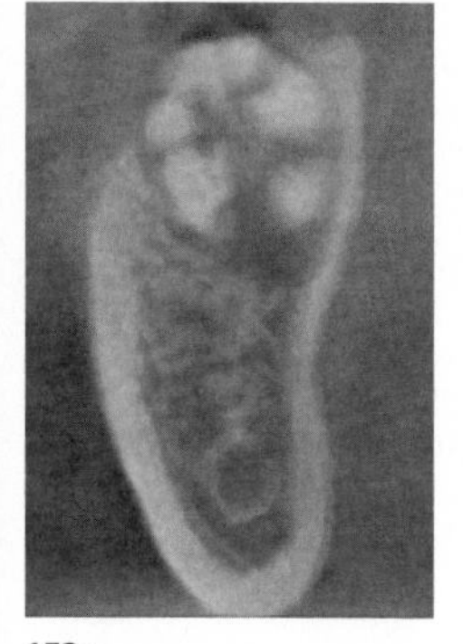

152 a

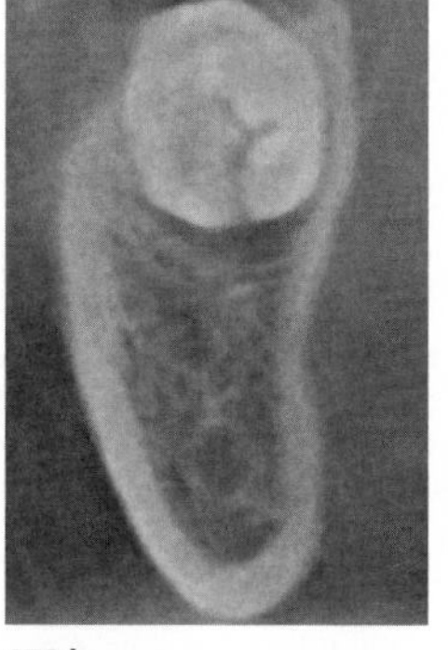

152 b

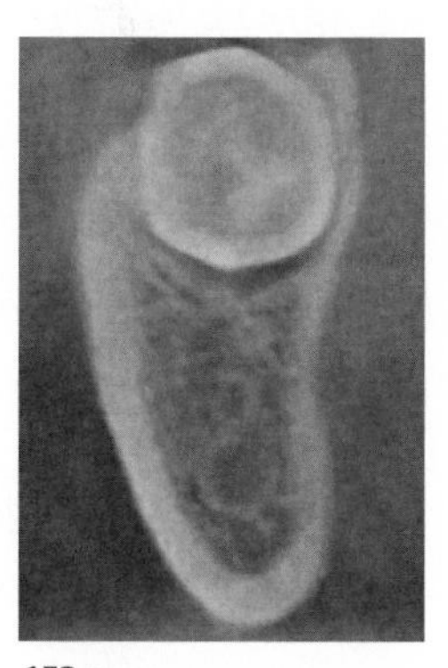

152 c

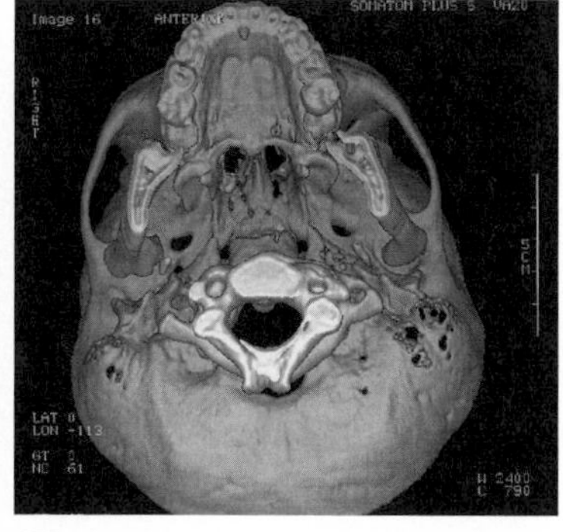

153 a

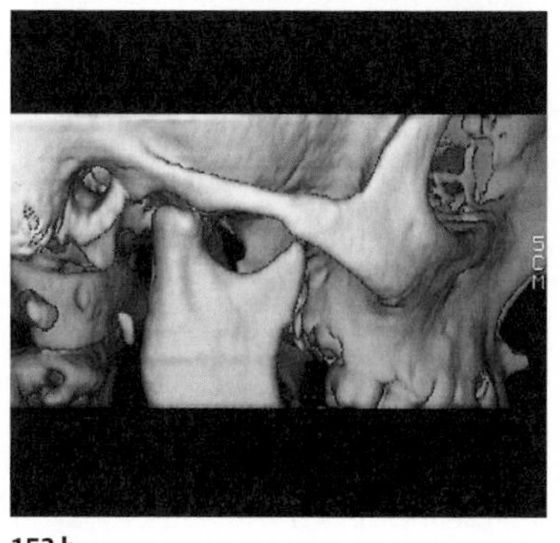

153 b

Magnetic resonance imaging, also known as magnetic resonance tomography (MRI and/or MRT, Bloch and Purcell 1946), is a procedure for creating images of internal body structures, but without the use of ionizing radiation. An MR image is made possible primarily because of the abundance of hydrogen in so many organic compounds. Because its nucleus has an uneven number of protons it exhibits a magnetic moment and an angular momentum. Within a stable external magnetic field, the nuclei behave like compass needles and are set into a spinning motion. By introduction of a high-frequency electromagnetic field perpendicular to the lines of force of the stationary magnet, the nuclei are tipped on their axes (nuclear magnetic resonance) and absorb energy. When the high-frequency electromagnetic field is shut off, the nuclei return to their original positions (relaxation) with release of a signal of the identical frequency. The tissue-specific and constant relaxation time is primarily responsible for the extraordinary soft-tissue contrast provided by the MRI procedure. The duration of the voltage of the induction field thus produced is measured from incoming and exiting pulses. From the collected data sets, images can be calculated and projected in every imaginable orientation; this also reduces the length of time the patient must actually be within the device. One domain that is particularly impacted by MRI is the depiction of joints; for this reason the TMJ was chosen to introduce and depict the anatomic structural signals of MRI.

Structure signals of the temporomandibular joint: MRI is the method of choice for determining the position of the articular disk and for examination of the intra-articular soft tissue structures whenever conservative therapy has been unsuccessful and it is necessary to define and clarify the indications for invasive therapy (surgery). In contrast to a conventional radiograph, the depiction of anatomic structures is characterized by a contrast reversal: Because of its scarcity of protons, bone is signal-poor and so is recorded as a dark structure, whereas soft tissues, because of their abundance of protons, are signal-intense, and therefore appear light. The articular disk, which under normal circumstances can be easily identified by its signal-poor structure, is however in degeneratively altered joints often very difficult to discern. Medial articular disk displacement/dislocation, while rare, can lead to incorrect interpretations with regard to the position of the bilaminar zone, and disk perforations are often less evident in the MRI compared to a more conventional arthrotomograph.

Fig. 154 Functional principle of MRI.

Fig. 155a **TMJ**, lateral view, mouth closed, showing the signal-producing anatomic structures.

Fig. 155b **TMJ**, frontal view, mouth closed, with signal-producing anatomic structures.

Fig. 156a **TMJ**, mouth closed, habitual intercuspation.

Fig. 156b **TMJ**, maximum mouth opening.

Legend for Figs. 155a, b:

1 Condyle
2 Lateral pterygoid muscle
3 Articular eminence (articular tubercle)
4 Glenoid fossa
5 Position of the articular disk in habitual intercuspation; the head of the condyle is partially overlapped
6 Bilaminar zone of the disk
7 External auditory meatus
8 Condyle, lateral pole
9 Condyle, medial pole

Magnetic field

Protons in the homogeneous magnetic field

Inciting nuclear spin

Magnetic field

Principle of the apparatus

154

155 a

155 b

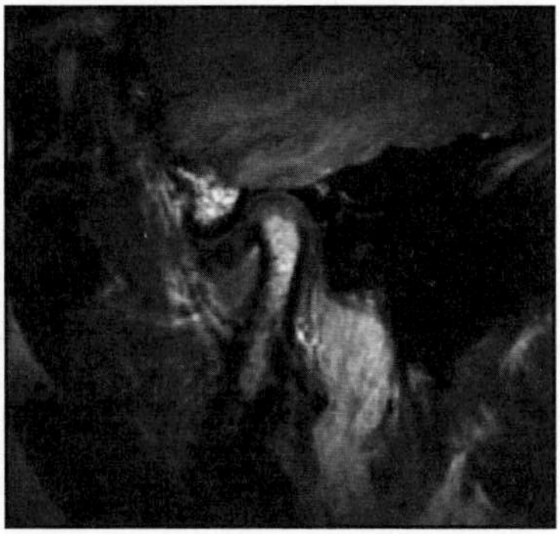

156 a

156 b

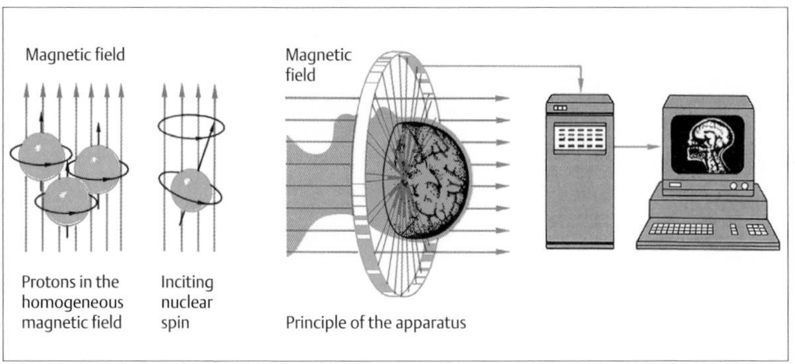

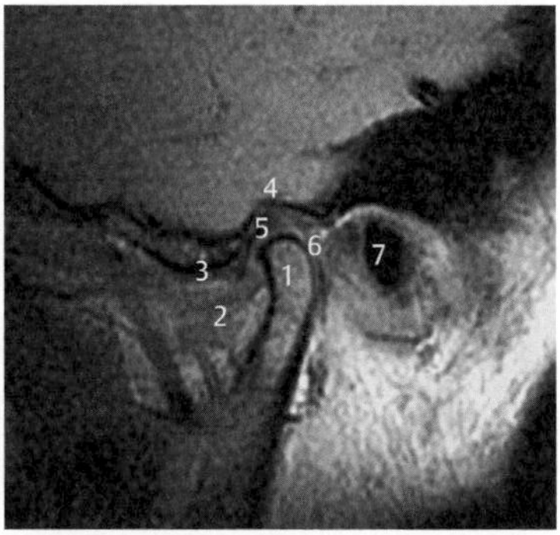

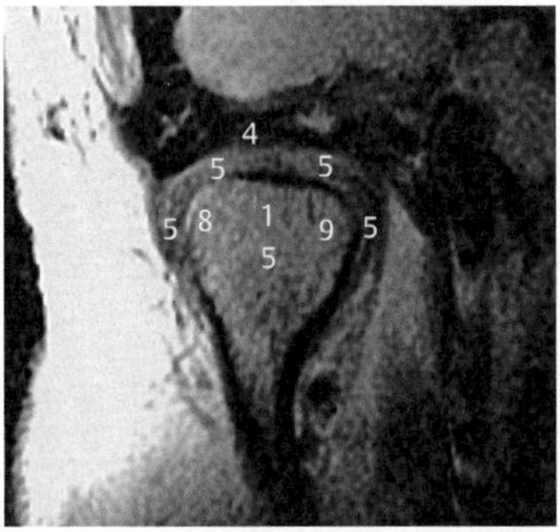

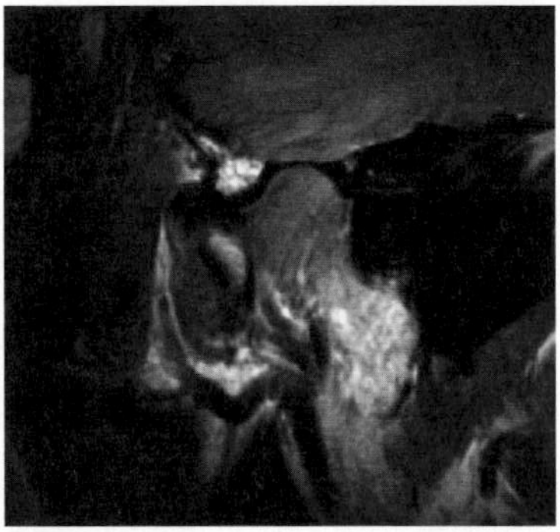

Localization Technique Using Equipment Common in the Dental Practice, and Conventional Radiographic Techniques

In the great majority of cases, it is impacted teeth, root fragments, and foreign bodies whose positional relationships to the adjacent teeth and anatomic structures must be examined and checked during the course of comprehensive dental treatment planning. In addition, it is also frequently necessary to depict individual root canals of multi-rooted teeth in order to successfully perform endodontic treatment. Thorough knowledge of radiographic localization techniques can also be very helpful in orthodontics and dental implantology.

Depending upon the treatment-related question and the equipment available, procedures for radiographic localization may be performed in the dental practice, or must be referred to a larger clinic or even a radiology center. In this chapter, the possibilities and limitations of dental radiographic examination methods are presented, which through the use of individual examples provide suggestions for their use in routine dental practice.

Generally speaking, the following methods for object localization are used in general dental practice:

- Comparisons of the clarity and size of the desired object to an appropriate reference object in conventional intraoral or panoramic radiographs.
- Excentric central ray projection in horizontal and vertical planes to observe any "wandering" of the desired object vis-à-vis the reference object, as viewed in intraoral radiographs (Clark).
- Altering the central ray targeting by 90° to the conventionally prepared initial radiograph in order to depict the desired object in the third dimension.
- Enhancing the panoramic radiograph in the third dimension using supplemental programs for the panoramic radiography units in the dental practice to depict transverse sections through the jaws with conventional linear or spiral tomography.

If it is necessary to refer the patient to a comprehensive clinic or a radiology center, the following methods for localization may be employed:

- Enhancement of the panoramic radiograph in the third dimension using conventional skull films.

Fig. 157 Possibilities and limitations of object localization using the panoramic radiograph. In the maxillary anterior region, a comparison of the desired object with the adjacent teeth permits conclusions about its localization. A size comparison between the completely impacted tooth 23 and tooth 13 as a reference object results here in an apparent enlargement of tooth 23, and this indicates that 23 is near to the plane of focus and therefore palatally positioned (example three in the schematic illustration).

Fig. 158 Schematic illustration of the possibilities for determination of object localization in a panoramic radiograph. Depending upon the actual location of the desired object in or on the plane of focus (**S**) or the distance from the image receptor (**BE**), entire teeth or portions of teeth will be depicted in both size and clarity (sharpness) with the central ray direction (**Z**) held constant. If the tooth is totally within the plane of focus (**O**) it will be depicted with clarity and correct size. If the tooth is in front of the plane of focus (**1**), it will be depicted smaller and less sharply. If the tooth is localized partially behind the plane of focus (**2** and **3**), the entire tooth or portions of the tooth will be depicted as larger than normal and blurred. On the other hand, if the panoramic radiograph reveals only an axial projection of the impacted tooth (**4** and **5**), extreme care in interpretation of the radiograph is indicated, and clarification using supplementary techniques must be performed.

Fig. 159 Possibilities and limitations of object localization using a panoramic radiograph. Impacted tooth 13 is positioned both obliquely and horizontally within the maxilla, and is depicted as enlarged and blurred in the image. On the other hand, its *root tip* is only slightly enlarged and is clearly depicted. These findings clearly indicate that tooth 13 has its crown located far palatal to teeth 11 and 12, and that its root tip is only slightly behind the plane of focus, in the region of the canine fossa (example two in the schematic illustration, Fig. **158**). Note also the root fragment of deciduous tooth 53.

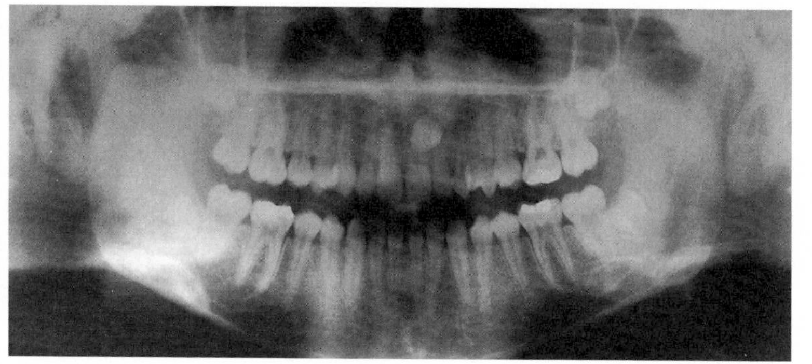

157

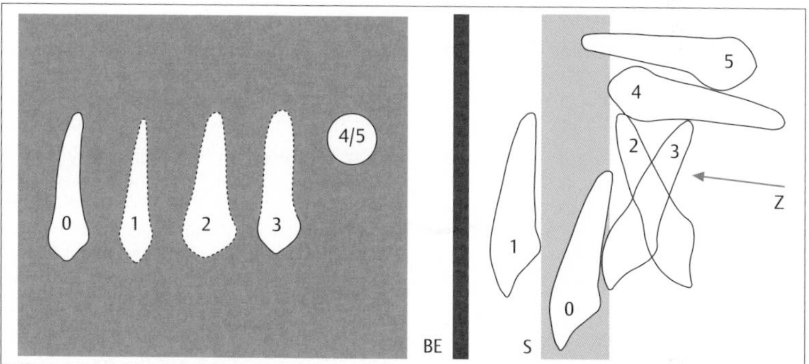

158

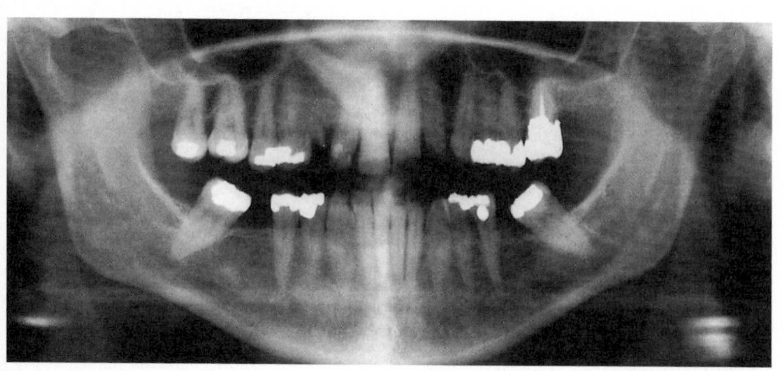

159

- Enhancement of the panoramic radiograph in the third dimension via axial or coronal computed tomography (CT) of the facial skeleton.
- Supplementing a panoramic radiograph with dental programs for CT, axial primary tomograms, and computed panoramic views and cross-sections of the jaws.

Already available on the commercial market is the first generation of dentally applicable high data volume computer tomographic equipment, providing images in a small format; during the course of the next few decades dental radiographic technique in terms of depicting the third dimension of structures will be dramatically and fundamentally changed.

Localization by means of image clarity and size comparisons: The varying distance of the desired object and the reference object from the plane of focus and from the image receptor (IR) permits the determination of location of the desired object vis-à-vis the (clinically visible) reference object.

The nearer an object is to the plane of focus, the further it is from the image receptor and will, as a consequence of the divergence of the roentgen rays, be enlarged and blurred as an image. The nearer an object is to the image receptor, the sharper and of more correct size will be the resultant image. Therefore any object which, in comparison to the reference object, is closer to the plane of focus (or further removed from the image receptor), will appear enlarged and blurred, while any object that is focus-far in comparison to the reference object will be depicted in proper size and sharper focus.

Fig. 160a Object localization using variation of horizontal direction of the central ray (Clark). The goal is to pinpoint the position of a completely impacted tooth 13. Initial periapical radiograph of the maxillary anterior region. In order to provide a better clinical view of the positioning, this film was taken without the use of an IRH.

Fig. 160b Object localization using variation of horizontal direction of the central ray (Clark). Using a distal-excentric modification of the central ray direction, the depiction of the positional relationship between the impacted tooth and the existing dental arch changes. In a departure from conventional rules, the second IR must not necessarily be positioned at exactly the same place as the initial radiograph. The single most important thing is that the relationship of the crown of the desired object (impacted third molar) to the roots of the teeth in the existing dental arch be depicted **completely**.

Fig. 161a,b Schematic depiction of the principles of horizontal central ray displacement. Dental arch (**1**), near-focus object (**2**), and far-focus object (**3**) overlap (**161 a/a**) in this projection and appear in the radiograph (**161 a/b**) in superimposition. By targeting the central ray at 20° distal (**161 b/a**), the desired objects can be depicted as separate structures: The focus-far object appears to move in the direction of the central ray deviation, while the focus-near object appears to move in the opposite direction (**161 b/b**). The image receptor should be positioned such that the crown of the impacted tooth and the roots of the adjacent teeth in the dental arch are completely depicted, in order to compare the “wandering” of the objects; contrary to the generally valid rules, the IR must not necessarily be positioned at precisely the same intraoral position (I and II).

Fig. 162a Periapical radiograph for localization via changing the horizontal targeting of the central ray. The orthoradial projection reveals the crown of impacted tooth 13 and the root of tooth 11 superimposed.

Fig. 162b Radiograph for localization by means of horizontal deviation of central ray targeting. The distal-excentric central ray projection now depicts the crown of the palatally positioned tooth 13 in superimposition with the root of tooth 12. Tooth 13 has “followed” the change in direction of the central ray.

Fig. 162c Schematic diagram of a vestibularly located tooth 13 using distal-excentric central targeting. The impacted tooth has “moved” contrary to the movement of the central ray, far from the projection surface, and therefore resides with its enlarged crown in superimposition over tooth 21.

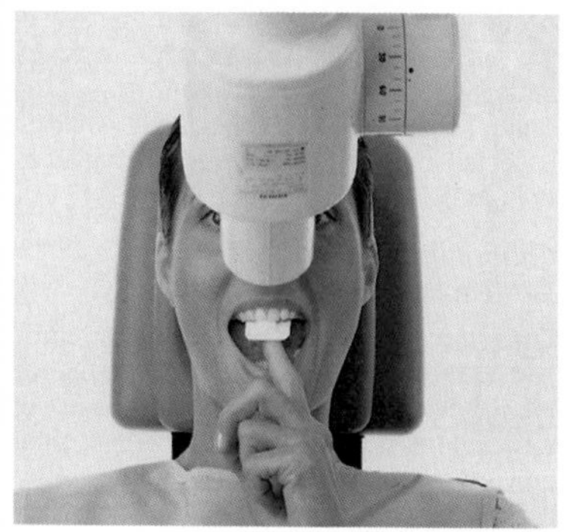
160 a

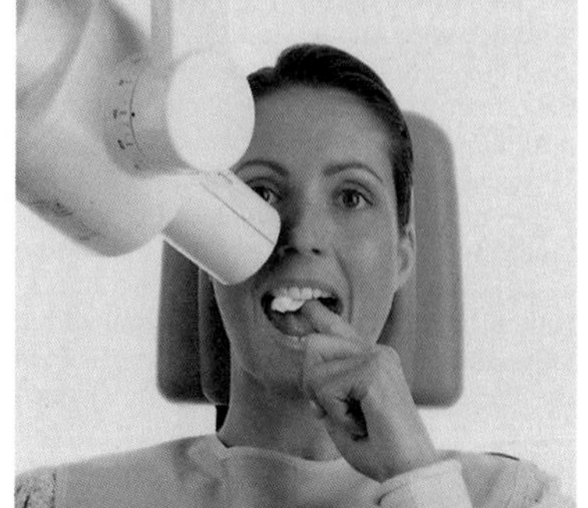
160 b

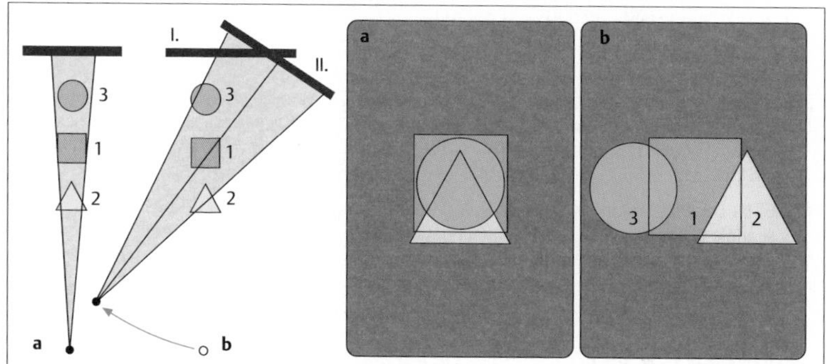

161 a

161 b

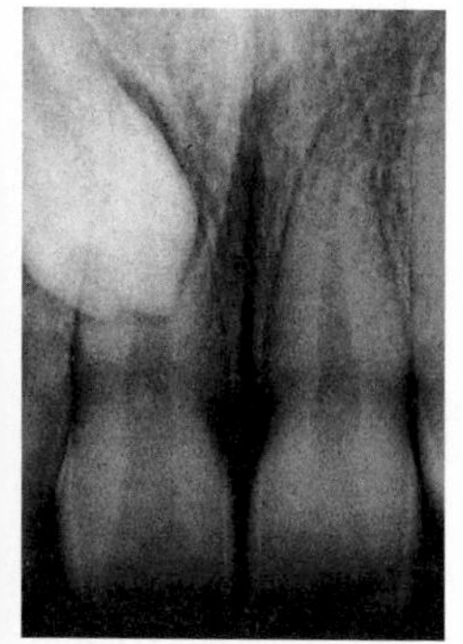
162 a

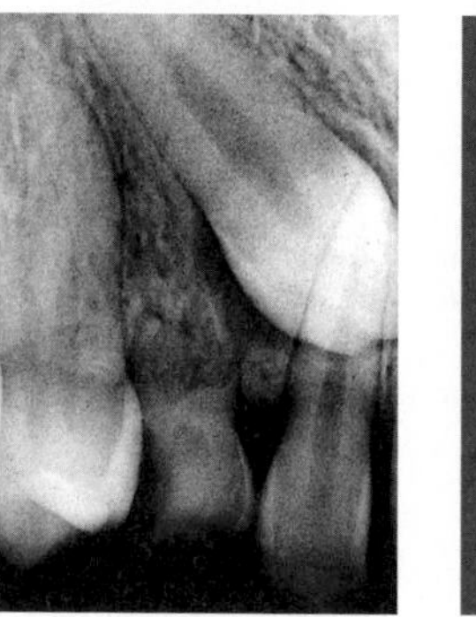
162 b

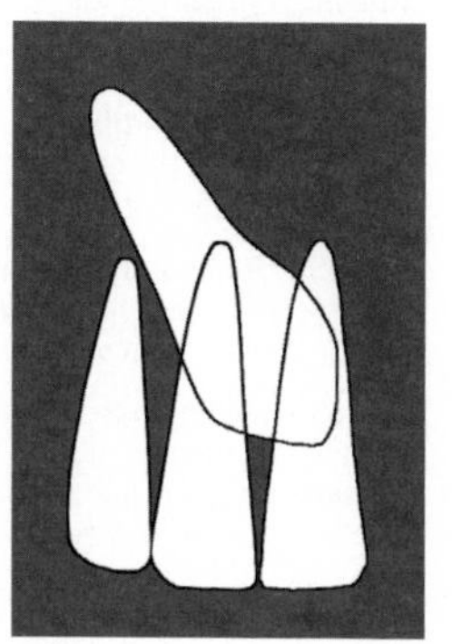
162 c

The application of this rule for positional determination can, however, only be usefully applied if the distance from the desired object to the reference object is large enough to permit resolution of differences in size and clarity.
This general rule can be applied primarily in the examination of intraoral and panoramic radiographs. Especially the panoramic radiograph offers the possibility to observe and examine the impacted tooth *in toto* and within its osseous environment. A tooth impacted in the maxilla, for example, may appear widened (palatal location) or decreased in size (vestibular location) and blurred. The crown and the root of the impacted tooth can, however, be depicted differently and thus provide information concerning an *oblique* localization within the maxilla. Any exceptions to this general rule will usually be observed only in the anterior region of the mandible. This is dependent upon the relationship of the base of the mandible to the alveolar ridge, so that a radiographically "widened" tooth (usually a canine) according to the general rule would be expected to be lingually positioned, but is actually positioned vestibularly (see p. **111**).

Changing the Direction of the Central Ray

Changing central ray targeting in the horizontal and vertical planes: This technique for localization is employed only with the use of intraoral image receptors. This method is not only valuable for determining the precise location of impacted teeth, but also for clear radiographic depiction of individual roots and root canals of multi-rooted teeth. This technique will complete the total spatial depiction provided by a two-dimensional, orthoradial projection.

Fig. 163a Localization by changing the vertical angle of the central ray (Clark). The object is to determine the position of the completely impacted tooth 13. Initial periapical radiograph of the anterior region. For reasons of photographic clarity, these clinical photographs were taken without the use of an IRH.

Fig. 163b Localization by changing the vertical angle of the central ray (Clark). By changing the vertical angle of the central ray, the spatial relationship between the desired (impacted) tooth and the existing dental arch will be different in the final radiograph. It is not absolutely necessary that the film be placed vertically in exactly the same angle as the original radiograph. Most important is that the relationship of the crown of the desired (impacted) tooth to the roots of the existing dental arch be **completely** depicted.

Fig. 164a,b Schematic diagram of the principles of vertical modification of central ray targeting. Dental arch (**1**), focus-near object (**2**), and focus-far object (**3**) are superimposed upon each other (**164 a/a**) in this projection, and in the final radiograph they will be depicted in superimposition (**164 b/a**). By changing the vertical angle of the central ray by 20° (**164 a/b**), the desired objects can be viewed as separate entities: The focus-far object appears to have moved in the direction of the change in the central ray, while the focus-near object "wanders" in the opposite direction and appears enlarged (**164 b/b**). The image receptor should be positioned so that the crown of the impacted tooth and the roots of the teeth in the dental arch are completely depicted, in order to compare the wandering of the objects.

Fig. 165a Radiographs for localization of an impacted canine using modified vertical central ray projection. The orthoradial projection shows a superimposition of the crown of impacted tooth 13 upon the root apex of tooth 11.

Fig. 165b Radiograph for localization by modifying the vertical angle of the central ray. By changing the vertical angle of the central ray, the crown of impacted tooth 13 has been effectively separated from the apex of tooth 11. Tooth 13 has traveled **with** the change of central ray, and is therefore palatally localized.

Fig. 165c Schematic representation of the vestibular position of tooth 13. The impacted tooth has apparently moved contrary to the movement of the central ray targeting, and appears enlarged and in obvious superimposition with tooth 11, i.e., in a vestibular position.

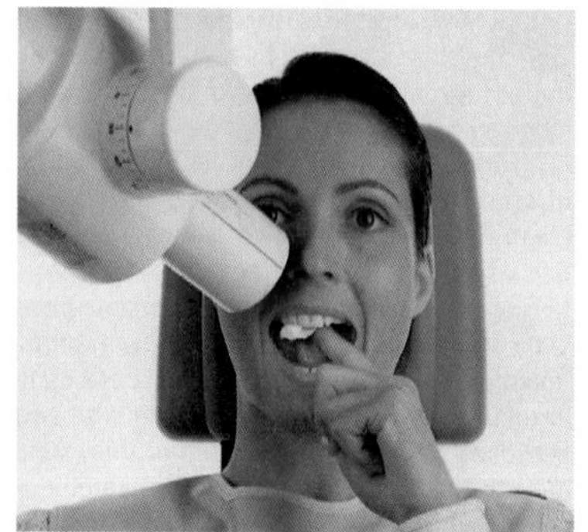

163 a

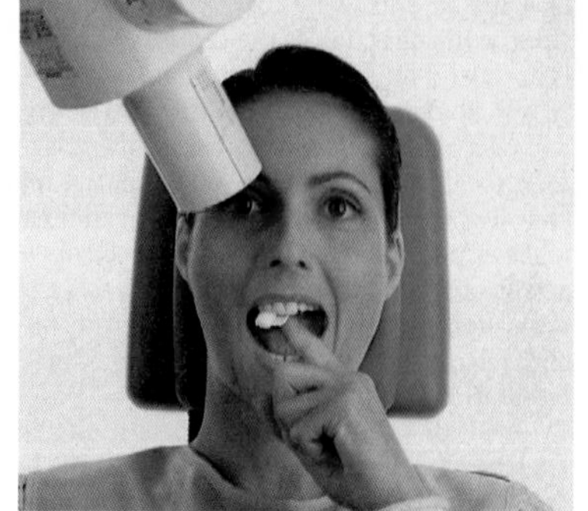

163 b

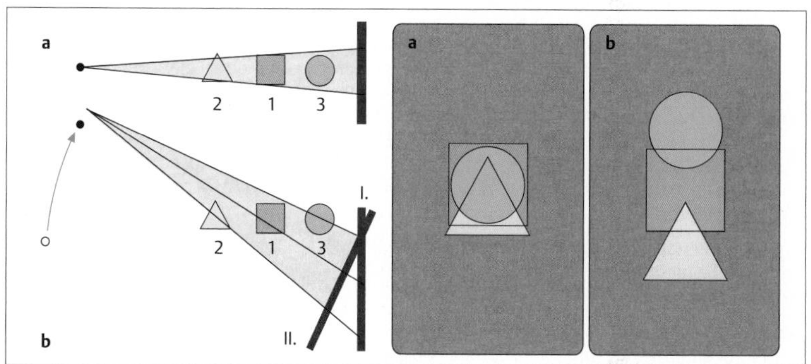

164 a

164 b

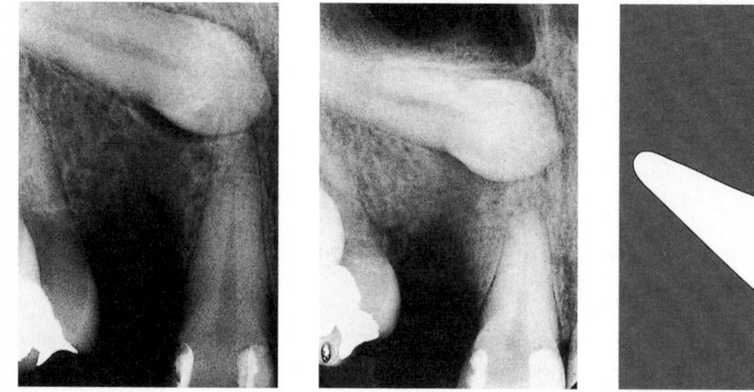

165 a

165 b

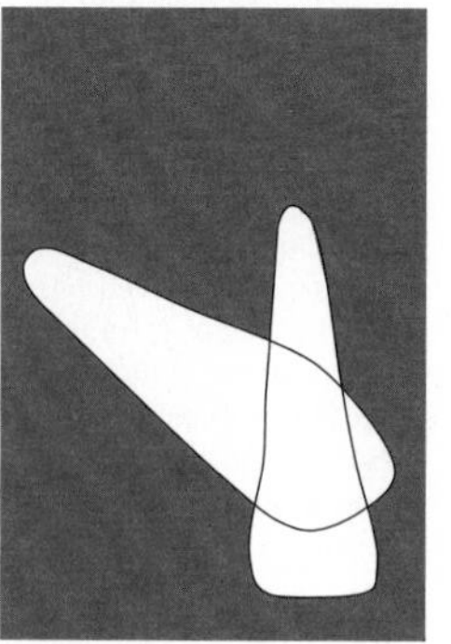

165 c

In order to effectively use the technique of shifting the direction of the central ray for localization of objects, an appropriate image receptor holder (IRH) is absolutely necessary, one which insures that the plane of the image receptor is at a right angle to the central ray (see Fig. **61b**). This right-angle technique makes it easy even for an inexperienced operator to properly target the desired objects and to ensure proper shifting of the central ray, and guarantee a fixed receptor-ray spatial orientation.

The principle of object location determination is simple: Objects that are located palatally or lingually to the dental arch and near the image receptor appear to "follow" any horizontal or vertical shifting of the radiographic central ray. Objects located vestibular to the dental arch and therefore further removed from the image receptor appear to "wander" on the radiograph contrary to the shifting of the central ray, and appear enlarged because of the larger distance to the plane of the image receptor.

Clear and separate projection of the root canals of multi-rooted teeth or single roots harboring two root canals follows the same principle. Worthy of note is that in addition to the maxillary first premolars, other teeth may also be two-rooted or possess roots with two root canals. Frequently included in this group are the mandibular canines, the mandibular premolars, and the mesial root of the mandibular first molar.

Fig. 166a Localization of individual roots and root canals. Schematic depiction of the technique for radiographic reproduction of individual roots on maxillary molar 26 (above). Orthoradial initial radiograph (**1**), depiction of the distobuccal root (**2**), and the mesiobuccal root (**3**). **m.e.** = Mesial-excentric projection; **d.e.** = distal-excentric projection. Below: Depiction for localization in two-rooted or roots with two canals, for example the maxillary premolars, the mandibular canine, and the mandibular premolars, situations that are not infrequently encountered during endodontic treatment. Depending upon the position of the tooth in the dental arch, either mesio- or distobuccal projections can be employed.

Fig. 166b Periapical radiograph depicting a single root. Artificial construct example for the depiction of the mesiobuccal root of tooth 26 using distal-excentric projection (see Fig. **166a**, above, 3 distal-excentric setup).

Fig. 166c Localization simulator for teaching and continuing education (Pasler). The simulator consists of an image receptor, an adjustable object holder, interchangeable acrylic models, and a special lamp with diaphragm; the simulator provides practical illustrations of dental object localization techniques for oral surgery and endodontics.

Fig. 167 Localization of lingually or vestibularly impacted mandibular third molars. The diagram represents an occlusal view of the left mandibular posterior segment. The possible positions of a completely impacted mandibular third molar are shown as **blue** (lingual) and **red** (vestibular). To precisely localize the position of the third molar, the initial orthoradial projection (**1**) is supplemented by a distal-excentric projection (**2**). Right: The results are depicted on the schematic radiograph. The initial image (**1**) is compared with the results of the distal-excentric projection (**2**). If the third molar is located lingually (**blue**), it will appear in the second IR to have moved away from adjacent tooth 37; it appears to have moved with the direction of shift of the central ray. If the tooth is located vestibularly (**red**), it will appear somewhat enlarged because of the greater distance to the image receptor and will appear superimposed over tooth 37 clearly; in other words, the tooth appears to have "wandered" in the opposite direction of the shift of the central ray projection. A mesial-excentric second radiograph (in which the film would be extremely difficult to properly position) would show the opposite result.

Fig. 168a, b Periapical radiographs for localization of a mandibular third molar. a. Orthoradial initial radiograph of tooth 38, showing a follicular cyst. **b.** The distal-excentric localization shows that tooth 38 appears to have moved contrary to the shift of the central ray, and must therefore be positioned vestibularly.

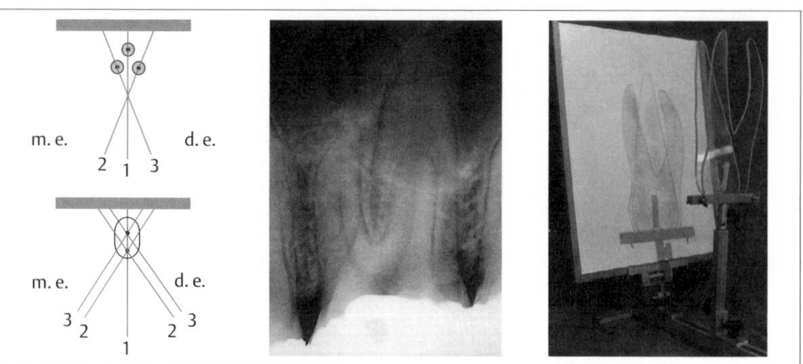

166 a

166 b

166 c

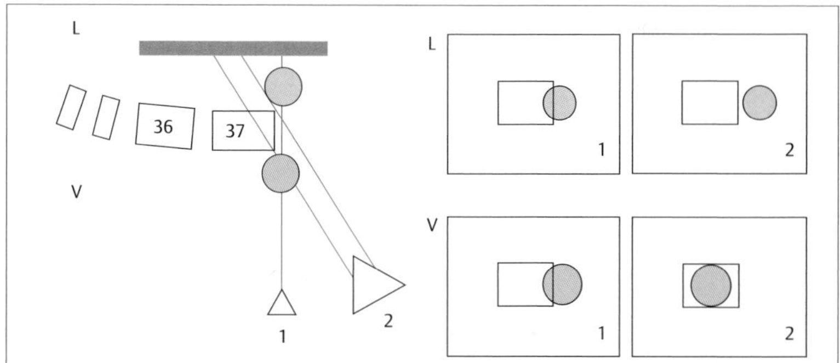

167

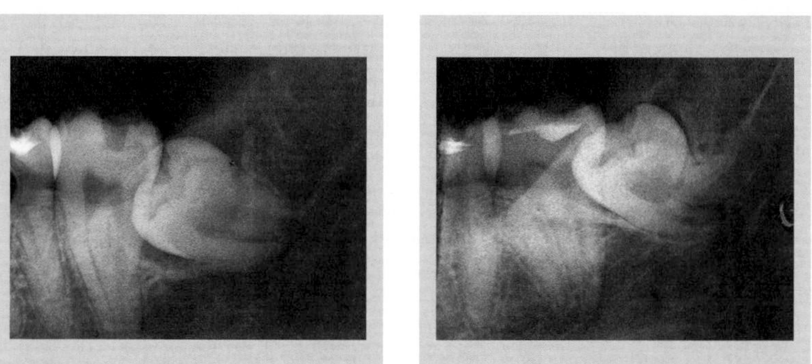

168 a

168 b

Depending upon the position of the impacted tooth in the dental arch, the anatomic peculiarities of roots and root canals can be captured and depicted using mesial- or distal-excentric projections of the central ray in the horizontal plane. Clear depiction and radiographic isolation of the buccal roots of maxillary molars using the technique of horizontally shifting the central ray projection follows the same rules. In comparison to the palatal root, the mesiobuccal root is nearer to the plane of focus and when radiographed from the distal-excentric direction, the tooth will appear to wander opposite to the direction of shift of the central ray. This permits it to be visualized and examined without any overlapping of the palatal root. If a mesial-excentric projection is employed, the distobuccal root will appear to wander further distally, and can also be successfully removed from any overlapping by the palatal root.

These techniques for "free projection" of craniofacial structures as practiced using the intraoral radiographic techniques that are common in dental practice and of significance can be vividly and graphically learned and practiced using a teaching device (see Fig. **166c**) for demonstrating the effects of correct and incorrect shifting of the central ray.

Changing the central ray projection by 90° to depict the third dimension: In those situations in which the anatomy permits targeting of the central ray absolutely parallel to the tooth long axis, it is possible using an orthoradial projection to depict the third dimension and therefore precisely localize the desired object. The image receptor (film or sensor) can be positioned at a right angle to the tooth long axis with the mouth closed. The anatomic situation in the maxilla is usually such that perfect arrangement of the IR vis-à-vis the central ray is often not possible, and therefore the radiographic techniques described above cannot always with 100% certainty provide a precise determination of the object's position. Therefore, especially in the maxilla it is frequently necessary to take supplemental radiographs such as lateral and frontal projections, cephalometric projections etc., to completely clarify spatial relationships of the desired object.

Fig. 169a Object localization by shifting the central ray direction by 90°. Periapical radiograph of the left mandibular posterior segment in a 9-year-old female. The completely impacted tooth 35 is depicted in this orthoradial projection.

Fig. 169b Localization by changing the target direction of the central ray by 90°. This second radiograph, taken with a 90° change in central ray projection, shows the position of tooth 35 (**arrow**) in an occlusal radiograph taken parallel to the long axis of the adjacent teeth (see Fig. **90a**). For patients traversing the mixed dentition stage, these types of images can also be obtained using large digital sensors. Of critical importance is that the central ray traverses the adjacent teeth axially.

Fig. 170 Object localization by changing the direction of the central ray. Clinical examination of this 46-year-old patient reveals that tooth 11 was missing. The panoramic radiograph reveals a radiopacity resembling a tooth at the level of the anterior nasal spine.

Fig. 171a Localization by changing the direction of the central ray. An occlusal radiograph of the maxilla, which can only be taken with an oblique projection because of anatomic constraints (see Fig. **85a**) clearly reveals the totally impacted tooth 11, depicted axially in this projection.

Fig. 171b Localization by changing the direction of the central ray. This lateral radiograph taken with extraoral and paramedian positioning of the image receptor reveals the ectopic position of the crown of tooth 11 within the anterior nasal spine, which has been displaced by a follicular cyst.

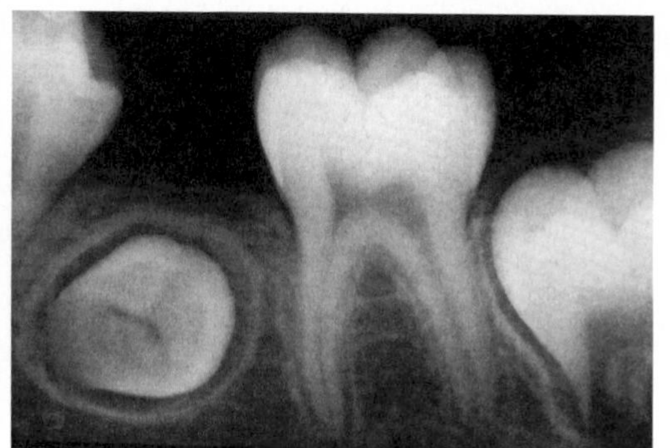

169 a

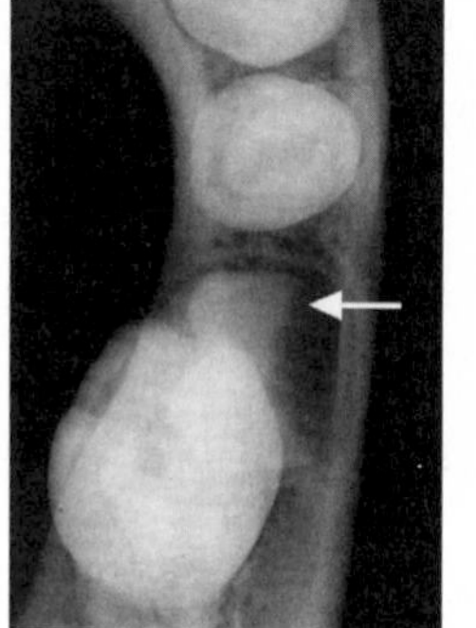

169 b

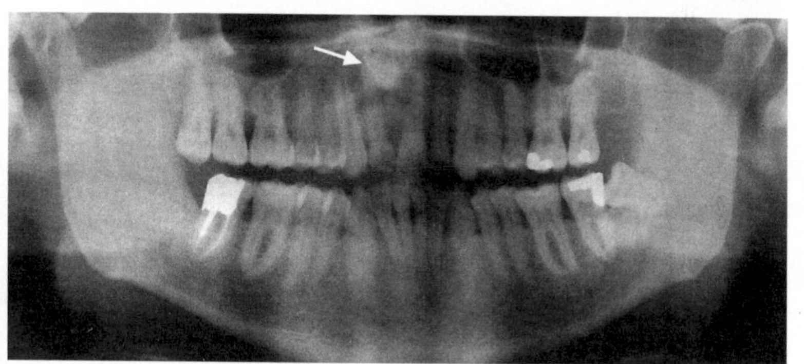

170

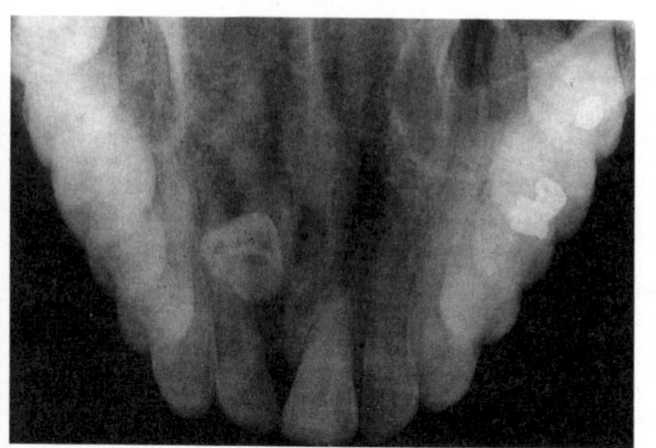

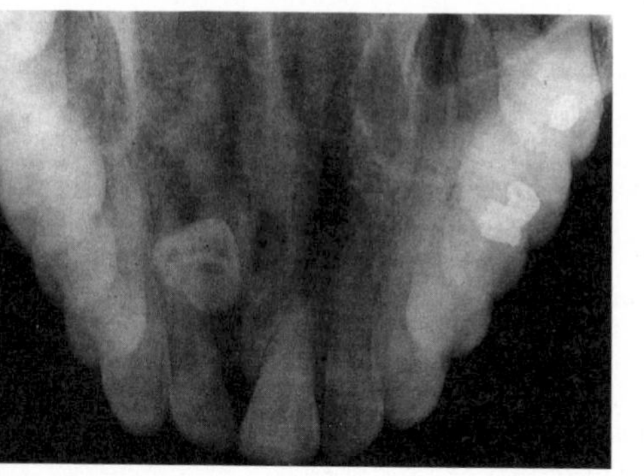

171 a

171 b

Cross-Sectional Depiction of the Jaw

For the most precise determination of the exact position of impacted and supernumerary teeth, roots and root fragments, dental implants and foreign bodies of all types, anatomic structures, and for depiction of the expanse of pathologic processes within the jaws, radiographic diagnostic examination in the third dimension is essential, indeed indispensable. The technological basis is a cross-sectional tomography of the jaw, which is indicated to eliminate any disturbing summation effect (volume artifacts) as completely as possible; for these reasons, computer-supported thin-layer tomographic procedures are superior to the more conventional thick-layer procedures of zonography.

For routine daily dental practice, supplementary programs for panoramic radiographic devices were developed, based upon the conventional technique of linear and spiral attenuation (see Fig. **1b**). The longer the paths that the image receptor and radiation source follow as they orbit the selected slice, the greater will be the slice angle and the blurring of images of tissues lying outside the slice (see Fig. **1a**). This results in a clearer image of the desired object with less apparent overlapping. Clearly then, complex spiral tomography is superior to simple linear attenuation.

There are, however, problems and potential difficulties with these conventional attempts at object localization, mainly proper and object-related adjustment of the planes of focus, and structure-related choice of exposure settings. It is for these reasons that any auxiliary personnel who are given the responsibility of performing these special radiographic techniques must be properly educated and continually up-dated with regard to advances in the field, in order to avoid unnecessary re-takes because of errors in the initial exposures, and ultimately to protect the patient from unnecessary radiation exposure. It is important to remember that the mandible, due to its wide-meshed trabecular osseous structure, is more often overexposed than the maxilla (exception: maxillary sinus). Transparent (radiolucent) lesions, for example, follicular cysts, are readily traversed by roentgen rays, and teeth that may be located within such cysts may be overexposed.

Fig. 172 Possibilities and limitations of object localization using panoramic radiography. This panoramic film depicts the completely impacted mandibular left canine; note that the area of the root appears very enlarged and blurred, while the tip of the crown is less enlarged and is quite sharply depicted. Upon cursory examination, the lower canine would appear to reside lingual to the mandibular anterior teeth, according to the rules described on p. **111**. In many cases, however, this interpretation proves to be false in cases of pathology in the mandibular anterior region, because the relationship of the tooth-supporting alveolar process to the base of the body of the mandible may be anatomically such that an impacted mandibular canine is indeed positioned vestibularly but nevertheless more focus-near than the incisors, therefore *simulating* a more lingual localization.

Fig. 173 a Possibilities and limitations of localization using the panoramic radiograph. This transversal linear tomograph of the mandibular anterior region of the same case (Fig. **172**) reveals the true, vestibular position of the impacted mandibular canine (Sirona Orthophos).

Fig 173 b Possibilities and limitations of localization using the panoramic radiograph. Same case as depicted in Fig. **174** shows the supplemental transversal radiograph of the right side of the mandible, and depicts the position of the both impacted and fully developed supernumerary premolar in the third dimension. The axially depicted supernumerary premolar is overexposed (arrow).

Fig. 174 Possibilities and limitations of localization using the panoramic radiograph. This radiograph of a 51-year-old female was the initial image taken, and reveals several supernumerary premolars (hyperodontia) as shown in the transversal layers above (Fig. **173 b**).

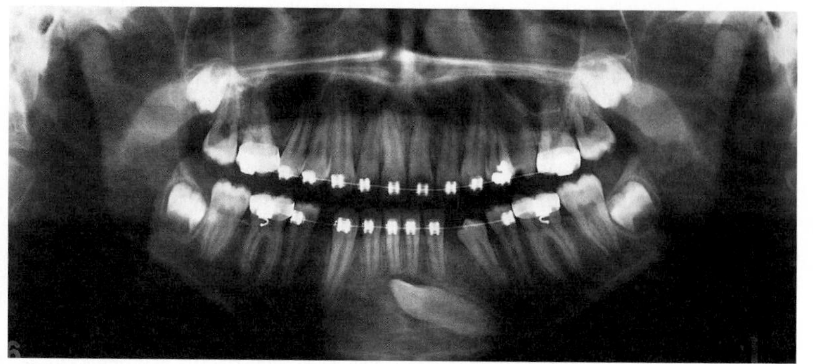

172

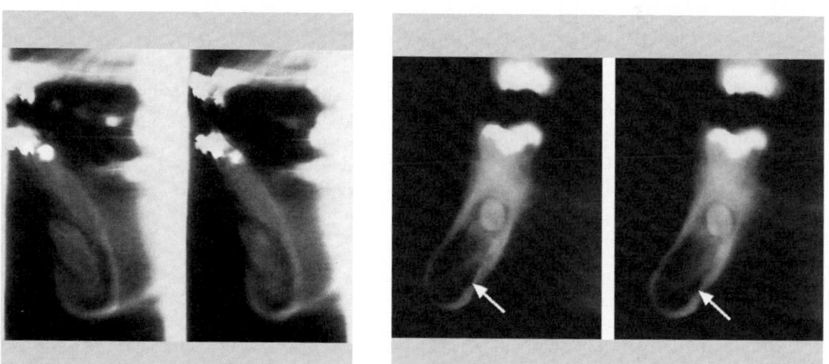

173 a

173 b

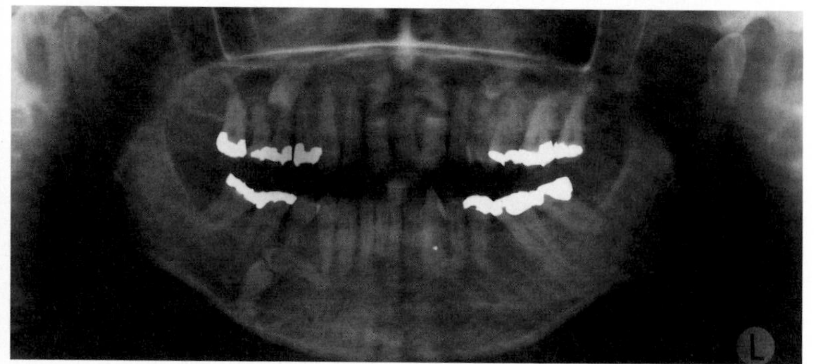

174

Supplementing the Panoramic Radiograph with Conventional Skull Images

Often the clinical examination and the dental history during an initial appointment provide the impetus to employ radiographic methods to locate an apparently missing tooth or a supernumerary tooth (diastema!). The two-dimensional intraoral or panoramic radiographs used for this purpose must, however, often be supplemented by examinations in the third-dimension, especially if unusual spatial relationships are initially encountered. This can be accomplished before any invasive clinical procedures through the use of conventional skull projections, which can be taken either in the private dental office using the cephalometric component of the panoramic radiography system, or can be referred to a radiology center or a university clinic, which may reduce radiation exposure for the patient and which may also be less costly. The indication for such supplemental radiographs is especially evident when, for example, maxillary or mandibular third molars are depicted in an axial view in the initial panoramic radiograph.

Supplementing the Panoramic Radiograph using Primary and Secondary Computed Tomography

As alternatives to the supplemental programs of the panoramic radiograph unit, axial and coronal CT offers images of greater clarity and higher resolution because they are thin-layer procedures. However, these radiographs do not permit transversal section views of the alveolar process.

By using dental CT programs, secondary cross sectional slices can be constructed from multiple panoramic views of different vertical slices, although the image clarity will be somewhat reduced. The graduations on the panoramic view and the numbered transversal layers permit a spatially precise identification of the depicted structures, as well as metric analysis in a ratio of 1:1.

Fig. 175a Localization of tooth 18, depicted axially in a panoramic radiograph. The initial panoramic radiograph of a 25-year-old patient revealed an axially depicted maxillary third molar with a follicular cyst. It is impossible, using this radiograph, to draw any exact conclusions concerning the position of the tooth. The superficial assessment of a "high position" of the impacted tooth 18 usually is not adequate for preoperative localization of a horizontally impacted third molar, and the clinician is well advised to clarify the precise position using a conventional skull film or CT preoperatively.

Fig. 175b Localization of a horizontally impacted maxillary third molar using conventional skull radiographs. This segment of a conventional skull radiograph ("reverse Towne"; see p. **91**) reveals that tooth 18 is not only horizontally impacted high in the maxilla, but also that the root tips are oriented vestibularly (**arrow**).

Fig. 176a Diagram for taking the conventional skull film, "mandible overview" (reverse Towne). This radiograph can be obtained with a lower radiation dose and usually less cost than a CT, and if performed properly will provide sufficient information to supplement the panoramic film. The precise desires and the special radiographic technique must be discussed with the radiologist in advance.

Fig. 176b Diagram for taking a conventional axial skull radiograph. As a supplement to the panoramic radiograph, this skull projection can depict the position of extreme medial or lateral impactions, as well as fractures of the zygomatic arches (see p. **87**).

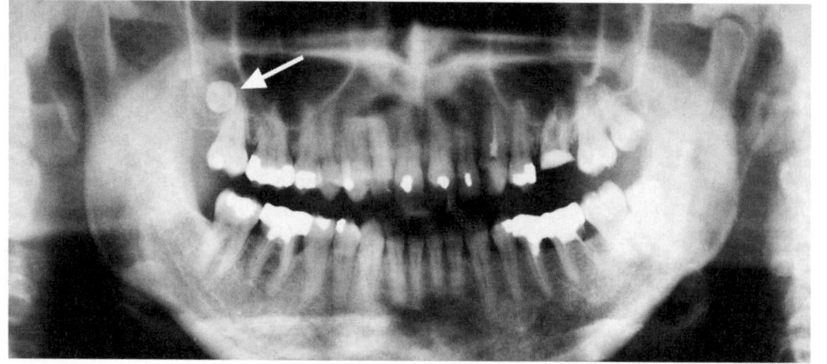

175 a

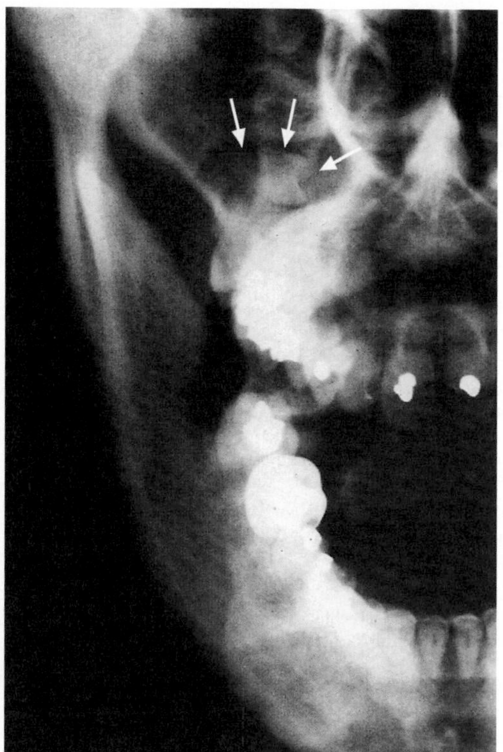

175 b

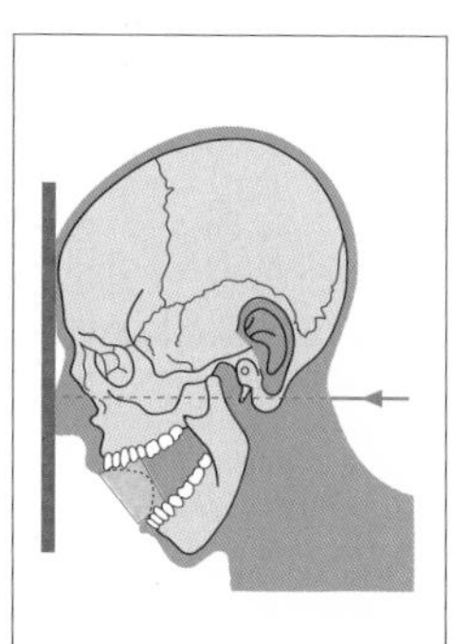

176 a

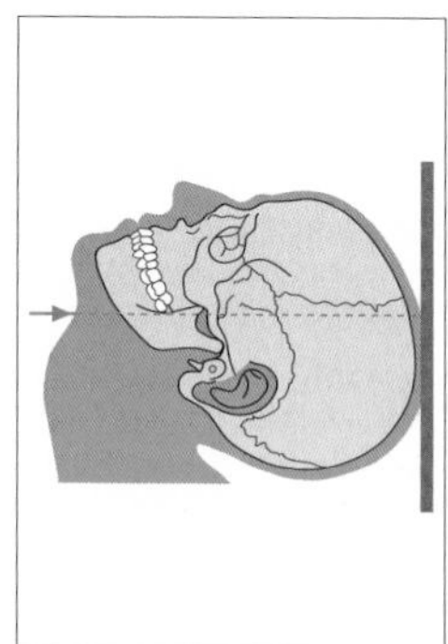

176 b

Even though today the depiction of the major salivary glands generally falls within the domain of sonography and no longer within the immediate treatment arena of dental medicine, in the daily practice of dentistry, it is not infrequent that serendipitous findings of sialoliths confront the dentist in intraoral and panoramic radiographs. Sialoliths consist primarily of calcium phosphate and calcium carbonate, and produce a summation effect overlapping teeth and jaw structures when viewed in two-dimensional intra- and extraoral radiographs; this can frequently lead to incorrect interpretation. In the mandibular area, sialoliths may cause blockage of salivary flow in the efferent ducts of the submandibular gland (Wharton's duct) and the sublingual gland. As seen in a panoramic radiograph, sialoliths in the parotid gland overlap the mandibular ascending ramus and may also be found in the efferent duct (Stensen's duct), which ends vestibularly in the mucosa near the maxillary second molar. For proper identification and interpretation of sialoliths, the observer must possess certain basic knowledge of the radiographic anatomy of the course of the various salivary ducts and their intraoral orifices. It is very important that the various ducts of the salivary glands be clearly projected in the third dimension.

Fig. 177a Localization of sialoliths in the dental practice. This radiograph, a type of "sialography," was prepared after injection of a water-soluble contrast medium and reveals the pathway of the duct (Wharton's duct) to the submandibular gland. Sialoliths are observed most often along the course of the duct from its "knee" to the intraoral orifice. In a panoramic radiograph of this region, sialoliths may be observed in the mandible from the first premolar up to the angle of the mandible, and can be misinterpreted as sclerosing pathologic alterations or even supernumerary teeth.

Fig. 177b Clinical positioning for localization of sialoliths in the sublingual gland and/or the submandibular gland. The IR is positioned identical to a half-arch occlusal radiograph of the mandible (see p. **61**). The central ray is targeted along the long axis of the mandibular molars, i.e., from caudal-lateral toward cranial-medial. With the patient's head tipped far backward, the entry point of the central ray is in the area of the angle of the mandible. The exposure settings should be reduced by 50%.

Fig. 178a Radiograph for localization of a sialolith in the duct of the submandibular gland. The sialolith clearly resides within Wharton's duct. Using this radiographic technique, and with dorsal-caudal toward ventral-cranial central ray targeting, any additional sialoliths in the area of the knee of the duct can also be observed.

Fig. 178b Localization of sialoliths in daily practice. Sialograph of the parotid gland with the arcuate course of Stensen's duct around the margin of the masseter muscle reveals a long, cranially directed accessory duct in the middle third of the major duct. Sialoliths may be observed within Stensen's duct and also in the numerous branches of that duct; these will be visible as radiopacities within the ascending ramus of the mandible as viewed in panoramic radiographs.

Fig. 179a Localization of sialoliths in daily practice. The radiograph reveals a sialolith in Stensen's duct (**arrow**), which becomes visible in the soft tissue when the patient puffs out the cheek during the exposure.

Fig. 179b Schematic diagram of a radiographic technique employing tangential targeting of the central ray. Using significantly reduced exposure settings and proper targeting of the central ray, this type of projection can be taken using large radiographic film packets, or digital sensors. Using such small image receptors, however, it is by no means easy to successfully capture the desired object; the effort may exceed the practical limitations of dental office equipment.

Fig. 179c Clinical positioning for tangential central ray targeting. Note that the patient has puffed out the right cheek, and that the central ray is targeted tangentially to the cheek but at a right angle to the film cassette.

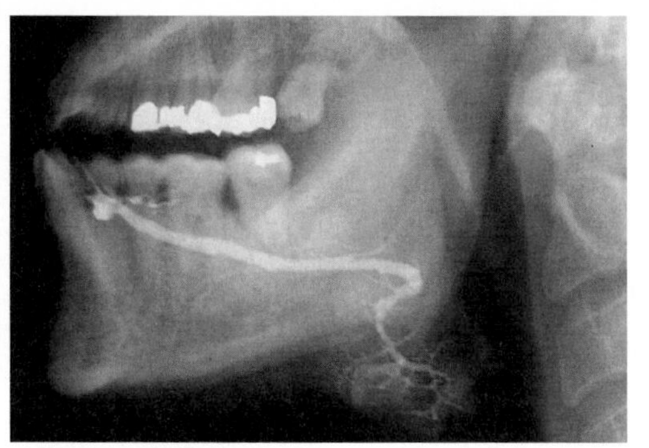
177 a

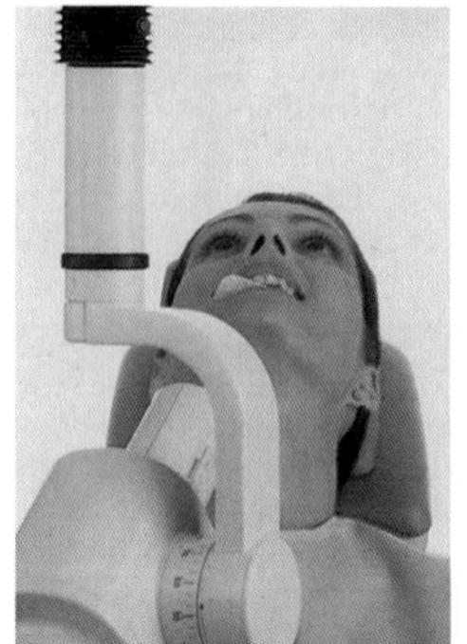
177 b

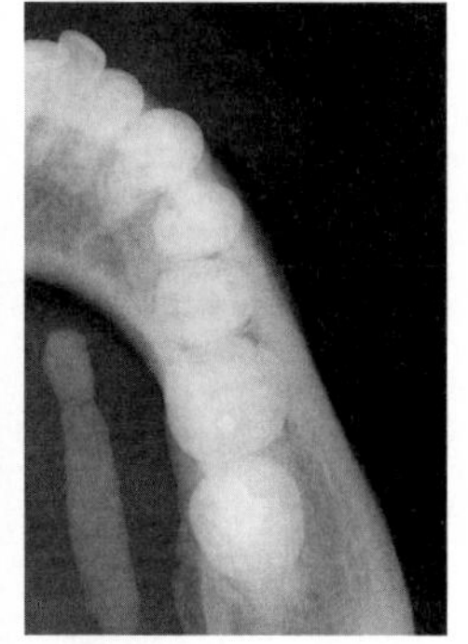
178 a

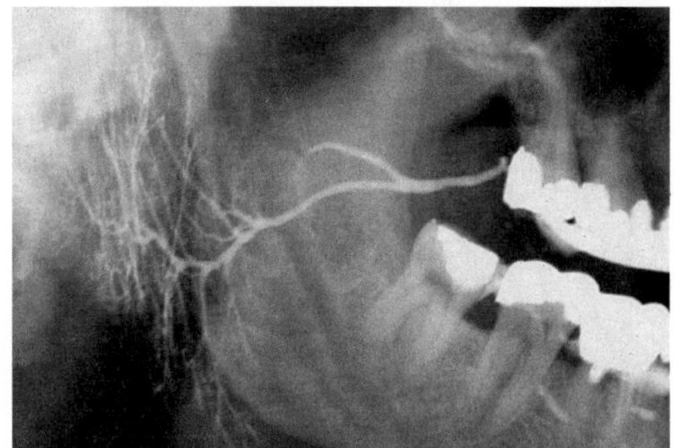
178 b

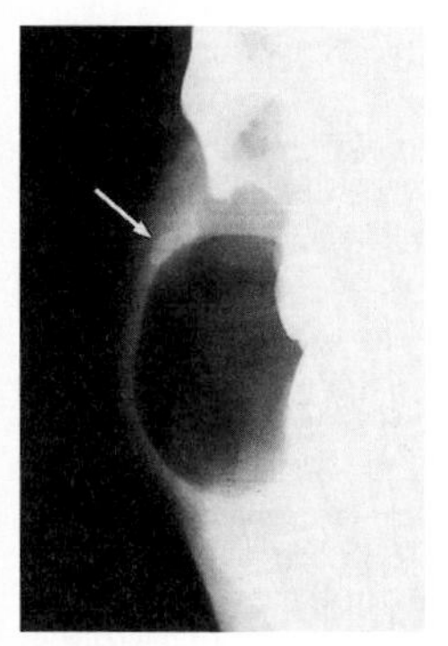
179 a

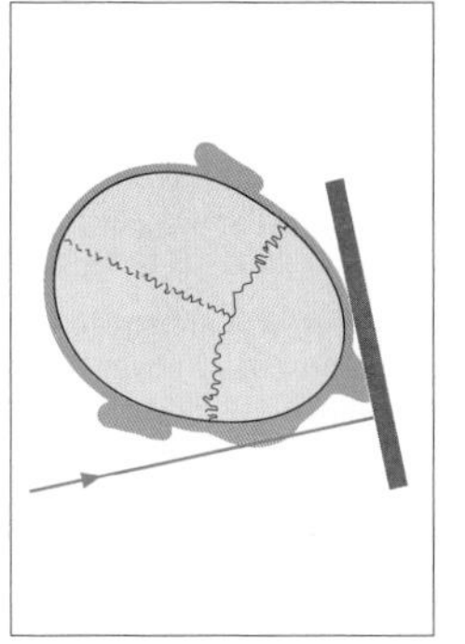
179 b

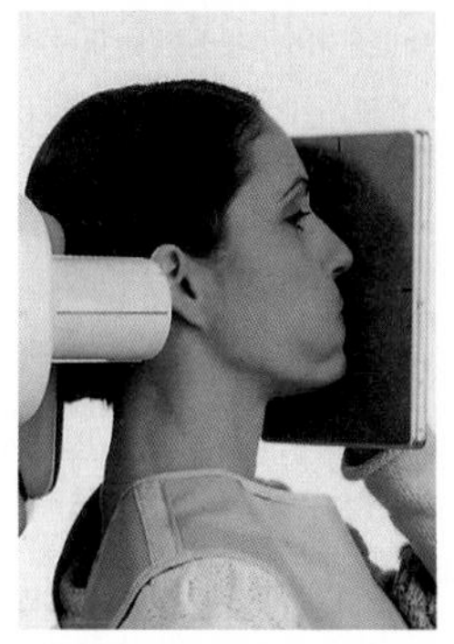
179 c

Depending upon each dentist's self-imposed demands in the arena of radiographic diagnostic capacity, the commercial marketplace today offers a large variety of radiographic units, image receptors, and image processing/developing systems. The quality of the equipment and supplies offered in this sector of the dental marketplace is very high, indeed. However, initial purchase costs can vary enormously, as do up-keep/maintenance costs; therefore very careful planning is indicated before making major purchases. Experience has demonstrated again and again that the prudent dentist will not simply choose a "convenient" mix of products, but rather a well-thought out and wherever possible an *expandable* product system.

Using modern roentgen generators, integrated exposure measurement, extremely high-sensitivity films and intensifying screens, it is possible to achieve high-quality images with an extraordinarily low radiation dose. Modern image receptors and digital image processing methods can enhance quality still further. There is absolutely no doubt that excessive radiation exposure results primarily from retakes necessitated by errors during the exposure, processing technical errors, incorrect indication, or illogical sequence of the steps in radiographic diagnostic examination.

With regard to intraoral dental films, both with and without intensifying screens, modern emulsion technology with homogeneously distributed tablet-shaped crystals (T-grain technique) has brought about great progress in the improvement of image sharpness and reproduction of detail. The luminescent emulsions of intensifying screens have likewise been improved by the use of rare earth elements, which enhance their sensitivity to the green and UV-blue regions of the spectrum in the 200 and 400 sensitivity classes. This has resulted in an elevation of the overall sensitivity of film-intensifying screen combinations and a reduction of the radiation dose measurable at the image receptor.

Fig. 180a Emulsion technique. In earlier conformations irregularly shaped AgBr crystals were randomly embedded in the emulsion layer.

Fig. 180b Emulsion technique. Discernment of details (resolution) and image sharpness/clarity could be significantly improved by regular distribution of sphere-shaped crystals of identical volume within the emulsion.

Fig. 180c Emulsion technique. With regular and consistent distribution of plate-like grains of uniform shape and size (T-grain technique), the detail resolution and image clarity is increased, while image "noise" is reduced.

Fig. 181a Structure of an intraoral film packet without intensifying screen. Cross-section through the modern, double-layered, film without intensifying screen. The emulsions and the overlying anatomic structures elicit the appearance of quality-degrading scattered radiation, especially in the highly sensitive regions.

Fig. 181b Architecture of a cassette film with enhancement foil. Only an enhancement screen (foil) that is evenly applied to the film will provide an image devoid of blurring. Screens must only be cleaned using special cleaning agents such as AGFA Curix Cleaner. Screens and cassette closure devices must be regularly inspected.

Fig. 182 Schematic depiction of the effects of intensifying screens. The roentgen rays impact the emulsion layers directly (**1** and **2** of the double-layered cassette film). Furthermore, the roentgen rays stimulate the fluorescing crystals of the front and back screens (**3** and **4**) to radiate long-wave light, thus enhancing the effect of the rays themselves. However, this also causes a simultaneous cross-over effect of scattered radiation (**5**) which diminishes image clarity.

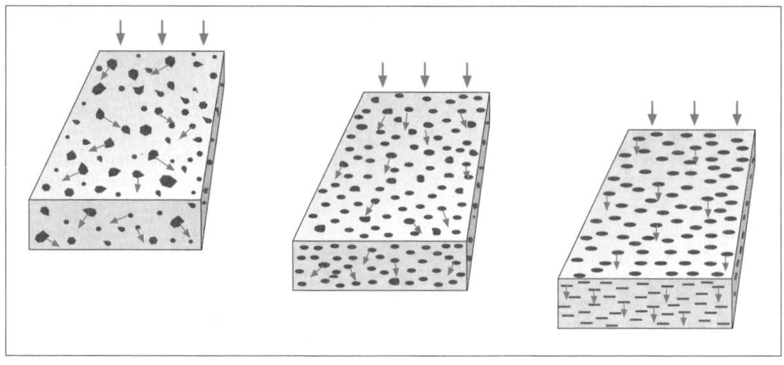

180 a 180 b 180 c

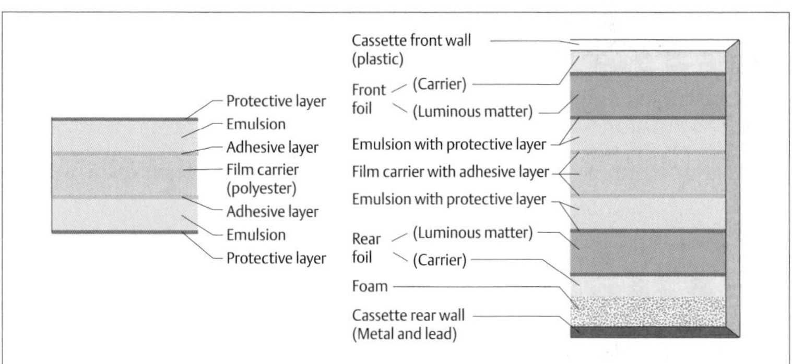

Protective layer
Emulsion
Adhesive layer
Film carrier
(polyester)
Adhesive layer
Emulsion
Protective layer
Cassette front wall
(plastic)
Front foil
(Carrier)
(Luminous matter)
Emulsion with protective layer
Film carrier with adhesive layer
Emulsion with protective layer
Rear foil
(Luminous matter)
(Carrier)
Foam
Cassette rear wall
(Metal and lead)

181 a 181 b

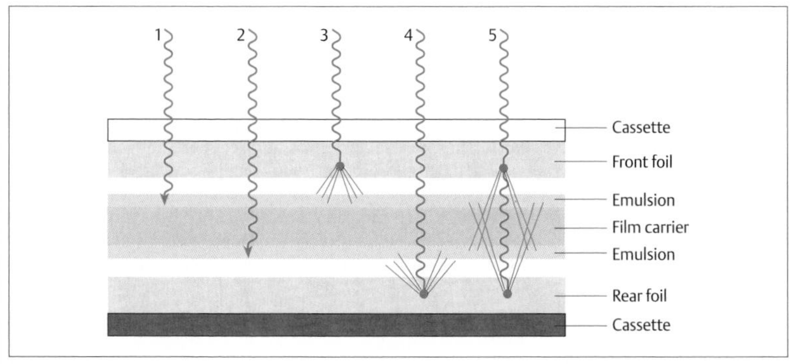

1
2
3
4
5
Cassette
Front foil
Emulsion
Film carrier
Emulsion
Rear foil
Cassette

182

But with these improvements, the manufacturers and diagnosticians alike have reached a limit, because any further increase in the intensification factor is bound to produce a decrease in image sharpness and contrast because of quantum noise, a grainier film, and increased cross-over effect, making recognition of details more difficult. All of these facts notwithstanding, cassettes of sensitivity 200 and 400 should be available in the dental practice, and clearly so-labeled, to permit examination of both adults and children with regard to the appropriate clinical/diagnostic questions while delivering the lowest possible radiation exposure dose.

Film developing/processing also plays an important role in quality assurance in radiographic diagnosis. Desired is a film development process without any variations in the quality of the chemical solutions, or the processing temperature, or the processing time; these are critical considerations with regard to the necessity to re-take radiographs, which always leads to elevated radiation exposure. For this reason, automated film processing equipment should be selected.

Radiographic films and enhancement screens: Radiographic films used universally today are almost without exception double, i.e., coated on both sides of the emulsion carrier. The emulsion carrier itself consists of polyester about 0.2 mm thick, which is frequently colored blue. Both sides of this material are coated with an adhesive layer of gelatin, which varies from 4–10 nm thick depending upon film type. With its imbedded layer of AgBr crystals in a flat arrangement and irregular distribution, modern emulsion technology provides a significantly increased resolution of detail. In the end, a hardened protective layer is formed, which can withstand higher processing temperatures and therefore permits more rapid developing procedures. In order to maintain the lowest possible exposure settings when using extraoral overview radiographs, enhancement screens are used in addition to the cassette film; these screens are coated with highly sensitive luminescent materials derived from rare earth elements, which far exceed the capabilities of the previously employed calcium-tungsten screens.

Fig. 183a Hand developing with tanks. The schematic shows the sequence of baths and the time in each tank, at a standard temperature of 20 °C. The duration of the final rinsing is of critical importance for the durability of the final radiograph.

Fig. 183b Principle of automated film processing. After entering the automatic device (**1**), the radiographic film is attached in the roller system and traverses in sequence the developing solutions, a rinsing interval, and the fixation bath (**2, 3, 4**), then through a film drying section (**5**), and is finally expelled (**6**) as a dry and final radiograph. Because of the “wringer” effect of the mechanical rollers and a sufficient intermediate rinsing procedure, the carry-over of chemicals from the developer bath to the fixation bath is reduced to an insignificant minimum.

Fig. 184a Partially automated device for intraoral radiograph developing. The “Periomat” device (Dürr Dental) can simultaneously process several films, and includes a drying procedure. The individual films are positioned in a holder and driven by a motor through the various baths, which must be changed from time to time by hand depending upon the frequency of use.

Fig. 184b Automatic developing for intraoral, panoramic, and cephalometric radiographs. This completely automatic developing apparatus (XR series, Dürr Dental) is a rolling device for large-format films, and provides attachments for changing films in daylight. It is outfitted with a device for automatically regenerating the chemicals as necessary, and provides rapid processing for all dental radiographs including large-format cassette films. When purchasing devices such as an automatic radiographic film processor, it is important to take special note of the service plan offered by the manufacturer.

Fig. 185a Film transport system. At each monthly change of chemicals, the movement mechanism of the machine is removed and cleaned with water or a spray.

Fig. 185b Chemical set. Concentrated developer and fixer guarantee simple and reliable use of chemicals.

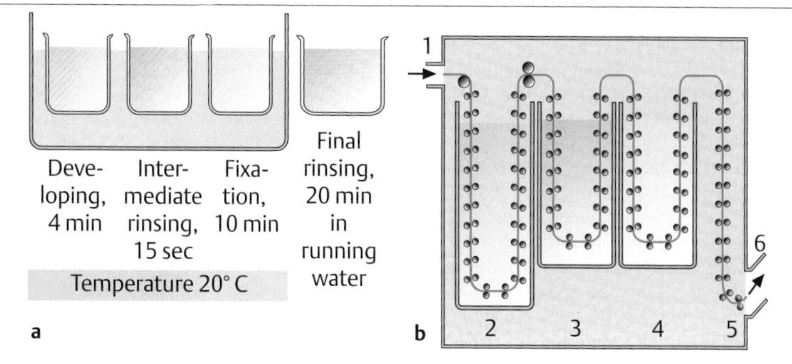

183 a

183 b

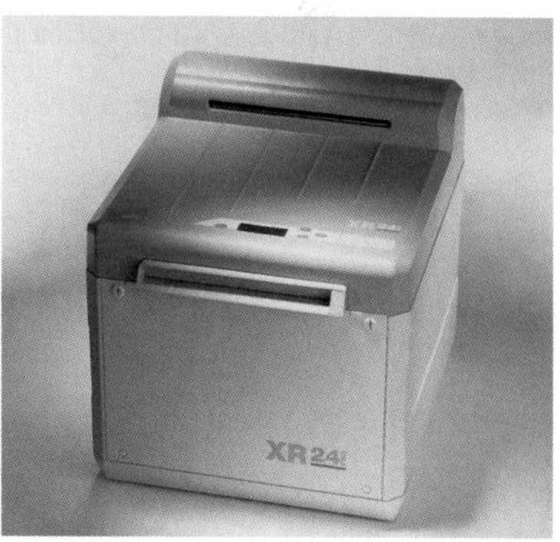

184 a

184 b

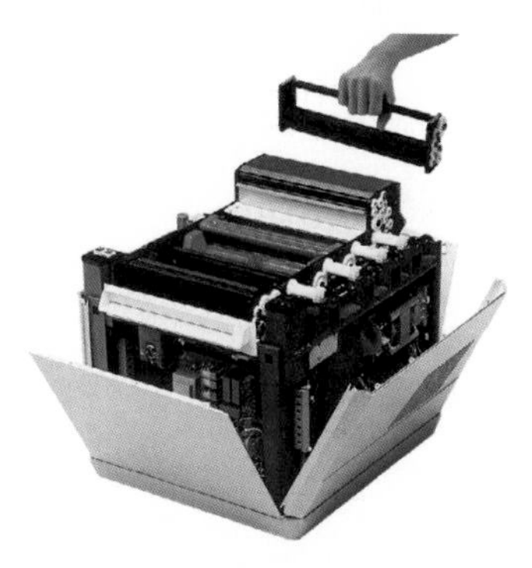

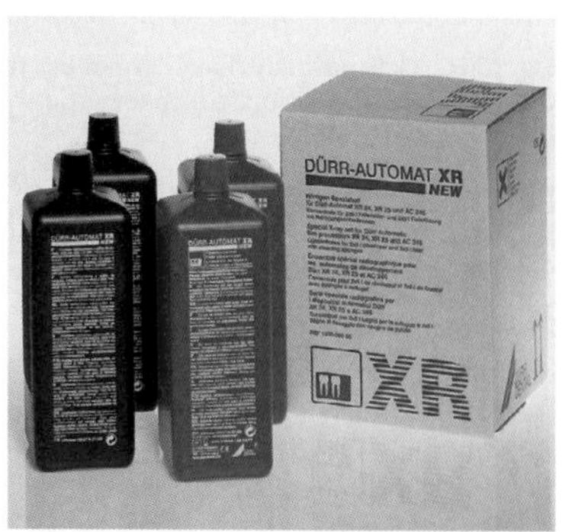

185 a

185 b

The enhancement screens are generally supplied as green-sensitive or UV blue-sensitive; combined with the appropriate film cassette they comprise the complete image receptor system. Combining components from various manufacturers is not recommended. Ninety-five percent of the image-producing darkening of the film is achieved by the luminescence of the enhancing screens, and only 5% by the roentgen rays. The so-called enhancement factor of the screens is a description of the relationship between exposure time versus a screen-free film, i.e., how much the exposure time can be reduced in order to produce a comparable result of image clarity in the final radiograph. The various classes of sensitivity indicate the exposure dose necessary to achieve the optical density 1.

It is important also to note that the enhancement screens only provide a regularly diffuse image clarity over the entire film when the cassette closure is intact, which insures even pressure exertion of the enhancement screens upon the cassette film.

Every type and brand of radiographic film must always be maintained cool and vertically in storage. Radiographic film must in no case be stored together with development chemicals, and must not be exposed to bright light sources or roentgen rays at any level. If the film with its emulsion is warmed or influenced by light, the emulsion will "mature" and this will result in elevation of background fog in the final radiograph. If the film intensifying screen system in the cassette is replaced by phosphor-coating imaging plates, the results of the data captured in the radiographic exposure can be further processed digitally after scanning (e.g., DenOptix Combo or Digora pct).

Frequent processing errors: In addition to the structure contrasts caused by variation of roentgen ray absorption, the actual film contrast is influenced not only by the characteristics of the radiographic film but also by its subsequent processing/developing; under developing, for example resulting from old or cold chemicals, and overdeveloping for exam-

Fig. 186a Use of cold chemicals. The radiograph appears faint and coarse-grained, because the proper temperature was not achieved during the developing process.

Fig. 186b Re-take, with proper temperatures during film developing. The chemicals used for developing an exposed radiographic film must be neither too cold nor too warm. The results of either error will be under- or overdeveloped radiographs exhibiting reduced contrast.

Fig. 186c Only partially filled developing tank. Evaporation reduced the amount of solution in the tank. Note here the undeveloped portion of the radiograph which was not exposed to the fixer solution.

Fig. 187a Inadequate tank filling. Too little liquid in the tanks.

Fig. 187b Contamination. Even before inserting the film into the developer solution, droplets of water touched the film. This weakened locally the effect of the developer solution.

Fig. 187c Contamination. Before the film was even dipped into the developer solution, droplets of developer contaminated the film, resulting in dark spots from overdevelopment.

Fig. 188a Contamination. This radiograph depicts artifacts in the form of "lightening bolts." Such artifacts result if the cassette film is removed too quickly from the film pack, especially in low humidity.

Fig. 188b Contamination. Note the impression of a fingernail along the long axis of the root of tooth 31, an artifact. Note also the transverse root fracture on tooth 42.

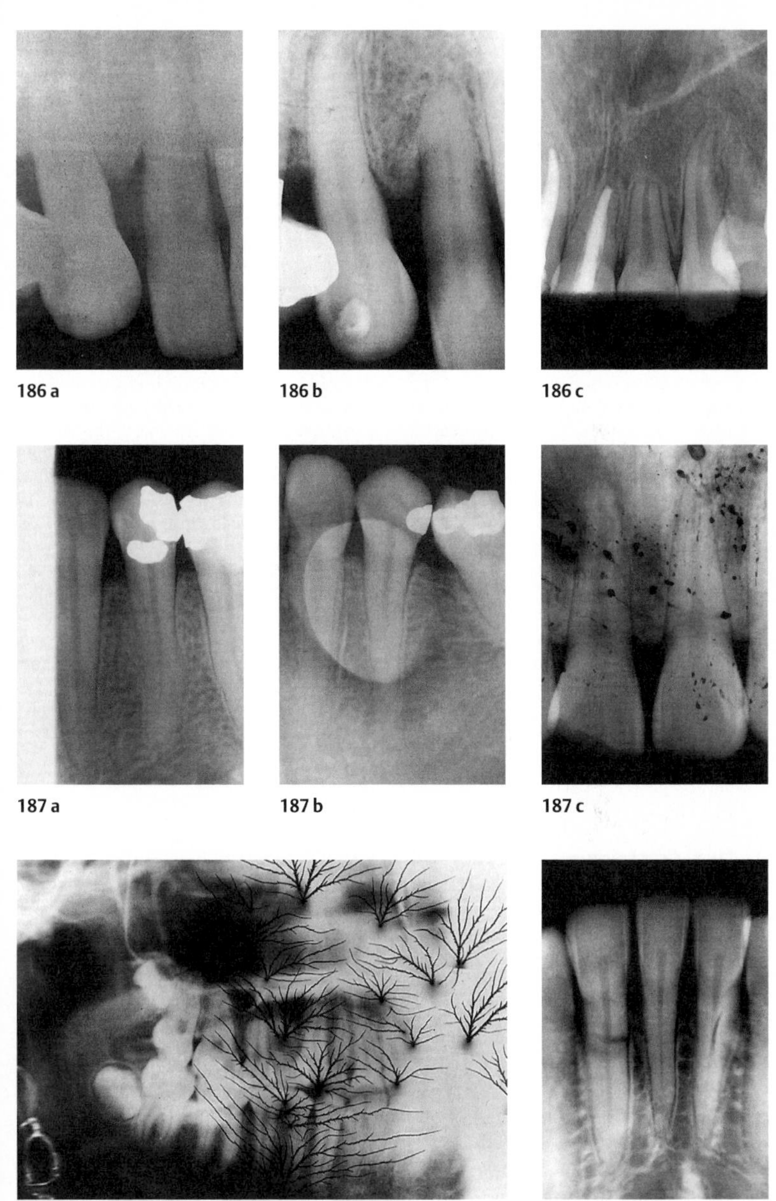

186 a 186 b 186 c

187 a 187 b 187 c

188 a 188 b

ple by excessive processing time in the developer solution will both reduce the optimum radiographic contrast in the final film. It is critical to keep in mind, that the directions for use of both developing chemicals and the radiographic equipment itself must be followed precisely in order to avoid errors and resulting useless films. "Premature aging" of radiographic film can occur if it is inappropriately stored, for example at temperatures above 20°C and in the vicinity of high intensity light (the sun!), as well as in proximity to active radiographic units. Radiographic film and film packets should not be stored flat one upon another, but rather vertically.

Inadvertent film exposures can occur if the film packet is opened in daylight, or through excessive manipulation of already opened film. Extracting a radiographic film rapidly out of a cassette can create static electricity that can produce artifacts in the final radiograph (see Fig. **188a**). Contamination of an opened film packet by water droplets or blasts of air will result in areas that appear to be overexposed because the developer solution is less effective in those contaminated areas. Even hand creams or lotions containing lipids will inhibit complete film development and leave behind bright fingerprints on the radiograph. Fixation solution sprays dissolve the not-yet-developed emulsion layer and leave behind obvious clear spots. Physical contact with other films awaiting processing, or excessively rapid introduction of films into the solutions can inhibit the sequential stages of the development process. If the technician's fingers become contaminated with developer solution, this will initiate an immediate start of the development process, and the result will be dark or black areas on the final radiograph.

If the development unit becomes contaminated with fixative solution, the entire radiograph will exhibit a gray haze. Inadequate fixation, for example due to old or cold fixation solution, as well as inadequate rinsing or drying will result in long term dichroic haze with brownish discoloration; over the long term, this can lead to destruction of the emulsion layer if the final radiographs are placed into plastic pouches when still moist; this is especially true for the panoramic films. If the fluid levels in the various tanks are too low, the upper sections of radiographic films will be completely undeveloped, with no visible image. Bending an intraoral film as well as the pressure of a fingernail will result in dark lines and half-moon-shaped artifacts on the final radiograph.

Contamination of the enhancement screens for cassette radiographic films always show up as artifacts on the final radiograph. Enhancement screens may only be cleaned using special solutions, and *never* with water or soap of any kind.

Fig. 189a Contamination. As the film was removed from its packaging, it was not handled exclusively on the edges, rather its surface was touched with a finger that was contaminated with developer solution.

Fig. 189b One film in contact with another during processing. If wet films come into contact with each other, for example hanging in a partially automated system or as a result of too rapid feeding of a fully automatic system, the result will be double images on which the contacting surfaces are underdeveloped.

Fig. 190a Excessive development temperature. Together with the pressures applied by the rollers in an automated development system, excessive temperature leads to "swimming" of the emulsion layer.

Fig. 190b Fracture of the emulsion layer. Before processing, the film was bent and the emulsion layer was severed; note the dark vertical line.

Fig. 191 Out-of-date cassette film. Out-of-date films will exhibit a clearly elevated background haze and produce final films with poor contrast. Similarly poor quality radiographs will result from overexposure or by the use of spent fixation solutions.

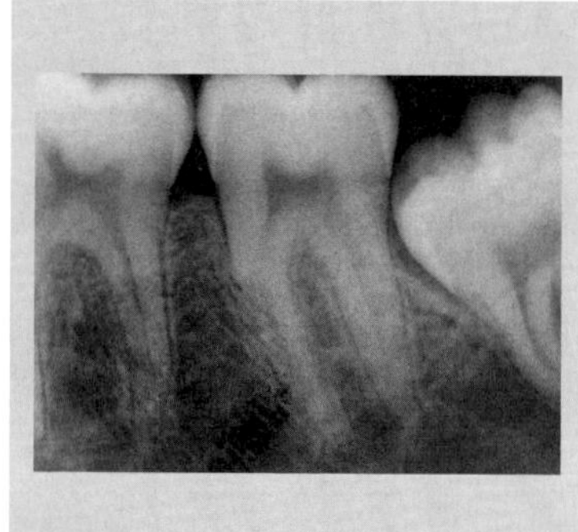

189 a

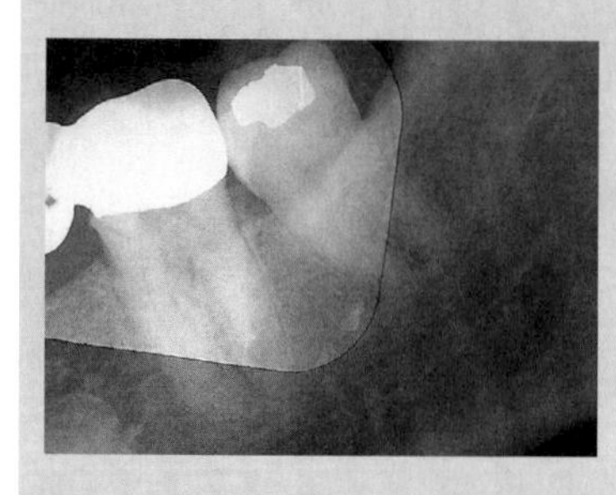

189 b

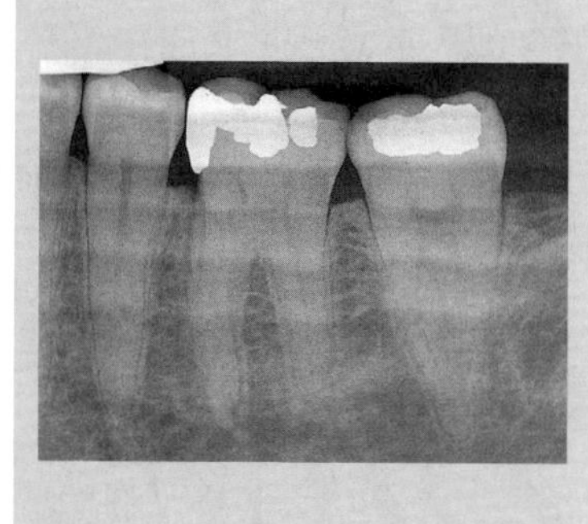

190 a

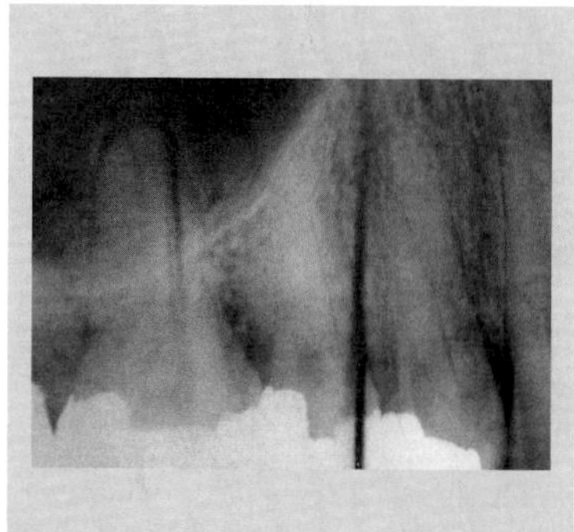

190 b

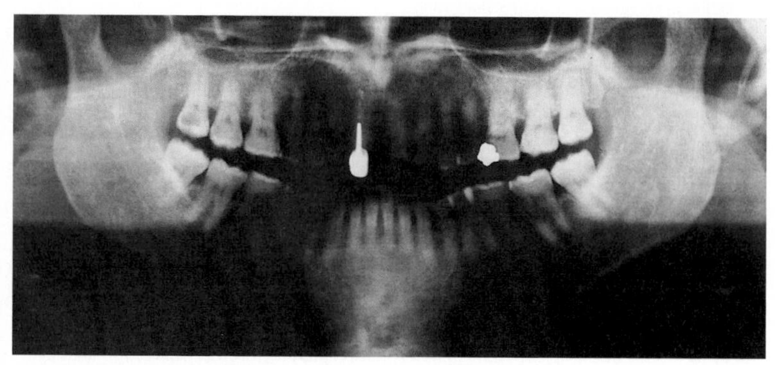

191

The digital radiograph: A digital image actually corresponds to the reduction of a conventional image into a prepared gridwork of image points, the so-called pixel (picture element). Each field of the grid is assigned a numerical value that represents a gray or color value from a pre-prepared and discrete palette. The discrete nature of the pixels in terms of both spatial location and gray scale permits the accumulation and storage of the image as data sets. TIFF (tagged interchange file format) and BMP (bitmap) are the most commonly used data formats.

In the field of digital imaging, there exist fundamental limitations regarding the data set in terms of spatial resolution and the gray and/or color nuances: Oblique lines are reproduced as "stair steps"; in addition, the absolute number of possible color and gray steps is predetermined. Intermediate shades or nuances are not reproduced. As long as the individual pixels are small enough and the available gray-stages and/or the color palette are expansive enough, these limitations will be of no consequence. The quality of a digital image depends upon the number, size, and depth of color of the grid points.

Pixel size: Persons with normal eyesight can discriminate with the naked eye structures down to ca. 0.1 mm in size (Jensen 1980). This fact leads to the conclusion that the pixel size—assuming a desired 1:1 size relationship—should not be larger than maximally 100 x 100 μ^2. From the absolute size of the image and the pixel size one can calculate the number of necessary image points. If an image in 3 x 4 cm format with square pixels 50 µm on each side is to be produced, an image matrix of 600 x 800 is necessary.

Gray-value palette: The available gray scale palette is determined by the computer storage capacity or the digitalization depth. With a storage depth of 8 bits (binary digits), for each pixel there is available a palette of $2^8 = 256$ shades of gray. Similarly, a storage capacity (depth) of 10 provides a palette of $2^{10} = 1024$ gray levels. It is important to point out that the human eye can only discern ca. 20 levels of gray simultaneously, therefore a reduced gray-value palette is of little consequence during superficial observation. For diagnostic purposes, on the other hand, images with a lower or poorer gray-value palette are less favorable. In dentistry, a gray-value palette of 256 levels of gray is the rule. In this system, black has a value of 0 and white a value of 255.

Histograms: A histogram is the graphic representation of the frequency distribution of the gray values in an image or a section of an image. In such a depiction, the frequency of appearance of each gray level in the image is counted. These types of histograms provide information about whether or not the available gray-value palette has been appropriately and optimally utilized for depicting the radiographic image. Linear histograms can be created by plotting the course of gray values graphically along a line on the digital image. This type of gray or density profile can be used to visualize the variation in intensity between contrast-poor structures.

Fig. 192a–c In a digital radiograph, the plane of the image is resolved into quadratic grid cells, the "pixels." Each pixel carries a gray- or color value from a predetermined, discrete, and finite palette. *Within* each grid cell there is no particular structure. The process of digitization renders the image visible when one overlays a conventional image with a pixel grid. For each pixel, an average gray value is determined and assigned a value from the standardized gray-value palette. This example has a pixel grid of 5 x 8 and a digitizing depth of $2^3 = 8$ gray levels (cf. Wenzel 1993).

Fig. 193a, b A gross pixel grid (**a** reduction to 69 x 109 image points) is more obvious than a less intense gray-level palette (**b** palette of 32 gray levels). For radiographic diagnosis, both parameters are important.

Fig. 194a Digital dental radiographs have a palette of at least 256 gray levels.

Fig. 194b The frequency of the various gray levels in a digital image can be depicted graphically in a histogram. Histograms are valuable aids for digital analysis and processing.

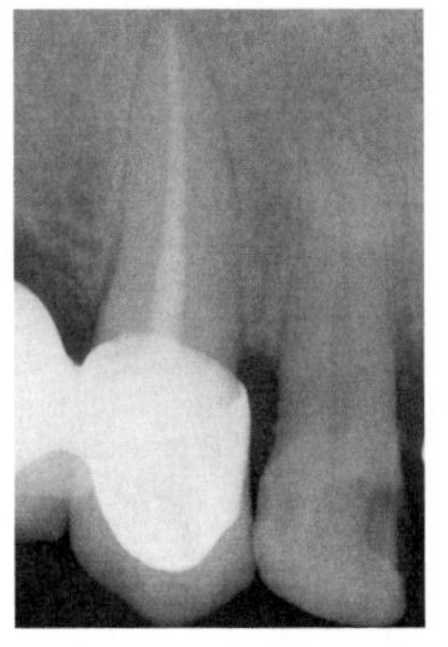

192 a

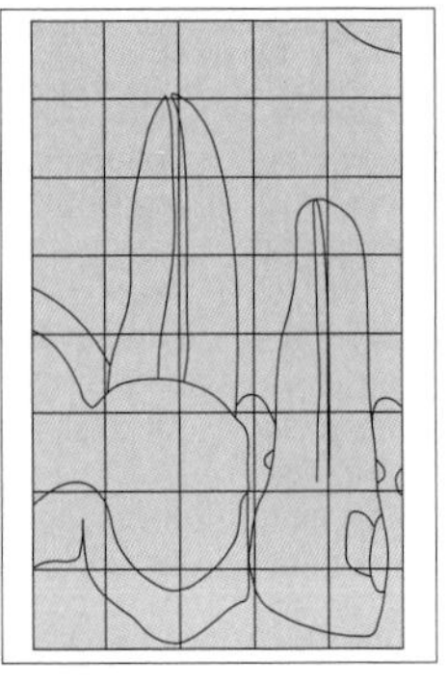

192 b

5	5	5	5	4
4	4	4	5	5
4	5	5	5	4
3	4	5	5	5
7	5	4	5	3
7	7	7	5	7
2	5	6	5	0
0	0	0	0	0

192 c

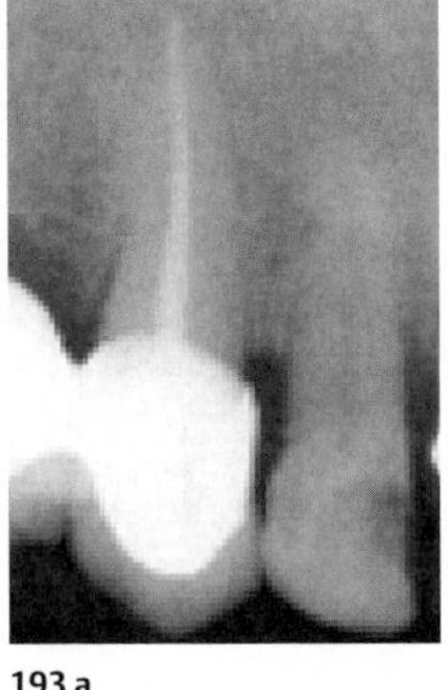

193 a

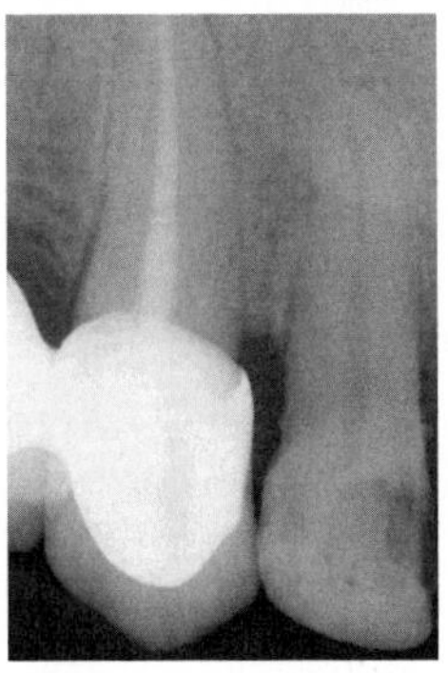

193 b

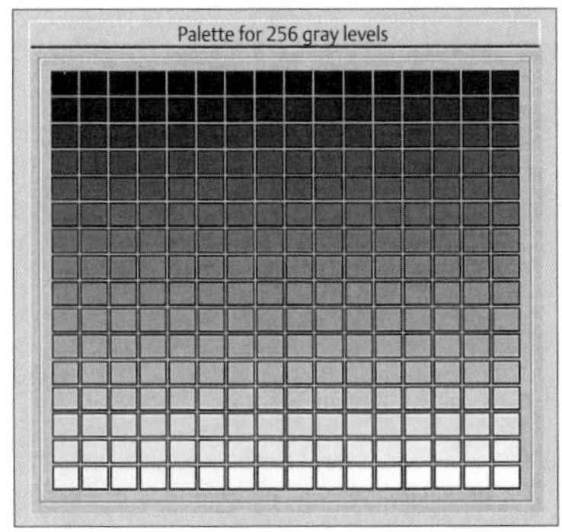

194 a

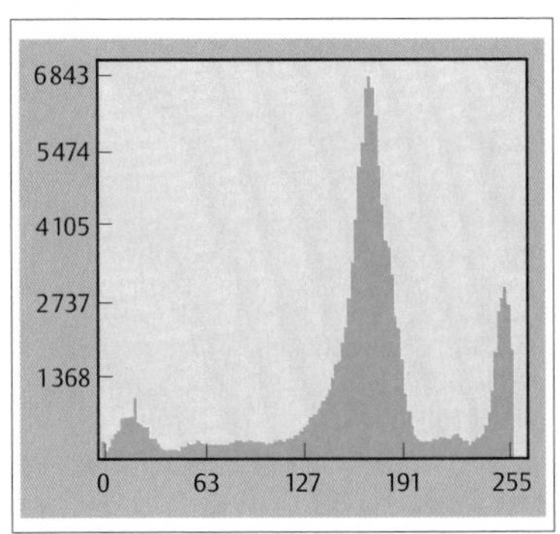

194 b

Digital imaging processing: From the purely technical point-of-view, a digital image is nothing more than a sequence of numbers stored in a database. Computer manipulation of the database can provide depictions other than the original level, or measurements within the digital image can be performed.

Variations of brightness and contrast: A digital image will become brighter if all of the gray level values are raised, for example, by addition of a constant, K, to all gray levels. Because the palette is limited there will be some loss of information: All pixels that have a gray value greater than or equal to (255-K) are depicted at the level of 255; pure white areas may exist (no gray value). By using a subtraction constant (K) from all of the gray values, any digital image can be darkened. Further, the contrast of a digital image can be influenced by the multiplication of all gray values by some constant, K. Factors larger than 1 effect an increase, while factors less than 1 cause a decrease in contrast. Through simultaneous alterations of brightness and contrast, the central area of the image expanse can be optimally depicted with the available gray-value palette. This process is referred to as windowing or histogram spreading.

Image processing with filters: One group of particularly effective image processing procedures is based upon fresh calculation of the gray levels of each pixel depending upon adjacent image points. The adjacent image areas used for the calculation are called "filter kernels." Using filters, it is possible, for example, to reduce image noise, increase image clarity, or elevate margins.

It should be noted that no type of image processing system or procedure can glean more information than was available in the original image. The situation may evolve into one in which certain portions of the original image are enhanced or quantified at the cost of other sections of the original image. Additional research is needed to define the areas of use as well as specific procedures for image processing necessary for dental radiographic diagnosis.

Fig. 195 Length measurements in a digital radiograph. The observer uses the mouse to click on reference points, and the computer program determines the combined lengths of the angled line segments from the pixel addresses (indicated dots).

Fig. 196 Enlargement of a section of the digital image. A 66 x 41 pixel size segment of the image has been enlarged to fill the image format. Enlargements in which the pixel structure of the digital image becomes visible are usually unproductive.

Fig. 197 Inverse digital image. The gray values are calculated according to y = 255 – x from the original values.

Fig. 198 Simultaneous alteration of brightness and contrast. The resulting image is contrast-rich, but lacking in detail; the edges of the original gray scale distribution are lost.

Fig. 199 Original image (digital radiographic system Sirona Sidexis, 412 x 658 pixels, 256 gray levels).

Fig. 200 Exchanging the gray level palette for a color palette produces interesting optical effects, but is virtually useless for diagnosis.

Fig. 201 Noise reduction by reconstruction of average gray values is a simple example of digital "filtering." Every pixel is adjusted to the average value of the gray level of its adjacent pixel. This type of filtering reduces image noise, but averages image detail.

Fig. 202 If the differences in the gray levels of adjacent image points are enhanced by an appropriate filter, this leads to a subjective increase of image sharpness. Simultaneously, however, image noise is enhanced.

Fig. 203 "Filtering with unsharp mask." A blurred image will be created from the original image by averaging (cf. Fig. **201**). By subtracting this image from the original image, a high-pass image is obtained that will represent the fine details especially well. This differential image is multiplied using an amplifying factor and added to the original image. The result is a visible accentuation of structural detail.

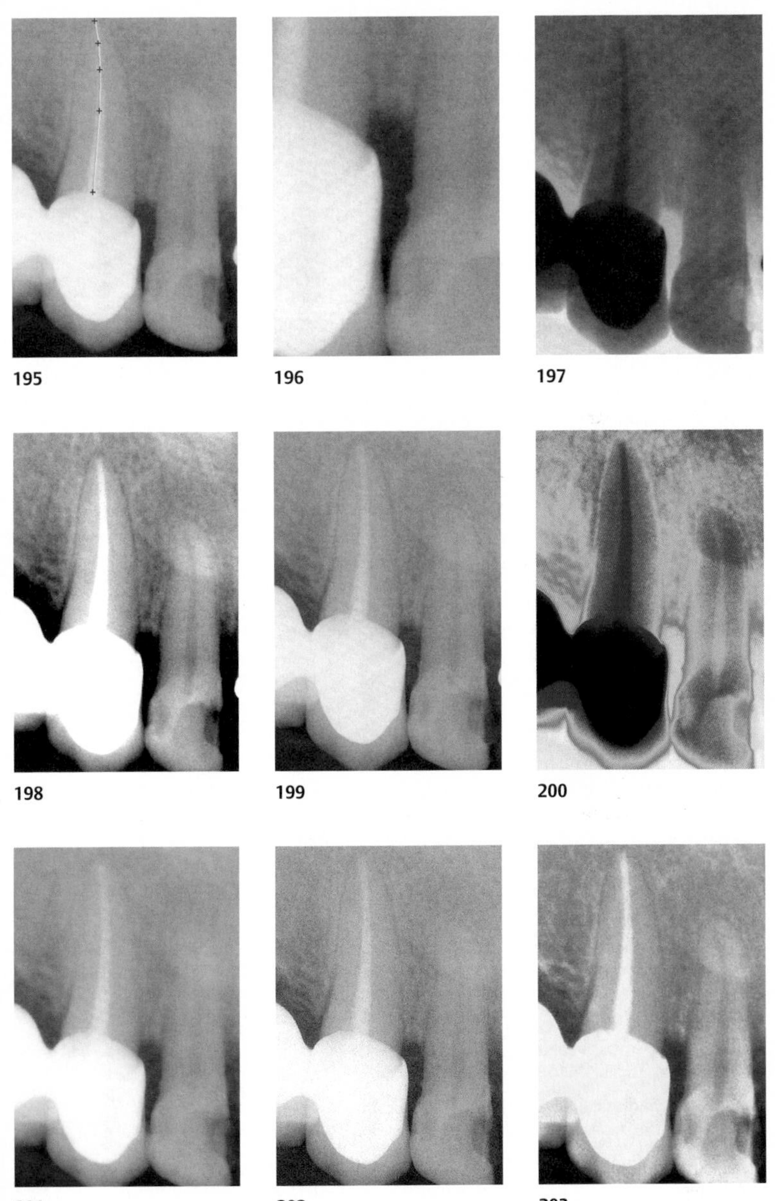

195

196

197

198

199

200

201

202

203

Conventional radiographs can be digitized using a scanner. In order to directly obtain digital radiographs, the conventional radiographic film must be replaced by a digital image receptor system. For this purpose, there are two different technologies available.

Systems with semiconductor sensors: The central element of these sensors is the semiconductor chip, which carries numerous miniaturized photo diodes on the surface (CCD- or CMOS-APS sensors). The photo diodes divide up the active receptor surface into image points. Thus, the resolution of the image into pixels occurs immediately, in the sensor itself. Semiconductor sensors have a high level of resolution. Pixel sizes down to 10 µm can be achieved. Different image formats require different sensors. For large-format extraoral radiographs, linear array sensors can be used, with which the surface can be scanned. The sensor is connected to the computer via a cable. The radiographic images can be viewed and examined immediately after the exposure (direct digital exposure technique).

Systems using storage phosphor plates: Light-excitable storage luminescent materials possess the characteristic that roentgen irradiation causes electrons to transfer into metastable conditions. Illumination with red or infrared light can again set them free. This causes them to emit light of a different wavelength (blue) whose intensity is proportional to the radiation dose. Using these materials it has been possible to construct multi-use storage plates to create images for radiographic diagnosis. Following radiation exposure, a latent image is stored in the plate. This image is read using a special laser scanner. For intraoral radiographs, the pixel size varies between 42 and 85 µm, depending upon the scanner that is used or the selected scan resolution. The typical time for the scanning procedure for a dental radiograph is 1–2 minutes. For a panoramic radiograph, depending upon the desired resolution (pixel size 85 to 170 µm) up to 6 minutes may be required. The storage plates can be regenerated by means of intensive illumination with visible light, and are quickly ready for the next radiographic exposure. They can be used for thousands of radiographs, until they are no longer usable because of purely mechanical wear and tear. For intraoral use, they must be housed for hygiene.

Fig. 204 **Intraoral radiographic sensors** (Trophy RVG) for the image formats, 2 x 3 cm^2 or 2.7 x 3.6 cm^2.

Fig. 205 **Construction schematic of a CCD-based radiographic sensor.** The roentgen rays elicit emission of light from the scintillator. This light is registered with a semiconductor chip upon which are attached numerous photo diodes. Each photo diode provides a single image point (cf. Horbaschek et al. 1996).

Fig. 206 The photo diodes of the CCD provide an analog intensity signal for every individual point, which is proportional to the incoming roentgen rays. The electrical signals from the CCD are amplified, digitized with an analog-digital converter, and then further processed into a digital radiograph. The radiographic image is immediately available on the computer screen.

Fig. 207 With the storage phosphor technique, reusable ones for intraoral radiographs and panoramic films are available in special scanners (DenOptix, Gendex Co.).

Fig. 208 **Schematic diagram of an image storage phosphor plate.** The crystals of the luminescent material are found in an emulsion that is layered upon a carrier substance made of polyester.

Fig. 209 **Reading in a scanner.** Reading is performed point for point with a laser beam. The luminescent light is registered with a photo multiplier whose signal is digitized and arranged into a pixel matrix (modified from Yaffe and Rowlands 1997).

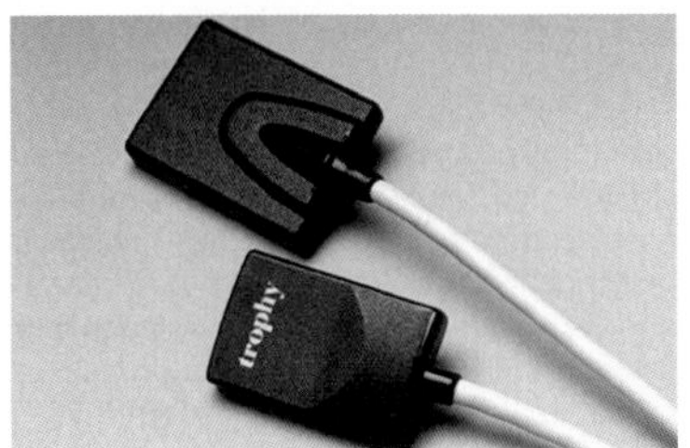

204

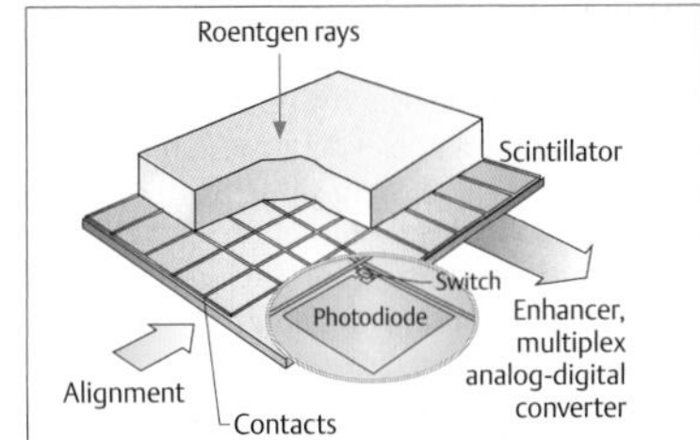

205

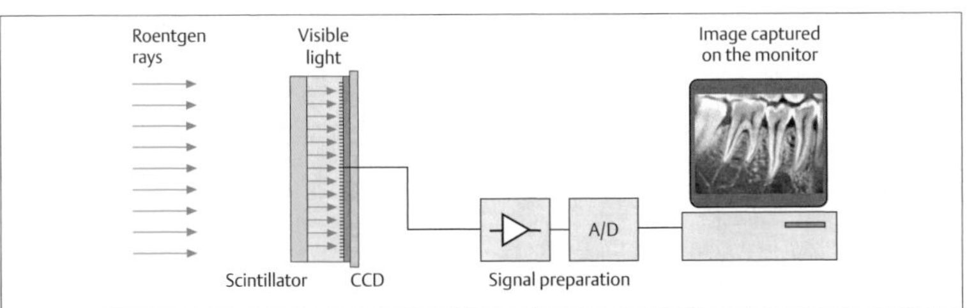

206

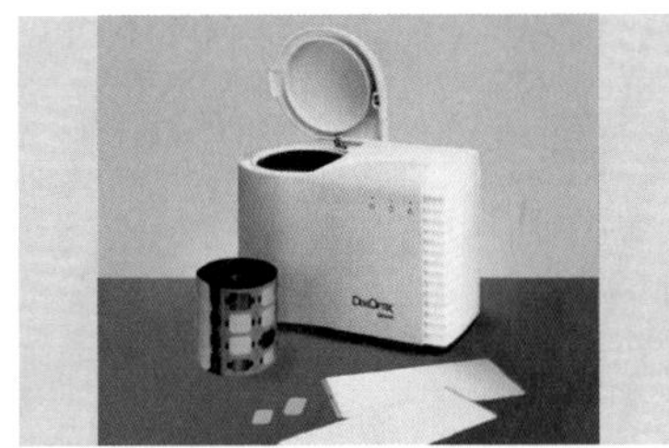

207

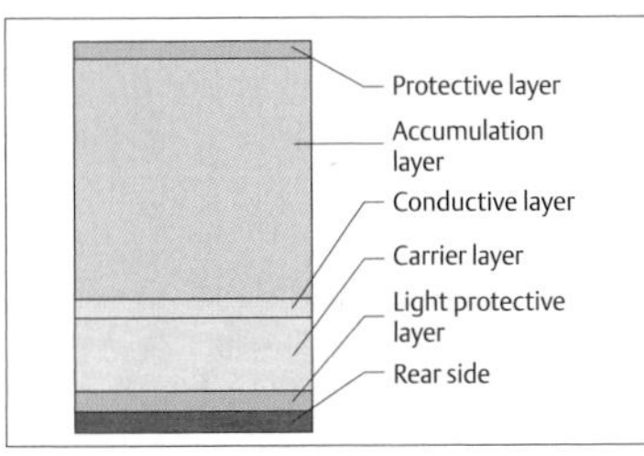

208

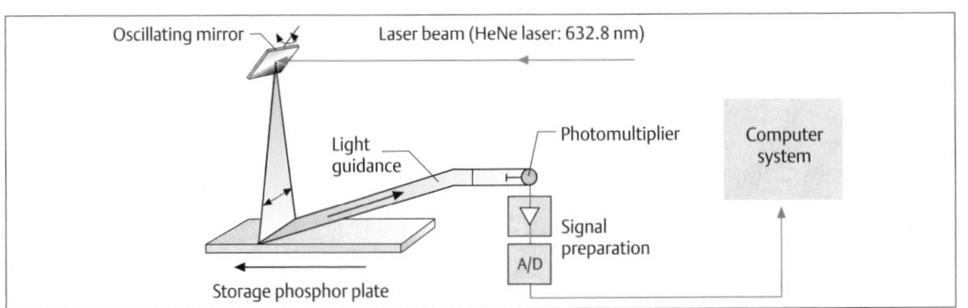

209

Exposure latitude: Digital image receptor systems have a large exposure latitude. The images are automatically processed by the system, so that it is not always noticeable whether they have been taken with an adequate radiation dose. Signs of excessive radiation dose (overexposure) include uniform black areas where gradations or a certain amount of image noise would be expected. Overexposure leads to a contrast-poor image with increased image noise.

Spatial resolution: The resolution capability can be estimated with the help of lead strip grids. A line pair consists of one transparent and one opaque line. With the naked eye, one can accurately discern up to 10 Lp/mm. Conventional dental radiographic films have a resolving capacity of 20 Lp/mm. With digital systems, the resolving capacity is limited by the pixel size. According to the so-called scanning or Nyquist theorem, only those structures can be best resolved that are twice as large as the pixels. This is expressed by the following equation:

$$\text{max. theor. resolution [Lp/mm]} < \frac{1}{2 \times \text{pixel size [mm]}}$$

A pixel size of 40 μm gives a theoretical resolution limit of 12.5 Lp/mm.

Subjective parameters of image quality: A purely technical description does not permit definitive conclusions concerning the effectiveness of a diagnostic procedure in a clinical situation. A simple characterization of diagnostic procedures (including the examining personnel) derives from the use of the terms *sensitivity* and *specificity.* The assumption here is that using an independent method (the so-called "gold standard") it can be determined with certainty that a given disease exists, or does not. The task of the clinical examiner is then to decide whether or not the disease exists using only the available diagnostic procedures to arrive at the conclusion. Given this set of circumstances, there are four possible results of the diagnostic test. From the results, *sensitivity* and *specificity* are calculated. Because, using this matrix, the examiner is forced to make a purely yes/no decision, her/his own individual and variable decision thresholds will have a significant influence on the result of the test.

This problem can be avoided if the examiner uses a *decision scale* with intermediate steps. An example is the ROC method (Receiver Operating Characteristic), a generalization of sensitivity and specificity (ICRU-54, 1996, Metz 1986). The better the results, the larger is the area under the ROC curve.

Fig. 210 Characteristic curves of conventional and digital radiographic systems. Radiographic films have an S-shaped gradation curve; for creating an image, the linear portion of the curve is used. Digital image receptor systems have linear characteristics. Their exposure range is considerably larger than with conventional films.

Fig. 211 Effect of varying the radiation dose upon image quality with conventional (right) and digital (left) systems. The exposure of the four film quadrants varies by a factor of two. Because of the automatic grade level accommodation of digital systems the optical density of digital films (**left**) is over a wide range independent of the exposure dose, but not image quality (Neitzel 1998).

Fig. 212 Estimating the local resolution using a lead line grid.

Fig. 213 When imaging periodic structures whose structural elements are smaller than the pixels, pseudopatterns may appear in the digital image. This phenomenon is referred to as undersampling, or the Moiré effect, and can lead to overestimation of the resolution capacity.

Fig. 214 Definition of the two related terms *sensitivity* and *specificity* for evaluating diagnostic procedures.

Fig. 215 Typical ROC curve. The area under the ROC curve is a measure of diagnostic performance. The larger this area is, the better the results agree with reality, i.e., the gold standard. With a purely serendipitous finding, the ROC curve would appear as a diagonal (surface: 0.5).

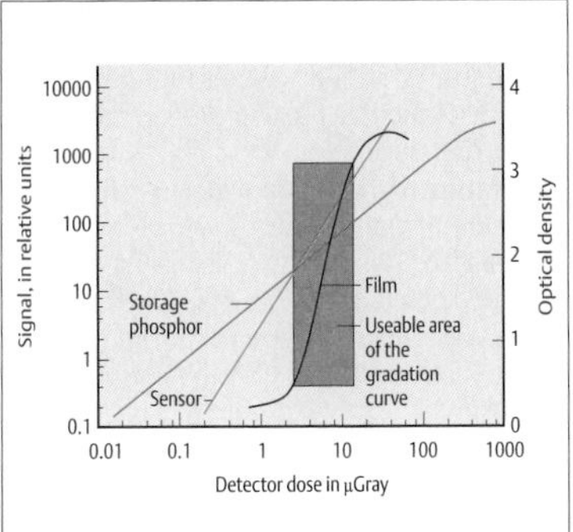

210

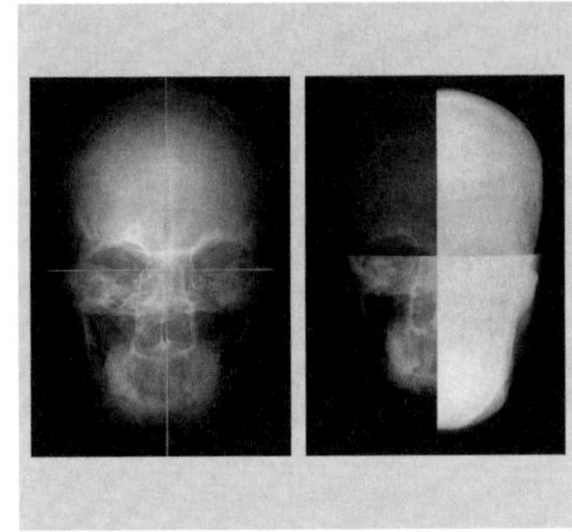

211

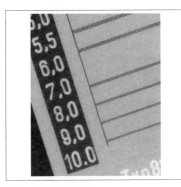

212

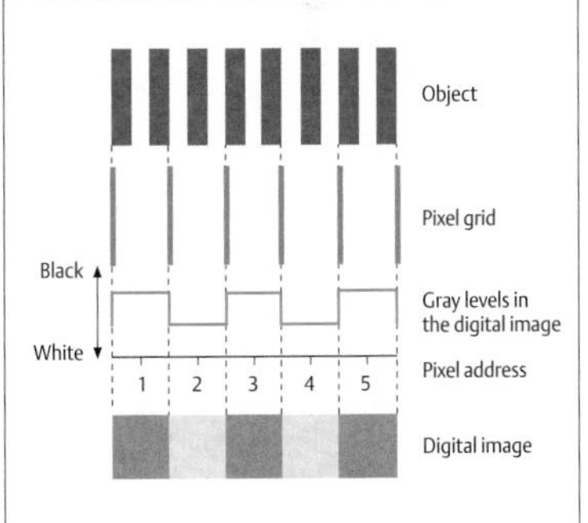

213

Sensitivity: TP/(TP + FN)
True-positive findings in relation to all diseased individuals; thus, a measure for the capability to detect a lesion when a lesion actually exists.

Specificity: TN/(TN + FP)
True-negative findings in relation to all healthy individuals; thus, a measure for the capability to eliminate a lesion when no lesion exists

True-positive findings: TP (true-positive)
False-negative findings: FN (false-negative)
False-positive findings: FP (false-positive)
True-negative findings: TN (true-negative)

214

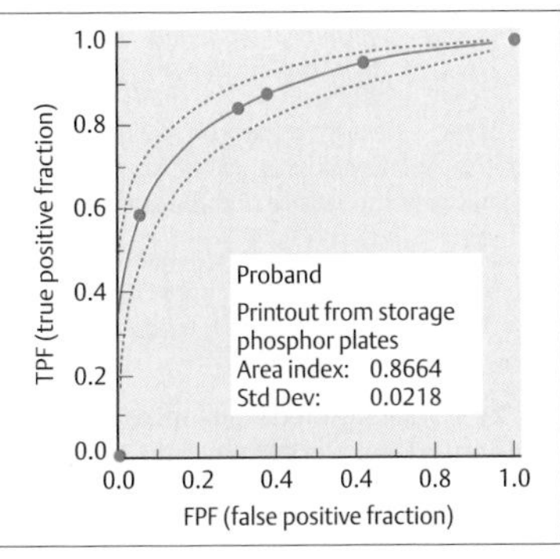

215

Radiation dose reduction by means of digital radiography: Digital image receptor systems have a high level of sensitivity and a broad dynamic scope. It is for this reason that a significant reduction of radiation dose can be achieved in contrast to conventional radiography.

Table **1** (below) presents the typical energy dose values in the at-risk organs of the head and neck, as well as an estimation of the effective doses with conventional and digital radiography. A radiation dose reduction vis-à-vis conventional technique will only be successfully achieved, however, when the conditions of exposure are properly synchronized with each other. For example, a small-format digital sensor (2 x 3 cm) should not be used in conjunction with a broad roentgen ray bundle (6-cm round cone).

Estimation of radiation exposure: Radiation exposure of the patient can be measured by skin surface dosimetry, or by using a radiographic "phantom" head. Such artificial test heads are, however, expensive. The dose per surface area product is easy to measure and is proportional to the exposure of a real patient. It is for this reason that the phantom head is used in the definition of dosage standards.

Table 1 Radiation exposure with typical conventional and digital radiographic examinations (Visser 2000).

Radiographic technique and exposure settings	**Energy dose in the at-risk organs (mGy)**			**Effective dose (μSv)**
Ø = Round cone □ = rectangular diaphragm	Lens of the eye	Parotid gland	Thyroid gland	
Intraoral films (70 kV/7 mA/1.5 mm Al)				
Intraoral film (3 × 4 cm, sensitivity E), Ø 6 cm (11 exposures/1.80 s/480 mGy cm²)	0.105	0.508	0.052	34.5
Intraoral film (3 × 4 cm, sensitivity E), □ 3 × 4 cm (11 exposures/1.80 s/320 mGy cm²)	0.088	0.246	0.049	18.5
CCD sensor chip (2 × 3 cm), Ø 6 cm (20 exposures/1.08 s/283 mGy cm²)	*0.106*	*0.682*	*0.018*	*21.7*
CCD sensor chip (2 × 3 cm), □ 3 × 4 cm (20 exposures/1.08 s/188 mGy cm²)	*0.033*	*0.137*	*0.012*	*10.3*
Storage phosphor (3 × 4 cm), □ 3 × 4 cm (11 exposures/0.37 s/67 mGy cm²)	*0.032*	*0.150*	*0.006*	*5.4*
Panoramic radiograph technique				
Orthopantomography 10E (75 kV/8 mA/15 s/71 mGy cm²)	0.014	0.406	0.017	19.1
Orthopantomography 100 digipan (Prg. I) (66–70 kV/5 mA/17.6 s/28 mGy cm²)	*0.003*	*0.223*	*0.006*	*4.9*

Fig. 216a The dose measured at a given point *decreases* with the square of the distance of the point from the radiation source. At the same time, the cross-sectional area of the effective radiation beam *increases* with the square of the distance. Their product, therefore, remains constant.

Fig. 216b The measurement chamber (in the figure, the Kerma X-C device; Wellhöfer Dosimetry Co., Schwarzenbruck) is positioned in the projected ray such that the entire cross-sectional area of the effective radiation beam is measured. The measurement read-out device can be installed outside of the radiography room.

Fig. 217 Radiation dosage measurement during digital intraoral radiography. A digital sensor is placed into the mouth of the phantom head. On the "skin" surface and inside the phantom head are numerous thermoluminescence (TL)-detectors (Visser 2000).

Fig. 218 The dose-surface product is especially well suited as a quantitative index. For a periapical film survey, bite-wing surveys, and panoramic radiographs, the effective dose is proportional to the dose-surface product (Visser 2000).

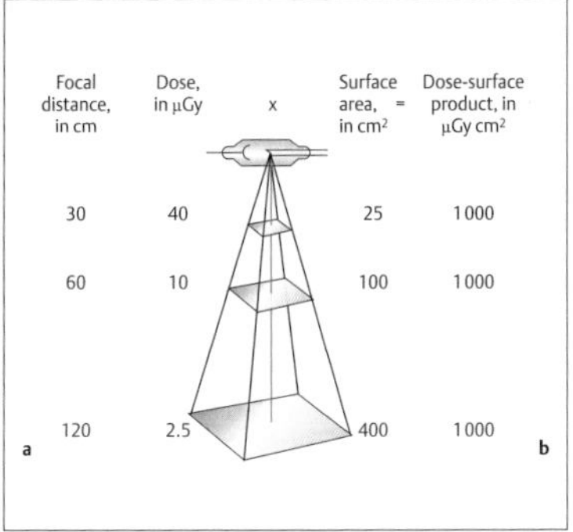

216 a

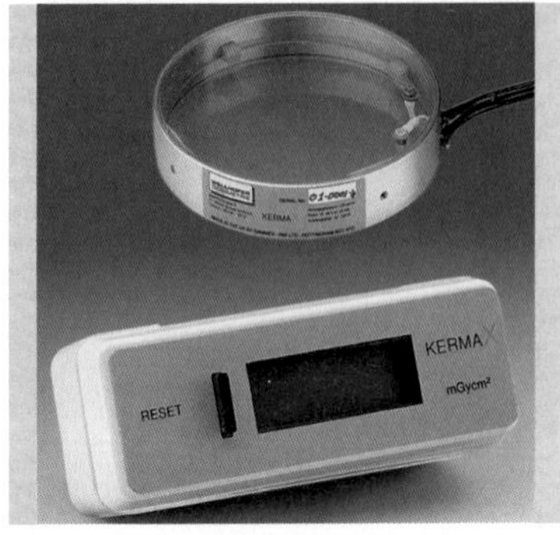

216 b

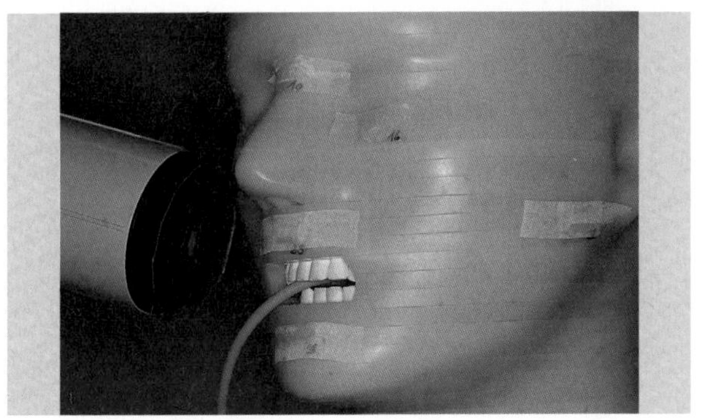

217

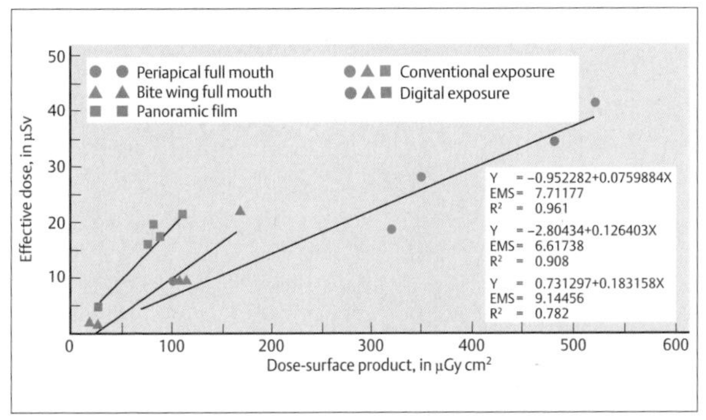

218

Radiographic Pathology

These chapters are structured around considerations in radiographic diagnosis. Presented are comprehensive depictions of a large variety of anomalies, dysmorphias, and regressive alterations of the teeth that confront each dentist in daily practice. The material is presented from a very practical point-of-view, which permits presentation of the most important radiographic findings in the relatively small space available. Because some of these pathologic alterations are genetically determined, the most important syndromes that may play a role are also briefly mentioned.

Hypodontia, Hyperodontia

Deviations from the normal number of teeth are referred to as anodontia, hypodontia, oligodontia, and hyperodontia. Complete absence of any teeth, as observed for example in ectodermal dysplasias, is referred to as anodontia. Both primary and permanent dentitions may be affected. It is worthy of note that a clinical appearance of anodontia may not be an appropriate diagnosis, and will demand the preparation of a panoramic radiograph. One example is the GAPO syndrome (genetically associated progeria syndrome), in which the partial symptom of clinical edentulousness is referred to as pseudoanodontia.

The term **hypodontia** is used to describe the congenital absence of teeth, which may be part of a phylogenetic dentition reduction. Included here are third molars, maxillary lateral incisors, mandibular central incisors, as well as second premolars. Hypodontia is also frequently observed in various syndromes, for example in chondroectodermal dysplasia (Ellis-van-Creveld syndrome) or premature graying of the hair.

The term **oligodontia** is used to describe a lower than normal number of teeth; this may be observed in various tooth groups with numerous congenitally missing elements. Oligodontia is also frequently a component of syndromes such as frontometaphyseal dysplasia (Gorlin–Cohen syndrome), the Marshall–Smith syndrome, iridodental dysplasia (Rieger syndrome), or in occulodentodigital dysplasia (Meyer–Schwickerath–Weyer syndrome).

Fig. 219 **Hypodontia**. The panoramic radiograph of a 7-year-old female reveals the congenital absence of second premolars in all four quadrants. This anomaly is pathognomonic for more than a dozen syndromes, frequently combined with nail and hair dysplasias. Note here also the delayed development of the maxillary and mandibular incisors.

Fig. 220 **Oligodontia**. The panoramic radiograph of a 12-year-old male clearly reveals the absence of numerous teeth from various tooth groups; this is a characteristic of oligodontia, which is one form of hypodontia. The definitive diagnosis clearly must not be made solely on the basis of a clinical examination. The differential diagnosis of the various forms of oligodontia and anodontia should not be made without a panoramic radiograph because of the frequency of concomitant tooth retention (impaction). Not infrequently, these anomalies represent the oral symptoms of a systemic syndrome.

Fig. 221 **Hyperodontia**. This panoramic radiograph of a 25-year-old male reveals supernumerary maxillary premolars, with persistence of the deciduous molars. Hyperodontia is often observed in cases of cleidocranial dysplasia (Scheuthauer–Marie–Sainton Syndrome [see Fig. **222**]), usually only in the permanent dentition, or in both primary and permanent dentitions in cases of intestinal polyposis III (Gardner Syndrome, see Fig. **435**).

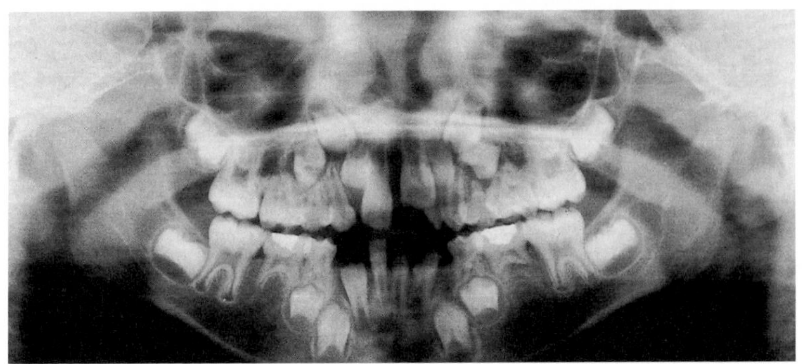

219

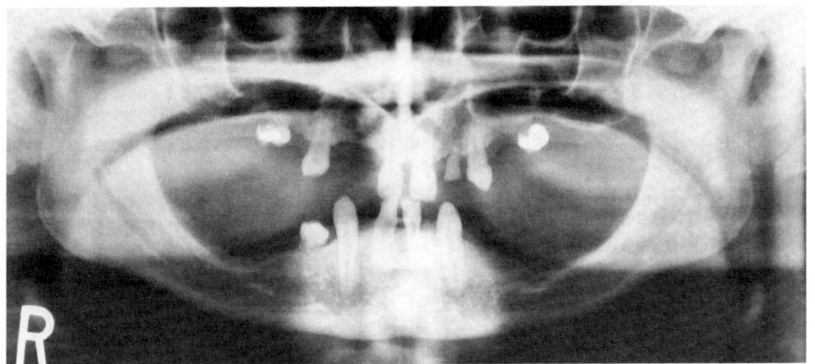

220

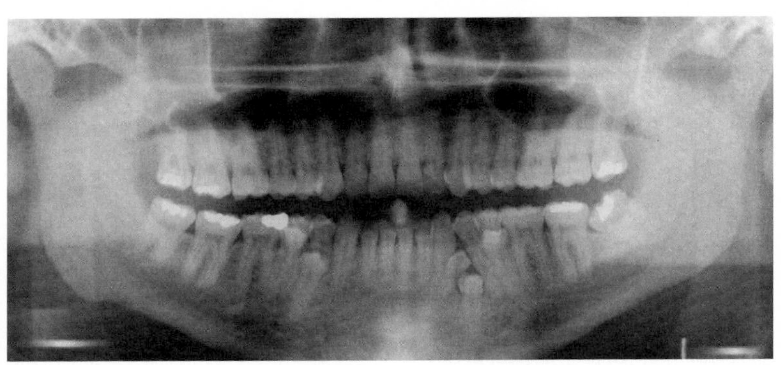

221

Hyperodontia is a term used to describe a condition in which there exists an excessive number of teeth. Included in this category is the mesiodens, which frequently occurs as a peg-shaped anterior tooth, or gemination (*twin teeth*) in the maxillary anterior region, supernumerary premolars or retromolars which, in the absence of any other explanation may be viewed as an overproduction by an irritated dental lamina. Hyperodontia is also observed in various syndromes, for example, cleidocranial dysplasia (Scheuthauer–Marie–Sainton syndrome), mandibulo-oculofacial dysmorphia (Hallermann–Streiff–François syndrome), or intestinal polyposis III (Gardner syndrome).

Clinically obvious over- or under-sized teeth represent conditions referred to as **macrodontia** or **microdontia** (see p. 159). Microdontia is often observed as rudimentary forms of third molars and retromolars, also as maxillary lateral incisors and other supernumerary teeth (e.g., mesiodens), and frequently exhibits a conically shaped crown. Microdontia is frequently observed as a component of the Marshall–Smith syndrome, the Johanson–Blizzard syndrome, and the Rothmund–Thomson syndrome, where it is often combined with oligodontia. Cases of pronounced macrodontia are extremely rare, and usually occur only through gemination (*twinning*) as in geminated maxillary central incisors. “Gigantism” of other teeth is rare (see Fig. **239a**). With some radiographic techniques, the boundaries between normal, oversized, and undersized teeth can be clearly perceived only when there is a striking discrepancy in size because, depending on whether the tooth in question is nearer the radiation source (further from the sensor) or further from the source (nearer the sensor) the tooth in question can appear either smaller or larger than its actual size (see Fig. **3a**).

Malformations of the Jaws

Cheilognathopalatoschisis (clefts of lip, jaw, palate) results from an inhibition of normal closure of the two halves of the maxillary process premaxilla from the 4th-9th week of embryogenesis. As the rate of malformations increases, so also does the number of combinations of these malformations. The cleft formations may be unilateral or bilateral, and the teeth near the clefts frequently appear as microdonts, with disturbances of mineralization of the dental enamel, aplasias, or as supernumerary teeth.

Fig. 222 Dysplasias and malformations of the jaws. This panoramic radiograph of a 13-year-old male is typical of cleidocranial dysplasia (Scheuthauer–Marie–Sainton Syndrome) with the classical primary symptoms of clavicular aplasia. The syndrome is also associated, however, with hypoplasias and dysplasias of the collar bone and is usually also associated with maxillary hypoplasia and microdontia. It is a genetic disorder, autosomal dominant with variable expressions, causing genetically based disturbances of ossification.

Fig. 223 Dysplasias and malformations of the jaws. This panoramic radiograph of a 19-year-old female reveals a bilateral cleft of palate and jaw (clinically, also the lip). The extraordinarily high number (beyond 100) of different clinical appearances of these clefts, with variable expression, leads to the conclusion that the cheilognathopalatoschisis can be an accompanying symptom in many different syndromes. Also identifiable in this radiograph are the dysplastic maxillary anterior teeth in the premaxilla, the microdont with enamel defects near to the cleft, the supernumerary microdont on the right side, the total absence of tooth 45 and the persistence of the remnants of tooth 85, chronic apical periodontitis on the nonvital and dysplastic tooth 35, and profound caries on nonvital tooth 36.

Fig. 224 Dysplasias and malformations of the jaws. This panoramic radiograph depicts a rare dysplasia of the mandible, with double-formation of the ascending ramus. The right side of the mandible encompasses numerous microdonts that resemble a compound odontoma. It is remarkable that the indentation or notch in the hypoplastic mandible is located precisely where the latent osseous cavern (Stafne cyst) is observed as a serendipitous finding below the mandibular canal. The basal compact bone is also significantly thickened at this site (cf. p. **281**).

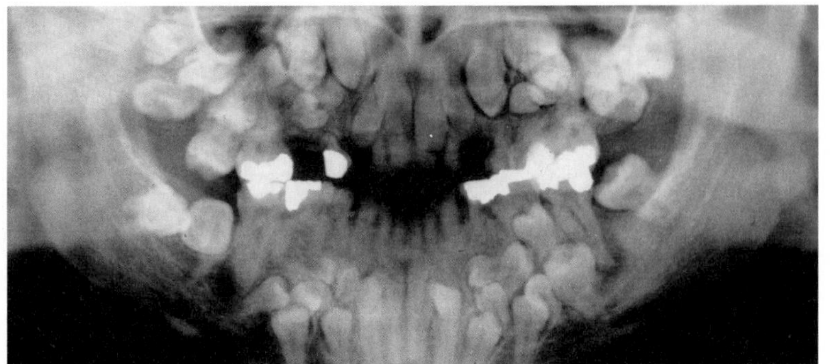

222

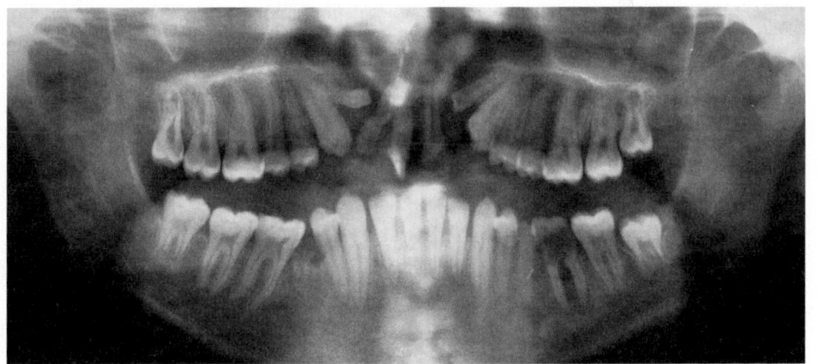

223

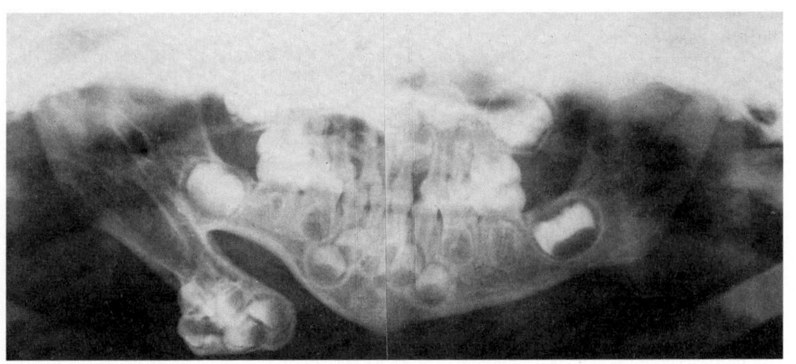

224

In addition to several genetically based facial clefts, such as those that occur in the context of the oculodentodigital syndrome (Meyer–Schwickerath–Weyer syndrome), the ectrodactyl-ectodermal dysplasia clefting syndrome (EEC), arthro-ophthalmopathy (Marshall–Smith–Stickler syndrome), and the cheilognathopalatoschisis with lower lip fistula (bilateral, Van-der-Woude syndrome), the heritability of the partial symptom of lip-jaw-palate clefting in the numerous combinations with other malformation complexes has not yet been clearly demonstrated.
The radiographic diagnosis is of extreme importance for the planning of any surgical procedure. In addition to a panoramic radiograph to provide basic information, other radiographs are usually required for accurate measurement of the width of the cleft, the teeth near the cleft, and the osseous environment. Supplemental intraoral radiographs possibly also combined with occlusal radiographs of appropriate sizes and wherever possible taken using an appropriate IRH, and with appropriate reduction of exposure settings will be required to provide supplemental radiographs with a high level of image clarity. Three-dimensional surface reconstructions using computer tomography (CT) can also be very helpful during surgical planning, if the higher radiation exposure is acceptable.
In cases of **malformations of the mandible** from the first pharyngeal arch, hemihypoplasia of the splanchnocranium can occur, with involvement of the mandible; these are mainly classified within oculoauriculovertebral dysplasia (Goldenhar–Cortin syndrome with oculoauricular and oculovertebral syndrome, Weyers–Thier syndrome). The clinical and radiographic symptoms can range from discrete hypoplasias with micromandibular retrognathia all the way to obvious facial asymmetries and double formation of the mandibular condyle (see Fig. **328**) and/or the ascending mandibular ramus.
In addition to panoramic radiography and targeted conventional skull projections, diagnosis today relies primarily on CT with three-dimensional surface reconstructions.

Fig. 225 Dentinogenesis imperfecta. This panoramic radiograph of a 17-year-old female depicts the incongruity between the tooth crowns that are still surrounded by intact enamel, and the hypoplastic roots, which exhibit obliterated pulp chambers and root canals; this is typical for the radicular type of dentinogenesis imperfecta.

Fig. 226 Dentinogenesis imperfecta. This panoramic radiograph of a 38-year-old female (Capdepont Syndrome) shows the typical picture of disproportionality between the tooth crowns and the hypoplastic roots in a less conspicuous form of dentinogenesis imperfecta; this is because there are also enamel defects caused by attrition, and this makes the tooth crowns appear smaller in the radiograph. Coronal type of dentinogenesis imperfecta.

Fig. 227 Taurodontism. In addition to the remaining tooth 85 and the fragment of tooth 75, this panoramic radiograph reveals impacted mandibular second premolars and a taurodont in the posterior segment of all four quadrants. Typical are the coronoapically elongated pulp chambers, the broad root canals, and the short roots of the first permanent molars, while second molars exhibit only a single and very wide root canal. The mandibular premolars often also exhibit very short roots in addition to the elongated pulp chamber. The appearance of a taurodont is inherited as an irregular dominant trait.

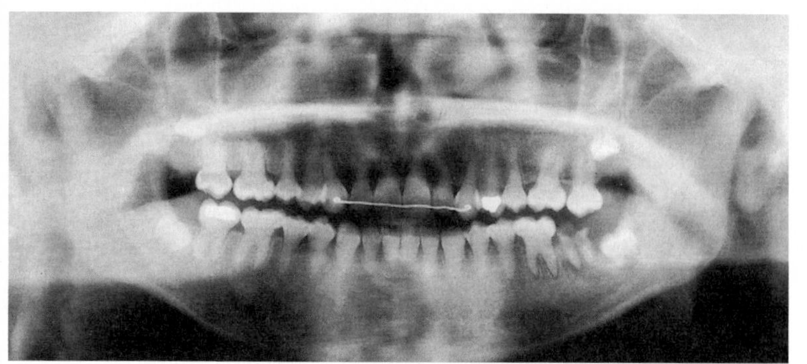

225

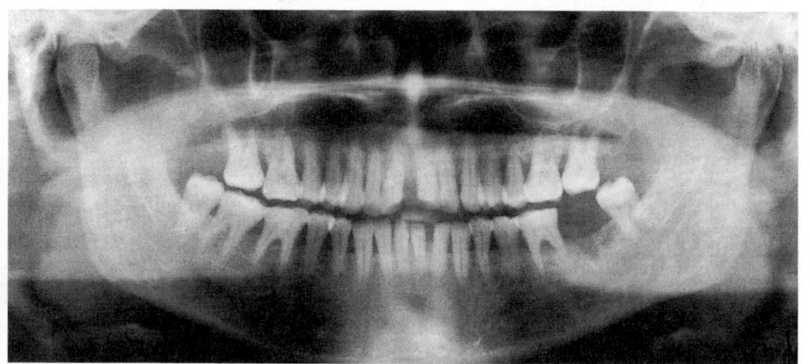

226

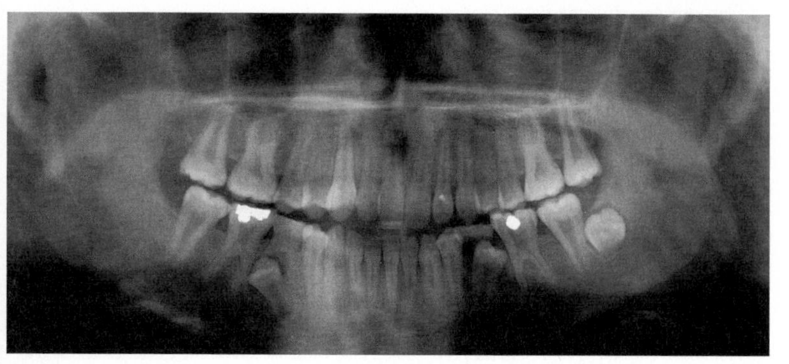

227

Dentinogenesis imperfecta and **dentin dysplasia** are not only heritable as autosomal dominant traits (*exception*: Goldblatt syndrome with autosomal recessive heredity), but can also be caused by environmental factors. Despite many similarities, these two conditions continue today to be viewed clinically as distinct entities, which are further classified into subtypes. The radiographic diagnosis of dentinogenesis imperfecta is primarily one of hypoplastic roots with obliterated root canals and pulp chambers, which appear in a disproportionate size relationship to the non-affected tooth crowns (Capdepont syndrome, or also in osteogenesis imperfecta, Lobstein types I–IV).

The radicular type of dentin dysplasia exhibits a similar radiographic appearance, with obliterations and possible denticle formation; the primary dentition is more severely affected. Fracture and abrasion of the dental enamel that is insufficiently bound to the pathologically altered dentin has been described for both dentinogenesis imperfecta as well as dentin dysplasia of the coronal type; this usually makes it impossible to achieve any radiographic differentiation.

Taurodont

Taurodonts may occur as individual teeth or entire groups of teeth (*taurodontism*). They are almost always characterized by a coronoapically elongated coronal pulp, and with short, horn-like roots, or also by a single very wide root canal. Taurodontism may be genetically based, also as a partial symptom of De-Barsy syndrome in both primary and permanent dentitions, or in cases of tricho-dento-osseous syndrome (TDO, or Robinson–Millerworth syndrome). Frequently the mandibular premolars are affected, as well as the molars in all four quadrants.

The panoramic radiograph provides an overview of all of the teeth. If endodontic therapy becomes necessary, additional supplemental intraoral radiographs will be required.

Amelogenesis Imperfecta

Amelogenesis imperfecta is a genetically based enamel dysplasia that may occur in both primary and permanent dentitions, but most commonly in the permanent dentition. From the clinical standpoint, one can differentiate among the following manifestations:

Fig. 228 Amelogenesis imperfecta. These bitewing radiographs depict a case of amelogenesis imperfecta type III, characterized by hypocalcification of the teeth (with intact enamel portions at the cementoenamel junction).

Fig. 229 Amelogenesis imperfecta. This 11-film intraoral radiographic survey of an 11-year-old female depicts hypocalcification of the teeth with transverse bands of radiolucency. The enamel of the undercalcified crowns ends as peg-shaped extensions that display radiopacity beneath the dentin density. The radiographic picture is similar to that frequently seen in cases of hypocalcemic vitamin D-dependent Ricketts, which is caused by a genetically based metabolic disease. In most cases the radiographs of this disorder serve primarily only for documentation; differentiation between and among the individual types of the disease is primarily a clinical endeavor. With regard to obtaining useful radiographic documentation, it is of technical importance that the exposure settings for the depiction of poorly calcified structures must be lower than would normally be used.

Fig. 230 a, b Hypercementosis. **a** Section from a panoramic radiograph revealing isolated hypercementosis on tooth 38. **b** Intraoral radiograph of the same case. Cemental dysplasias in the form of hypercementosis sometimes occur as the result of trauma or chronic apical periodontitis, and only rarely on vital teeth (for example in Gardner Syndrome). But they may also be observed as a generalized finding in elderly males, where they represent a radiographic sign for the existence of osteodystrophy deformans (Paget disease of bone).

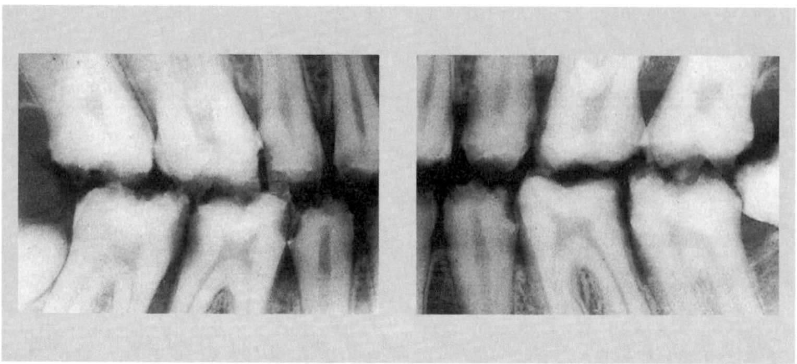

228

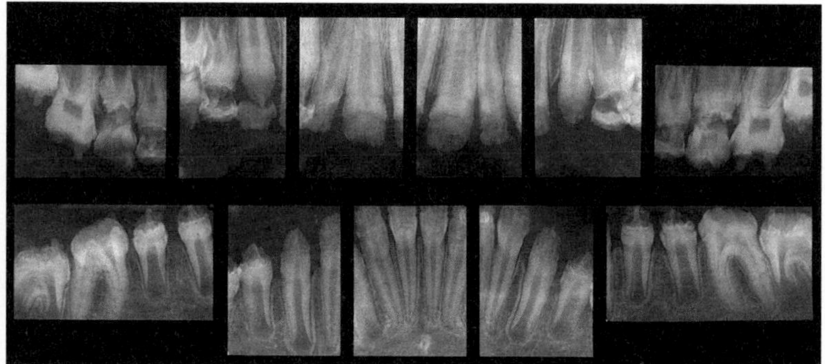

229

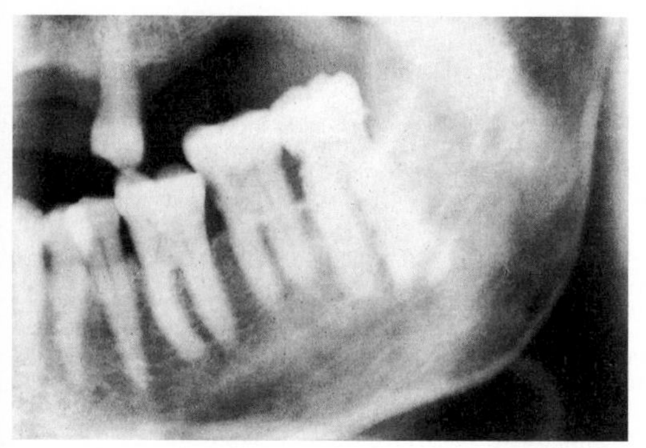

230 a

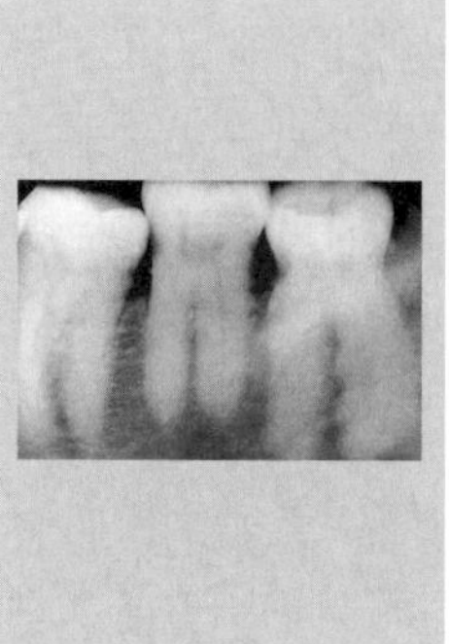

230 b

- Dental enamel hypoplasias of various types range from small and locally demarcated hypoplastic enamel defects and thin enamel caps all the way to total aplasia of the enamel; even sex-linked genetic forms are known. Enamel hypoplasias have been described in conjunction with the Costello syndrome and the tricho-dento-osseous syndrome (Robinson–Millerworth syndrome, often accompanied by taurodontism).
- The underlying cause of clinically observed tooth crown attrition is likely the various types of hypomaturation and mineralization deficiencies in the face of otherwise normally thick but soft (immature) dental enamel. Sex-linked genetic forms are known. For example, hypomaturation has also been observed in cases of hypohidrotic ectodermal dysplasia.
- Hypocalcification occurs in various types through faulty calcification of tooth enamel where the enamel mantel was originally of normal thickness but very soft. The cervical portions of the enamel cap may nevertheless remain intact. Combinations of hypocalcification with seborrhea (sebaceous gland hyperfunction, Witkop–Brearley–Gentry syndrome) and onycholysis have been described. Yellowish discoloration of teeth due to hypocalcification is endemic in Switzerland (Kohlschütter–Tönz syndrome).

In cases such as this the primary value of radiographs are forensic and for insurance purposes, because it is rarely possible to arrive at true diagnostic differentiation on the basis of radiographic examination. The panoramic radiograph is the overview of choice in disease types that include osteodystrophy and impacted dysplastic teeth. Periapical radiographs remain absolutely necessary, taken using reduced exposure settings and supplemented in the posterior segments with bitewing radiographs. It must be kept uppermost in mind that when taking radiographs of patients suffering from enamel defects, the exposure settings must be reduced in comparison to normal, in order to achieve perfect documentation.

Cemental Dysplasias

Cemental dysplasias occur in many variations and also as characteristic components of many disorders such as periapical dysplasia (see p. **269/271**), cementoblastoma, cementoblastic fibroma, in cases of hypophosphatasia

Fig. 231 Odontodysplasia. The panoramic radiograph of a 15-year-old female presents a rare form of unilateral odontodysplasia in the region of teeth 41–47; the etiology was never clarified.

Fig. 232a *Dens in dente*. The periapical radiograph of tooth 23 reveals a dysplastic root and the appearance of a tooth-like structure *within* tooth 23; the tooth also exhibits chronic apical periodontitis. This rare case, which affected a maxillary canine and not a maxillary lateral incisor, is a case of true duplicature—a true *dens in dente*—which may be closely related to an odontoma. With the related *dens invaginatus*, which much more frequently occurs on maxillary lateral incisors, the defect is different in that it results from an effective invagination of the enamel organ. This results in various shapes and sizes of coronal invagination emanating from the cingulum. Such manifestations of coronal invaginations may also rarely originate from deep fissures, especially in mandibular premolars.

Fig. 232b *Dentes confusi* (a true macrodont is shown in Fig. 239a). This section from a panoramic radiograph depicts two maxillary central incisors which, as a result of gemination, have developed into "fused teeth" or "composite teeth." The clinical appearance is one of extremely wide tooth crowns that are not infrequently characterized by a varyingly deep groove in the middle of the incisal edge of the tooth. The radiographic appearance depicts very wide roots and broad pulp chambers, which often exhibit two pronounced pulp horns.

Fig. 233 Gemination. This panoramic radiograph of a 53-year-old female exhibits a rare form of gemination in which the crowns of both completely developed mandibular molars reside in a common follicular sac, which appears in the radiograph to be a large follicular cyst emanating from the cemento-enamel junctions (CEJ) of both impacted molars. The slow-growing lesion caused compression and a typical displacement of the mandibular canal.

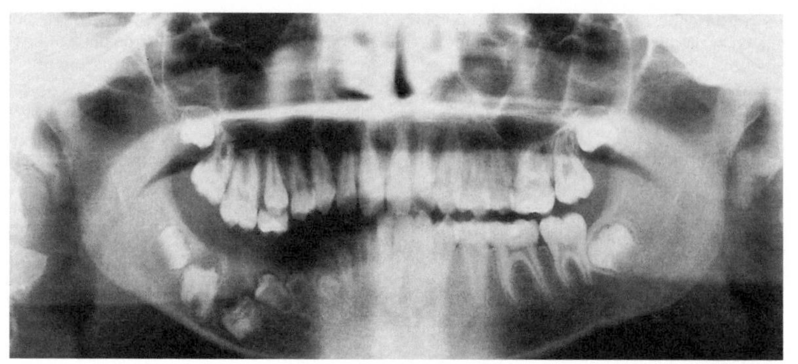

231

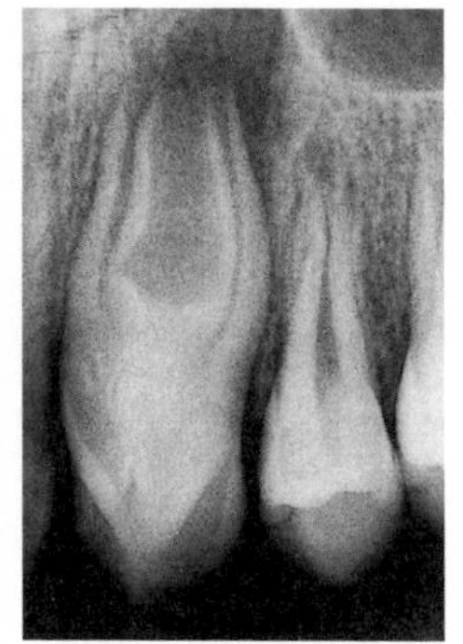

232 a

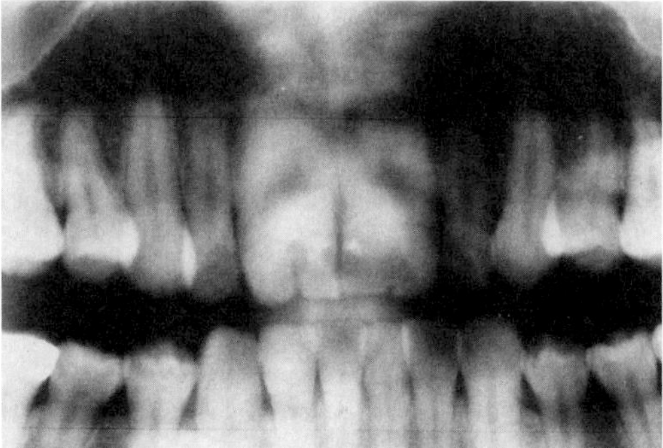

232 b

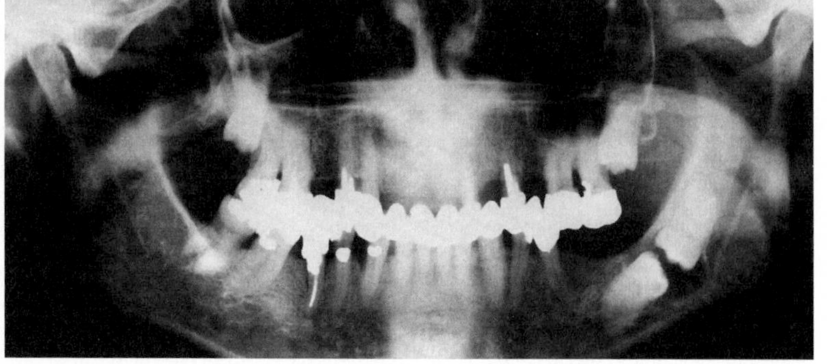

233

(Rathbun syndrome), and with osteitis deformans (Paget disease of bone, p. **291**). Hypercementosis is characterized by excessive formation of cementum, which can be caused by periapical inflammation or traumatic occlusion.

In cases of vital teeth with hypercementosis, the periodontal ligament space is maintained, but may not always be clearly visible, depending upon the resolution capacity of the radiographic equipment employed.

Odontodysplasias

Odontodysplasias present as malformations of ecto- and mesodermal portions of the affected teeth, so that enamel, dentin, as well as root cementum may be affected. The normal eruption of such malformed teeth is disturbed or delayed. Dysplastic and impacted teeth and portions of teeth can develop follicular cysts, and are frequently resorbed. Dental dysplasia may be observed as a manifestation of osteogenesis imperfecta (Lobstein type). The etiology can involve early trauma, radiotherapy, and tumors or tumor-like lesions that developed in early childhood.

Gemination, *dens in dente*, duplicature (*twinning*): A deep palatal pit (cingulum; foramen caecum) on a maxillary lateral incisor, or a deep occlusal fissure on a mandibular first premolar can be the clinical signs of enamel invagination, which can best be depicted using periapical radiographs. **Gemination** refers to the double formation of a tooth bud or the incomplete division of same. The rare occurrence of a ***dens in dente*** or also **duplicature** with complete division of the tooth bud is found most often with maxillary canines, and may be considered similar to the odontoma (see p. **265**). With large invaginations or a full *dens in dente*, pulpal necrosis frequently occurs, with subsequent periapical inflammation. The ***dentes confusi*** (fused teeth) occurs through the union of two tooth buds or separation of a single bud; the clinical appearance is referred to as the **macrodont.** Radiographic diagnosis reveals a united, plump root with a greatly enlarged pulp chamber. Most often affected are the maxillary central incisors of both primary and permanent dentitions. ***Dentes concreti*** (coalesced teeth) is a term that refers to teeth that are fused together only in the root segments. Most often involved are the maxillary second and third molars. A rare instance of duplicature can sometimes be observed in the molar region of the mandible where the crowns of two impacted molars exist within the same follicular sac (Fig. **233**). The occlusal surfaces of the involved molars always approximate each other closely.

Fig. 234 a, b ***Dentes concreti.*** **a** The intraoral, periapical radiograph of the left maxillary tuberosity region depicts tooth 27, whose root tip appears overlapped by the roots of the deeply horizontally impacted tooth 28. The intraoral radiograph provides a summation effect that does *not* provide information about whether the two teeth are actually fused to each other or not, but suspicion of tooth fusion in such cases cannot be ruled out. **b** This radiograph of the extracted molars reveals that teeth 27 and 28 were actually fused together via a bridge of cementum.

Fig. 235a **Denticle.** Denticles are the so-called "pulp stones" that exist as free entities or near the wall of the pulp chamber or within root canals. It is not possible from a radiographic diagnostic point-of-view to determine whether the radiopaque bodies are free within the pulpal tissue or actually attached to the internal root canal wall. This bitewing radiograph of a young patient reveals not only proximal caries on tooth 25, but also denticles within the coronal pulp of teeth 26, 35, and 36.

Fig. 235b **Denticle.** This periapical radiograph of the region of tooth 13 also reveals numerous denticles within the root canals of tooth 14. Note also the proximal caries on the mesial surface.

Fig. 236a, b **Enamel pearls.** **a** The periapical radiograph reveals a roundish radiopacity apical to the pulp chamber of tooth 36. Note that this radiograph was taken with a slightly distal-excentric projection in which the central ray was targeted on tooth 37. **b** This section from a panoramic radiograph of the same tooth reveals that the roundish and well-demarcated radiopacity was caused by an *addition effect* (overlapping) of the two roots of tooth 36, thus simulating the presence of an enamel pearl.

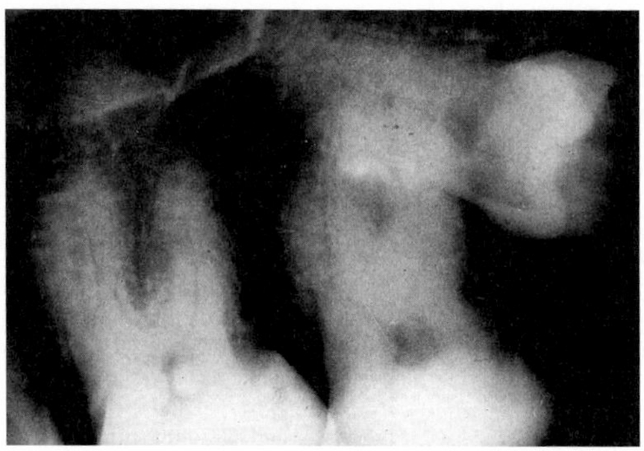

234 a

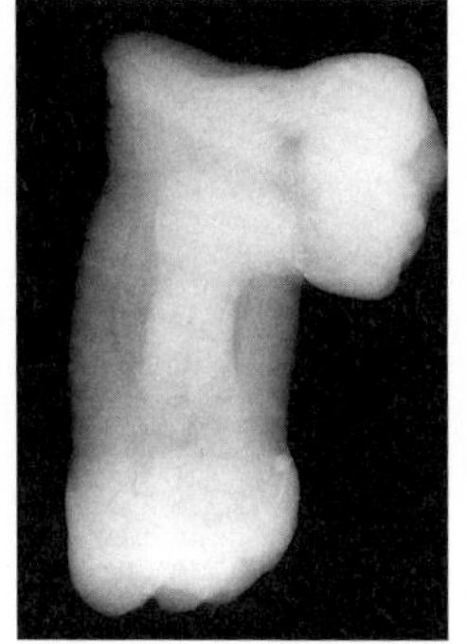

234 b

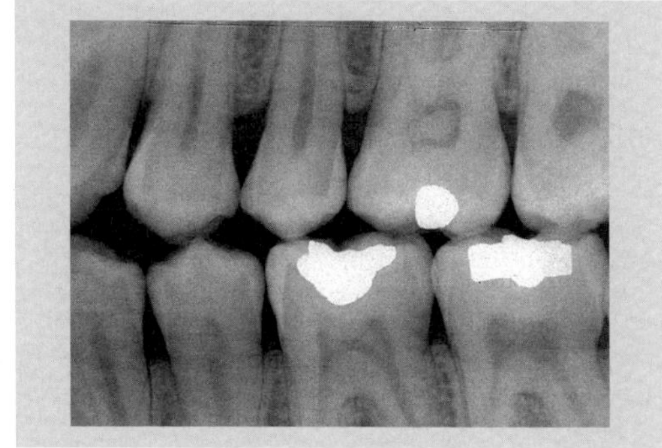

235 a

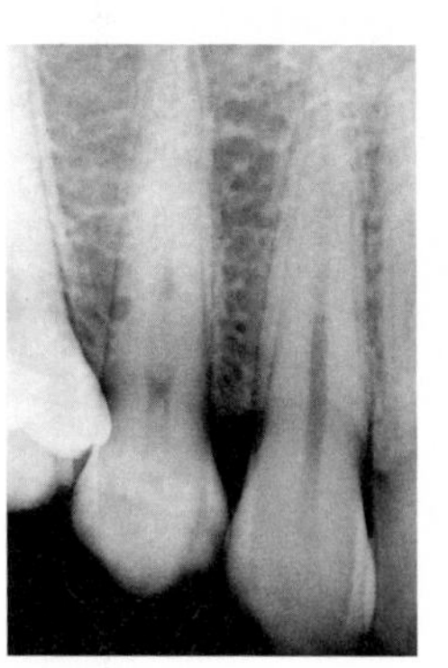

235 b

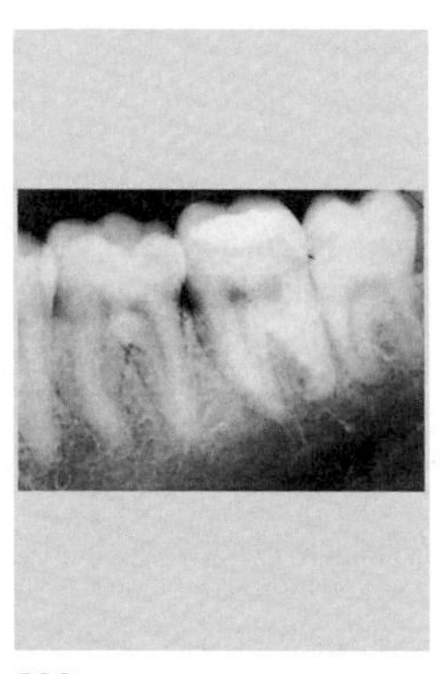

236 a

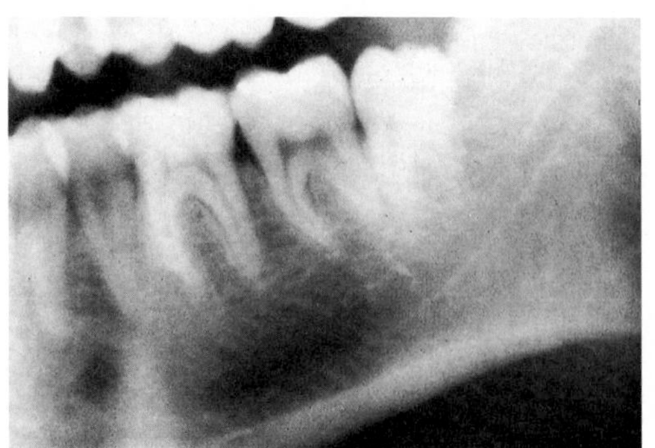

236 b

Denticles or "**pulp stones**" are radiopaque hard tissue structures within the coronal pulp chamber and/or the root canal pulp. In the literature, one finds differentiations between adherent (near the hard tissue wall) and non-adherent (free), as well as between true and sham denticles. These calcified structures may be of developmental etiology or may be a reaction of the pulp to thermal or bacterial irritation. Some patients may complain of neuralgia. Denticles may be a sub-symptom of the Ehlers–Danlos syndrome. Radiographic diagnosis cannot provide differentiation between and among the various forms of denticles.

Enamel Pearls

Enamel pearls are islands of enamel tissue located distant from the normal enamel cap, usually at the cementoenamel junction or upon the cervical root surface. They can be clearly visualized in the radiograph only when they are located in the proximal regions. The round or roundish radiopacities frequently observed in radiographs of molar regions and furcations are almost always the result of overlapping (addition effect) of the molar roots where they meet the crown of the tooth. This can be visualized by tracing the periodontal ligament space into the interradicular area (see Fig. **236a**).

Impacted Teeth

Impacted teeth: Impediments to normal tooth eruption, as well as ankylosis of a tooth to the alveolar bone are often impossible to depict using individual radiographs, bitewing radiographs, or even a complete intraoral survey, or may be depicted only incompletely. Impacted teeth that are not discovered by the examining dentist represent an extraordinary security and trust risk vis-à-vis the patient. Even though the panoramic radiograph will provide a complete overview of the jaws, it is important to note that because it is a zonographic summation radiograph it must be analyzed with particular care in order to, for example, detect a mesiodens within the overlapping shadow of the cervical vertebrate, or a microdont hidden in the tuberosity and/or retromolar region. It is important to remember that the clinical examination of an edentulous jaw that is recorded and designated as such, can be regarded as *malpractice* if the clinician does not perform a radiographic examination. A dentist may feel that radiographs are unnecessary for a clinically edentulous patient, and may choose to "protect the patient" from radiation exposure. **Wrong** choice! For etiologic reasons that cannot always be deciphered, improperly targeted eruption forces or hindrances to tooth eruption can displace tooth buds and developing teeth into abnormal positions and locations. Any hindrance to normal tooth eruption can cause not only tooth impaction but also pathologic deformation of the affected tooth, which is frequently developing. On the other hand, the forces caused by tooth eruption can also impinge upon adjacent teeth, eliciting inclusions and even tooth resorption; all of these may be associated with neuralgiform pain. The possibility of cystic development and growth of the involved dental sac because of hematogenic infection or exogenous irritation cannot be excluded.

Fig. 237 **Impacted teeth**. The panoramic radiograph of a 22-year-old male clearly depicts impacted third molars in both maxilla and mandible. The eruption of tooth 28 is inhibited by a microdont (micromolar), and is associated with an eruption cyst. The pressure caused by development and eruption of the partially impacted tooth 48 has forced tooth 47 into a horizontal position.

Fig. 238 **Impacted teeth**. The panoramic radiograph of this 42-year-old female depicts an axial projection of microdont 18. It is located high in the maxillary tuberosity (**arrow**), and is quite difficult to discern in this underexposed radiograph because of overlapping by the soft palate. Note also the osteoma on the floor of the right maxillary sinus (compare to p.**123**).

Fig. 239a **Impacted teeth**. This section from a panoramic radiograph of a 9-year-old female depicts the rare macrodont 35.

Fig. 239b **Impacted teeth**. The periapical radiograph of the region of the left maxillary canine exhibits total impaction of tooth 22. The root formation of tooth 23 made its way around the impacted tooth 22 and effectively closed the space between 21 and 24 with its canine crown!

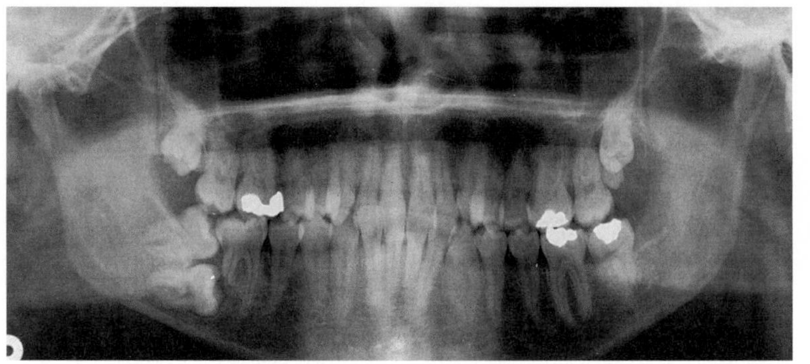

237

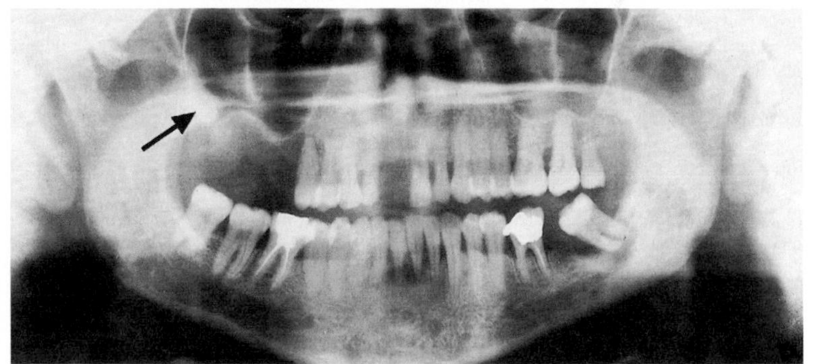

238

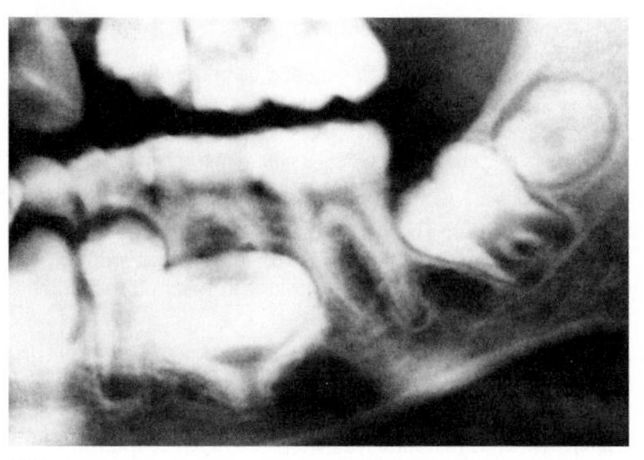

239 a

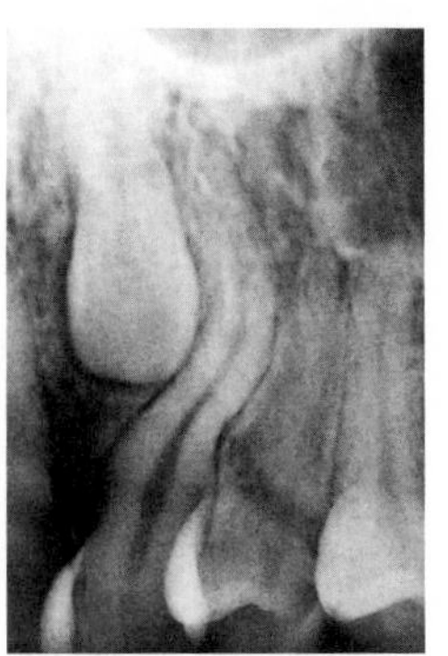

239 b

Impacted/retained teeth often represent a symptom of or manifestation of various syndromes:

- Inherited multiple tooth impaction
- Cleidocranial dysplasia (Scheuthauer–Marie–Sainton syndrome)
- GAPO (genetically associated progeria syndrome)
- Albright's hereditary osteodystrophy
- Gardner syndrome
- Gorlin–Chaudry–Moss syndrome
- Oto-palato-digital syndrome (Taybi syndrome)

Resorption of impacted teeth can also occur as a manifestation of the Rutherford syndrome.

Regressive Alterations, Resorptions

Regressive alterations of the teeth and in the jaws represent involution (degeneration) of biologic structures. In addition to the normal and physiologic resorption of deciduous teeth, resorption may also be observed on impacted teeth that are surrounded partially or entirely by bone; persistent and unphysiologic overloading or injuries resulting from loss of mechanical integrity often instigate such resorption. Tooth resorption may also signal the presence of a syndrome. Resorption and dissolution of teeth and other calcified structures may also occur due to as yet unexplained phenomena that may include growth pressures in the mixed dentition stage, retained deciduous molars, or even endogenic damage of tooth buds of the permanent dentition.

Today, still, we use the term "idiopathic root resorption" to describe all of those cases in which neither a pre-existing trauma, radiation therapy, nor orthodontic therapy can be identified as the etiology. Root resorptions often occur following re-implantation and transplantation of individual teeth.

Following tooth loss, the alveolar ridge becomes severely reduced in size and height, and "alveolar ridge atrophy" is classified under the involutive periodontal diseases, in so far as they are not elicited by any syndrome.

Fig. 240 a Impacted teeth, impediment to tooth eruption. This section from a panoramic radiograph of a 57-year-old male shows a rare instance of impaction of tooth 47, which appears to have completely traversed the body of the mandible, passing lateral to the mandibular canal and even penetrating the basal cortical bone.

Fig. 240 b Impacted teeth, hindrance to eruption. The periapical radiograph reveals the dysplastic tooth 36 with its widely diverging roots, which impinge upon the mandibular canal and appear to be ankylosed to the basal cortical bone of the mandible.

Fig. 241 a Impacted teeth, hindrance to eruption. The periapical radiograph was taken to clarify the diastema between teeth 14 and 12 and the absence of a permanent canine. It clearly shows a complex odontoma inhibiting eruption of the totally impacted tooth 13.

Fig. 241 b Impacted teeth, hindrance to tooth eruption. This section from the panoramic radiograph of a 44-year-old female reveals that the carious and obviously resorbing tooth 75 represents a hindrance to eruption of the impacted tooth 35, which also appears to be ankylosed to the basal compact bone. Radiographic evaluation does not always make it possible to ascertain the existence of ankylosis.

Fig. 242 a Impacted teeth, hindrance to eruption. This periapical radiograph reveals that tooth 35 is completely inhibited from eruption by the adjacent teeth 34 and 36. Note also the eruption cyst and apparent distal reactive sclerosis around the distal root fragment of tooth 75, another hindrance to normal eruption.

Fig. 242 b Impacted teeth, hindrance to eruption. The periapical radiograph reveals a partially impacted tooth 38. As a result of its horizontal impaction position, and the developing periodontal pocket distal to tooth 37, dental caries has developed at the distal cementoenamel junction. Resorption and eruption forces have undermined the nonvital tooth 37, leading ultimately to fracture of the mesial root.

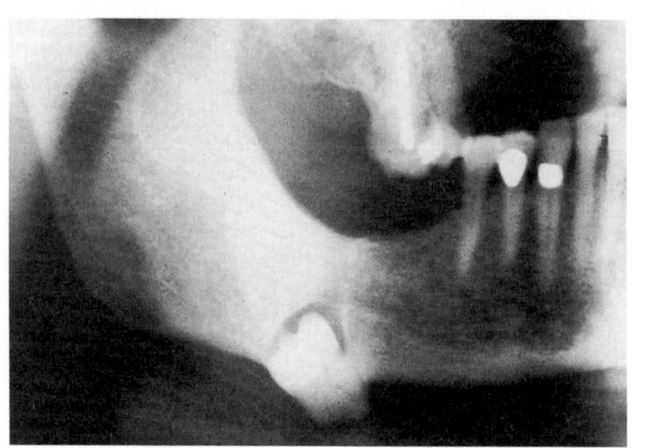
240 a

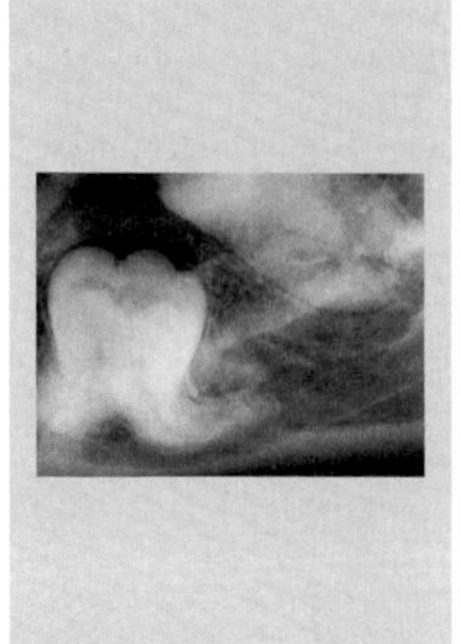
240 b

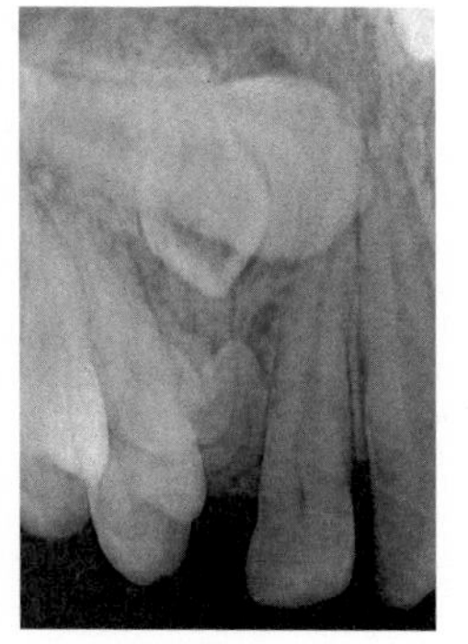
241 a

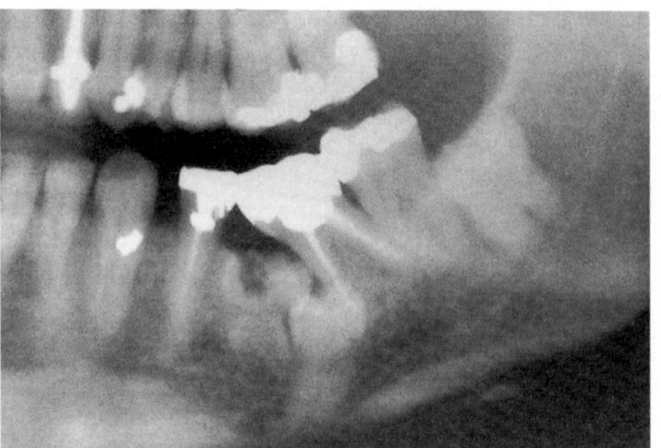
241 b

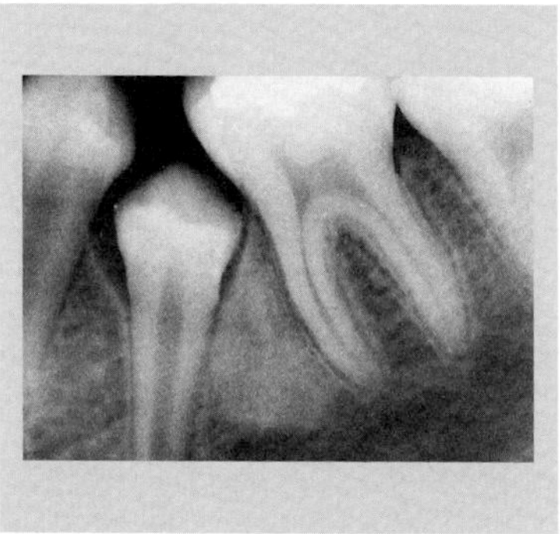
242 a

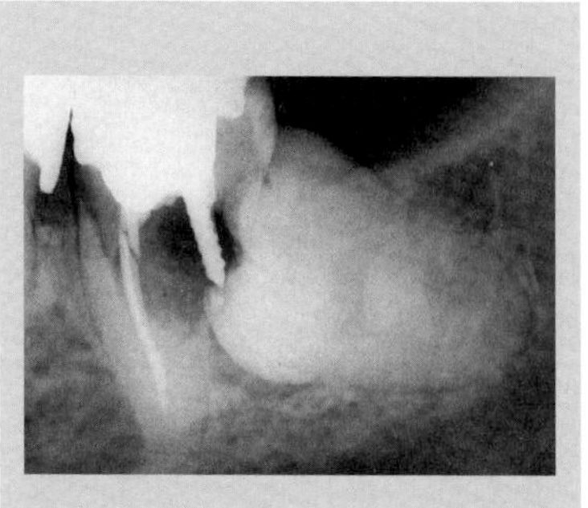
242 b

Tooth resorptions are frequently encountered and can be associated with a myriad of etiologies. A comprehensive summary of the most likely causes would include:

- Physiologic root resorption during the mixed dentition stage
- Resorption of teeth due to endogenic or exogenic irritation
- Root resorption due to chronic periapical inflammation
- Idiopathic resorption
- "Resorptions" resulting from pathologic dentin dysplasias
- *Apparent* "resorptions" caused by subtraction effects and overexposure of radiographs

The eruption forces emanating from the tooth buds of the permanent dentition are responsible for the **physiologic resorption** of the deciduous teeth. Nonvital, infected, or missing deciduous teeth can disturb the normal process of permanent tooth eruption, causing late eruption or altering the direction of eruption leading eventually to tooth positional anomalies.

Numerous endogenic and exogenic influences can lead to **unphysiologic resorption** of teeth. Missing permanent tooth buds or malpositioning of permanent teeth can lead to impaction of deciduous teeth (primarily deciduous molars) or inhibit their normal exfoliation, leading to their eventual resorption.

Delayed eruption, deciduous tooth retention, and resorption of impacted teeth are often also observed in the autosomal-dominant hereditary Rutherford syndrome. Congenitally missing (or resorbed?) premolars are also characteristic of the PHC (*premature hereditary canities*) or Böök syndrome.

If deciduous teeth (especially in the anterior region) persist rather than being normally exfoliated, root resorption is frequent, sometimes followed by substitution with new bone formation.

Internal resorptions of teeth are sometimes observed in retained/impacted and ankylosed molars in the maxilla and, less often, in the mandible; these are almost always the result of pulpal irritations. "Internal granuloma," seen primarily in the maxillary anterior region, may also occur following pulpal irritation (e.g., iatrogenic irritation caused by trauma of tooth preparation or through advancing bacterial infections).

Fig. 243 Regressive alterations of the teeth. This panoramic radiograph of a 22-year-old female reveals idiopathic resorption of submerged deciduous teeth 75 and 85. Note also the direction of the long axes of teeth 35 and 36, as well as the eruption cyst around tooth 18.

Fig. 244 Regressive alterations of the teeth. This panoramic radiograph of a 7-year-old male reveals an idiopathic resorption of the tooth crowns of the unerupted premolars, 35 and 45. Note also the stage of development of tooth buds 34 and 44, where root development has already begun.

Fig. 245a Regressive alterations of the teeth. The periapical radiograph reveals root resorption with new bone formation around the persisting deciduous tooth 53.

Fig. 245b Regressive alterations of the teeth. This section from a panoramic radiograph reveals the almost total resorption of the traumatized bridge abutment, tooth 47, with osseous deposition.

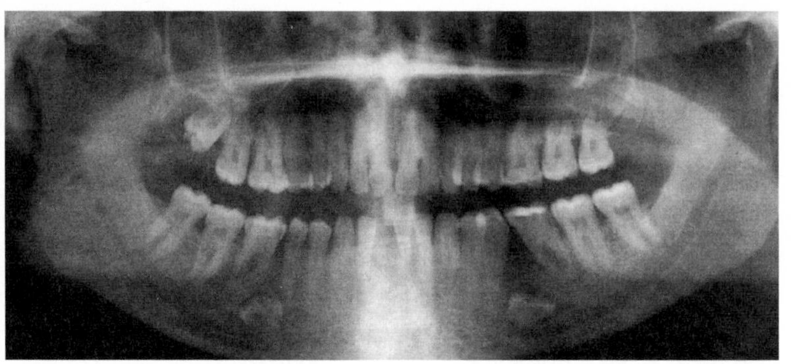

243

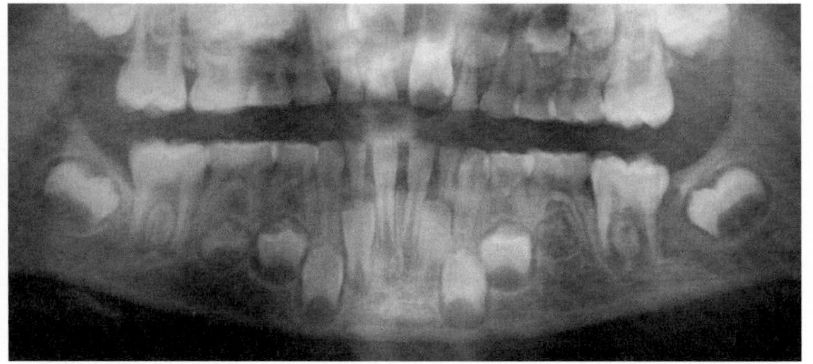

244

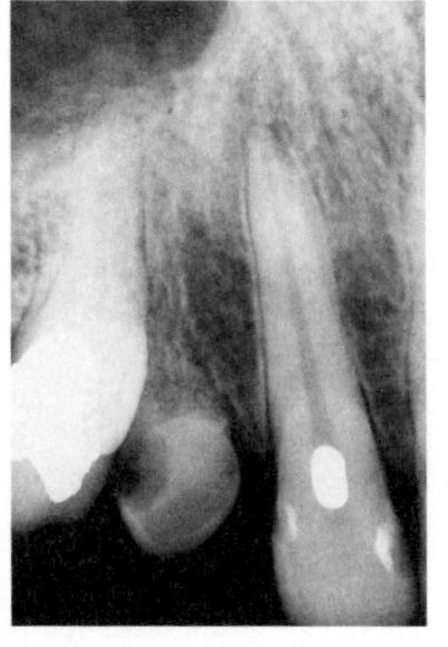

245 a

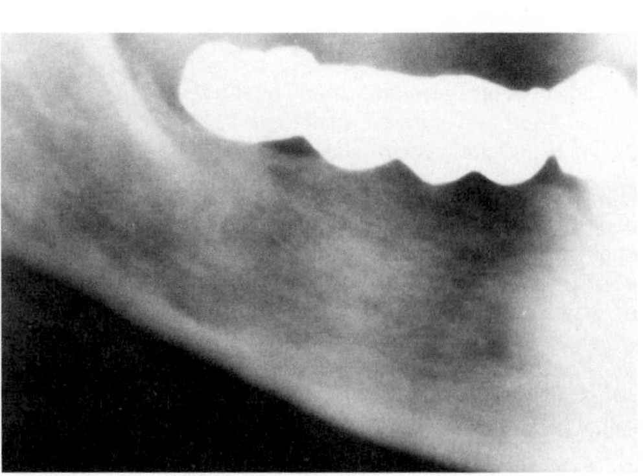

245 b

The internal granuloma originates from the pulpal tissues and can ultimately result in spontaneous fracture of the affected tooth.

External tooth resorption always begins first in the area of the root, and proceeds from the periodontal ligament. Such resorption may be caused iatrogenically, for example through excessive force application during orthodontic treatment or through overloading of abutment teeth by fixed or removable bridgework. External resorption can, however, also occur as the result of accident/trauma, for example, following incomplete tooth luxation, or by the eruption forces exerted by a partially impacted adjacent tooth. Resorptions occur frequently with ankylosed teeth. Root resorption can also occur as a consequence of chronic periapical inflammation.

If a thorough medical and dental history cannot ascertain any etiology for the condition, the loss of tooth substance has to be described as "idiopathic resorption."

Dentin hypoplasia of genetically based etiology (Capdedont syndrome) is often referred to, *incorrectly*, as "resorption." The radiographic picture of radicular dentin hypoplasia occurs not due to resorption but due to insufficient new dentin production. This can be of importance when formulating the radiographic differential diagnosis.

Fig. 246a Regressive alterations of the teeth. This routine periapical radiograph reveals advanced internal resorption of tooth 38; this is not infrequently observed in impacted teeth. Note also the hypercementosis on the mesial root.

Fig. 246b Regressive alterations of the teeth. This section of a panoramic radiograph of a 25-year-old male reveals that tooth 37, following loss of tooth 36, has been tipped mesially by pressure from the third molar; 37 also appears to be ankylosed. This is an advanced case, with internal resorption extending to the area of the root apices.

Fig. 247a Regressive alterations of the teeth. This section from a panoramic radiograph of a 47-year-old female depicts central resorption (internal granuloma) of bridge abutment tooth 13, which, in addition, exhibits secondary caries at the cervical area. Of note also is the profound caries on teeth 11 and 22 (both of which also exhibit radiographic signs of chronic apical periodontitis), the secondary caries distally on tooth 46, and the destruction of the crowns of teeth 33 and 44 by the carious process.

Fig. 247b Regressive alterations of the teeth. The periapical radiograph clearly shows the advanced resorption of the crown of tooth 23, which resulted from trauma to the palatal root of tooth 24 due to perforation of a metal root post.

Fig. 248a, b Regressive alterations of the teeth. **a** This periapical radiograph clearly reveals the peripheral (external) root resorption distally on tooth 11, that was without doubt elicited by trauma during tooth preparation. Peripheral tooth resorptions can only be clearly identified if the hard tissue defect is traversed tangentially by the roentgen rays, which is often the case when the substance loss occurs proximally. A "central granuloma," based upon radiographic diagnosis, is not necessarily always centrally located because of the two-dimensional summation effect of roentgen rays. **b** The same case depicts the radiographic appearance of obvious root resorption that could be termed "internal or central granuloma," following tooth preparation. The pulpal boundary remains easily identifiable. Tooth 21 remained clinically viable.

Fig. 248c Regressive alterations of the teeth. The periapical radiograph depicts a nonvital tooth 42, with apical root resorption resulting from chronic apical periodontitis.

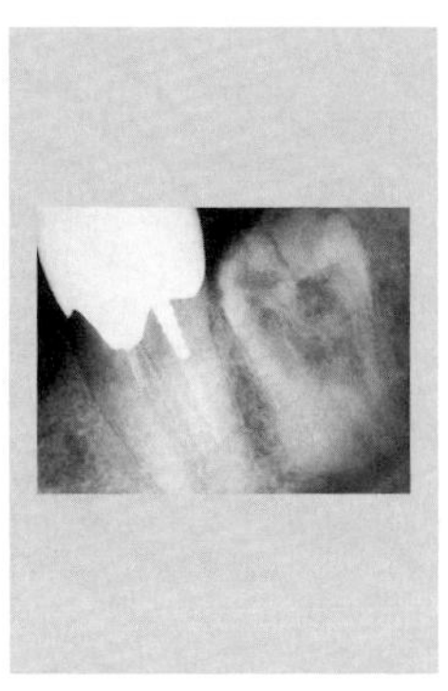
246 a

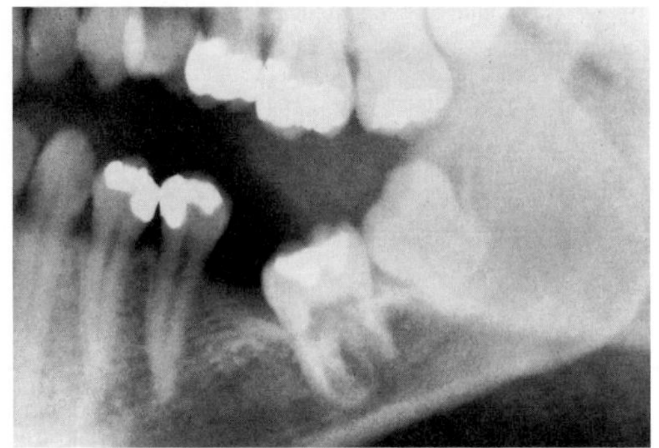
246 b

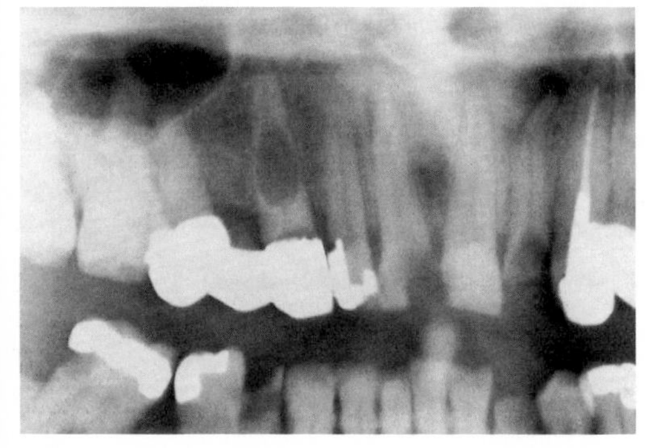
247 a

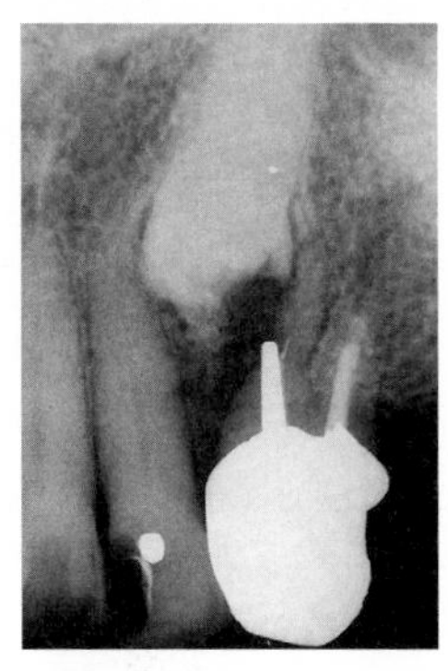
247 b

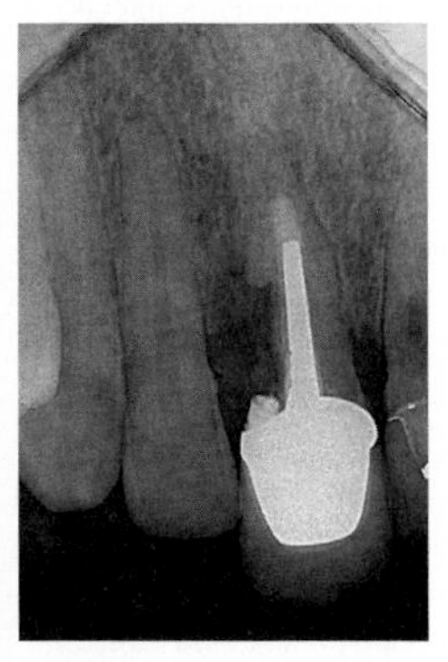
248 a

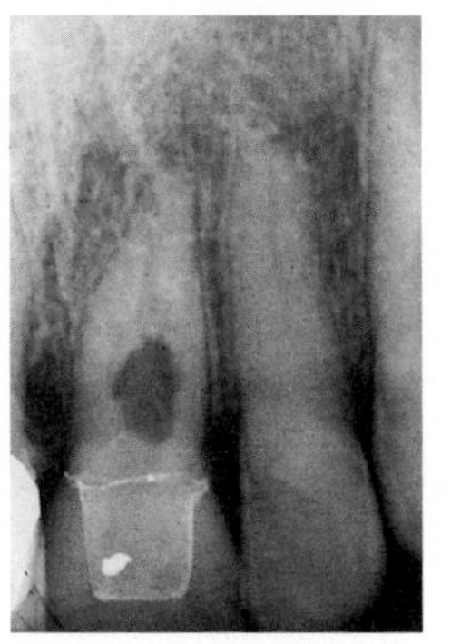
248 b

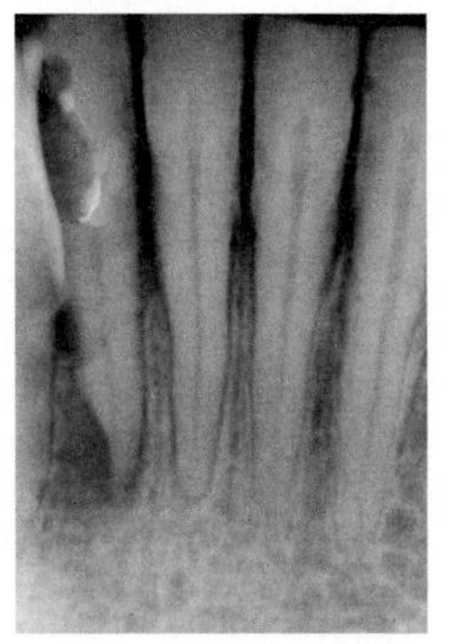
248 c

The terms "calculus and concrements" refer—radiographically—to radiopacities observed in or on the teeth and jaws, or which are superimposed upon the teeth or jaws (addition effect, overlapping). Because all intraoral and panoramic radiographs provide in fact only two-dimensional summation views, all structure-elicited radiopacities that are projected onto the image receptor as overlapped upon each other will be depicted as such on the final image. These types of overlapping effects are often not easy to interpret; the final analysis will depend upon the experience of the interpreter of such radiographs, and her/his ability to properly evaluate any masking summation effects on the basis of knowledge of radiographic anatomy and spatial relationships as viewed in two dimensions. There exist very real dangers of incorrect radiographic interpretation; in many cases, this can only be overcome by additional, supplemental radiographs to project the true third dimension. The dental practice team must realize that in questionable situations, intraoral projections or a panoramic radiograph may need to be supplemented by occlusal images or even computed tomography (CT).

Dental Calculus

Dental calculus is most often detected on those tooth surfaces that are near to the efferent ducts of the major salivary glands. Salivary secretions from the submandibular and sublingual glands lead primarily to calculus accumulations on the lingual surfaces of the mandibular anterior teeth, while the intraoral duct (Stensen's duct) of the parotid gland occasions calculus on the buccal surfaces of the maxillary first permanent molars. Upon the cervical aspects of the tooth crowns and any exposed root surfaces, mineralization of bacterial plaque leads to the formation of dental calculus, which consists primarily of calcium phosphate, and which can be easily detected proximally in bitewing radiographs. In intraoral and panoramic radiographs, massive accumulations of calculus lead to addition effects at cervical areas and tooth crowns. In cases of advanced periodontitis with pockets of significant depth, calculus is also formed from the components of inflammatory pocket secretions, which are mineralized into hard concrements by physiologic mineralization; these adhere tenaciously to root cementum (so-called *subgingival calculus*).

Fig. 249 a Calcifications and concrements. The bitewing radiograph reveals subgingival calculus, which is mineralized dental plaque, and is often visible radiographically as cervical "spurs" upon the proximal tooth surfaces in the posterior segments. Note also the generalized horizontal periodontal bone loss.

Fig. 249 b Calcifications and concrements. This periapical radiograph in a case of advanced periodontitis reveals concrements representing subgingival calculus that derive from the inflammatory pocket secretions.

Fig. 250 a Calcifications and concrements. This section from a panoramic radiograph depicts calcification of the cervical lymph nodes.

Fig. 250 b Calcifications and concrements. This section from a panoramic radiograph of a 79-year-old male reveals calcified cervical lymph nodes as well as calcifications within the common carotid artery.

Fig. 251 a Calcifications and concrements. This tangential cheek radiograph reveals a phlebolith. Depending upon its size it may also be visible on intraoral or panoramic radiographs as an addition effect.

Fig. 251 b Calcifications and concrements. This section from a panoramic radiograph reveals calcification in the frontal lobe of the parotid gland following mumps in a juvenile.

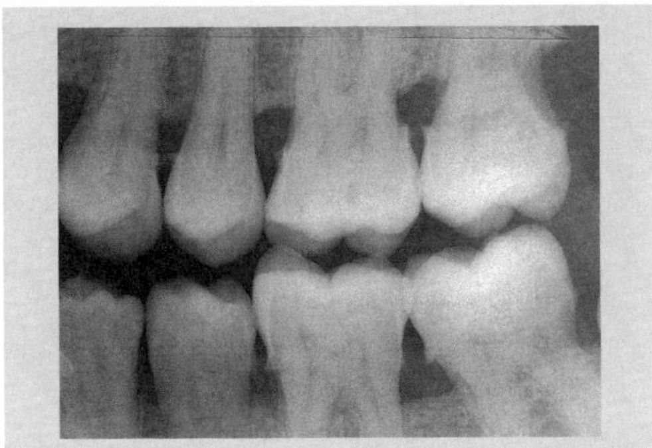

249 a

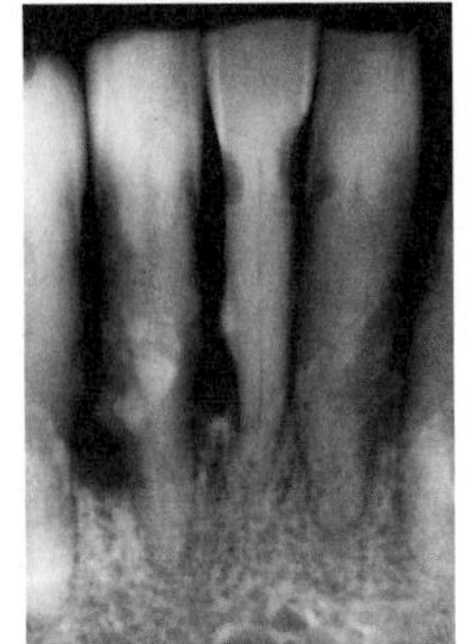

249 b

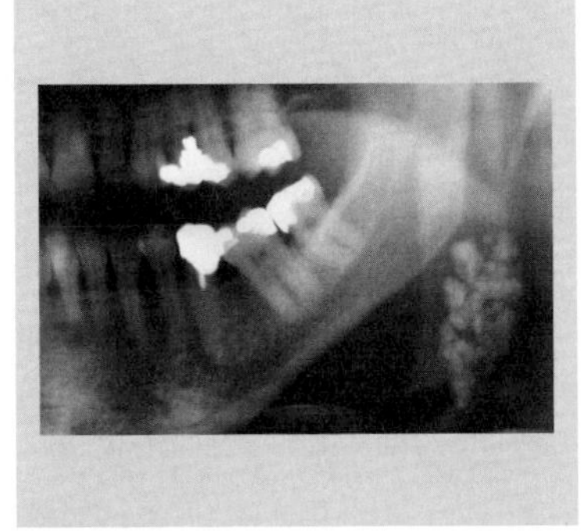

250 a

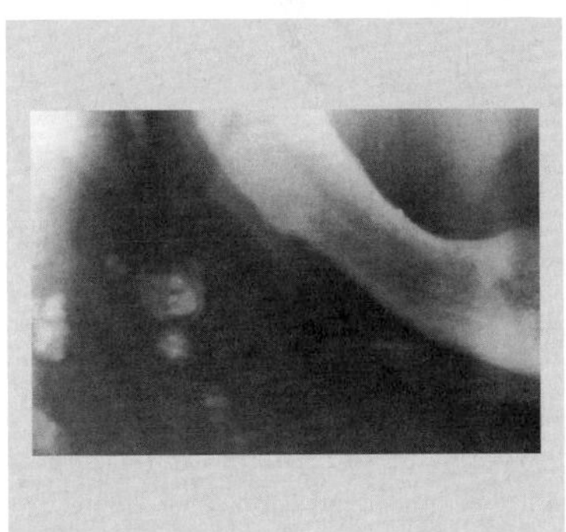

250 b

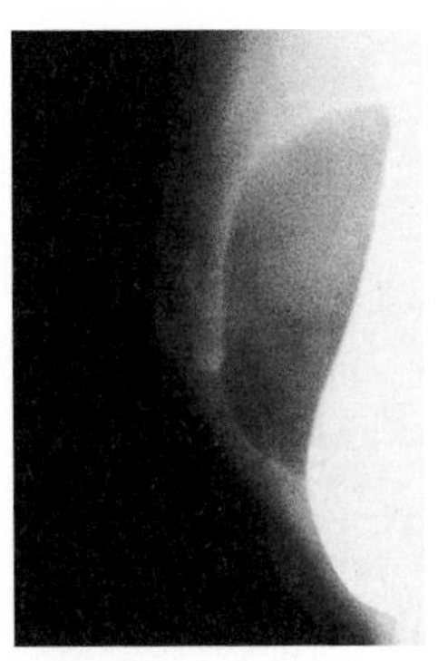

251 a

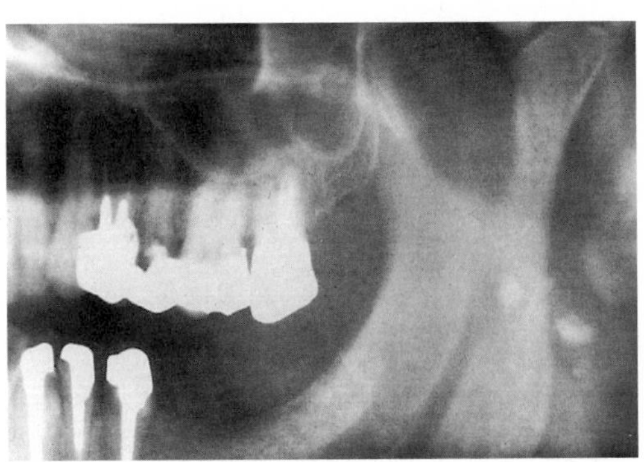

251 b

Calcified cervical lymph nodes may be found along and ventral to the sternocleidomastoid muscle and are easy to discern in a panoramic radiograph as a continuation of the dorsal border of the ascending ramus of the mandible. The rare occurrence today of calcifications of the regional lymph nodes can be traced primarily to healing following tuberculous lymphadenopathy (bovine type), which was formerly transferred via milk from diseased cows.

Arteriosclerosis

True **calcification of arteries** is rare, seen most often in cases of nicotine abuse. This phenomenon may be visible in a panoramic radiograph below the angle of the mandible as a reaction of the vascular walls, with calcifications mainly in the carotid sinus and plexus, and in the branches of the common carotid artery.

Phleboliths

Phleboliths are “venous stones” that are actually calcified areas of venous thrombosis. Radiographically these are usually projected from soft tissue hemangiomas onto the jaw or the maxillary sinuses (see Fig. **442**).

Rhinoliths

Rhinoliths are foreign bodies encrusted with calcium salts, found within the nasal cavity but also in the maxillary sinus; these can often be seen in periapical and also in panoramic radiographs.

Calcifications within the Parotid Gland

Calcification within the parotid gland following mumps will be seen in the panoramic radiograph projected partially onto the mandibular ramus; these originate in the frontal lobe of the gland. They are located above the dorsal portion of the attachment of the masseter muscle at the angle of the mandible.

Ossifications

Ossifications appear as calcium-rich radiopacities, sometimes with evidence of bone structure. They are observed in cases of ossifying myositis, following injury to the periosteum, in some metabolic disturbances as well as hereditary connective tissue disorders. The region of the masseter muscle with its expansive insertions represents the favored localization of this rare disorder.

Ossifications of the stylohyoid chain are clearly visible in the panoramic radiograph, without any overlapping structures. These can be observed either as an extended styloid process or as ossifications of the entire stylohyoid ligament. Within these fragile formations, fractures, pseudoarthroses, or even necrosis may be found, frequently as a consequence of whiplash injury, and may also cause neuralgiform symptoms, headaches, and functional disturbances with head movement.

Fig. 252 Calcifications and concrements. This panoramic radiograph of a 53-year-old male reveals a sialolith near to the orifice of Wharton’s duct; it appears as an addition effect over the roots of teeth 34 and 35. Such a radiographic appearance could easily be confused with a supernumerary premolar.

Fig. 253 a, b Calcifications and concrements. a This periapical radiograph from a 31-year-old male reveals a well-demarcated radiopacity situated over the apex of tooth 35. **b** This unilateral occlusal radiograph of the mandible clearly reveals in the third dimension the 26-mm long sialolith within Wharton’s duct of the right submandibular gland.

Fig. 254 a, b Calcifications and concrements. a This section from a panoramic radiograph of a 70-year-old female reveals an extremely discrete radiopacity distal to tooth 45 at the level of the alveolar crest (**arrow**). **b** The unilateral mandibular radiograph, taken with the film fixed to the occlusal surfaces, depicts the round, layered sialolith near the orifice of the right Wharton duct. Because the stone was near to the plane of focus, its spherical configuration is distorted in the panoramic radiograph and appears more oval in shape.

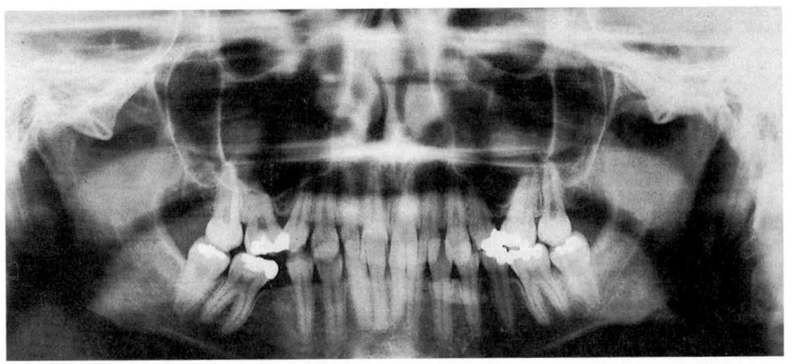

252

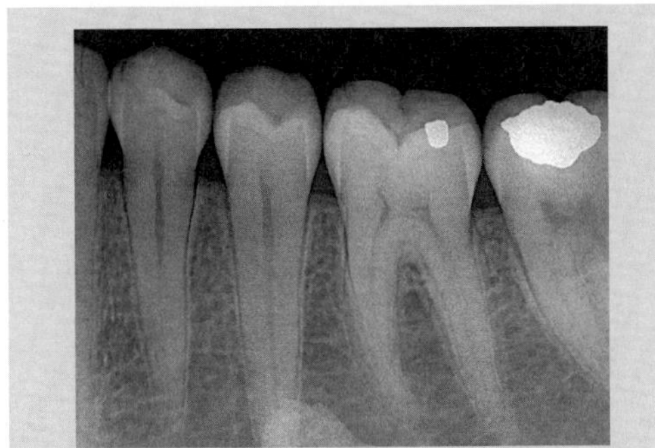

253 a

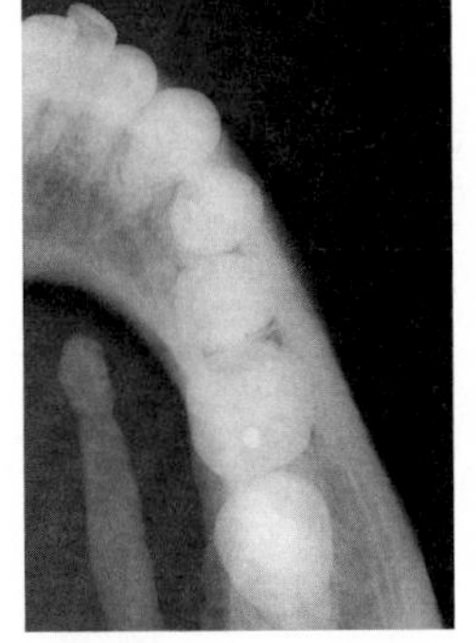

253 b

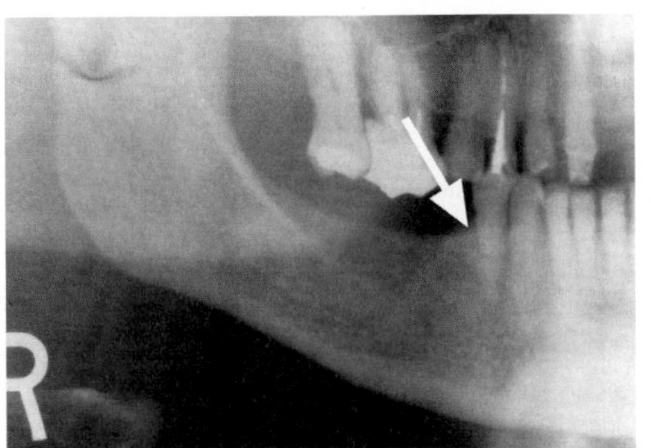

254 a

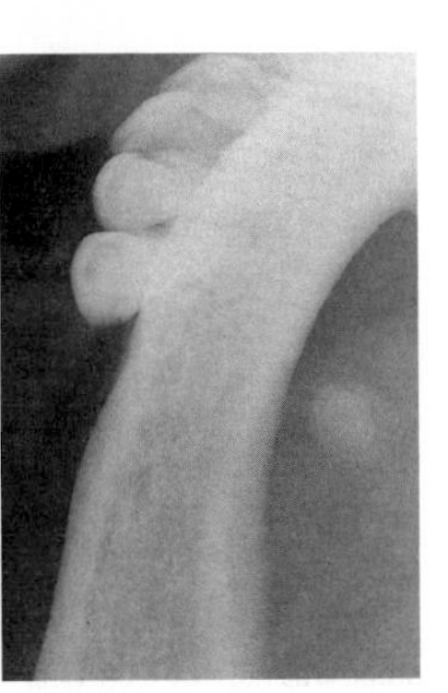

254 b

It is reasonable to suspect the existence of sialoliths if the patient presents a history of intermittent pain and swelling immediately before and during meals, in the region of the major salivary glands. In periapical radiographs and especially in the panoramic view it is frequently possible to serendipitously discover circumscribed radiopacities that appear as summation effects overlapping the angle of the mandible, the body of the mandible, or the ascending ramus. Such radiographically visible sialoliths prevent the normal flow of saliva in the various salivary ducts. Sialoliths consist of inorganic layers of calcium phosphate or calcium carbonate, with an organic substrate of mucopolysaccharides, amino acids, cholesterol, and uric acid. Sialoliths can appear in extremely variable radiopaque shapes and sizes, but also as radiolucent structures, so that additional examination using sialography or, preferably, sonography may be indicated. Children are only extremely rarely affected, and in adults the preponderance is in males age 30–50. Sialoliths are detected commonly in the knee of Wharton's duct and less frequently in the sublingual or parotid glands (see also p. **125**). Sialoliths may develop without any symptoms, or only vague symptoms, to significant size, and for this reason are quite often detected only quite late.

It is not uncommon that the lack of salivary flow from the duct orifices leads to xerostomia and resultant interdental papillary (gingival) inflammation, which enhances the clinical signs and symptoms.

Fig. 255 a, b Calcifications and concrements. a This section from a panoramic radiograph of a 62-year-old male reveals in the area of the right mandibular angle an oval, irregularly demarcated radiopacity in the region of the bend of the afferent duct (see p. **125**) of the submandibular gland that is reminiscent of an osteoma (not infrequently observed in that region; caution: possibility of Paget disease of bone). **b** The properly underexposed unilateral occlusal radiograph of the same case reveals a large, layered, and irregularly shaped sialolith that formed at the bend of Wharton's duct.

Fig. 256 a, b Calcifications and concrements. a This section from a panoramic radiograph of a 41-year-old female reveals a round radiopacity in the left angle of the mandible. **b** The unilateral occlusal radiograph of the mandible clearly depicts the round and layered sialolith with a localization that demanded experienced radiographic technique to depict the third dimension (see p. **61**).

Fig. 257 Ossification. This panoramic radiograph is presented as an example of the possible ossifications of soft tissue structures. The ossification, which originates from the collagenous chordal tissue between the styloid process of the sphenoid bone and the minor horn of the hyoid bone can lead to necrosis (**arrow, right**) and to the formation of pseudoarthroses (**arrow, left**) after trauma, especially whiplash trauma.

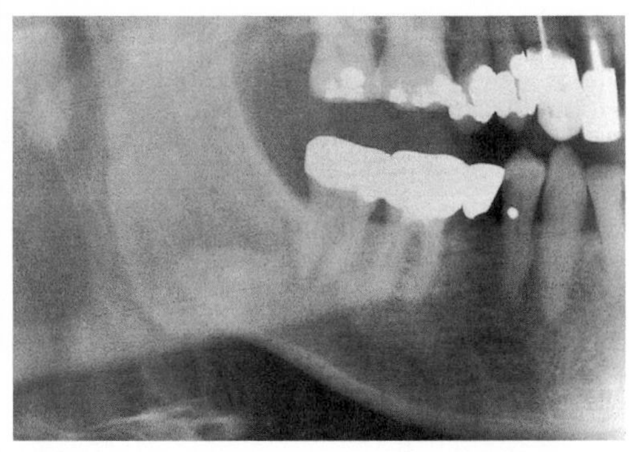

255 a

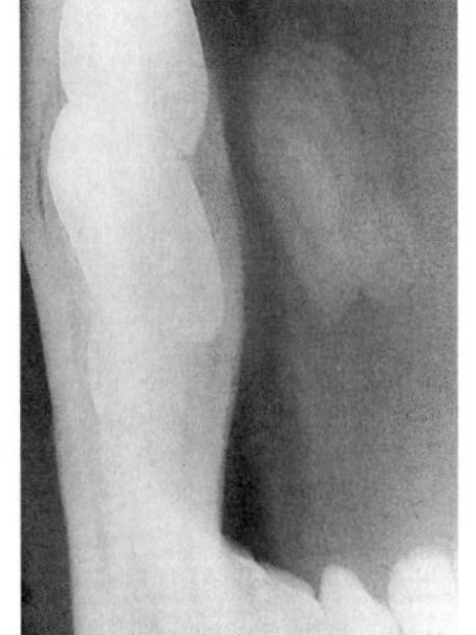

255 b

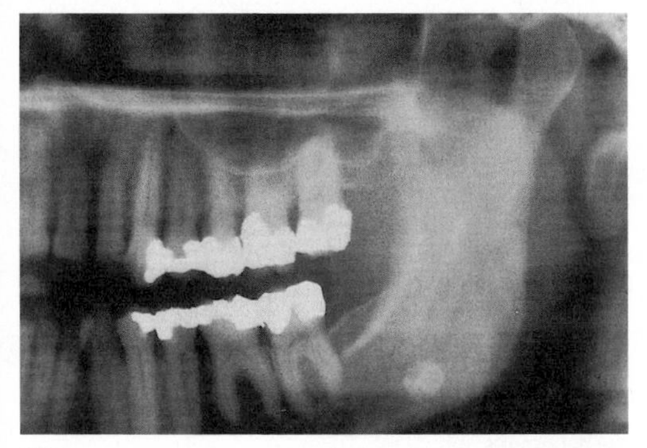

256 a

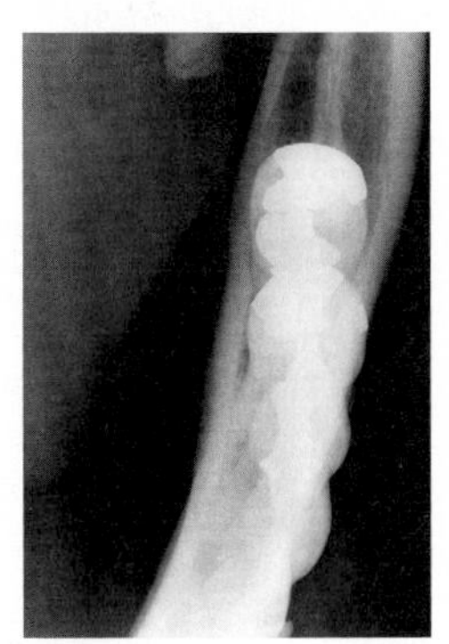

256 b

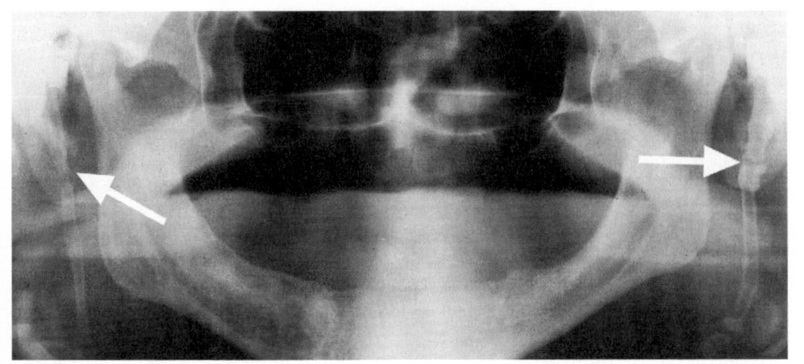

257

Dental caries is without doubt the most frequently encountered dental disease. If dental caries is not detected early and treated by appropriate restorative therapy, the result can be loss of vitality of the affected tooth, and subsequent periapical inflammatory reactions and local osteomyelitis, which can represent etiologic factors for a variety of other diseases. A genetic predisposition toward susceptibility for dental caries can no longer be denied. Tooth position, tooth shape, enamel quality, and the viscosity of saliva are all genetically determined, and in terms of caries susceptibility the quality of the enamel matrix and the degree of maturity of the enamel itself, as well as disturbances of calcium metabolism likely play important roles. The most common genetically based syndromes and dysplasias that include caries susceptibility are:

- Amelogenesis imperfecta
- Ectodermal dysplasia (Rapp–Hodgkin syndrome)
- Lacrimoauriculodentodigital syndrome (LADD, Levy–Hollister syndrome), with hypo- or aplasia of the salivary glands
- Naegeli's incontinentia pigmenti (Naegeli syndrome, Franceschetti–Jadassohn syndrome)
- Orofaciodigital syndrome (OFD syndrome, Papillon–Léage–Psaume syndrome)
- Pyknodysostosis (Maroteaux–Lamy syndrome)
- Rothmund–Thomson syndrome
- Shwachman syndrome, with pancreatic lipomatosis

In addition to reduction of sugar consumption, caries inhibition is associated primarily with good oral hygiene and a regular program of examining for caries incidence in children and adolescents, with radiographic examinations at intervals appropriate to individual caries risk parameters.

Early detection of *initial* carious lesions greatly improves the chance for perfect restorative therapy. The (bitewing) radiographic examination for detection of initial carious lesions remains even today superior to all other examination methods including, for example, transillumination or the measurement of electrical resistance, especially in the posterior dental segments.

Fig. 258 Caries as observed in the panoramic radiograph. This extraordinarily clear panoramic radiograph (taken with the OP 10 Siemens unit) clearly reveals profound caries on teeth 14, 22 distal, 25 mesial, 45 mesial, and 47. With regard to possible caries on teeth 24 distal, 34 mesial and distal, 35 distal, and 44 mesial, as well as the possibility of secondary caries on the occlusal surface of tooth 46, even a panoramic radiograph of this quality cannot permit unambiguous diagnostic conclusions. The panoramic overview radiograph provides an initial diagnostic base for both teeth and jaws, that must in most cases be supplemented by bitewing radiographs. A high-quality panoramic radiograph provides zonography for detecting expansive and profound dental caries, but is insufficient for detection of initial carious lesions.

Fig. 259 a, b Early caries diagnosis using bitewing radiographs. Caries check for a 17-year-old female. Noteworthy are the symmetrical restorations on the occlusal surfaces of teeth 36 and 46. It is common in dental practice to observe symmetrical caries occurrence in young persons.

Fig. 260 a, b Caries diagnosis with bitewing radiographs. These are the bitewing radiographs of a 20-year-old male, who had presented regularly every 6 months over a long period of years for clinical examination. These radiographs review the *totally inadequate* results of clinical examination with mirror and explorer in a patient with high caries frequency and susceptibility: Note profound caries on teeth 16 distal, 15 distal and mesial, 14 distal, 24 distal, 25 mesial and distal, 26 distal, 27 mesial, and 36 distal. The carious process has invaded the dentin of teeth 17, 24, 36, and 45. The most recent *clinical* examination by a dentist had been performed only 6 months before these radiographs were taken!

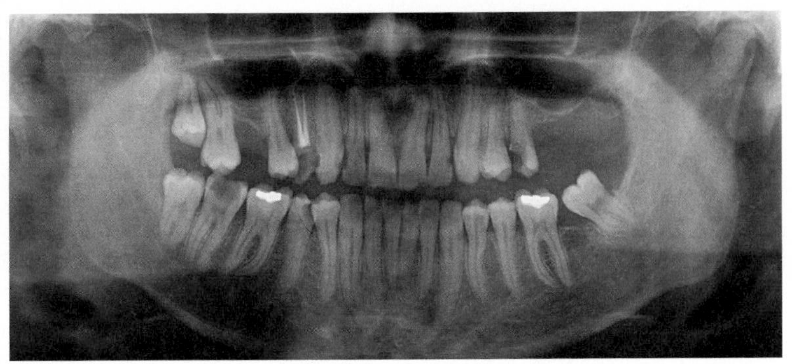

258

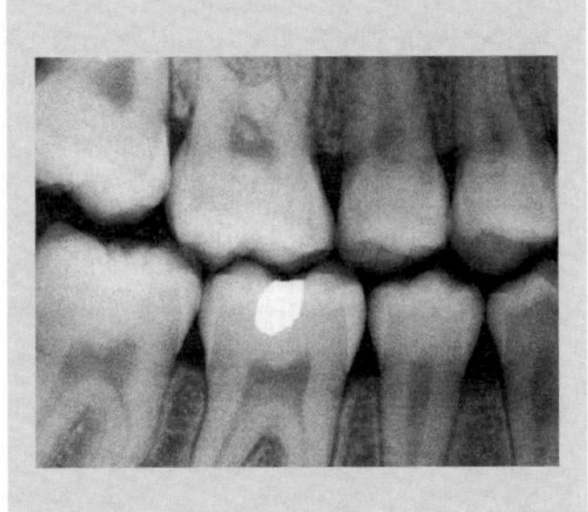

259 a

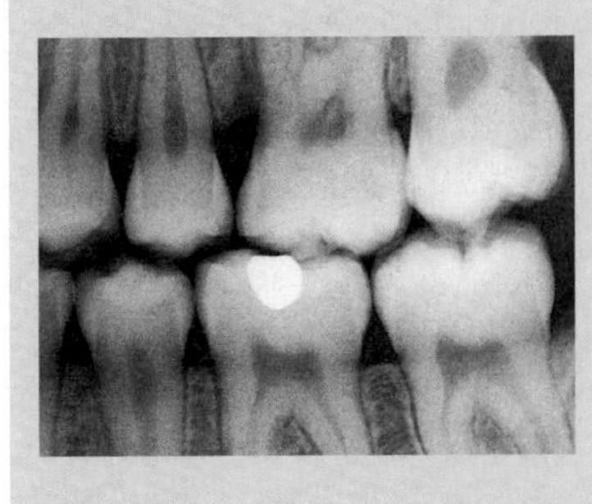

259 b

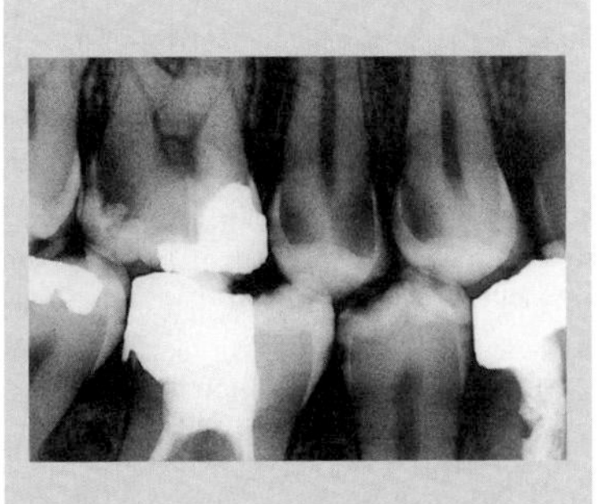

260 a

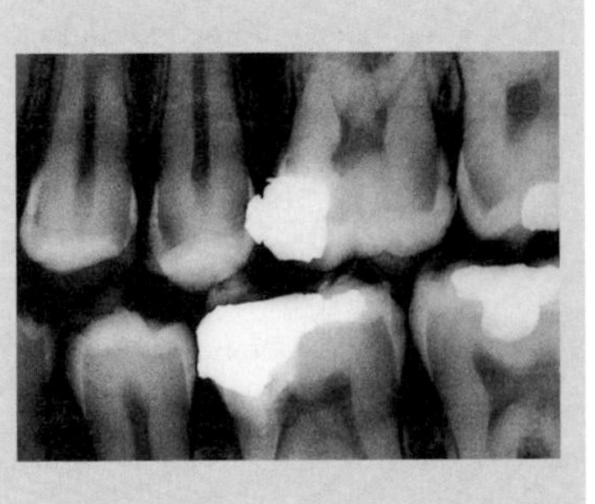

269 b

It has been acknowledged for many decades that clinical examination with a mouth mirror and explorer is inadequate for the diagnosis of initial dental caries; this knowledge leads to the fact that radiographic early diagnosis must be part of the overall examination scheme. It is nevertheless important to keep uppermost in mind that radiographic examination must always be performed with full knowledge of radiographic anatomy, proper radiographic projection technique, and the biological effects of irradiation. These considerations are primary to prevent any distortion of the true anatomic/pathologic situation, and resultant incorrect diagnosis leading to inappropriate treatment.

In virtually every modern dental practice today, the radiographic equipment that is available on a routine daily basis will provide both overview radiographs (e.g., panoramic views) as well as targeted intraoral projections for the depiction of the jaws and individual teeth. For the early diagnosis of (proximal) dental caries, still today the bitewing radiograph taken with a coronally targeted central ray and retrocoronal position of the image receptor at right angles to each other remains the method of choice. To re-state the obvious: The bitewing radiograph remains the sole technique for reliable and early detection of interdental caries in the posterior dental segments. Radiographic examination for dental caries must be performed in all age categories, but with consideration for individual caries frequency and susceptibility. For this purpose, patient-friendly image receptors must be available for all age groups, and today this can only be guaranteed through the use of conventional radiographic IR assortments. Appropriately sized intraoral image receptors simplify the correct and as far as possible pain-fee positioning in the oral cavity, and therefore improved ultimate radiographic quality.

The use of ionizing radiation for diagnostic purposes must be achieved with the lowest possible radiation dose, especially in children and adolescents; this must ensure perfect and reliable early caries diagnosis. A calculable minimal radiation exposure dose must be used to ensure diagnostic ability to discern details, which is also subsumed in the term "radiographic quality," and this minimal dose must not reduce diagnostic quality if the very purpose of the examination is to be fulfilled. The bottom line here is the timely identification of enamel demineralization or other injury to the tooth.

Fig. 261 a, b Caries in the deciduous teeth. The bitewing radiographs reveal severe caries on virtually all deciduous teeth in this 5-year-old male. Such radiographic findings are also common in certain syndromes or dysplasias.

Fig. 262 a, b Caries in the deciduous dentition. These two bitewing radiographs were selected in order to compare and contrast the existing true proximal caries on the mesial surface of tooth 55 with the apparent (but nonexistent) caries on the mesial surface of tooth 65. The latter is caused by the shape of the deciduous tooth crown. Because of the varying size of the Carabelli cusp of the maxillary second deciduous molar, and depending upon the exposure settings, a pronounced addition effect can occur in the middle of the tooth crown, and the mesial—or also the distal—portion of the crown will exhibit a caries-like radiolucency. The intact enamel surface on the mesial of tooth 65 and the erupted enamel cap mesial of tooth 55 confirm the diagnosis in the 6-year-old male.

Fig. 263 a, b Proximal caries in the mixed dentition. Proximal caries near the contact point of tooth 75 with tooth 36, and also the contact between tooth 85 and permanent tooth 46. Noteworthy also is that the persistence of deciduous tooth 85 appears to have elicited an oblique development and eruption pathway of the root of permanent tooth 45 in this 10-year-old male. It is also possible that the radiographic underexposure caused primarily by the use of extremely sensitive film, and the overlapping of the initial carious lesion by intact enamel, would lead to underestimating the caries or that it would be rendered completely invisible (nondiagnosable).

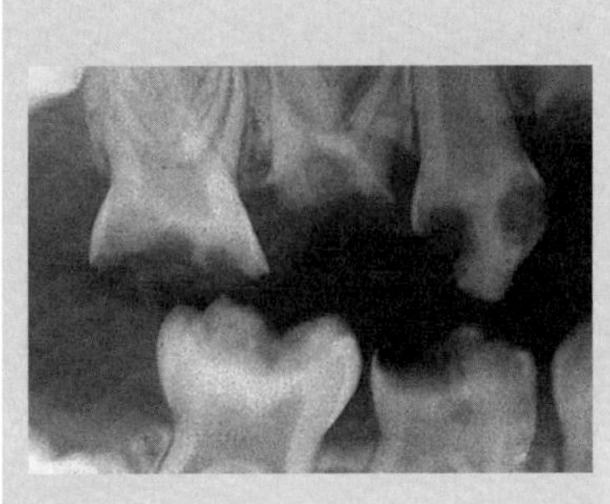

261 a

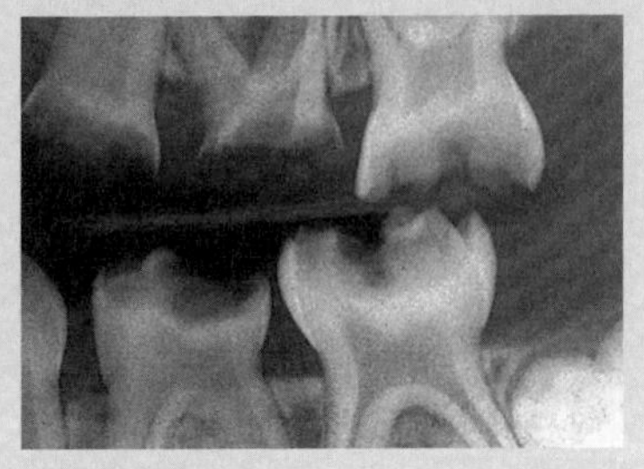

261 b

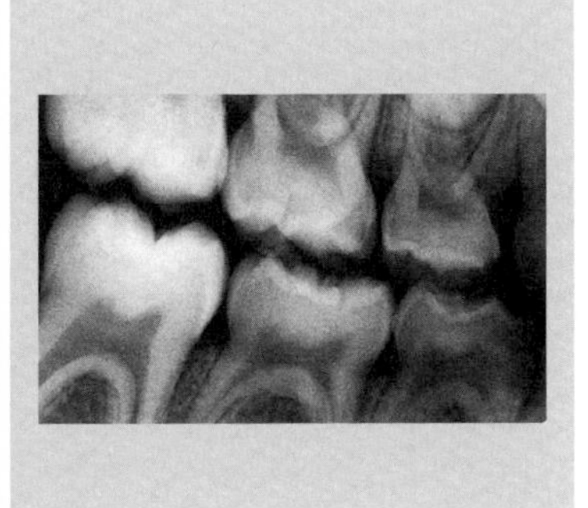

262 a

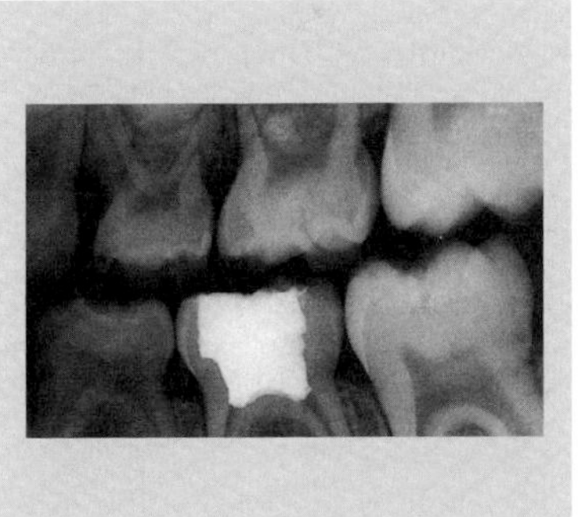

262 b

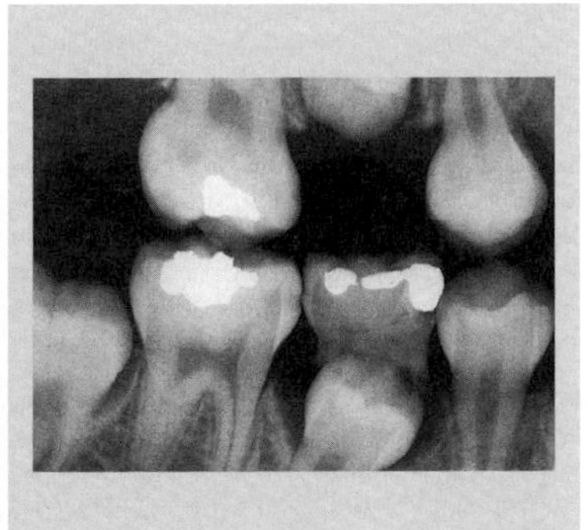

263 a

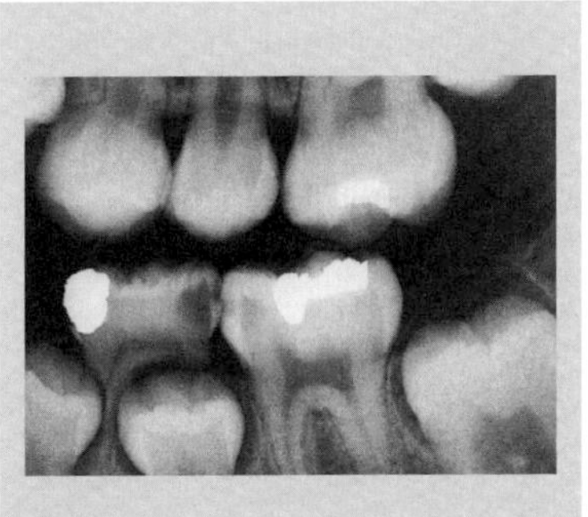

263 b

In cases exhibiting severe apical lesions or advanced periodontitis, the anatomic relationships in the oral cavity often make it impossible to use a parallel or right-angle technique to depict tooth roots without distortion; with coronal lesions, however, it should always be possible to direct the central ray perpendicular to the long axis of the tooth. In virtually all such situations, the ideal projection with the image receptor positioned parallel to the crown's axis and the central ray targeted perpendicular to it coronally or interocclusally will provide an ideal radiograph. This is not only desirable but an absolute necessity because apical-oblique projections or carelessly prepared parallel projections will depict carious lesions only unclearly or not at all, even when the carious process is quite advanced; such errors could result in incorrect diagnosis and eventual harm to the patient. The enamel cap of the tooth crown will only be clearly and definably depicted when it is perpendicular to the central ray projection. The greater the distance of the irradiation source from the image receptor, the clearer will be the final image. The initial radiographic picture of the carious process will reveal the area of the demineralization (or also a developmentally related enamel defect) clearly, if the demineralization is located on the proximal enamel surfaces and is tangentially traversed by the roentgen rays. Carious lesions located on the buccal or oral (palatal/lingual) surface will only be seen on a radiograph when the lesions are quite advanced; such lesions should be detected by the *clinical* examination.

The diagnosis of recurrent caries or secondary caries is only seldom possible radiographically.

Radiation effects such as the tangential effect and summation effects must also be considered when taking radiographs for caries diagnosis.

Intraoral radiographs provide two-dimensional images, with the third dimension represented by summation effects caused by the various anatomic structures. Depending upon whether a superimposition leads to enhanced radiopacity or enhanced radiolucency upon the desired object, one speaks of an "addition effect" or a "subtraction effect." Depending upon the intensity (density) of the superimposed structure(s), any existing pathologic defects or lesions will be rendered smaller and blurred by the addition effect, or brighter and washed-out in appearance by the subtraction effect.

Fig. 264 a, b Caries diagnosis in adults. The bitewing radiographs of a 17-year-old female clearly reveal caries on teeth 17 mesial, 16 distal, 25 distal, 26 distal, 37 distal and mesial, 36 mesial, 35 mesial, 34 distal, 46 mesial, 47 mesial, and 47 occlusal. Note also the burn-out effect at the cervical areas of teeth 47 distal and 27 distal, the undercontoured restoration margin on tooth 26 distal, caries at the level of the contact point (!) on tooth 37 distal with the position of tooth 38 impeding its own eruption, and the scarcely visible occlusal fissure caries on tooth 47.

Fig. 265 a, b Depiction of proximal caries using intraoral periapical radiographs and intraoral bitewing (coronally projected) radiographs. This comparison reveals the varying quality and interpretability following apical or coronal central ray projection in terms of the profound caries on tooth 25 mesial and distal as well as the expanse of the residual (secondary) caries on the mesial of tooth 26. Targeting the central ray perpendicular to the tooth crowns depicts proximal caries clearly and without distortion. Note also the differences in depiction of the maxillary alveolar crest.

Fig. 266 a, b Caries diagnosis using periapical radiographs and coronally projected bitewing radiographs. While the periapical radiograph depicts what appears to be a completely intact marginal closure of the gold crown on the distal aspect of tooth 46, the coronally projected bitewing radiograph clearly reveals not only an advanced area of secondary caries, but also an inadequate crown margin. Note also the proximal restoration overhangs in the maxilla and the amalgam residue in the extraction site of tooth 16.

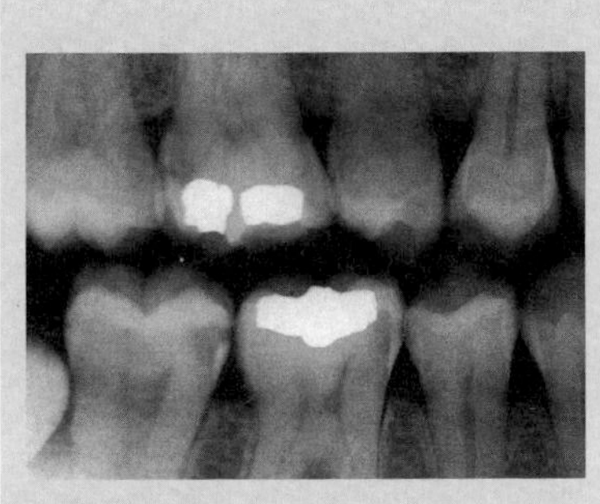

264 a

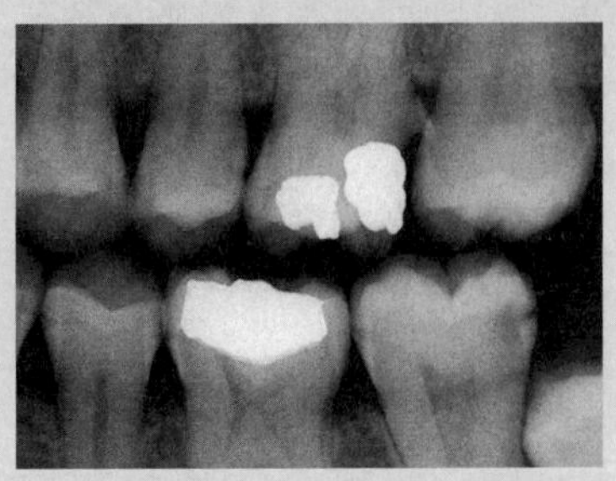

264 b

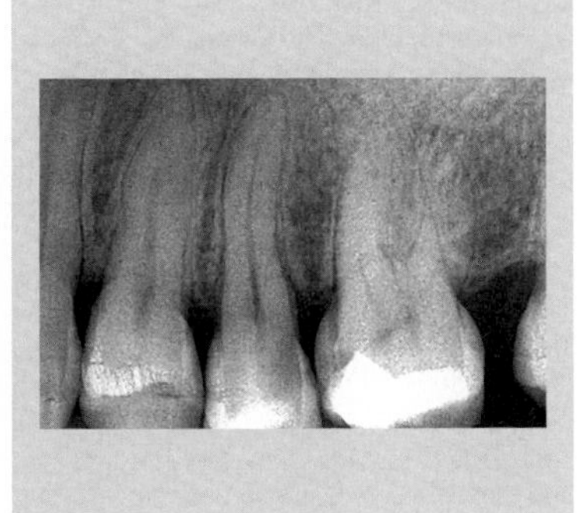

265 a

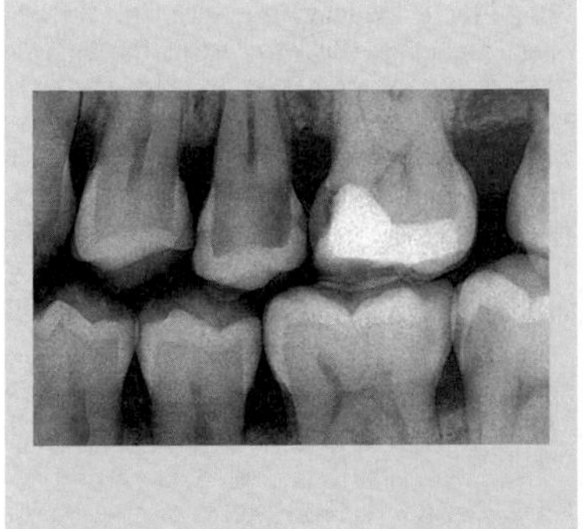

265 b

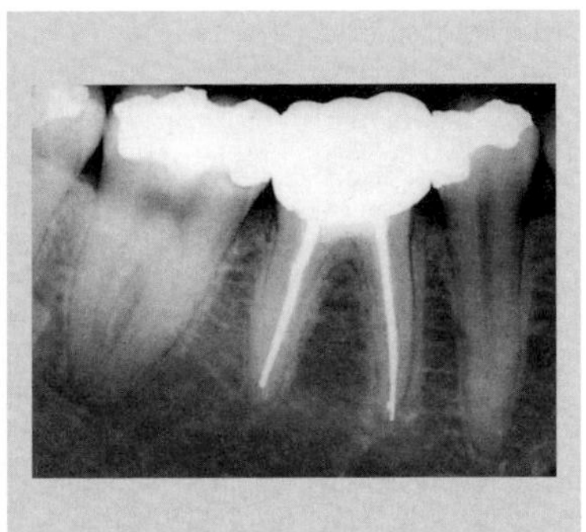

266 a

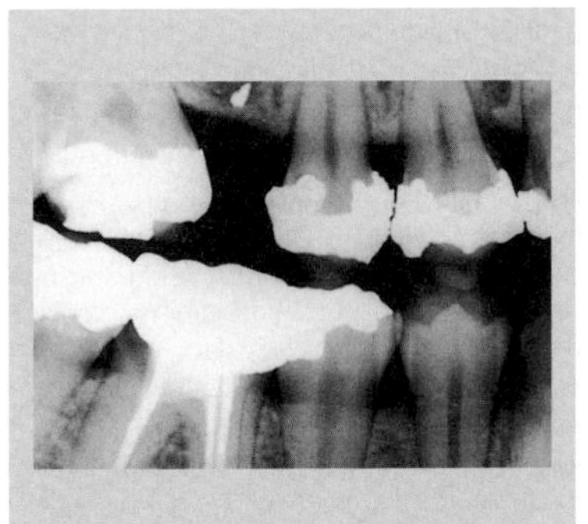

266 b

The end result is that incipient caries will almost always be *underestimated* in radiographic diagnosis because the proximal lesions are superimposed (overlapped) by intact enamel and dentin, and even the weak radiopacity of the soft tissues of the cheek play a role in this regard. Portions of the tooth crowns and the cervical area of each tooth may exhibit radiolucencies that could lead to an incorrect diagnosis of carious lesions (burn-out effect); this occurs primarily in teeth that are rotated in the arch or because the horizontal structure and location of the alveolar ridge "exposes" the cervical area to the radiation. These types of addition and/or subtraction effects will be enhanced by under- or overexposure.

In most cases, a carious lesion that has penetrated into dentin exhibits a poorly demarcated periphery, and in cases of deep (profound) caries one frequently observes a thickened reaction zone around the endangered and physiologically retracting pulpal tissues.

Developmentally elicited irregularities or pits-fissures in the enamel cap will only be visible in the proximal segments due to the tangential effect of the roentgen rays. Because such developmental anomalies are generally sharply demarcated radiolucencies, they can usually be differentiated from incipient caries. However, it is often impossible at this stage.

Fig. 267a Occlusal or fissure caries. Even advanced caries in occlusal fissures cannot always be depicted radiographically because of the oblique projection normally utilized for periapical images, and furthermore cannot always be discerned because of the addition effect of the remaining intact enamel mantel, even in bitewing radiographs. And even careful clinical examination often reveals what appears to be intact enamel, especially if it has been hardened by topical fluoride application over an extended period of time. Even expansive dentin caries can often only be detected clinically by the presence of enamel discoloration or frank enamel breach. This bitewing radiograph clearly reveals profound, deep occlusal caries on teeth 16 and 46. A more discrete appearance of occlusal fissure caries in various stages can be observed on teeth 17 and 47, and proximal caries is clearly visible on teeth 16, 15, 45, and 46.

Fig. 267b Cervical (tooth neck) caries. This periapical radiograph reveals deep caries on tooth 37 mesial. Tooth 36 distal reveals dentin caries at the cementoenamel junction, likely caused by food impaction.

Fig. 268a Cervical caries. Deep cervical caries at the cementoenamel junction on the distal surface of tooth 13. The radiographic differential diagnosis could also include peripheral (external) granuloma elicited by trauma from tooth preparation, for example preparation for the restoration in tooth 14 (see also Fig. **248a**).

Fig. 268b Cervical caries. This periapical radiograph reveals expansive and circumferential cervical caries on the mandibular incisors.

Fig. 268c Caries on impacted teeth. Partially impacted teeth exposed to the oral cavity frequently exhibit carious lesions, and may cause clinical symptoms of pulpitis in advanced stages.

Fig. 269a Cervical caries. The supererupted third molar exhibits an inaccessible contact with its adjacent tooth that led to persistent food impaction; note the expansive proximal cervical caries at the cementoenamel junction. The bitewing radiographic techniques currently in use often are associated with failure to diagnose proximal carious lesions on third molars. It is not infrequent that the buccal surfaces of maxillary third molars exhibit symmetrical cervical caries that both clinically and with bitewing radiographs can only be diagnosed in the initial stages with extremely careful examination.

Fig. 269b Cervical caries. Interdental contact point discrepancies and poor marginal closure of restorations in the proximal area, and crowns, frequently represent the etiology for carious lesions at the cementoenamel junction. Radiographically, such lesions are difficult to differentiate from secondary caries or improper cavity preparations.

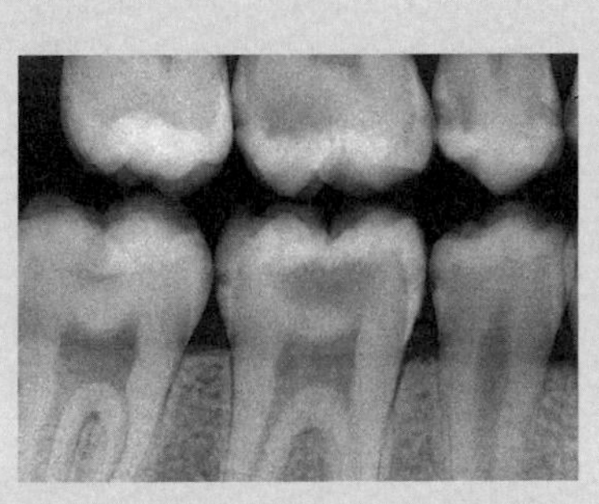

267 a

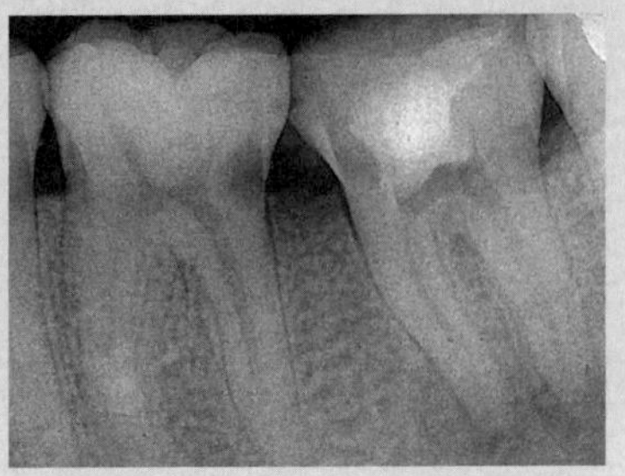

267 b

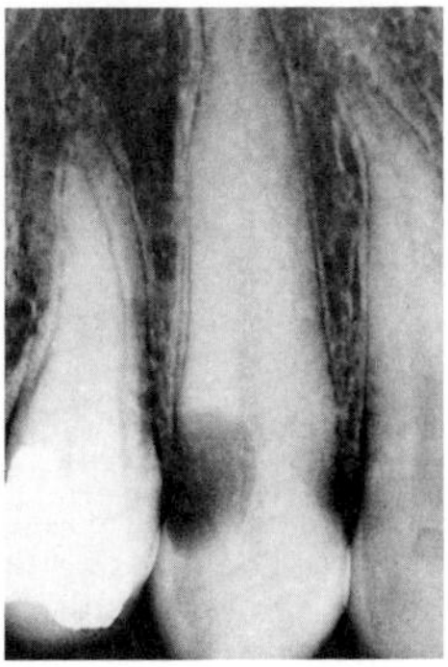

268 a

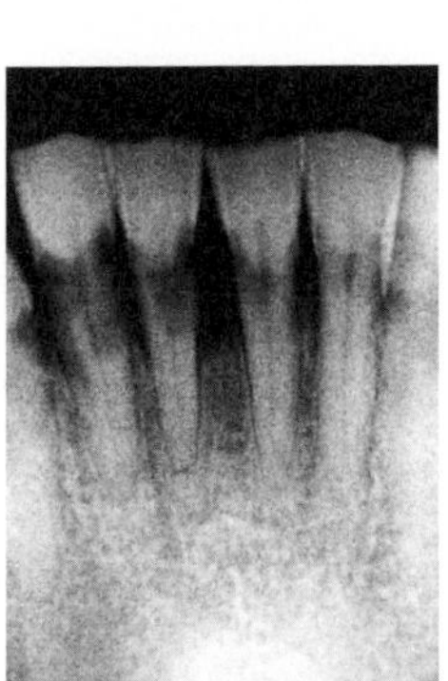

268 b

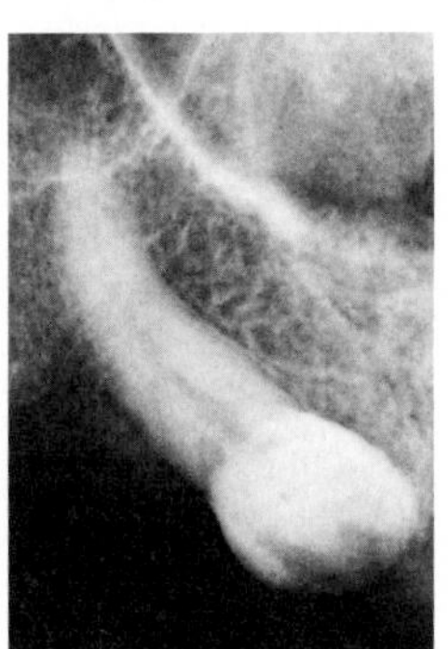

268 c

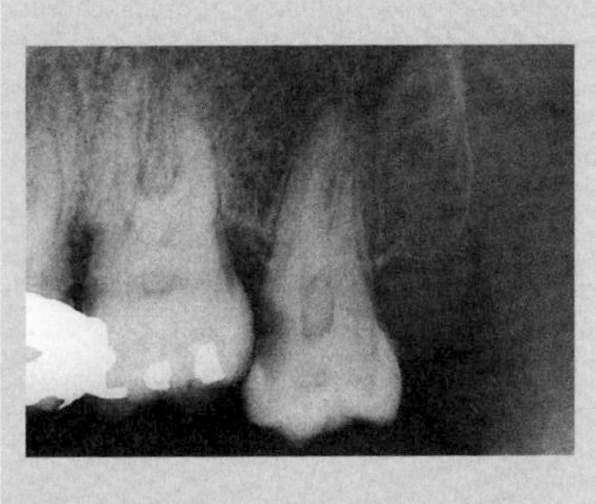

269 a

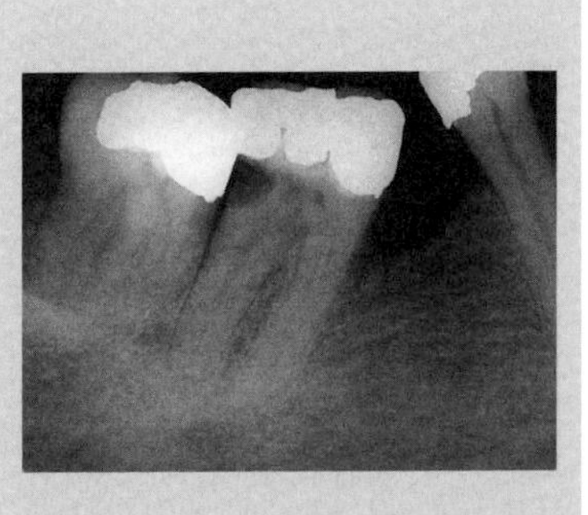

269 b

to differentiate between developmentally elicited enamel defects and initial demineralization, so these types of radiolucencies must be repeatedly examined over a period of at least one year.

Recurrent caries beneath radiopaque crowns and restorations is often difficult or impossible to detect radiographically. In such cases, coronal projection of the central ray will provide results superior to those achieved with other methods. The future of early caries diagnosis belongs to thin-slice techniques, which have the capability to depict the crowns of individual teeth, especially in the posterior segments, in any desired plane without any overlapping.

An important radiation phenomenon in dental radiographic interpretation and diagnosis is the often so-called "transition phenomenon" (*edge effect*); the radiograph often exhibits a band of radiolucency at the transition between the margins of a gold crown or amalgam restoration and tooth structure. In many cases it is difficult to differentiate this from secondary or recurrent caries.

Fig. 270a Secondary caries. The bitewing radiograph reveals profound secondary caries (recurrent caries) on abutment tooth 37, which also exhibits endodontic treatment and supports a full cast crown bridge abutment. If the central ray projection were to be directed steeply caudally, the caries would be overlapped by the lingual crown margin and therefore completely undetectable on the radiograph. For this reason, an intraoral (periapical) radiographic survey without supplemental bitewings is not indicated for caries diagnosis. Note also the burn-out effect on the distal aspect of bridge abutment tooth 35. In the original image, the lingual periodontal ligament space was clearly evident, and therefore this is a subtraction effect distally on a tooth that is rotated in the arch.

Fig. 270b Secondary caries. This (mouth open!) bitewing radiograph reveals secondary caries distally on tooth 46, and apparent fracture of an amalgam restoration in the distal proximal box. Tooth 48 exhibits pronounced occlusal caries (fissure caries). It is easy to see that clinical technical errors made when taking this projection led to significant loss of radiographic information (see p. **57**).

Fig. 271 a, b Secondary caries. These bitewing radiographs reveal not only multiple missing teeth but also numerous amalgam restorations with extraordinarily poor marginal adaptation, as well as several endodontically treated teeth, exhibiting secondary caries on teeth 17 mesial, 15 mesial, 27 mesial, and 35 distal. In such a radiographic depiction, however, there exists the possibility and even probability that additional carious lesions exist that were impossible to depict on the radiograph because of overlapping by the metal restorations themselves.

Fig. 272a Burn-out effects. In that area of each tooth where the cervical region is not overlapped by the enamel cap or by the alveolar bone, a zone of radiolucency will be visible because the roentgen rays are less dampened, and the less radiopaque cementum/dentin of the tooth cervix is effectively overexposed. This burn-out effect must not be confused with the radiolucencies exhibited by true carious lesions. This periapical radiograph permits an actual comparison of the burn-out effect with typical anterior tooth caries (teeth 12 mesial and 11 distal).

Fig. 272b Burn-out effects. Maxillary anterior teeth and also first premolars that are malpositioned (rotated) in the dental arch also exhibit burn-out effect in those areas where the roentgen rays are less dampened. In this image, tooth 22 is rotated (malpositioned) with its mesial aspect buccally and the resulting burn-out effects both mesially and distally are apparent around the tooth crown (see also chapter "Radiographic Anatomy" page **72**).

Fig. 272c Burn-out effects. Mandibular incisors and also premolars that are rotated along the tooth long axis will also exhibit a burn-out effect, which is enhanced especially in the presence of recession of the alveolar crest. With more advanced osseous recession, even the cervical areas of premolars and molars in both arches will exhibit the burn-out effect. In this radiograph, one notes especially the burn-out effects around teeth 42 distal and 31 distal.

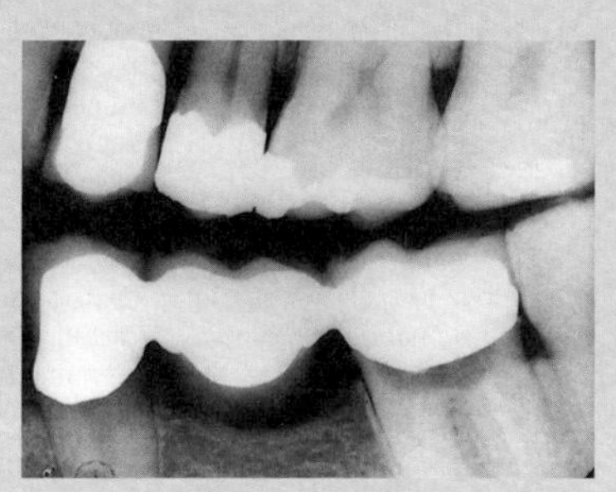

270 a

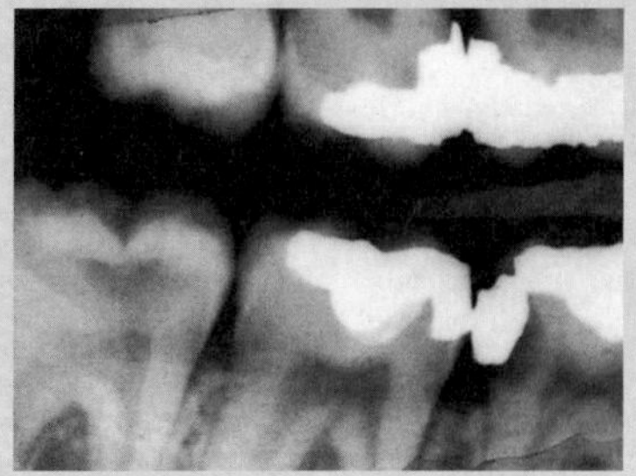
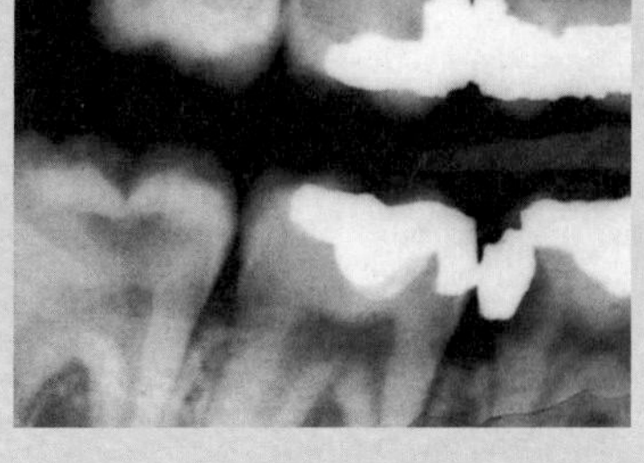

270 b

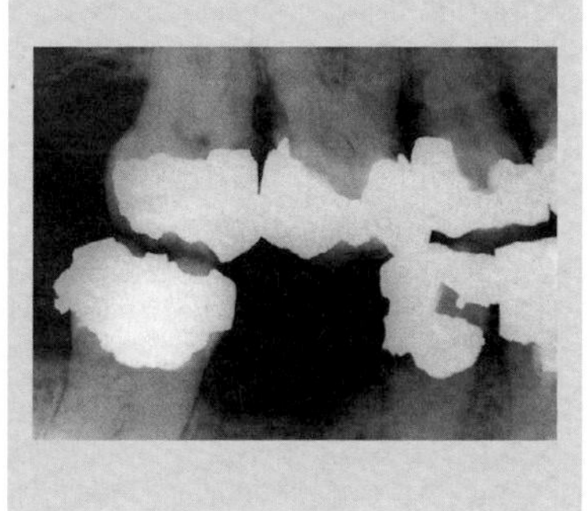

271 a

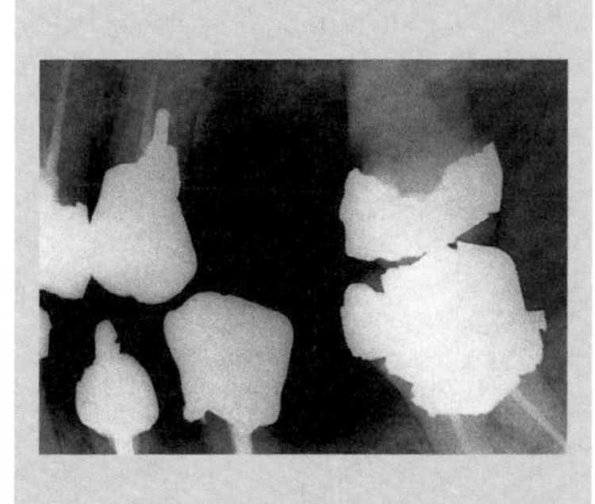

271 b

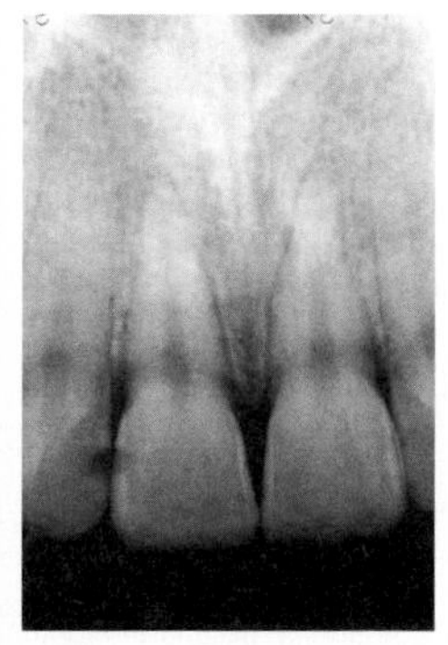

272 a

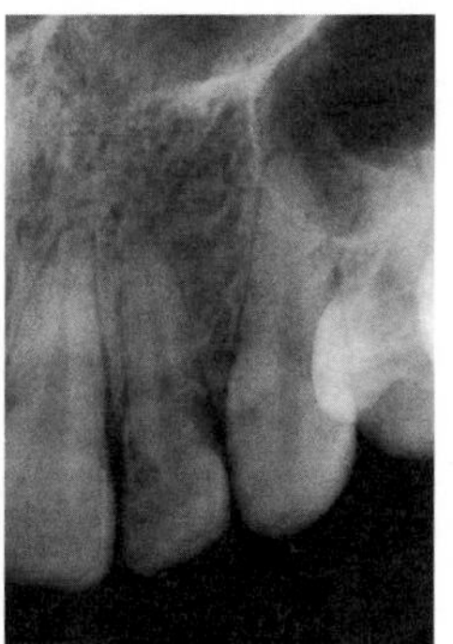

272 b

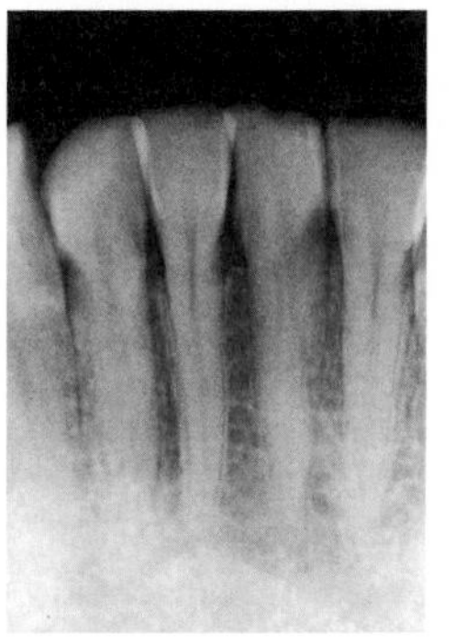

272 c

In order to obtain a complete and thorough radiographic diagnosis at the initial appointment for each patient, a panoramic radiograph is indicated, also for patients manifesting clinical signs of periodontitis; the correct position of the jaw should be established according to the guidelines presented on pages **10/11**.

Even though a panoramic radiograph presents only two-dimensional zonography (thick-slice scan) and a two-dimensional summation process, if it is taken correctly it can to a great extent replace the "traditional" complete intraoral periodontal survey. This represents time-saving for the dental practice team, as well as more comfort and significant reduction of radiation exposure for the patient. The predetermined angle of projection with the panoramic apparatus and the orofacially targeted central ray along the dental arch with very nearly the same object-projection surface distances are clearly superior to a radiographic survey taken with individual periapical images using various projection angles in both vertical and horizontal planes. In addition, a panoramic radiograph provides an overview of the course of the entire alveolar ridge crest. In special cases, where particular details have not been optimally depicted, the panoramic radiograph can be supplemented with targeted intraoral projections, such as bitewings in the posterior segments or special projections in the anterior regions. Such supplemental images can usually be taken without consideration for depicting the entire tooth crown, using an appropriate image receptor holder (IRH) and employing the right-angle technique.

Fig. 273 **Marginal periodontitis**. This extremely high-quality panoramic radiograph of a 44-year-old female resulted from precise positioning (see p. **11**) and properly selected exposure data and clearly depicts moderate to severe adult periodontitis (chronic periodontitis). From a radiographic diagnostic point-of-view, one observes the ravages of advanced periodontitis on numerous teeth, with bone loss up to two-thirds of the root length and virtually all furcations in both maxillary and mandibular molars involved. Even though a panoramic radiograph is only a two-dimensional picture, this view of the alveolar ridge provides a central ray projection angle that is the same in all arch segments, in contrast to a periodontal survey taken using individual periapical radiographs; the image even provides, at least to a certain degree, depiction of the maxillary anterior region and also the mandibular anterior segment in a single projection.

Fig. 274 **Marginal periodontitis**. This panoramic radiograph of a 54-year-old female reveals the consequences of adult (chronic) periodontitis, with multiple tooth loss. Because of the lack of any timely and appropriate prosthetic treatment, teeth 25, 26, 28, and 38 have become elongated (supererupted). The existing traumatic occlusion between 28 and 38 has led to severe vertical osseous defects around these teeth due to periodontal ligament trauma. Both of these teeth, but especially tooth 38, exhibit poorly demarcated alveolar walls, with local sclerosing ostitis. A dentogenic pseudocyst is obvious in the left maxillary sinus, likely of inflammatory etiology.

Fig. 275 **Marginal periodontitis**. The panoramic radiograph of a 46-year-old female reveals advanced (progressive) periodontitis. In addition to generalized bone loss all along the alveolar crest, note also severe vertical defects around the roots of many affected teeth. From these initial osseous lesions, which can be very well observed on teeth 44 and 45, the bony pockets progress vertically to the root apices, and this can be visualized in a more advanced stage between teeth 25 and 26, and in "terminal" stages on teeth 26, 27, 38, 37, 36, 32, and 46. Visible also is the inflammatory mucosal swelling and the radiopacity in the left maxillary sinus, as well as the reactive, chronic, and diffuse sclerosing osteomyelitis with its typical "cotton wool" appearance in the region of the affected tooth roots.

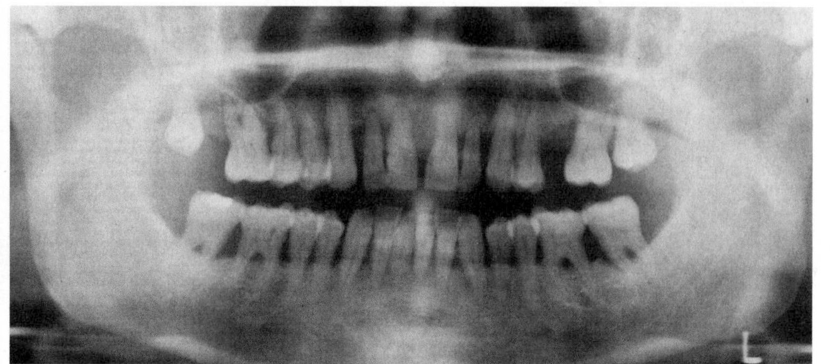

273

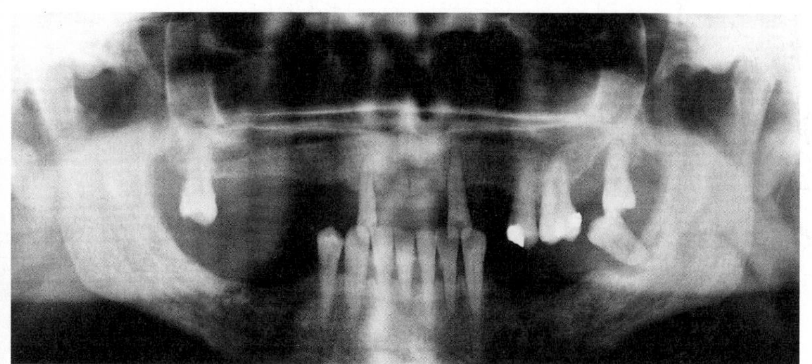

274

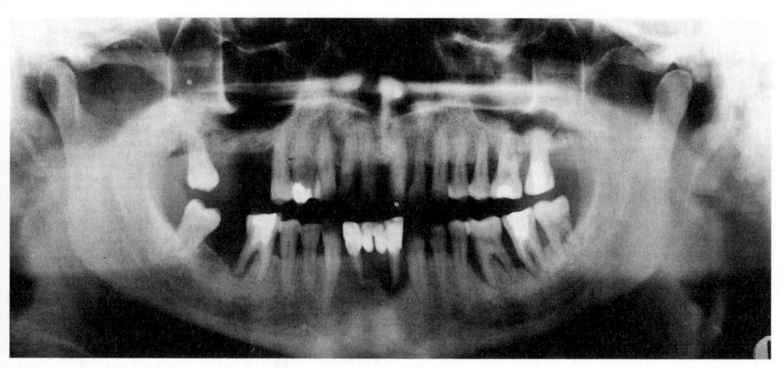

275

Fig. 276a Depicting the course of the alveolar ridge using periapical radiographs. This enlarged periapical radiograph, taken of the region of maxillary teeth 11–13 using the bisecting angle technique, depicts the course of the vestibular (or buccal) and the palatal (or lingual) portions of the alveolar crest because of the oblique projection of the central ray. With apically projected intraoral (periapical) radiographs of the maxilla and mandible, the vestibular (or buccal) portion of the alveolar ridge with be depicted without any overlapping. For this reason, if such radiographs are taken using the normal and routine exposure settings, these structures are frequently overexposed and may be rendered virtually invisible; an important additional consideration is the role played by the distance of the image receptor from the radiation source. The palatal (or lingual) portion of the alveolar crest is not only nearer to the image receptor (IR), it is also superimposed by the alveolar bone proper. The addition effect thus created causes the lingual/palatal segments of the alveolar crest to be more clearly depicted (**arrow**). It is for this reason that in periodontitis patients with vertical defects and multi-walled bony pockets the periapical radiographic technique with its unavoidable summation effects cannot provide or guarantee an exact radiographic diagnostic conclusion concerning the true shape and depth of a bony periodontal pocket.

Fig. 276b Depiction of the course of the alveolar ridge using periapical radiographs. Apically projected radiographs of the premolar and molar regions of the maxilla clearly depict the palatal aspect of the alveolar ridge (**arrow**). Especially in the maxilla, because of purely anatomic circumstances, attempts at parallel and right-angle techniques usually only achieve an oblique projection; therefore, a spatially and dimensionally accurate depiction of the shape and extent of bone loss cannot be guaranteed using intraoral projections in all segments of the dental arch. Any radiographic diagnosis that attempts to quantitate the stages of periodontal bone loss using periapical radiographs demands extreme caution and restraint because the roots of the teeth will be projected as radiopacities overlapping the alveolar ridge and any existing osseous defects.

Fig. 277 Depicting the course of the alveolar crest using periapical and bitewing radiographs. The very oversimplified schematic diagrams above and below demonstrate the advantages of a perfectly horizontal projection (**blue**) as opposed to an oblique projection (**red**) in both maxilla and mandible when taking radiographs to evaluate generalized horizontal bone loss. With an oblique central ray projection (**red**), any existing bone loss will appear less severe than is actually the case because the vestibular portion of the alveolar crest will be projected onto the palatal/lingual cementoenamel junction causing object distortion. The four periapical radiographs are apically projected pictures of the posterior segments of the maxilla (**above**) and the mandible (**below**). For purposes of comparison, the bitewing radiographs of the same case were taken with a perfectly horizontally targeted central ray. It becomes quickly obvious that the location of the alveolar crest in relation to the cementoenamel junctions is falsely depicted in the periapical projections. Only the bitewing radiographs reveal the true extent of bone loss. Particularly striking are the comparisons of apparent bone loss between teeth 16 and 15, 25 and 26, as well as 35 and 36. Even intraoral radiographs taken to evaluate periodontal bone loss and attempting to employ the parallel or right-angle technique must frequently (especially in the maxilla) be taken with a slightly oblique projection for anatomic reasons, especially if the entire tooth is to be depicted. This can often lead to results similar to those achieved with a standard oblique apical projection. In cases of advanced periodontitis, a properly projected panoramic radiograph is frequently sufficient, and if necessary can be supplemented by targeted intraoral projections, which can consciously neglect complete depiction of the tooth crown. For particular complicated cases, primary or secondary CT (computed tomography) scans or VT (volume tomography) may be indicated.

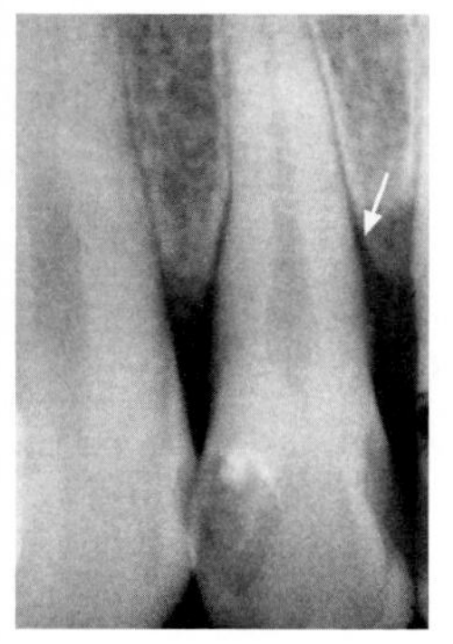

276 a

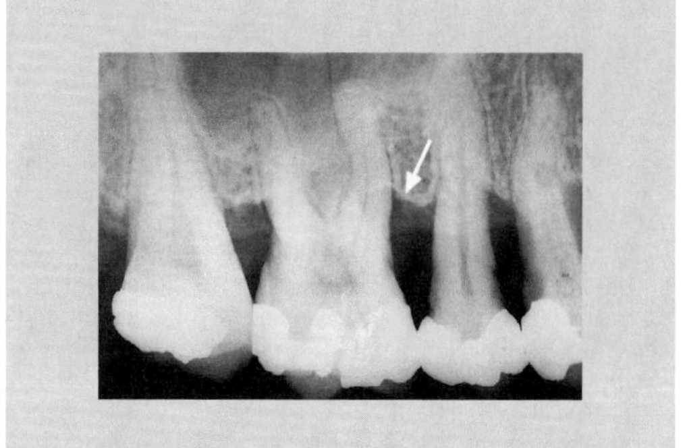

276 b

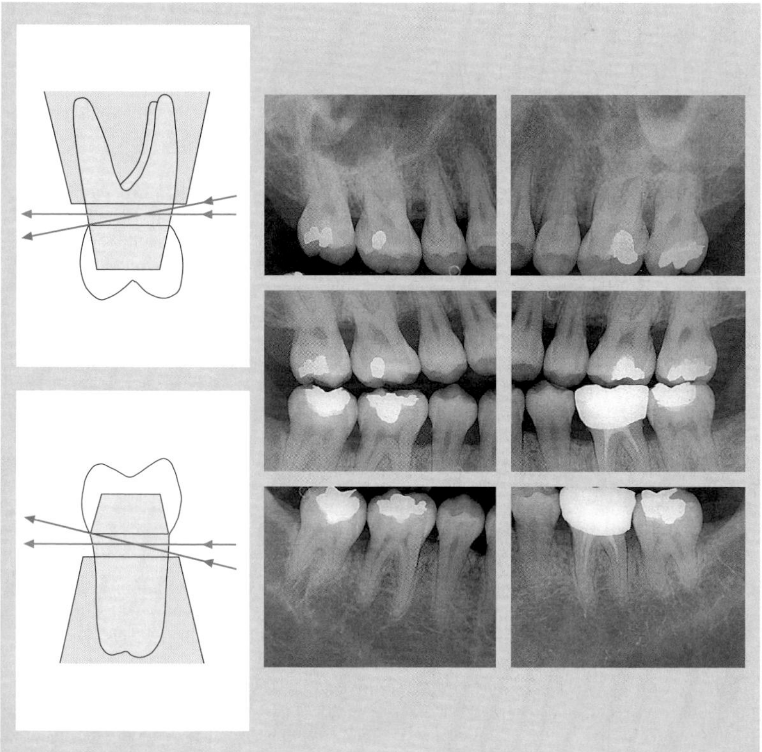

277

For treatment planning and for therapeutic success, it is important to gather concrete information, and this demands anatomically perfect depiction of bone loss in comparison to the level of the cementoenamel junction in order to permit correct interpretation of the shape and depth of periodontal pockets. When evaluating multi-walled bony pockets using a two-dimensional radiographic procedure, it is important to keep in mind that thin osseous walls or those that have been rendered more radiolucent by the effects of acute inflammatory conditions may be rendered radiographically invisible if the exposure settings are too high. Also of significance is an evaluation of the osseous reactions in the remaining bone surrounding the periodontally affected tooth roots, and this cannot be fully and completely ascertained using intraoral dental radiographs.

Especially in advanced cases, these and similar questions can be approached and answered today much more precisely using computed tomography (CT), which by means of primary axial thin-layer tomography or secondary jaw cross-sectional views, can depict the desired structures in a relationship of 1:1. The further development of cone beam computed tomography with volume measurement capability (see Fig. **151/152**) provides improved depiction of individual tooth roots and their surrounding alveolar bone in all possible planes of section. The oft-mentioned "subtraction radiography" technique, which permits precise repositioning over time and measurement of osseous resorption and osseous apposition, is indicated only for specific research purposes and is not suitable for general dental practice use.

Fig. 278a Depicting the course of the alveolar crest using supplemental intraoral targeted radiographs. The diagram shows the correct (blue) and the incorrect (red) central ray projections for proper depiction of the osseous septum between teeth 13 and 12. Only precise orthoradial targeting of the central ray to the desired interdental space will provide an optimum radiograph with a high level of interpretability (see also p. **45**).

Fig. 278b Depicting the course of the alveolar crest using supplemental intraoral targeted radiographs. The skull preparation shows how the osseous septum between teeth 13 and 12 must be targeted in order to achieve an orthoradial depiction. Noteworthy also are the interdental septa between teeth 14 and 13 as well as between 12 and 11, which are not appropriately projected with the orthoradial central ray (see p. **45**).

Fig. 278c Depicting the course of the alveolar crest using supplemental intraoral targeted radiographs. The periapical radiograph not only optimally depicts the targeted interdental septum, it also reveals the periodontal ligament spaces of the adjacent teeth without any overlapping. To facilitate proper taking of such special projections, the use of an appropriate IR holder is recommended, which will properly position the IR in the middle of the palatal vault. This tip concerning IRH devices is often also applicable to other anatomically problematic regions of the dental arches.

Fig. 279 Depicting the course of the alveolar ridge using a panoramic radiograph and a supplemental targeted intraoral radiograph. This panoramic radiograph of a 58-year-old male was the initial radiograph, and provides a useful basis for radiographic diagnostic examination. Only on tooth 31 is the course of the alveolar ridge distorted and unclear. The periapical radiograph (Fig. **280a**) was taken to clarify the preliminary findings.

Fig. 280a Depicting the course of the alveolar ridge using supplemental and targeted intraoral radiographs. To supplement the panoramic radiograph depicted above (Fig. **279**), a single intraoral (periapical) targeted radiograph was taken for clear depiction of the alveolar crest in the region of tooth 31.

Fig. 280b Caries, restoration overhang, calculus, and periodontal pathology. Section from a panoramic radiograph of a 44-year-old male with adult periodontitis and traumatic occlusion between teeth 17 and 47. Caries 25 mesial and distal, and 26 mesial. Note also elongation (supereruption) of teeth 25, 26, and 27. Calculus on teeth 33, 32, 31, 41, 42, and 43, and a grossly overcontoured MOD restoration on tooth 24.

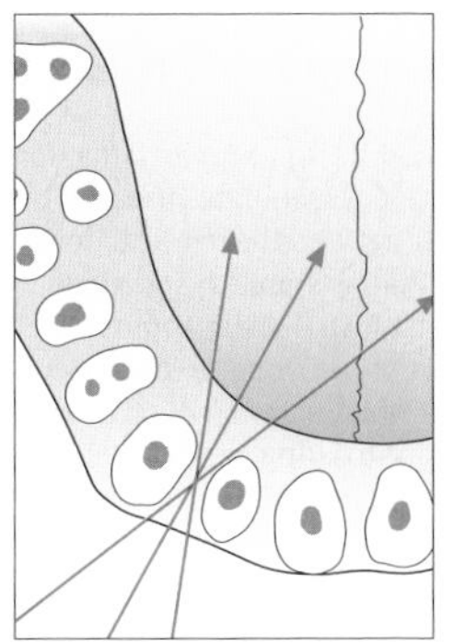

278 a

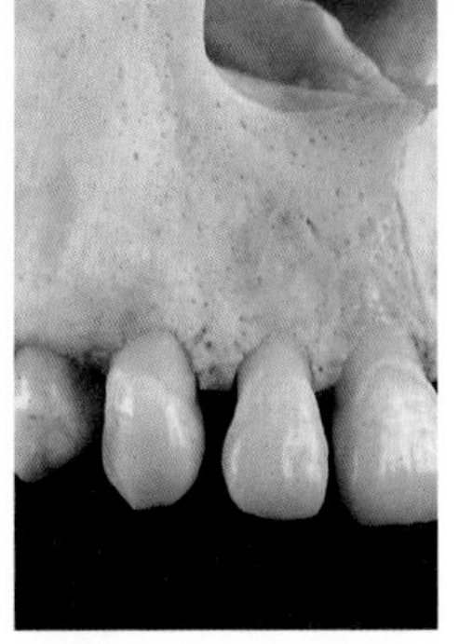

278 b

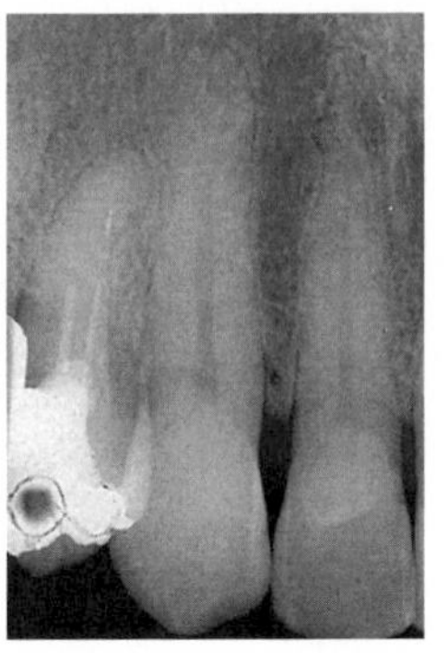

278 c

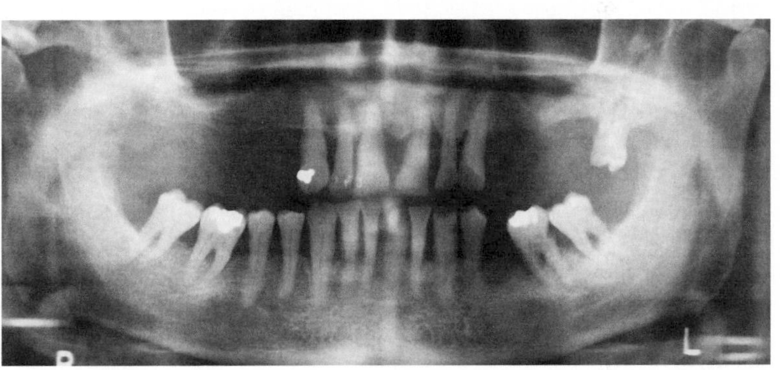

279

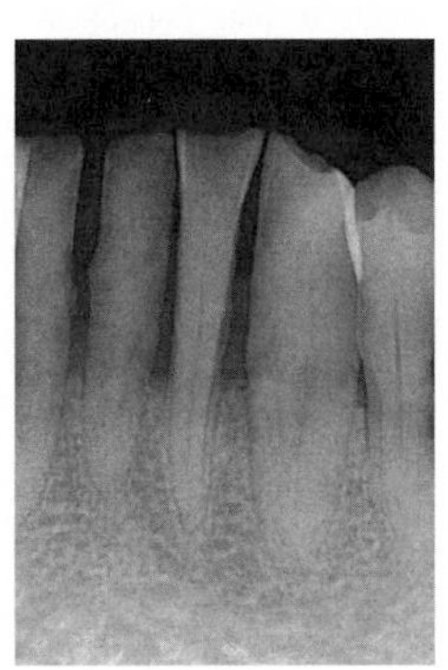

280 a

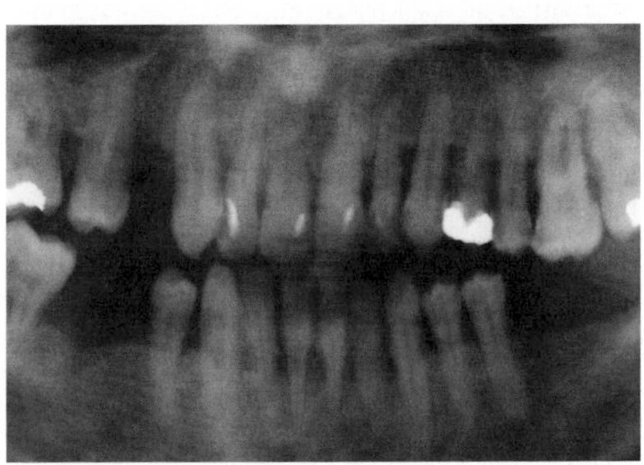

280 b

The **etiologies of radiographically visible periodontal diseases** are numerous. Unfortunately, the clinical classification of these diseases is not always helpful for a diagnostically valuable radiographic description, because the radiographic examination and diagnosis evolves only from the two-dimensional image, which cannot always be precisely correlated to the results of a thorough clinical examination. On the other hand, experience in diagnostic radiography may contribute to the detection of other disease processes that may *simulate* periodontal disease (clinically), or even disease processes that may elicit periodontal disease secondarily; this can therefore contribute to more appropriate therapeutic approaches.

Two important criteria for proper detection and classification of periodontal diseases include the patient's age and the medical/dental history; this information should be provided to the diagnosing radiologist where appropriate.

The clinical aspect of periodontal diseases relate primarily to inflammation, which usually develops from a pre-existing gingivitis. Bacterial plaque (biofilm), improper or inadequate oral hygiene, and calculus accumulation are important etiologic factors (see p. **166**).

Fig. 281 Possibilities with CT in the radiographic diagnosis of periodontal diseases. Initial panoramic radiograph of a 21-year-old male. Aggressive periodontitis with isolated severe bone loss between teeth 14–15, 11–23, 41–42, and 43–46. Spherical radiopacity in the right maxillary sinus. The following figures indicate the importance of proper patient positioning.

Fig. 282a Axial CT of the maxilla. Here the plane of the selected slice is a bit too high dorsally and shows the anterior teeth at the level of the cementoenamel junction and the molars at the apical third of the roots. Obvious is the lack of any vestibular osseous lamella on the alveolar process, and osteolysis in the region of teeth 13 mesial–23 distal. The bone loss between teeth 14 and 15 has achieved the level of the middle third of the root. Note also the slightly oblique positioning of the selected slice, wherein the right side is somewhat higher than the left.

Fig. 282b Axial CT of the maxilla. The slightly asymmetric section through the maxilla (see above) portrays the right maxillary sinus in its full dimension, and with a pseudocyst on the lateral wall that likely derived from an inflammatory process. The bone loss on the vestibular aspect of teeth 21–22 is not portrayed at its deepest point. The other areas of bone loss (visible in the adjacent figure) exhibit a partially intact vestibular osseous lamella by teeth 13–21. There, and also around tooth 22, the osteolytic process has reached the border, and one can observe a reaction zone with sclerosing ostitis and individual lacunae, all of which announce further progressing of the bone loss.

Fig. 283a Axial CT of the mandible. This somewhat asymmetric slice through the mandible (see above) provides a section that depicts the level of the furcations of the molars on the right side, and approximately the apical third of the roots of the mandibular teeth on the left side. Between the roots of teeth 41 and 42, one notes the absence of a vestibular osseous lamella of the alveolar process, as well as the typical trabecular pattern of the interradicular osseous septum. Distal to tooth 43 one observes remnants of the septum; there is a total lack of covering osseous lamellae on the vestibular aspect and on the lingual it is visible if somewhat shadowy because it extends somewhat higher.

Fig. 283b Axial CT of the mandible. This somewhat asymmetric slice through the mandible (see above) provides a layer that traverses the middle third of the roots of the right mandibular molars, and the apical third of those molars on the left side. Between teeth 41 and 42 the floor of the osteolytic process is obvious (see adjacent image), with remaining vestibular osseous lamellae as well as signs of normal bone structure. Between 43 and 45, the overlying lamella on the vestibular aspect is partially intact. From the distal of tooth 43 to the distal of tooth 44, the floor of the bony pocket is clear. Mesial to tooth 45, bone destruction has progressed into the apical region of the root of tooth 45. The osseous resorption of the vestibular compact bone at the level of the partially impacted tooth 48 anticipates the eruption of this third molar in the buccal direction. Quite in contrast to conventional intraoral radiographs, pocket depths can be accurately measured 1:1 with both axial primary tomographies as well as with transverse secondary tomography, provided by most commercially available dental CT programs.

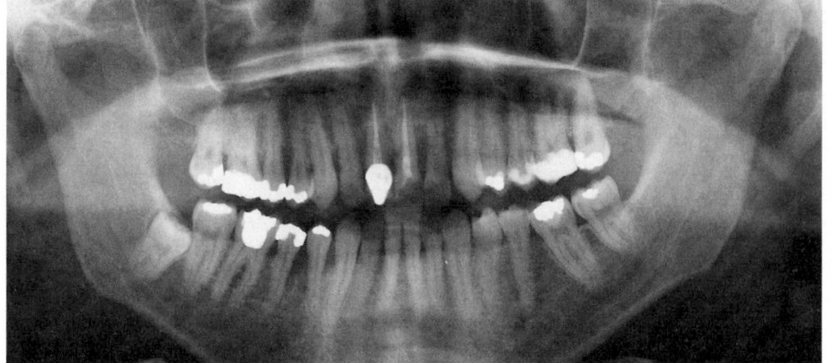
281

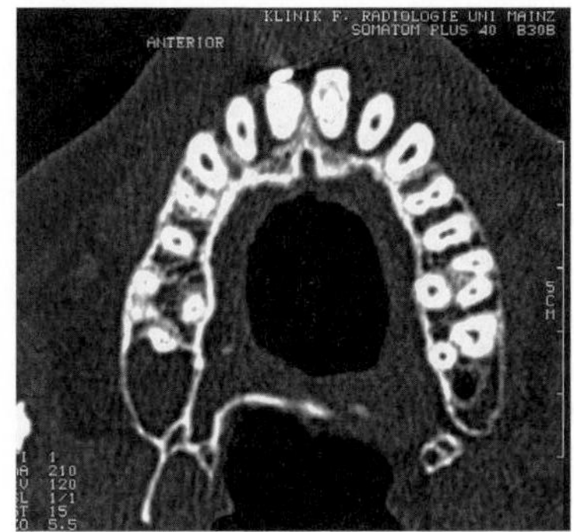

282 a

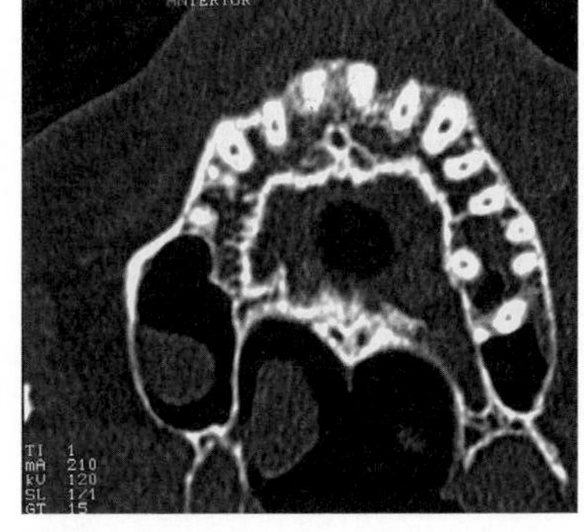

282 b

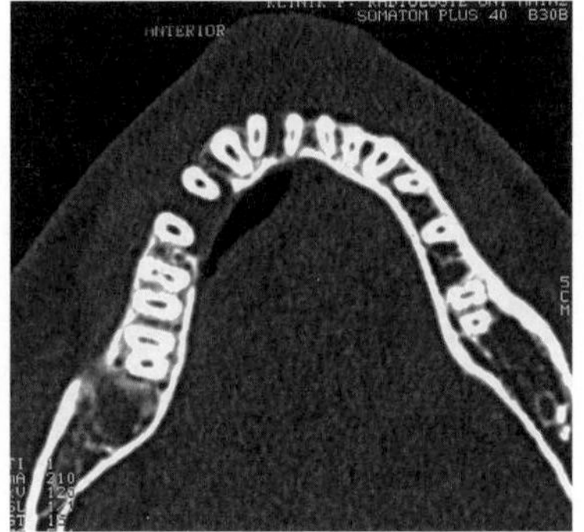

283 a

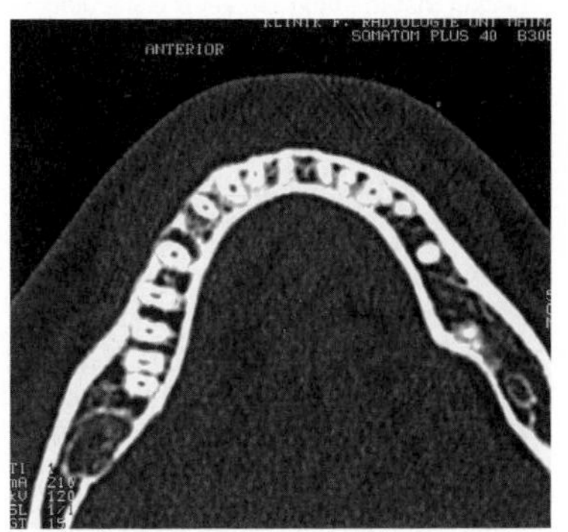

283 b

The rough surface of dental calculus serves as a nidus for plaque formation and accumulation. In the mandible, the most common site is the lingual surfaces of the anterior teeth. In the maxilla, calculus is usually only detected on the buccal surfaces of the molars.

Fig. 284a Advanced periodontitis. The periapical radiograph clearly depicts an isolated bony pocket between teeth 31 and 32. Clinically there was an obvious periodontal abscess emanating from tooth 31. The acute inflammation becomes apparent within bone only after a latent period of many days; it can be identified here already as a blurred demarcation at the base of the pocket. Distal to tooth 32 one observes triangulation at the entrance to the alveolus, with lacunae in the osseous structure of the septum; this is the radiographic expression of an expanding area of inflammation.

Fig. 284b Advanced periodontitis. Terminal stage of advanced periodontitis, with periodontal abscess. Following an extended period of time under the influence of the inflammatory process, the normal osseous structures have effectively disappeared and there are zones of radiolucency in the periapical regions that are surrounded by sclerosed reaction zones.

Fig. 284c Advanced chronic periodontitis. Horizontal bone loss in the anterior segment of the mandible. Subgingival calculus is clearly visible on the coronal third of the roots of the anterior teeth. The obviously widened vascular canals in the remaining interdental bone are often evidence of increased vascularization in the slowly progressing adult periodontitis. The clearly visible sclerosis of the interdental septa indicates that this is a case of chronic, slowly progressing inflammatory disease.

Fig. 285a Advanced periodontitis. Note the deep funnel-shaped bony pocket distal to tooth 23; the pocket has expanded into the periapical region of the alveolar process. The bone in this region exhibits a washed-out appearance and lack of normal osseous structure. The clinical examination revealed a periodontal abscess. Note also the lacunae in the sclerosed structure of the alveolar ridge around the root of tooth 22 as evidence of an advancing acute inflammatory process.

Fig. 285b Advanced periodontitis. The periapical radiograph of the maxillary anterior region demonstrates that with recurring episodes (*bursts*) of inflammation, osseous destruction can advance spirally around the affected root in the apical direction. The radiographic diagnosis leads to the suspicion that the bony pocket is expanding along the root surface, because the radiopacity of the root of tooth 11 overlaps any bony pocket in a two-dimensional summation image.

Fig. 285c Chronic advanced periodontitis. Horizontal bone loss in the maxillary anterior region, without radiographic signs of acute inflammation in this case of generalized, involutive periodontal disease.

Fig. 286a Central hemangioma. Serendipitous radiographic finding in a 19-year-old female. The radiograph was taken because of clinical signs of tooth mobility (25) without any visible pathologic alterations of the gingiva. In comparison to an isolated, vertical osseous defect, this periapical radiograph reveals irregular osseous structure between teeth 24 and 25; the honeycomb-like and here scarcely visible radiolucency is reminiscent of the early form of ameloblastoma (see Fig. **379b**).

Fig. 286b Eosinophilic granuloma. This mild form of a Langerhans cell granulomatosis (eosinophilic granuloma) in a 43-year-old female exhibits a sharply demarcated, garland-shaped radiolucency, which extends from the mesial root of tooth 16 to the mesial aspect of tooth 14. The osteolytic process in the alveolar bone leads only quite late to any clinical mobility of the affected teeth. In the later stages of development of this lesion, the affected teeth as viewed in a periapical radiograph appear to "hang in mid-air."

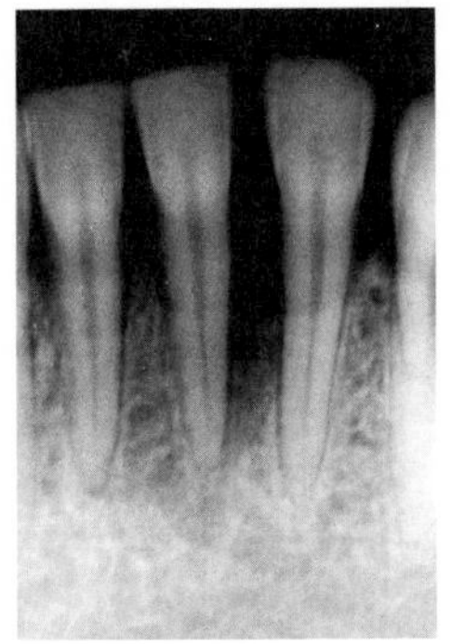
284 a

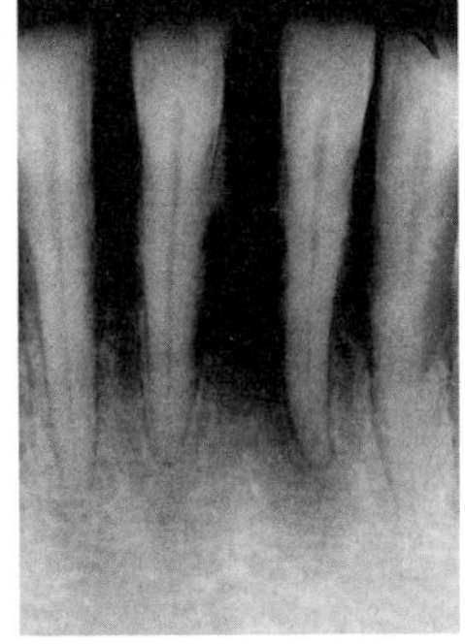
284 b

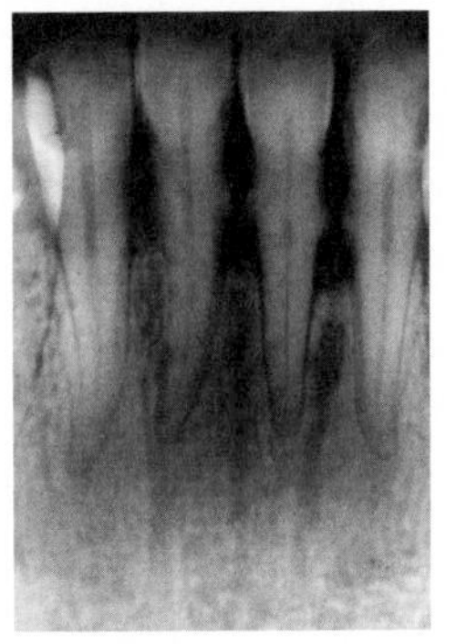
284 c

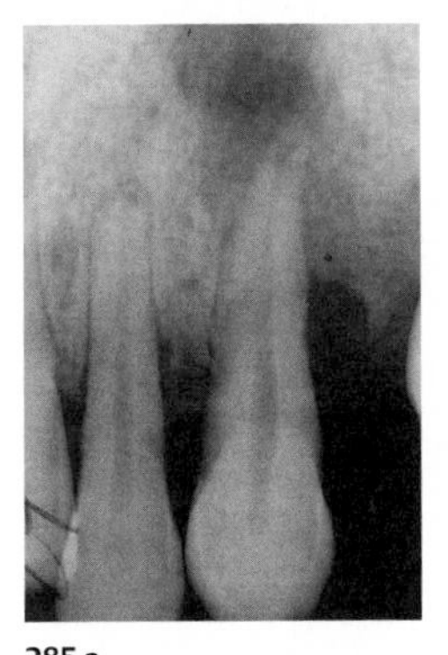
285 a

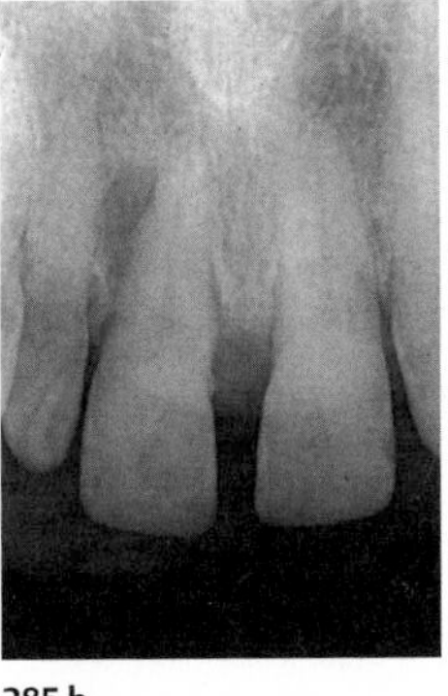
285 b

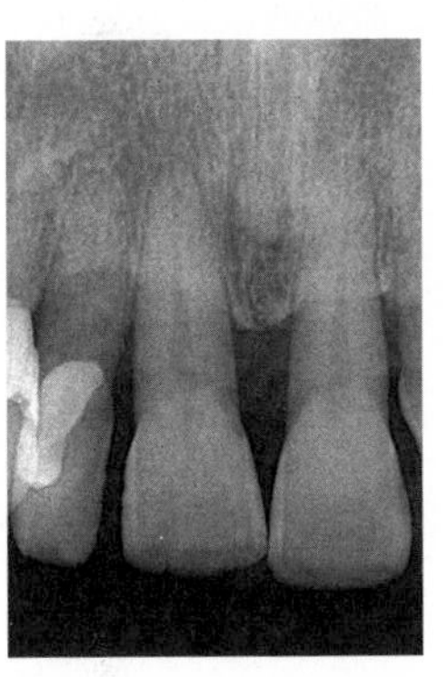
285 c

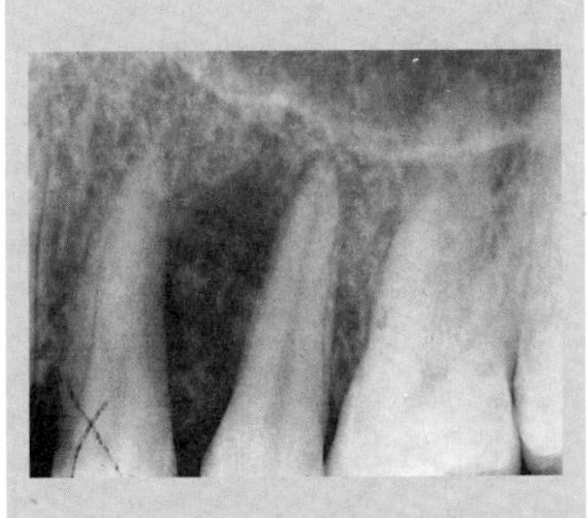
286 a

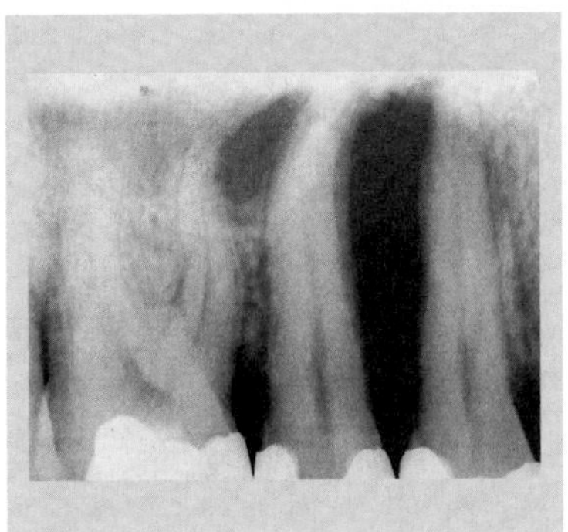
286 b

In addition to the inflammation elicited by dental plaque biofilm, there are additional etiologic factors and risk factors:

- Positional anomalies of the teeth, above all caused by untreated extraction spaces, impacted teeth, expanding or expansive cysts and tumors, as well as genetically based hypodontia or hyperodontia (e.g., supernumerary teeth)
- Macroglossia
- Trauma caused by occlusal disharmonies as a result of restorations, crowns, and bridges. Inadequate margin closure, poor contact points, recurrent caries with food impaction, or as the result of occlusal disturbances elicited by full-mouth restorative rehabilitation, or forced orthodontic treatment
- Accidental trauma with injury to the periodontal ligament of the involved teeth, or periodontal ligament injury during preparation of adjacent teeth, or during endodontic therapy
- Effects of hematologic diseases/disorders.
- Effect of job-related diseases
- Smoking
- As accompanying symptoms of various syndromes

A special form of marginal periodontitis with pocket formation may be observed with partially impacted mandibular third molars; this is referred to as **pericoronitis**.

Numerous medical (systemic) syndromes are associated with tooth positional anomalies and this can also lead to periodontal pathology, especially because oral hygiene is frequently unsatisfactory in such cases. The following syndromes and/or diseases may be involved:

- Diabetes mellitus, especially the genetically based, noninsulin-dependent variant (Type IIa)
- Ehlers–Danlos syndrome (elastic fibrodysplasia, type VIII with autosomal dominant inheritance and premature tooth loss)
- Eosinophilic granuloma, a variant of the Abt–Letterer–Siwe syndrome (earlier: histiocytosis X), which is also referred to as the Hand–Schüller–Christian disease
- Neutropenia, a chronic benign disorder elicited by a genetically based disturbance of granulocyte formation
- Neutrophil functional disturbances caused by leukocyte adhesion defects beginning prepubertally

Fig. 287 Eosinophilic granuloma. This panoramic radiograph of a 66-year-old male reveals a mild form of Langerhans cell granulomatosis (earlier referred to as histiocytosis X). In comparison to the end stage of advanced periodontitis (see Fig. **288a**), the radiograph (especially noticeable on teeth 47 and 46) reveals the pathognomonically typical picture of "teeth suspended in mid-air," with confluent radiolucencies, and the garland-shaped boundaries of sclerosed bone. The Hand–Schüller–Christian disease affects adolescent boys above all, but also older males, and for this reason any residual dentition with "suspended teeth" always elicits the suspicion of an eosinophilic granuloma.

Fig. 288a Advanced periodontitis. The periapical radiograph reveals the terminal stage of advanced periodontitis; upon cursory inspection one notes certain similarities with the above-depicted eosinophilic granuloma. Here also, the affected teeth appear "suspended" in the jaw; however, the circumapical expansion of the osteolysis caused by bacterial infection along with the sclerotic reaction zones provides a comparatively different radiographic image.

Fig. 288b Neutropenia. Chronic familial neutropenia is a genetically related disorder of granulocyte formation, and leads to periodontal pathology; the radiographic picture may lead to confusion vis-à-vis severe generalized juvenile periodontitis. Eleven-year-old male.

Fig. 289 Diabetes mellitus. This panoramic radiograph of a 43-year-old female reveals periodontitis with furcation invasion on teeth 36 and 46. This is likely a case of genetically related, noninsulin-dependent adult diabetes.

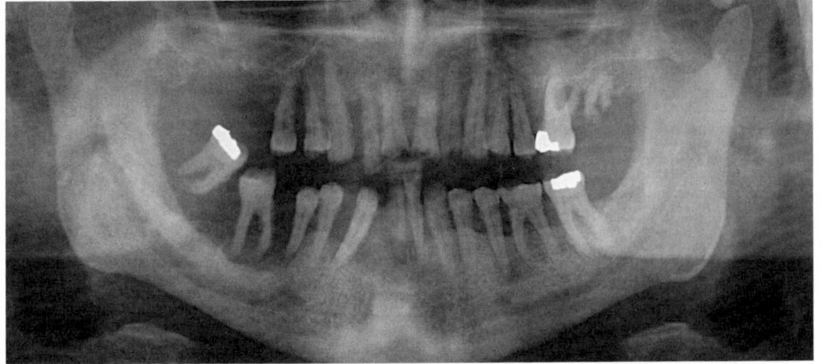

287

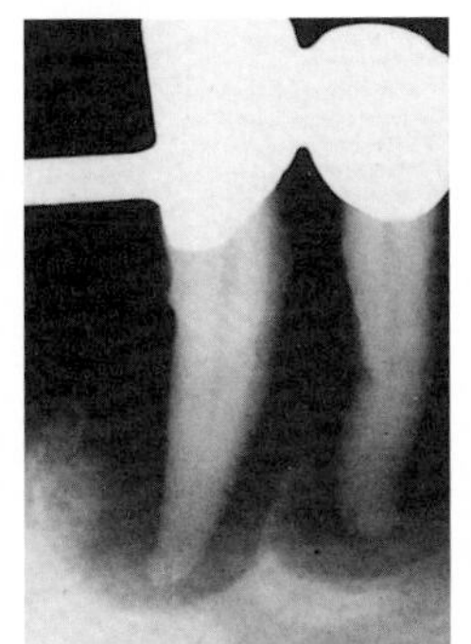

288 a

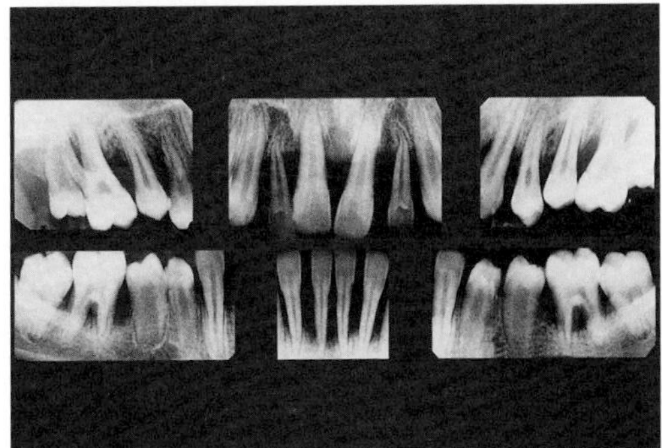

288 b

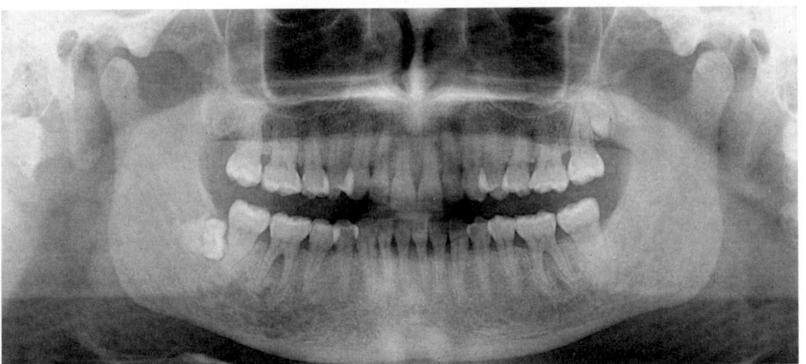

289

- Papillon–Lefèvre syndrome (keratosis palmoplantaris), with gingivitis, periodontitis, and gingival recession
- Idiopathic periodontal pathology (juvenile periodontitis), possibly with neutrophil dysfunction and pre-pubertal onset
- Robinow syndrome with multiple dysplasias and the accompanying symptom of gingival hypoplasia

The following diseases may also simulate inflammatory periodontal diseases:

- Peripheral giant cell granuloma with cup-shaped defects and destruction of the surrounding alveolar process (see Fig. **410 a**)
- Intraosseous (central) hemangioma
- Carcinoma and sarcoma with destruction of the periodontal ligament (attachment loss)

In the realm of periodontal pathology, the following types present characteristic radiographic images:

- The extremely rare pre-pubertal periodontitis of early childhood
- Localized juvenile periodontitis (LJP) which begins at around puberty and affects primarily the first permanent molars and incisors, predominantly in females
- Rapidly progressive periodontitis (RPP) now known as aggressive periodontitis in young adults
- Slowing progressing periodontitis of adults (chronic periodontitis)

Worthy of consideration also are traumatogenic and involutive forms of periodontal disease, which may be localized or generalized.

Radiographic signs of acute and chronic inflammations of the jaws: Acute intraosseous inflammation only becomes visible in a radiograph after a period of latency, when the poorly demarcated radiolucency becomes visible following demineralization and serous imbibition.

If the virulence of the causative microflora is low or if the host defense reaction is strong, slowly progressing chronic inflammations begin to exhibit the typical signs of chronic diffuse osteomyelitis, with poorly demarcated radiopacities (cotton wool effect). A radiographic picture shows only a single point in time during the advancing disease process.

Fig. 290 a Periodontal pathology caused by trauma. The periapical radiograph reveals a gross extrusion of root canal filling material at the furcation of tooth 36. Noteworthy is the damage to the periodontal ligament and the furcal area of the mesial root, which was caused by the creation of a false canal during endodontic instrumentation. The consequence has been the development of interradicular bone resorption. Note also the massive recurrent caries on the mesial surface of tooth 37.

Fig. 290 b Periodontal pathology caused by trauma. This periapical radiograph reveals interdental bone resorption between teeth 35 and 37, caused by the grotesque amalgam overhang on the mesial of tooth 37. Noteworthy also is the deep proximal caries on the distal of tooth 34, and the undercontour of the restoration on the distal of tooth 37, with recurrent caries, as well as the distinct carious lesion on the distal of 38.

Fig. 291 a Periodontal pathology caused by trauma. The periapical radiograph depicts tooth 11, which exhibits a central (internal) granuloma that developed following trauma. It is also interesting to observe that the dentin lining of the pulp chamber remains intact. In addition, tooth 11 exhibits a bony pocket on the mesial surface (accident-related).

Fig. 291 b Periodontal pathology caused by trauma. This section from a panoramic radiograph reveals the consequences of traumatic occlusion, caused by the maxillary three-unit fixed bridge. Note the massive bone resorption in the mandible following occlusal trauma to the periodontium. Note also the sclerosed reaction zones at the apices of the roots of teeth 36 and 37.

Fig. 292 Involutive periodontal pathology (alveolar atrophy). The panoramic radiograph of a 77-year-old female reveals age-related involution of the alveolar ridge and the body of the mandible; this was earlier referred to as alveolar ridge atrophy.

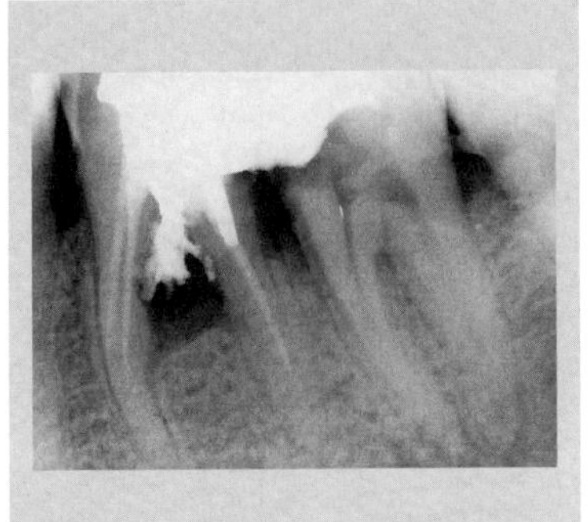

290 a

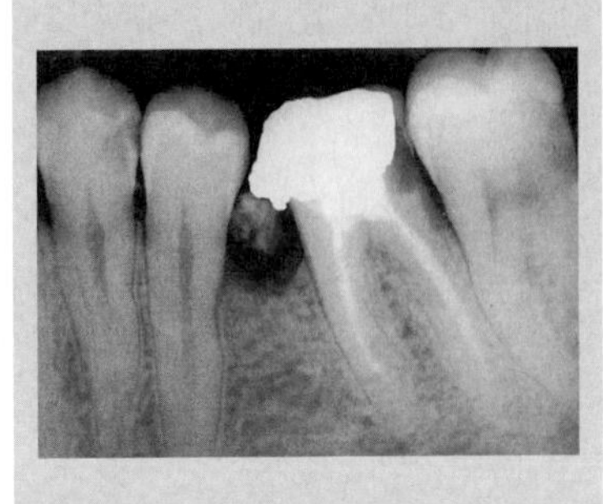

290 b

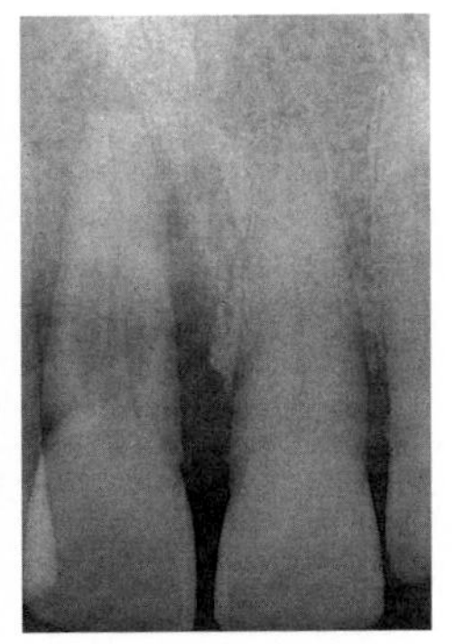

291 a

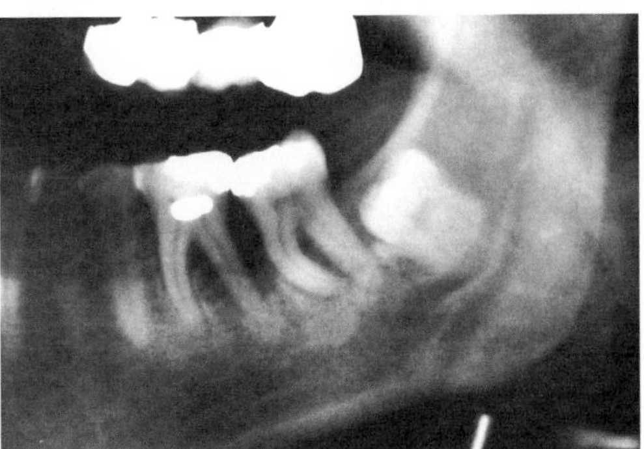

291 b

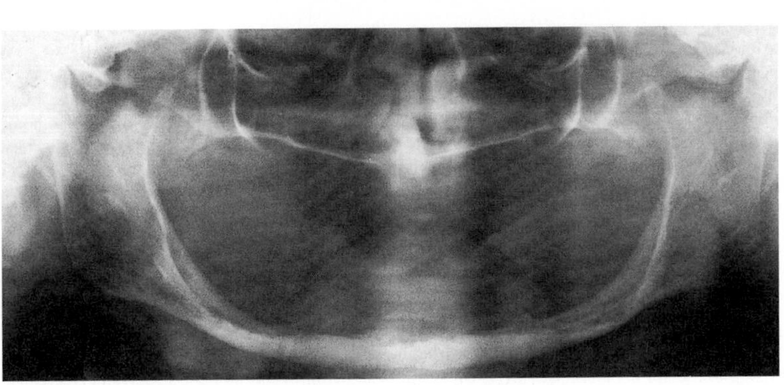

292

Even if the patient is experiencing severe clinical symptoms of pulpitis, the radiograph will not depict any interpretable pathologic alterations if there have been no osseous structural alterations in the periapical region. Only when the advancing pulpal inflammation exits the apical foramen will radiographic signs become evident, including a widened periodontal ligament space and a poorly demarcated periapical radiolucency, the latter caused by demineralization and serous imbibition; these signs generally occur only after a certain period of latency. Because the bone matrix remains viable at this stage, remineralization can occur following appropriate treatment with ultimate healing of the previous osseous defect; such healing can be seen on the radiograph. Also in cases of acute apical periodontitis the radiograph provides only the *current condition* in terms of structural alterations caused by the advancing inflammatory process, and therefore without thorough knowledge of the *clinical* situation radiographic diagnosis will not always provide a comprehensive interpretation.

Fig. 293a Apical periodontitis in periapical radiographs. Clinically, tooth 22 exhibited a subperiosteal abscess and was endodontically trephined; despite severe clinical symptoms, the periapical radiograph reveals no periapical lesion.

Fig. 293b Apical periodontitis in periapical radiographs. In another patient, tooth 22 exhibited a subperiosteal abscess clinically following recurrent caries with pulpal necrosis; the periapical radiograph reveals a widened periodontal ligament space, especially apically, and a poorly demarcated periapical radiolucency.

Fig. 293c Apical periodontitis in periapical radiographs. In still another patient, the radiograph of tooth 22 reveals that the periodontal ligament space and the lamina dura end at the apex as a poorly demarcated radiolucency. The tooth was clinically nonvital and exhibited symptoms of chronic apical periodontitis as well as a periapical granuloma.

Fig. 294a Apical periodontitis in periapical radiographs. In a fourth patient, the radiograph of tooth 22 reveals an encapsulated granuloma. The lamina dura extends into the easily discerned and sclerotic reaction zone surrounding the tooth. At this stage, it is radiographically impossible to definitively decide whether the lesion represents an encapsulated granuloma or a small radicular cyst. Only the diameter of the lesion may give clues; the critical boundary is at about 6 mm. The radiolucency at the apex of tooth 21 is caused by the overlapping of the incisive foramen.

Fig. 294b Apical periodontitis in periapical radiographs. Tooth 36 supports a full cast crown and exhibits the radiographic signs of chronic apical periodontitis and focal sclerosing osteomyelitis in an acute stage. The obvious bone loss between the two roots is also an indication of localized periodontitis with furcation invasion, but this could have been occasioned by occlusal trauma. The lamina dura at both root apices is resorbed, the distal root exhibits a poorly demarcated periapical radiolucency that is a sign of an acute inflammatory process. Despite deep pulp amputation, tooth 35 exhibits an intact periodontal ligament space. As with the root of tooth 36, one can also note signs of focal sclerosing osteomyelitis.

Fig. 295a Apical periodontitis in periapical radiographs. The periapical radiograph of tooth 36 reveals chronic apical periodontitis that resulted from trauma during tooth preparation; note also the inadequate marginal closure of the crown (distal).

Fig. 295b Apical periodontitis, panoramic radiograph. This section from a panoramic radiograph of the same case (Fig. **295a**) reveals the overall situation. The comparison makes it clear that zonography not only makes possible a bilateral comparison of osseous structures, but also larger marginal and apical defects can be portrayed in their environment more realistically than with individual periapical radiographs.

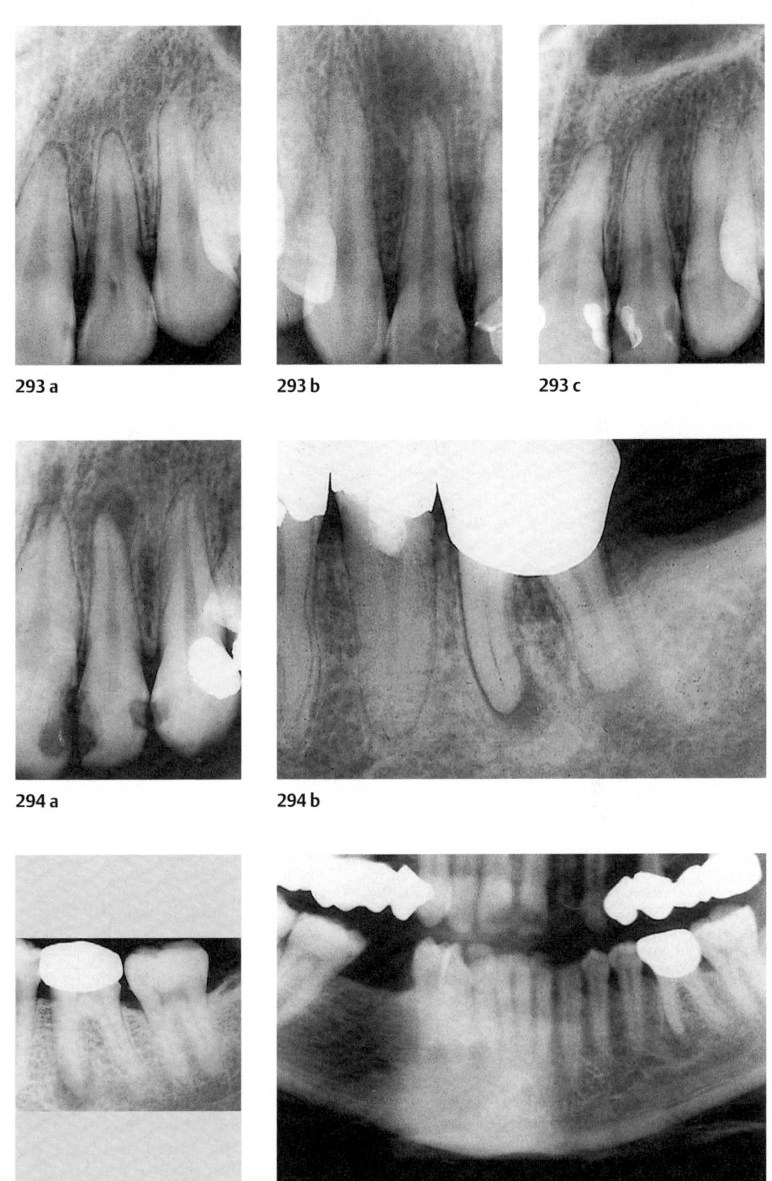

293 a

293 b

293 c

294 a

294 b

295 a

295 b

The development and progression of chronic forms of apical periodontitis depend upon the virulence of the microbial etiology as well as the effectiveness of the host immune response; in the course of disease development and progression, structural alterations become manifest, which can be evaluated radiographically. The initial and most important radiographic symptom is resorption of the lamina dura, which renders the periodontal ligament space at the periapical region no longer discernable. The lamina dura that remains intact around the coronal portions of the root extend to the periapical radiolucency, which is referred to as a **granuloma**, i. e., a chronic granulating inflammation. A granuloma that is surrounded by an expanding reaction zone that appears in the radiograph to be a radiopaque continuation of the lamina dura is described as an encapsulated granuloma. The apex of the root usually appears free within the radiolucency, but it is also possible for a granuloma to develop from a *lateral* branch of the pulpal arborization. In the final stages, usually following repeated acute phases, there is resorption of the affected root and the formation of hypercementosis. During acute stages of chronic apical periodontitis, one observes in the radiograph that the affected structures appear blurred in comparison to surrounding tissues. The sclerosing reaction zone surrounding encapsulated granulomas can mimic a radicular cyst, and in terms of radiographic diagnosis up to a diameter of about 6 mm cannot be differentiated from a cyst (see Fig. **370**).

With further regard to periapical radiolucencies, periapical cemental dysplasia (see p. **269**) in its fibroblastic stage may also resemble chronic apical periodontitis. In such cases, however, the tooth remains vital, and vitality must therefore be tested before the initiation of any therapeutic measures.

Fig. 296 Chronic apical periodontitis and focal sclerosing osteomyelitis as viewed in a panoramic radiograph. This panoramic radiograph of an 18-year-old male reveals chronic focal sclerosing osteomyelitis emanating from nonvital tooth 46, which exhibits broad furcation invasion as well as a bony pocket. In comparison to the left side of the mandible, the clearly discernible and well demarcated reactive sclerosis at the apical regions of teeth 45 and 46 is accompanied by a diffuse radiopacity on the right side. The distal root of tooth 46 has begun to resorb. Distally on teeth 36 and 46 one notes symmetrical dental caries. Note also that in younger patients it is frequently virtually impossible to discern the mandibular canal, but on the right side in this radiograph it is clearly visible as a result of the diffuse sclerosis.

Fig. 297 Chronic apical periodontitis and focal sclerosing osteomyelitis as viewed in the panoramic radiograph. This panoramic radiograph of a 34-year-old female reveals a chronic and diffuse sclerosing osteomyelitis emanating from teeth 17 and 26. Clearly visible are the periapical radiolucencies with sclerosed boundaries toward the maxillary sinuses, which are intensified by the radiopacity of a sinusitis especially on the right side. These types of addition effects in the radiograph render visible the osseous structures with the typical overlapping of areas of osteolysis and osteoblastic activity. Note also the poorly demarcated boundary to the alveolar lobe of the right maxillary sinus.

Fig. 298 Acute osteomyelitis. This panoramic radiograph of a 34-year-old female depicts an acute exacerbation of chronic focal sclerosing osteomyelitis. The alveoli of extracted tooth 46 still exhibit remnants of the lamina dura in a stage of delayed wound healing. The expanding osteomyelitis, with its areas of osteolysis and reactive sclerosis, is perpetuated primarily by the nonvital tooth 47 with its marginal and apical periodontitis and an obvious apical lesion. These radiographic signs became visible only following a latency period of 1–2 weeks.

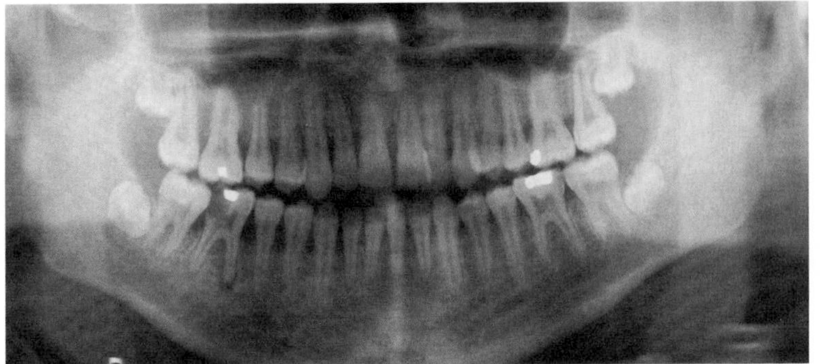

296

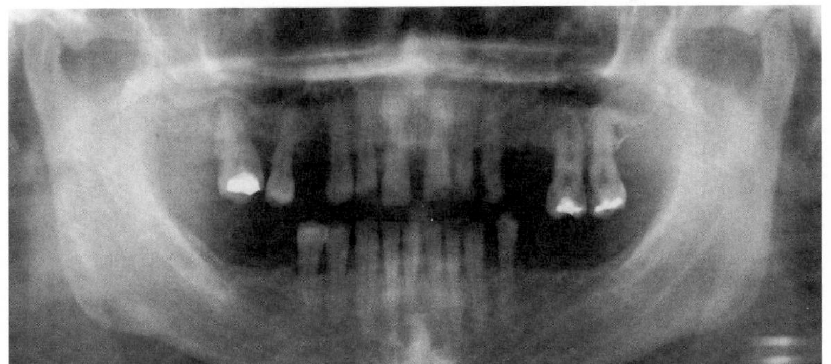

297

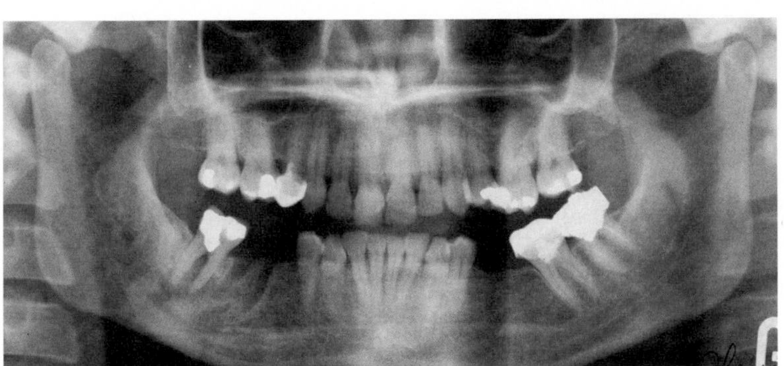

298

In patients suffering from Paget disease of bone, osteolysis may be radiographically evident in the initial stages even with maintained vitality of affected teeth. As viewed radiographically, the course of osteomyelitis includes adjacent zones of osseous resorption and osseous apposition. The radiographic picture is one of cloudy radiopacities (cotton wool effect) with apparent enlargement of the jaw, and thus the radiographic picture resembles chronic, diffuse osteomyelitis.

During the progression of apical or marginal periodontitis, as well as following tooth extraction or irritation relating to medicaments used during endodontic therapy, microbial agents will be introduced into the bone and may lead to host defense reactions and bone marrow inflammation that are visible on a radiograph. In general, one differentiates between acute and chronic forms of osteomyelitis, and both the virulence of the microbial etiologic agent and the host defense posture of the organism are determining factors concerning the course and severity of the disease. Because of its anatomic structure, the mandible is significantly more frequently affected than the maxilla. On the basis of the differences in osseous structure in the maxilla (close trabeculation) and in the mandible (widely spaced trabeculation in the body of the mandible), and the vascularization, it is possible to diagnose the varying forms radiographically. Already existing pathologic structural alterations such as those caused by ostitis deformans or fibrous dysplasia will complicate the radiographic diagnostic evaluation of suspected osteomyelitis. Furthermore, it is not always possible to differentiate radiographically between acute and/or chronic, and primary chronic versus secondary chronic forms of osteomyelitis, without prior knowledge of the medical/dental history and the findings from clinical examination.

Early clinical symptoms of acute osteomyelitis include pain and high fever, paresthesia of the inferior alveolar nerve, maxillary sinusitis, and mobility of numerous teeth, which upon percussion elicit a dull sound. Any structural (osseous) alterations resulting from these osteomyelitic etiologies will be visible radiographically only after a latency period of 1–2 weeks. The radiograph is a two-dimensional summation picture that reveals the osteolysis as manifested by demineralization of the osseous trabeculae. Uninhibited progression of the inflammation, with persistence of undemineralized trabeculae as viewed in the third dimension may impart to the radiographic picture the semblance of multiple small osseous sequesters.

An exceptionally difficult disease picture is provided by the hematogenically induced acute osteomyelitis neonatorum, which usually effects the mandible, because the host de-

Fig. 299 **Acute osteomyelitis.** In the early stages of acute osteomyelitis, despite the presence of clinical signs and symptoms, there are no radiographically discernable features. Only 1–2 weeks after initiation of the disease can spot-like osteolysis and osteosclerosis be detected radiographically, and it is for this reason that the clinical signs are of extreme importance.

Fig. 300 **Acute osteomyelitis.** In contrast to the panoramic radiograph of the same patient (Fig. **299**), this scintigraphy reveals an elevation of activity in the body of the mandible and its ramus on the right side, and shows the true expansion of the existing acute osteomyelitis.

Fig. 301 **Chronic osteomyelitis.** This panoramic radiograph of a 75-year-old male reveals chronic osteomyelitis. Obvious are the spotty areas of osteolysis and reactive sclerosis, which are rendered even more visible along the course of the mandibular canal. For a patient of this age, the vertical dimension of the body of the mandible and its astonishing volume enlargement is pathognomonic. The orofacial expansion, on the other hand, is only discernible via axial CT. In a patient of this age and gender, however, one must always consider Paget disease of bone (see p. **290**).

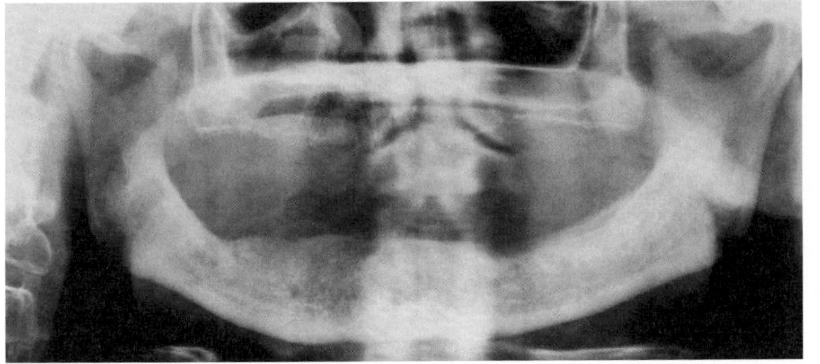

299

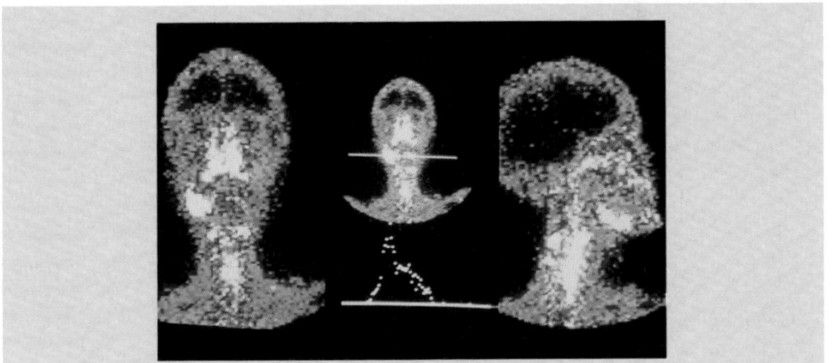

300

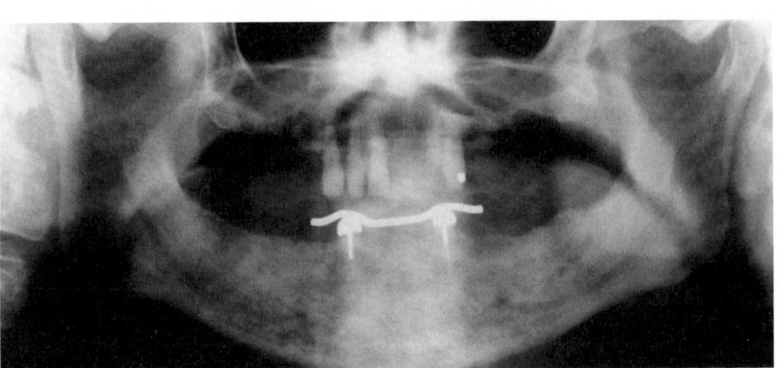

301

fense of newborn infants is always deficient. The clinical symptoms include high fever, chills, severe pain, swelling, and paresthesia of the inferior alveolar nerve with effects in the area served by the mental nerve. At the apex of severity of the disease, the inflammation of the dental sac leads to its eventual sequestration. Sonography is indicated as a possibility for diagnostic imaging, because the effects of the fulminating and progressive acute inflammation in the early stages cannot be depicted with conventional radiographs. The prognosis is unfavorable because of the danger of sepsis, if high doses of antibiotics are not given already in the early stages.

If the appropriate therapy is not provided, acute, suppurative forms of osteomyelitis emanating from apical periodontitis during the first decade of life will evolve into chronic suppurative osteomyelitis. Sequestration of tooth buds with periosteal new bone formation and osseous sequesters occur in late stages and can be detected radiographically. Later consequences can involve resorption of the tooth buds of the permanent dentition or developmental disturbances (dysplasias) in the mandible, which is most often affected. For visual early diagnosis, sonography is indicated, as well as leukocyte scintigraphy.

It is difficult to initially differentiate clinically between an acute osteomyelitis and the rare Ewing sarcoma that occurs in children in the first decade of life.

If untreated, the acute forms of osteomyelitis will develop into secondary forms of osteomyelitis, although this has become very seldom today because of modern antibiotic therapy.

Much more common is primary chronic osteomyelitis, which manifests itself by infrequently occurring, recurring and relatively mild pain and paresthesia because of the altered host defense. Depending upon the virulence of the microflora and the intensity of the host defense response, the radiograph will reveal changes in osseous structure with reactive new bone formation and osseous sequesters that are either resorbed or sloughed.

Following pulpitis and pulpal necrosis, well-demarcated endosteal new bone formation will occur, primarily in the mandible, as a reaction to a recurring, sub-threshold bacterial infection; this is referred to as focal sclerosing osteomyelitis and can be seen in the radiograph concentrically around the apex of the affected tooth. The clinical course is usually asymptomatic.

Fig. 302 Chronic osteomyelitis. These two sections taken from the panoramic radiograph of a 19-year-old male depict chronic osteomyelitis following extraction of tooth 38 and disturbed/delayed wound healing. This radiograph provided a comparison of the typical radiographic appearance of chronic osteomyelitis (left mandibular ramus) in comparison to the healthy mandibular ramus on the right side (**left** radiograph). The radiograph on the **right** section reveals that the extraction wound of tooth 38 has healed. Only weeks later were the typical alterations of osseous structure captured in the radiograph. Irregular areas of radiolucency and reactive sclerosis provide a picture with cloudy shadows (cotton wool effect). In the right picture, the course of the mandibular canal can no longer be definitively followed (paresthesia). On the other hand, the articular process is only seldom involved in the inflammatory process. This case is one of diffuse sclerosing osteomyelitis.

Fig. 303 Chronic osteomyelitis. These two illustrations are sections from the panoramic radiograph of a 48-year-old male, which reveal a poorly demarcated, osteolytically expanded extraction site at tooth 47, that is overlapped massively by inflammatory swelling of the soft tissues (**left illustration**). Within the soft tissue shadow, one can identify vague small sequesters. The spotty radiolucencies and radiopacities provide the typical picture of chronic osteomyelitis. The course of the mandibular canal in the direction of the mental foramen cannot be discerned.

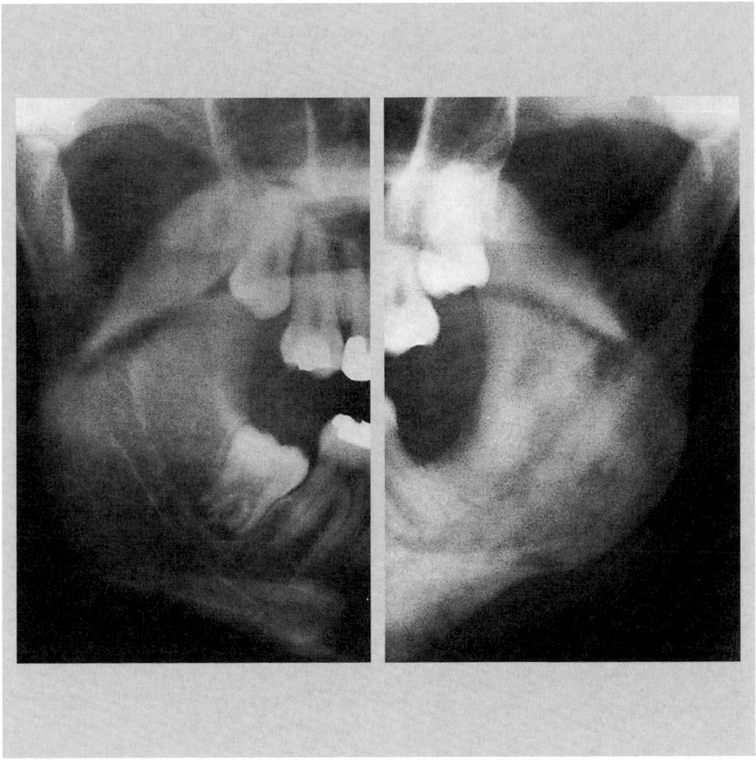

302

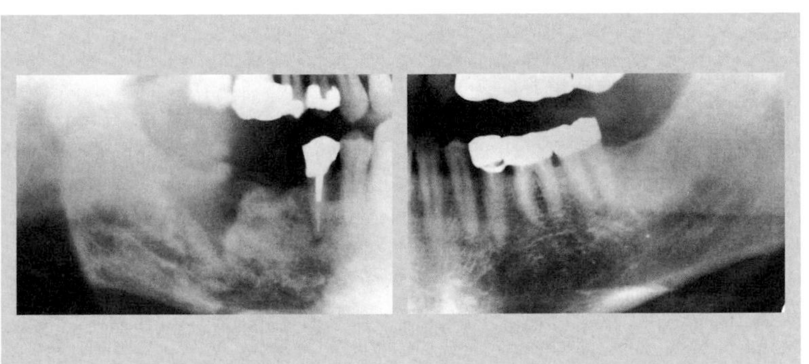

303

Not infrequently, following extraction of teeth manifesting chronic apical periodontitis and a local osteoblastic reaction, and usually following delayed wound healing, an intraosseous hyperostosis occurs, which is also referred to as "bone scars." Depending upon the virulence of the microflora and the individual host response, the radiographic picture will be one of tightly woven trabecularization or osteosclerotic hyperostosis, which are frequently irregular in shape but sharply demarcated.

Repeated recurrences with subthreshold infections lead to an expansion of the reactive new bone formation, which is visible in a panoramic radiograph as diffuse and poorly demarcated sclerosis. This chronic, diffuse sclerosing form of osteomyelitis with endosteal new bone formation is most often observed in the mandible and appears in the radiograph—again depending upon the virulence of the microflora, the host response, and the duration of the infection—as varying degrees of cloudy radiopacities with areas of radiolucencies (cotton wool effect). In a panoramic radiograph, a left-right comparison will reveal the mandibular canal prominently on the unaffected side. This disease occurs primarily in elderly individuals and mostly in men, which renders more difficult the radiographically important differentiation with Paget disease of bone (see p. **290**).

A special form of diffuse sclerosing osteomyelitis may be observed primarily in younger patients. Its course is slow, with relatively mild pain, and emanates frequently from a pericoronitis of the mandibular third molars, especially following extraction and open wound healing. The radiograph will show dense but cloudy radiopacities and frequently destruction of the structure of the mandibular canal (clinical paresthesia) and virtual disappearance of the border between trabecular and compact bone. This osteoblastic, nonsuppurative form of osteomyelitis, which is also known by the term Osteomyelitis Garré, will lead with time to an increase in volume that cannot always be captured in a two-dimensional panoramic radiograph; however, both axial CT and scintigraphy showing increased metabolic activity can provide appropriate images for diagnosis.

Fig. 304 Reactive intraosseous hyperostosis following inflammation of dentogenic origin. This panoramic radiograph of a 50-year-old female reveals a desolate and periodontally severely involved dentition with numerous missing teeth in both arches. Distal and apical to the supererupted and periodontally involved tooth 47, one notes an irregular and poorly demarcated area of very high radiopacity. These and similar hypermineralized or osteosclerotic areas usually develop as a consequence of chronic marginal and apical periodontitis, or as the result of an extraction with delayed wound healing. Such lesions are found almost exclusively in the mandible. This is a classic case of intraosseous sclerosis or hyperostosis.

Fig. 305 Reactive intraosseous hyperostosis following inflammation of dentogenic origin. The panoramic radiograph of a 50-year-old female reveals a reactive intraosseous hyperostosis within the extraction wound of tooth 46, following delayed wound healing (dry socket); it is entirely possible that this lesion was also caused by and is being maintained by chronic marginal and apical periodontitis around teeth 45 and 47.

Fig. 306 Fracture line osteomyelitis. The panoramic radiograph of a 67-year-old female reveals bilateral fractures at the angle of the mandible, with fracture line osteomyelitis, following extraction of the mandibular third molars. The patient suffered from osteoporosis. Noteworthy is the poorly demarcated fracture line, which is a sign that the incident occurred some time previously. At the left mandibular angle, osseous destruction predominates, while on the right side bone apposition and a periosteal reaction can be observed.

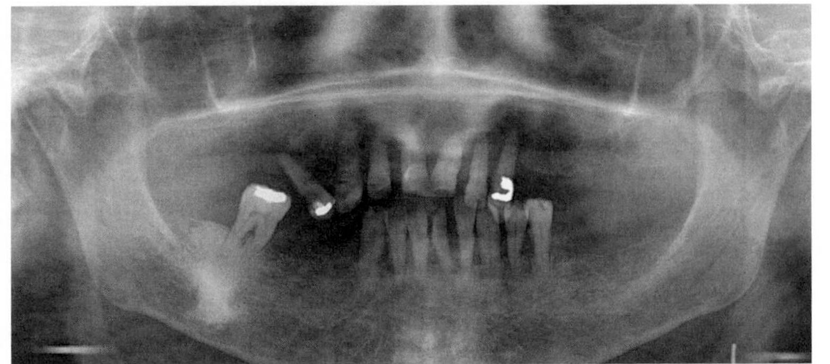

304

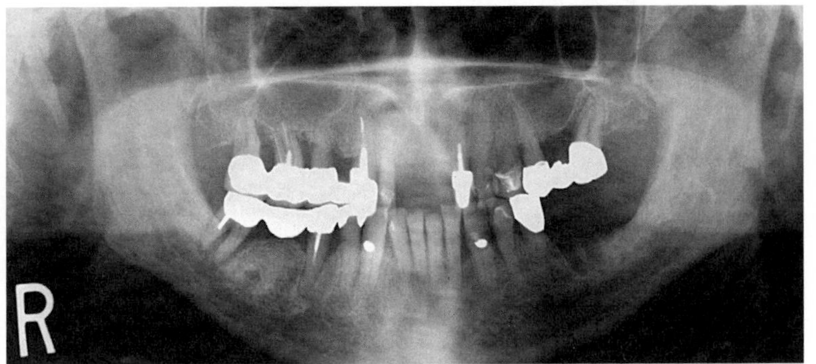

305

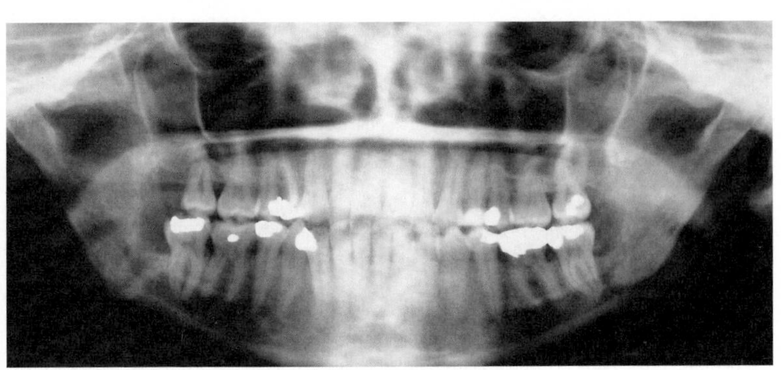

306

In its advanced stages, chronic osteomyelitis as viewed in the radiograph will also exhibit periosteal osseous new bone formation, sequesters, and spontaneous fractures. Radiographic diagnosis will also discern double contours in the compact bone of the mandible. The various shapes and lobes of the maxillary sinuses are of significance in the maxilla as the origination points for chronic osteomyelitis. The increase in volume of the affected jaw can be depicted in the vertical dimension with a panoramic radiograph, but not in the orofacial direction; for this reason, a supplemental axial CT is recommended.

Depending upon the dose that is delivered during a course of radiation therapy (e.g., for malignant tumors), damage to the vascular system within the field of irradiation will occur resulting in vascular injuries, so that the blood supply to irradiated areas of bone becomes insufficient. In addition to thickening of the trabeculae, a prominent radiographic observation is a loss of structural detail (osteonecrosis). If secondarily infected, radio-osteomyelitis will develop within the damaged bone; this is usually only discovered following a spontaneous fracture. It is very important that all dental or surgical treatment that is necessary be performed *before* entering into a necessary course of radiation therapy. Even routine dental procedures performed following radiation therapy and without consideration of the previous procedures can bring very unpleasant consequences.

If osteosynthesis is insufficient following closure of fractures of the jaw, especially the more frequently affected mandible, the ingress of microflora can lead to fracture line osteomyelitis. Even in the most favorable circumstances, delayed healing will result and the patient will experience pain. However, in most cases there will be osseous necrosis, reactive new bone formation, sequesters, and pseudoarthroses. Furthermore, fractures of the alveolar ridge can occur following tooth extraction, and lead to osseous reactions and sequester formation.

Facial trauma may be associated with aseptic osseous necrosis, as is often observed as a consequence of forced orthodontic treatment, associated with local circulatory disturbances. Also in these cases, bacterial contamination can induce osteomyelitis.

It is, in fact, highly likely that circulatory disturbances are the ultimate cause of most cases of so-called "idiopathic" osseous necrosis.

Additional possible causes for osteomyelitis include specific inflammations such as tuberculosis, actinomycosis, or even the syphilitic gumma.

Fig. 307 Osteomyelitis, with sequestration. This type of panoramic radiograph (Status-X Siemens) of the mandible reveals a sequester in the anterior region of the mandible in a case of chronic osteomyelitis (this type of radiograph is seldom used today). Note especially the thickened osseous structure, which is a sign of diffuse, chronic osteomyelitis.

Fig. 308 a, b Osteomyelitis, with sequester formation. This presentation of a periapical radiograph of the molar region of the mandible on the left side (**a**) and a section from the panoramic radiograph of the same patient (**b**) clearly show the significance of an overview radiograph in terms of radiographic diagnosis. The panoramic radiograph clearly reveals osteomyelitis with sequester formation and a spontaneous fracture (**arrows**) in a 53-year-old male.

Fig. 309 Osteoradionecrosis. The panoramic radiograph of a 58-year-old male reveals the terminal condition of osteoradionecrosis, with spontaneous fractures following radiation therapy. Dependent upon and in relationship to the radiation dose, there will be disturbance of vascular supply due to vascular fibrosis in irradiated segments of the bone, and this subsequently leads to a reduction of host defense mechanisms. Before initiating any necessary course of radiation therapy, all marginal and apical periodontitis as well as nonvital teeth and remaining root fragments must be treated or eliminated in order to avoid the risk of osteoradionecrosis. Following successful radiation therapy, any and all dental treatment must be performed extremely carefully in order to avoid subsequent microbial infections.

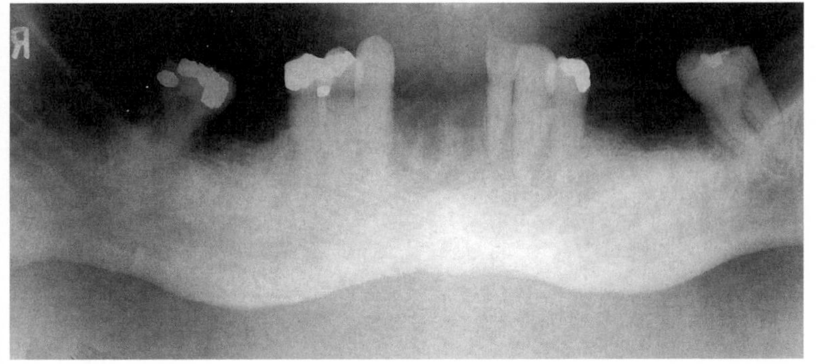

307

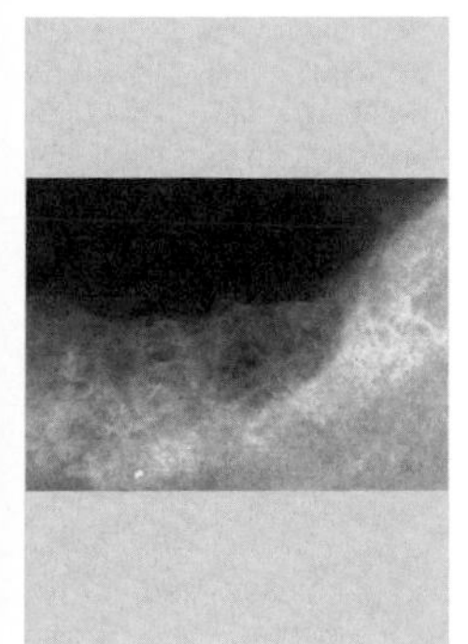

308 a

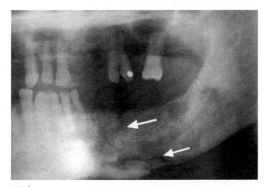

308 b

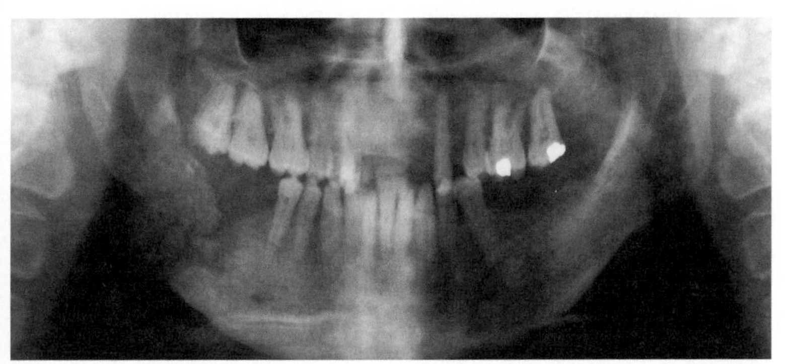

309

Anatomy of the maxillary sinuses: Even within the first year of life, unilateral or bilateral air-containing maxillary sinuses can be observed radiographically. The greatest width of the maxillary sinuses in the frontal plane is achieved following eruption of the permanent dentition, and the greatest height around age 40. It is noteworthy, however, that if posterior teeth are extracted early in life deep alveolar recesses often form from the sinuses, and following later tooth extractions these recesses may also expand in the direction of the alveolar ridge. Smaller maxillary sinuses usually extend from the second premolars to the second molars, while larger sinuses extend from the first premolars or even from the canine and even beyond the third molars.

The shape of the maxillary sinus is commonly described as a pyramid with the wall of the nasal cavity as its base and its apex inclined toward the zygomatic bone. The paranasal sinuses and often also the maxillary sinuses are quite frequently of asymmetric shape. This general consideration is also applicable with regard to the possible size differences as well as for the overall shape of the sinus, and particularly for the configuration of the floor of the sinus. With regard specifically to the size of the maxillary sinuses, one may not infrequently observe significant differences in the size of the left and right sinuses, with one side exhibiting greater than average size or a very small sinus. Abnormally large size is usually accompanied by a perceptible thinning of the sinus walls, and an abnormally small sinus is often accompanied by thickening of the surrounding osseous lamellae. A small sinus may result from a developmentally induced depression and thickening of the facial wall, which can give a false impression of a pathologic radiopacity in a panoramic radiograph.

Hypoplasia or aplasia of the maxillary sinuses can also be an accompanying symptom in syndromes such as cranio-osseous dysplasia or Voorhoeve's disease. In such cases, the thickened sinus walls meet prematurely in the caudal area forming a sharp angle, or even at the level of the floor of the nasal cavity. The resultant "high" sinus "floor" is therefore often scarcely visible in a panoramic radiograph, and can lead to a diagnosis of aplasia of the maxillary sinuses (see Fig. **312b**). In especially pronounced cases, the clinical examination will reveal actual facial asymmetry. Impacted teeth, especially the canines and the third molars can also be the cause of smaller maxillary sinuses.

Fig. 310a Anatomy of the maxillary sinuses. Section through the mesiobuccal root of the maxillary right first molar, exhibiting normal distance from the root apex to the broad and flat sinus floor.

Fig. 310b Anatomy of the maxillary sinuses. Section through the right maxillary first molar exhibiting a very large maxillary sinus that descends almost to the apex of the palatal root.

Fig. 310c Anatomy of the maxillary sinuses. Cross section at the level of the floor of the sinus. The deeply located sinus floor is perforated by the apices of the maxillary molars. The anterior recess and the canine root are also depicted as sectioned.

Fig. 311a Anatomy of the maxillary sinuses. Section at the level of the sinus floor. On the right side, note the broad, smooth sinus floor, but on the left side the floor is divided into three segments by crescent-shaped septa, and the sinus floor is perforated by the buccal root apices of tooth 27.

Fig. 311b Anatomy of the maxillary sinuses. Section at the level of the sinus floor. The right side reveals a sinus in three segments divided by crescent-shaped septa; the left side reveals numerous septa dividing the sinus into numerous distinct recesses.

Fig. 312a Anatomy of the maxillary sinuses. Lateral view of the normal anatomic relationship of the tooth roots to the floor of the sinus.

Fig. 312b Anatomy of the maxillary sinuses. This frontal section at the level of the maxillary hiatus depicts the possible combination of a distended sinus (**right**), and on the **left** side a small sinus deformed by a widened nasal passage with depression of the facial sinus wall and a narrow, high "floor."

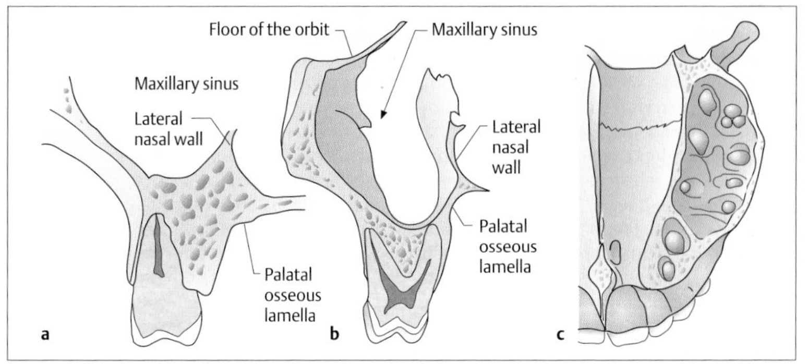
Floor of the orbit
Maxillary sinus
Maxillary sinus
Lateral nasal wall
Lateral nasal wall
Palatal osseous lamella
Palatal osseous lamella
a
b
c

310

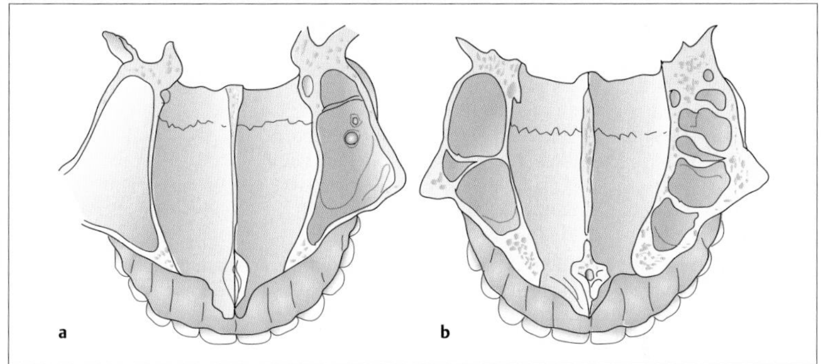
a
b

311

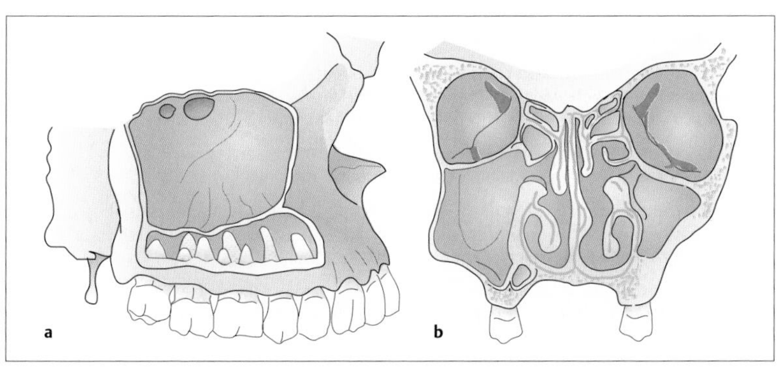
a
b

312

The shape and configuration of the floor of the alveolar recess of the maxillary sinus are also extremely variable. Virtually all shapes and sizes are possible (see Fig. **311**), ranging from a wide open space with no divisions all the way to a multi-chambered sinus and a sinus floor exhibiting high septa with asymmetric shapes. In general one observes that the alveolar recess usually exhibits a small anterior lobe that extends over the first premolar and not infrequently also up to the canine. One usually observes a crescent-shaped osseous septum above the second premolars that separates the anterior from the primary sinus recess; this may also extend over the first and second molars, and often even above the third molars. Not infrequently, however, an additional osseous septum above the second molar separates the primary recess from a posterior one, which is usually observed to be in intimate contact with the subjacent third molar.

Depending upon the expanse of the alveolar recess in the direction of the alveolar process, the spatial relationship to the roots of the posterior teeth will be more or less intimate. The root tips are usually separated from the maxillary sinus by bone of varying thickness and by an adjacent lamella that clearly demarcates the floor of the sinus from the sinus itself (see Fig. **312a**). In the case of very large maxillary sinuses, however, the individual apices of the posterior teeth may appear to push up against the floor of the sinus, and are often only covered by the most external osseous lamellae and the lining sinus mucosa (see Fig. **310c**).

Fig. 313a Dentogenic irritation of the sinus. Residual caries is apparent beneath the amalgam restoration on tooth 24. The angle of projection has somewhat "elongated" the palatal root, which exhibits a slight widening of the periodontal ligament space in the periapical region, immediately below the anterior recess of the sinus. The clinical picture was one of full-blown pulpitis without obvious sinus involvement.

Fig. 313b Dentogenic irritation of the sinus. Tooth 25 exhibits a full crown, and is nonvital. The periodontal ligament space is widened and the border of the sinus exhibits an apparent breach caused by pressure atrophy. The clinical examination revealed percussion sensitivity with acute apical periodontitis.

Fig. 313c Dentogenic irritation of the sinus. The root apex of tooth 23 is superimposed upon the anterior sinus recess. Note widening of the periodontal ligament space and an apical radiolucency. The clinical picture was one of subperiosteal abscess without obvious sinus involvement.

Fig. 314a Dentogenic irritation of the sinus. Tooth 25 exhibits a full crown and endodontic treatment. The root apex is clearly completely covered by bone, without any evidence of sinus alteration.

Fig. 314b Dentogenic irritation of the sinus. The apical granuloma on the mesiobuccal root of tooth 26 has penetrated the floor of the sinus and elicited a reactive swelling of the sinus mucosa; this is clearly indicated by the mild radiopacity at the sinus floor.

Fig. 315 Dentogenic irritation of the sinus. This panoramic radiograph exhibits root fragments, deep caries, proximal caries, and occlusal carious lesions. In the left maxillary sinus one observes a dentogenic pseudocyst emanating from the nonvital tooth 27 (**arrow**). The right maxillary sinus exhibits reactive mucosal swelling (**arrow**) above nonvital teeth 25 and 26. Bilateral dentogenic infections of the maxillary sinuses in a 20-year-old female.

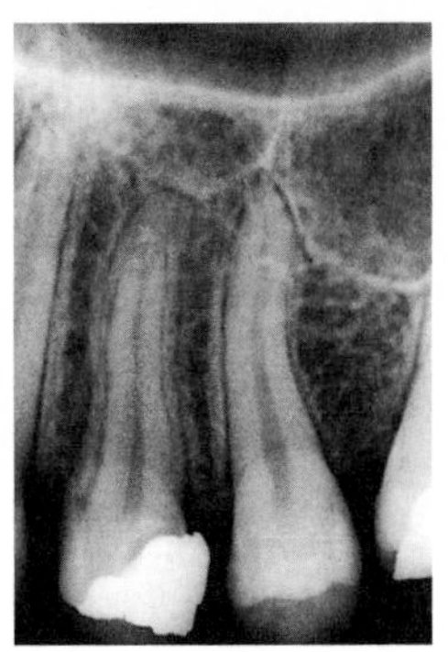

313 a

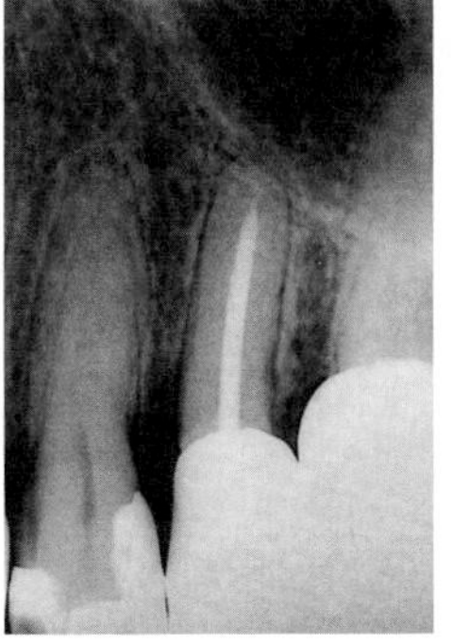

313 b

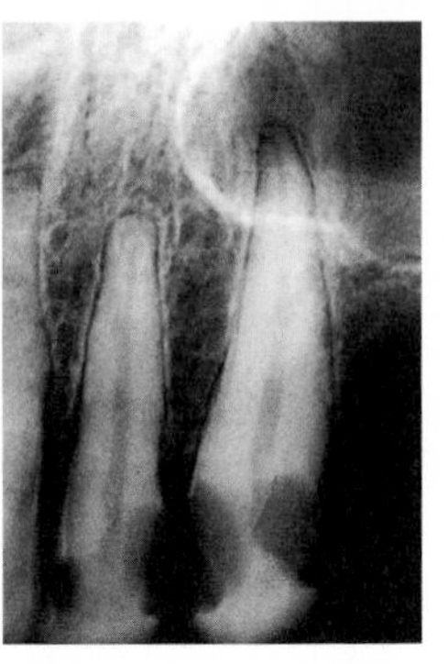

313 c

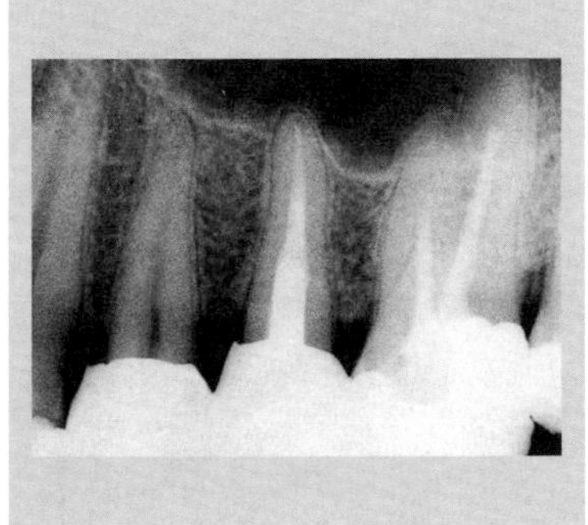

314 a

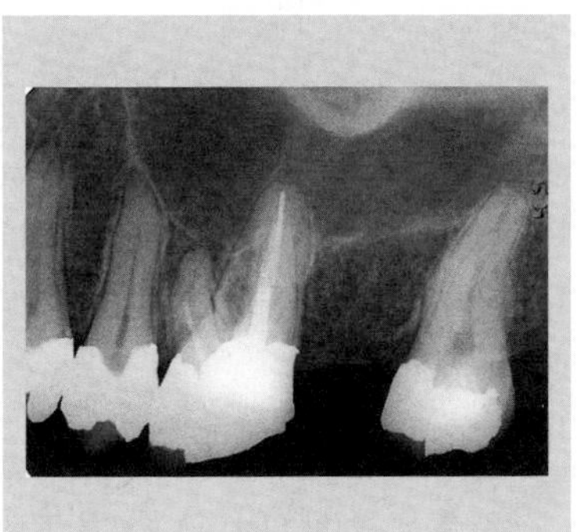

314 b

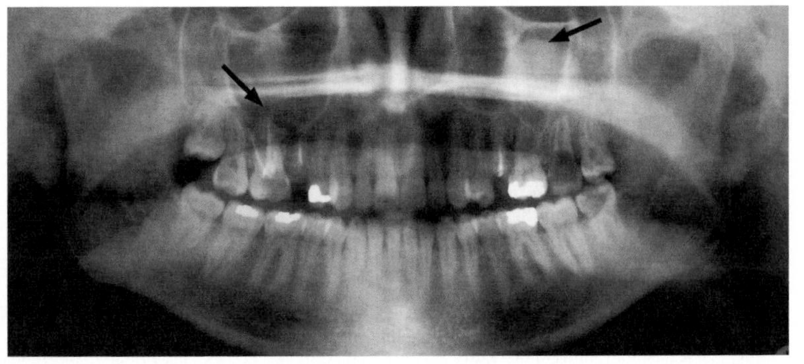

315

The root apices of individual teeth, especially the second premolars and the first molars may actually penetrate completely into the maxillary sinus (see Fig. **310c**), where they are covered only by the mucosa that lines the sinus; the result is that the vascular elements and nerve fiber bundles serving the affected teeth via the apices will also be affected by rhinogenic inflammation of the maxillary sinus mucosa, and such teeth will react subjectively and/or objectively upon clinical examination. On the other hand, it is also possible that a purely dentogenic infection can proceed along the vascular canals to involve the maxillary sinus; in this sense, it is even possible for dentogenic infections of the anterior teeth to play an etiologic role in inflammation of the maxillary sinuses.

While extensive recesses are common in the paranasal sinuses, these are less frequently observed in the maxillary sinuses. These can nevertheless delay the healing processes following chronic rhinogenic and dentogenic inflammation, and therefore may frequently elicit radiopacities at representative stages in the process. In addition to expansion of the alveolar recess, one frequently encounters an additional recess in the region of the body of the zygoma, which is known as the zygomatic recess. Less common are infraorbital and nasal recess formations, and very rarely one may observe a palatal recess that (radiographically) separates the hard palate into two lamellae. In cases where the maxillary sinuses are extremely distended, the condition is referred to as **Pneumosinus dilatans**. Within the roof of the maxillary sinus, which also represents the floor of the orbits, and in the ventral wall of the maxillary sinus, the canine fossa, one may encounter dehiscences, i.e., the maxillary sinus mucosa is in direct contact with the soft tissues of the floor of the orbit and the canine fossa in the region of the canines, without any osseous separation. Such anatomic relationships can result in irritations and persistent rhinogenic and dentogenic inflammation of the maxillary sinus mucosa leading to collateral swelling within the orbits or also in the area of the canine fossa. Depending upon the clinical status of the canine, such conditions can lead to various "suspected" diagnoses that cannot always be completely clarified or verified with the means and methods available in a private dental practice.

Within the dental office, the panoramic radiograph is without doubt the examination method of choice to provide a clearer overview of the jaws. The standard panoramic radiograph provides an overview of the maxilla, including the maxillary sinuses up to the floor of the orbit. Because the depicted slice represents zonography (see Fig. **2b**) and basically follows the course of the dental arch, the roots of the maxillary posterior teeth and therefore also the alveolar recess of the maxillary sinuses are captured in the plane of focus, and if the patient and his tongue are properly positioned (p. **17**), the resultant radiograph will provide interpretable data.

Fig. 316 Sinus pathology caused by chronic apical periodontitis. The radiographs on this page reveal a dentogenic pseudocyst, which resulted from chronic apical periodontitis emanating from the nonvital teeth 24 and 26. Note the irregular radiolucencies above the apices of the affected teeth. Forty-one-year-old female; trauma from tooth preparation.

Fig. 317 Sinus pathology caused by chronic apical periodontitis. The panoramic radiograph of the same case reveals a spherical radiolucency (arrows) in the left maxillary sinus. Both of the sinuses are small, with a high sinus floor. The medial boundaries of the sinuses, i.e., the lateral walls of the nasal cavity, cannot be discerned. Note the ill-adapted crown margins.

Fig. 318 Sinus pathology caused by chronic apical periodontitis. The Waters posteroanterior projection, which was taken for further examination of the sinuses, reveals the spherical pseudocyst on the left side (**arrows**), whose surface was struck tangentially by the central ray and is therefore clearly visible. The remainder of both the left and right sinus is air-containing, i.e., they do not exhibit any pathologic alteration. The lateral walls of the nasal cavity extend toward the maxillary sinuses. The right sinus exhibits infraorbital recesses and a large zygomatic recess. These radiographic findings do not provide signs that would lead to a diagnosis of maxillary sinusitis.

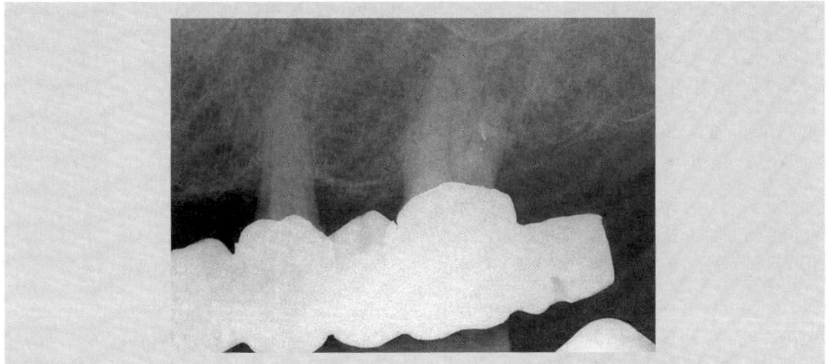

316

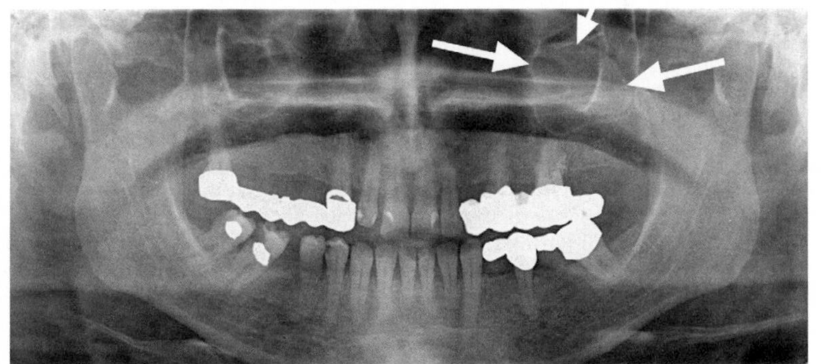

317

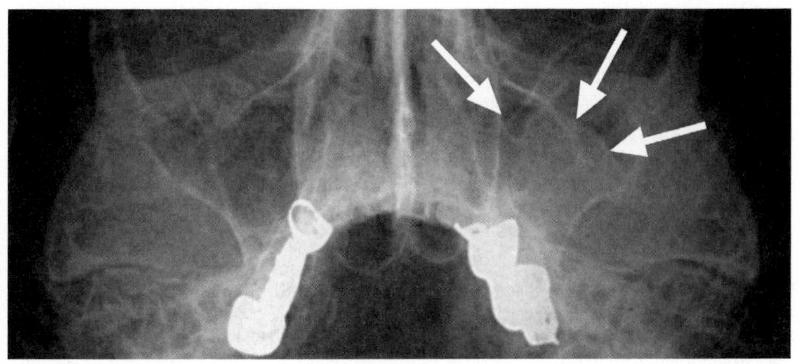

318

The anatomic characteristics, the exposure settings, and the radiographic projection technique may combine to render radiographic views of the maxillary sinuses that are diagnostically inadequate, for example soft tissue shadowing and bordering osseous lamellae, especially medially, as well as fluid levels in cases of empyema or hematosinus that can only seldom be appropriately depicted. The medial portions of the maxillary sinuses are almost always overexposed because the central ray in this region as it progresses toward the image receptor traverses the hollow cavities of the epipharynx, the posterior naris, and the nasal cavity and is therefore not dampened by any osseous structures. Reactive mucosal swelling caused by apical or periodontal infection, as well as exudate-filled pseudocysts will be depicted in the radiograph as shadowing similar to soft tissue differentiated from the rest of the air-filled sinus by a Mach-effect because they are not surrounded by an osseous bordering lamella as is the case with dentogenic cysts; such lamellae are often lost in the case of infected cysts. The Mach-effect is defined as "an artifical linear radiolucency seen along the edge of a superimposed radiodensity." If the sinus is totally shadowed by mucosal swelling, exudate, or empyema, these are radiographic signs of an acute or chronic maxillary sinusitis. In a panoramic radiograph, however, only a partial shadowing will be visible in the dorsal segment of the sinus where the central ray is weakened by the superimposition of radiopaque structures of the facial skeleton. Fluid levels, which are often observed in cases of acute and chronic sinus pathology and also following zygomatic fractures, are often not visible in a panoramic radiograph because the equipment permits projection of the central ray upward and the tangential effect of the rays along the horizontal surface of the fluid level cannot be taken advantage of.

An additional important radiographic sign is signaled by the condition of the bordering osseous lamellae on the floor of the alveolar recess. Osteolysis and osteosclerosis caused by expanding dentogenic or rhinogenic inflammation or by tumors in the maxilla often lead to dissolution of the opaque bordering osseous lamellae on the floor of the alveolar sinus recess. Such structural changes are usually easy to observe in a panoramic radiograph, and should always be an indication for consultation with an ENT (Ear, Nose and Throat) specialist.

Fig. 319 Sinus pathology caused by chronic apical periodontitis. This panoramic view depicts the condition of an acute exacerbation of a chronic apical periodontitis in a 57-year-old female, emanating from the endodontically treated tooth 17. The right maxillary sinus exhibits shadowing only in the dorsal segment because the medial portions of the maxillary sinuses are not depicted as radiopaque in a panoramic radiograph due to the subtraction effect in that area.

Fig. 320 Sinus pathology caused by chronic apical periodontitis. This section from a Waters posteroanterior projection, which was taken to evaluate the maxillary sinus in the case depicted above, reveals an almost completely radiopaque right maxillary sinus. In contrast to chronic rhinogenic inflammation of the maxillary sinus, one observes no thickening of the sinus mucosa on the sinus walls. The left sinus is normal and air-containing. Typical acute, unilateral sinusitis of dentogenic origin.

Fig. 321 Acute catarrhal maxillary sinusitis. This section from a Waters posteroanterior projection reveals the radiographic signs (**right**) of an incipient, bilateral acute catarrhal sinusitis. The 17-year-old female with vital teeth presented with the clinical picture of acute rhinogenic sinusitis and typical dental pain (percussion sensitivity) in the posterior teeth of the maxilla. Note also the likely inappropriate selection of radiographic exposure settings.

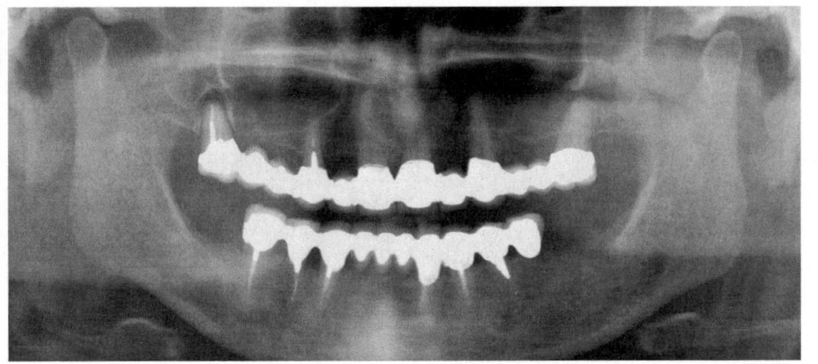

319

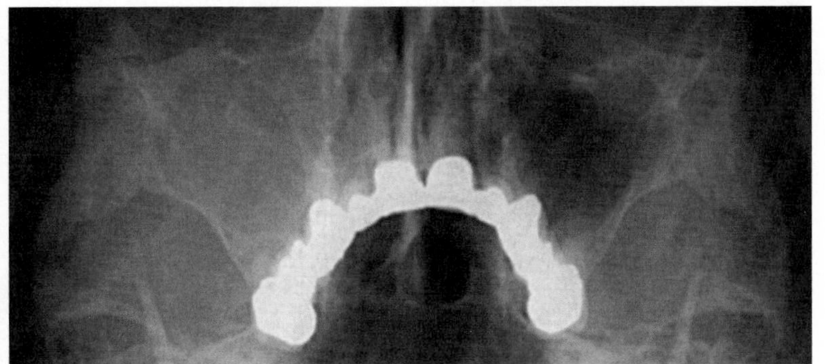

320

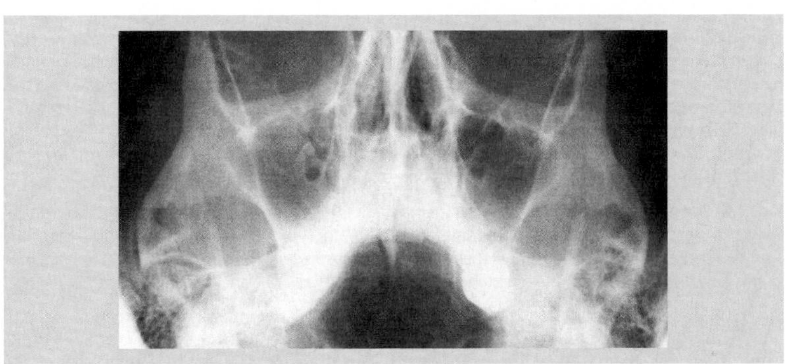

321

Intraoral radiographs only depict the mediobasal portion of the alveolar sinus recess because of the variable shape and course of the sinus floor and the projection angle of the central ray; noteworthy, however, is that the almost always clearly visible laterobasal bordering lamella is often *incorrectly* regarded as the "sinus floor." It is not always possible to ascertain with certainty whether the root apex of the affected tooth remains covered by the osseous lamella of the floor of the sinus, and only seldom is it possible to determine whether the bony lamella has only been deformed or completely perforated due to the pressure atrophy exerted by an expanding granuloma. Because of the angle of central ray projection, an apical granuloma will often appear to be "within the sinus," but this is seldom the case. In patients exhibiting nonvital teeth on only one side of the maxilla, a complete radiographic survey will permit comparison of the affected side with the healthy side and often reveal that the maxillary sinus on the affected side is less radiolucent. If this is the case, dentogenic involvement of the sinus is to be suspected. If vitality testing procedures have not provided definitive evidence for the existence of a nonvital tooth, the clinician can suspect a rhinogenically elicited mucosal swelling or must consider the possibility of an anatomically narrow sinus.

Conventional and digital radiographs: One can examine the maxillary sinuses conventionally using a standard panoramic radiograph (see p. **5**) with the patient positioned according to the indication; the examination can also be performed using additional programs for zonography (thick layer tomography), or with transverse projections of the maxilla in which the slice thickness usually equals or exceeds that of zonography. However, thick layer tomographies are not free from the volume artifacts that reduce image quality, such as metals or radiolucencies and radiopacities adjacent to the slice, and are therefore not actually indicated for comprehensive maxillary sinus diagnosis unless one limits the demands of the procedure to depiction of the shape and thickness of the alveolar ridge or the localization of foreign bodies, root fragments, or the localization of impacted teeth. Precise patient positioning for these types of zonographies is difficult and time-consuming, is demanding for the technical personnel, and despite the most careful positioning does not always lead to satisfactory depiction of the desired structures.

Using the technique of thin layer-computed tomography (CT), one can obtain sharp axial sections of the maxilla, free of superimpositions; from the digital data so-obtained, reconstructions of the anatomic structures in all planes can be generated without any further radiation exposure for the patient. Such data can furthermore be precisely measured with the use of special computer programs (see also Figs. **149**/**150**).

Fig. 322 Pseudocysts in the maxillary sinuses. This panoramic radiograph reveals a large pseudocyst (**arrows**) in the right maxillary sinus positioned broadly upon the mucosa; this lesion cannot be of dentogenic origin because all teeth in the arch proved to be clinically vital. In contrast to this cystoid formation, whose borders can be clearly delineated by the tangential ingress of the rays, a diffuse shadowing is also apparent in the left sinus, but the borders are not clearly defined because of the angle of projection. Pseudocysts filled with inflammatory exudate often occur during stages of a catarrhal sinusitis, and are therefore of rhinogenic origin.

Fig. 323 Pseudocysts in the maxillary sinuses. Left: Lateral topogram showing the vertical marking lines to delineate the desired layer for depiction of rhinogenic pseudocysts in the maxillary sinus. **Right:** Axial slice at the level of the maxillary sinuses with markings to assist selecting a panoramic view. Also marked are the position and signs of the maxillary transverse section.

Fig. 324 Pseudocysts in the maxillary sinuses. Above: Panoramic view with section through both nasal and maxillary sinuses. **Below:** These slices from the series of secondarily obtained transverse sections of the maxilla depict accurately measurable position and shape of the right pseudocyst in a 1:1 relationship.

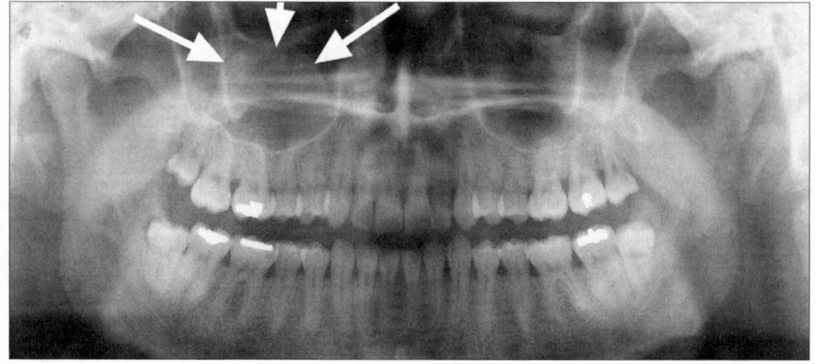

322

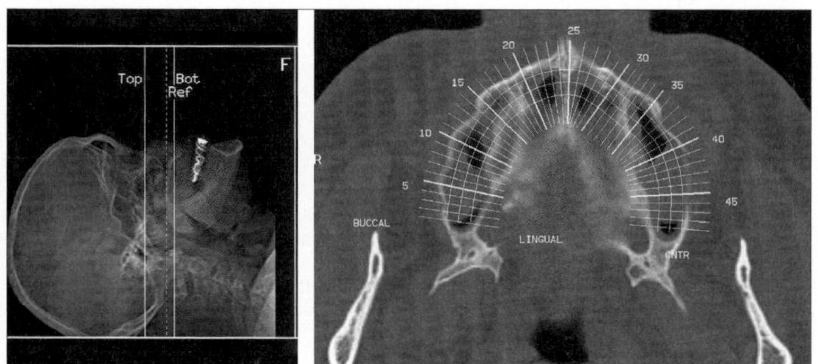
Top
Bot
Ref
F
R
5
10
15
20
25
30
35
40
45
BUCCAL
LINGUAL
CNTR

323

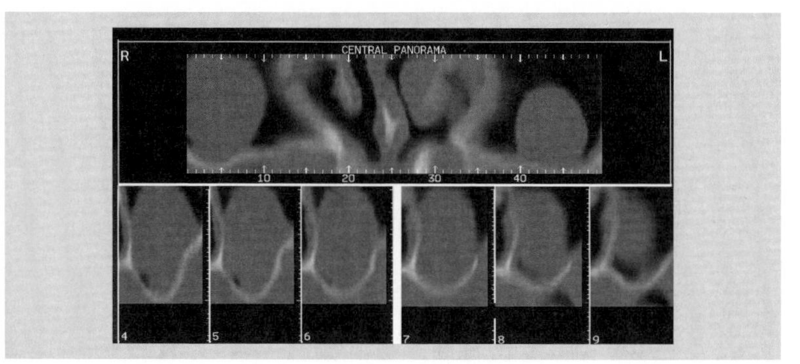
R
CENTRAL PANORAMA
L
10
20
30
40
4
5
6
7
8
9

324

However, there is a significant disadvantage associated with observation of dentogenic sinus disorders because the system-related resolution capacity of the computed tomograph is incapable of accurately depicting structures with a thickness of less than ca. 0.3 mm; for this reason, it is not possible to accurately examine the condition of the periodontal ligament space or narrow fracture lines in fractured teeth.

To summarize, it is worthy of note that inflammation of the sinus mucosa can occur not only in cases of dentogenic infections, but also with benign and malignant tumors. Any radiographic differentiation between inflammation and osteolytic as well as progressing malignant tumors will be extremely difficult, especially in the initial stages.

When considering inflammation of the maxillary sinuses, the medical history and the intraoral clinical examination play very important roles. Even specialists from related medical/dental disciplines not infrequently encounter difficulties because in many instances patients with a true rhinogenic maxillary sinus disorder present in the dental practice and complain of pain in one or several vital teeth in the maxillary posterior segment. The patient can often precisely identify the apparently affected teeth because chewing elicits pain and they are percussion sensitive. The teeth often react only mildly positively to standard vitality tests. In virgin teeth or those with only small restorations, a periapical radiograph or a panoramic view will provide no evidence of alterations in the periapical regions. If, in such a situation, the dentist progresses to a diagnosis of pulpitis and proceeds with appropriate (endodontic) therapy, it is entirely possible (and likely) that a mistake has been made, which can no longer be rectified! Clinical symptoms that appear to be emanating from teeth can occur as a result of acute and/or chronic maxillary sinus inflammation during all stages of the disease process. In many cases, additional tests by the dentist are indicated, such as percussion sensitivity of the body of the zygoma, pressure sensitivity at the infraorbital foramen, as well as any increase in facial pain. If nonvital or endodontically treated teeth are present in the area of the sinus floor, it is possible that a dentogenically elicited maxillary sinusitis is present, and such a condition can be both diagnosed and treated using common dental practice procedures.

Fig. 325 **Polyposis in the maxillary sinuses**. The panoramic radiograph clearly reveals a tooth-like polyp that appears to hang from the roof of the sinus (**black arrow**). In the region of the left maxillary sinus, one observes an additional "hanging" polyp (**black arrow**) as well as a pseudocyst (**white arrow**) on the sinus floor. Chronic, hyperplastic catarrhal inflammation of both maxillary sinuses. Polyposis in a 30-year-old male.

Fig. 326 **Root fragment within the maxillary sinus**. This panoramic radiograph reveals the condition several weeks following attempted extraction of maxillary third molar, 16. The root fragment (**arrow**) is only poorly discernible due to the addition effect with the thickened and altered mucosa resulting from inflammation. An oro-antral fistula exists. The sinus on the right side also exhibits shadowing. The alveoli remain clearly visible, and exhibit the disturbed and delayed healing process. Thirty-three-year-old male.

Fig. 327 **Root canal filling material in the maxillary sinus**. This panoramic radiograph reveals the root canal filling material (**arrow**) that was compressed into the maxillary sinus from the root of tooth 25; the material appears to lie within the orbit. In fact, the material is located infraorbitally in the craniodorsal recess of the left maxillary sinus, which is superimposed upon the floor of the orbit by the projection angle. Thirty-year-old female.

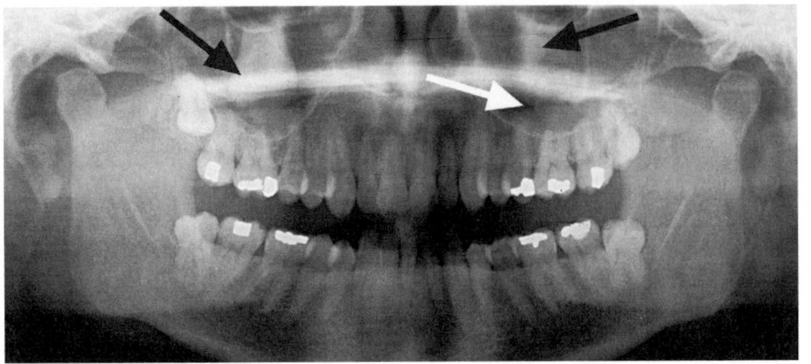

325

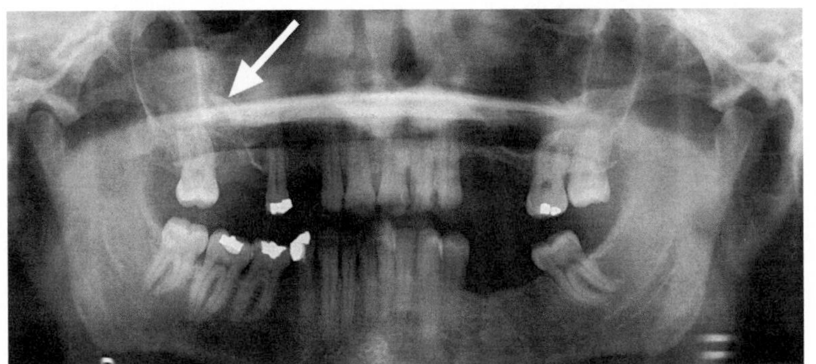

326

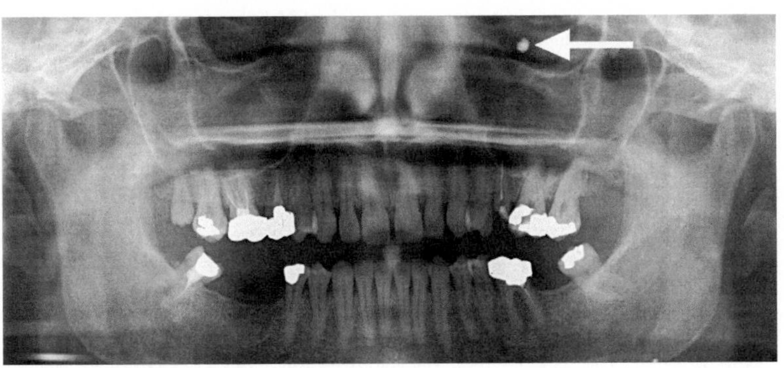

327

The simplest classification of disorders of the temporomandibular joints (TMJ) describes them as either primary or secondary arthropathy:

- Primary arthropathies are associated with etiologies within the joint itself, or trauma, which lead to functional disturbances.
- Secondary arthropathies occur on the basis of diseases not associated directly with the joints, or are caused by destabilization of occlusoarticular relationships.

However, this mnemonically helpful classification must not conceal the fact that the primary and secondary arthropathies which elicit functional disturbances often have overlapping or mutually enhancing effects; therefore, from the point-of-view of radiographic diagnosis, this simple classification is not always applicable or meaningful in the individual case.

A distinct category is comprised of systemic syndromes with TMJ manifestations, both primary joint alterations such as TMJ aplasia in the Nager-de-Reynier syndrome, or secondary arthropathies such as loose articulation within the TMJ capsule in cases of neurogenic acro-osteolysis, or with motion inhibition resulting from fibro-ostotic dysplasia of the jaws.

In the arena of radiographic diagnosis, TMJ arthropathies can only be detected if pathologic alterations of hard tissues have occurred, resulting in radiographically discernible pathology or positional anomalies of the condyles.

Fig. 328 TMJ Dysplasia. This panoramic radiograph reveals gemination of the condyle (left side). Gemination of the condyle on the right side was also visible in an original radiograph, but in this view the two heads of the geminated condyle are scarcely visible because they are located one behind the other and thus subject to the radiographic summation effect. Using this radiographic technique it is therefore not often possible to definitively determine whether the case is one of bifid condyle or a true gemination. Particularly visible on the left side is the flat, elongated fossa with its articular tubercule, a sign that the dysplasia occurred even before the patient's 12th year of life. The findings were serendipitous as the clinician attempted to document pericoronitis on tooth 48.

Fig. 329 TMJ Dysplasia. The panoramic radiograph depicts on the left side hyperplasia of the condyle with elongation of the mandibular collum (neck) and the ramus, as well as a left-side widening of the body of the mandible in a patient who exhibited facial asymmetry; this condition could only be documented radiographically following precise positioning of the patient. The various manifestations of asymmetries of the facial skeleton occur during various growth phases. The coracoid process on the left condyle can easily be confused with an arthrosis (see Fig. **339b**), and the size increase with an osteochondroma (see p. 283).

Fig. 330 TMJ Dysplasia. This panoramic radiograph of a 36-year-old male reveals hypoplasia of the TMJ, the ramus, and the body of the mandible on the right side in a case of Nager syndrome (acrofacial dysostosis, Nager type), with the Pierre-Robin sequence, which can also appear with the Franceschetti syndrome.

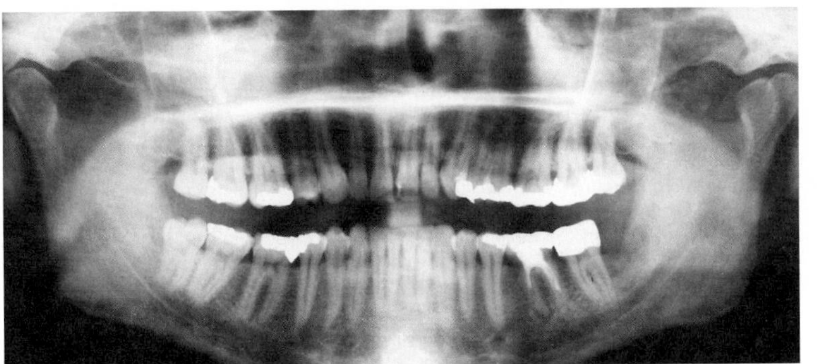

328

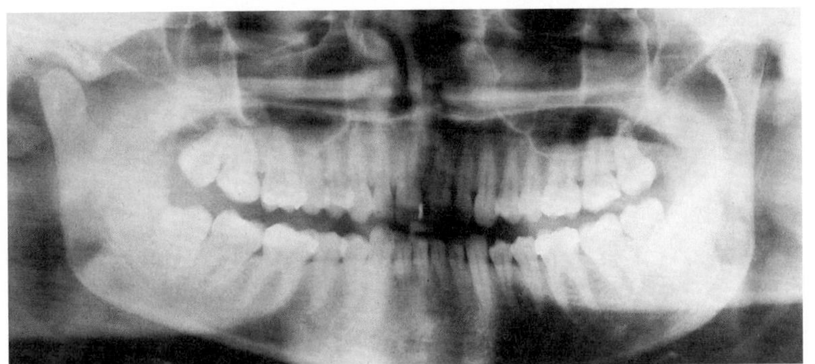

329

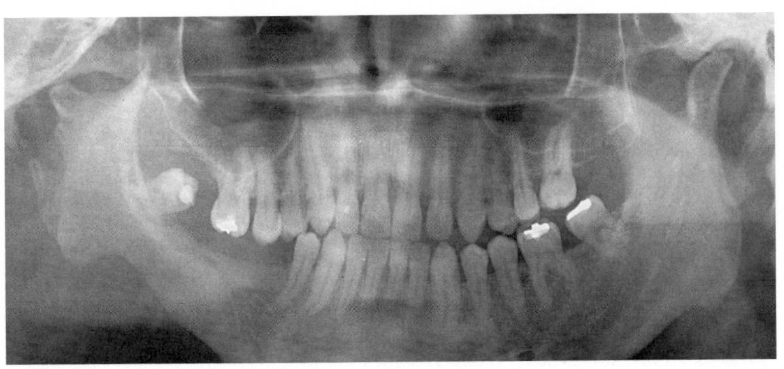

330

Pathologic alterations of the radiolucent soft tissues of the TMJ, for example lesions of the articular disk, can only be visualized using magnetic resonance imaging (MRI) as a noninvasive procedure. In dental practice, the panoramic radiograph is the examination method of choice to obtain initial information concerning TMJ morphology or positional anomalies of the condyles (radiograph taken in edge-to-edge anterior occlusion or in habitual occlusion).

Primary Arthropathies

Primary arthropathies can be classified as follows:

- Dysplasias of the TMJ that are manifestations of syndromes
- Arthritis of the TMJ as a manifestation of various forms of polyarthritis
- Tumors and tumor-like lesions
- Trauma

Dysplasia, hypo-, and hyperplasia: Dysplasia, hypoplasia, and/or hyperplasia of the temporomandibular joints usually occur as manifestations of syndromes that are often associated also with dysplasias of the jaws. Included here are acrofacial dysostosis (mandibulofacial dysostosis, Nager type), the Franceschetti syndrome (mandibulofacial dysostosis), and the Goldenhar syndrome (oculoauriculovertebral dysplasia) with hypoplasia of the facial skeleton.

Hypoplasia of the condyles is often associated with various forms of micro- and retrognathia, occurring not infrequently in the first decade of life as the result of trauma to or inflammation within the TMJ.

Fig. 331 **TMJ Dysplasia**. This panoramic radiograph depicts Nager syndrome with aplasia of the right TMJ and a compensatory elongation (active hyperplasia) of the coronoid process on the right side. Delayed eruption of teeth 45 and 46, with possible ankylosis of these teeth. Retrognathia and micrognathia, with deviation of the mandibular midline toward the right side upon mouth opening. The arrows indicate: (**1**) oblique line of the ascending ramus, (**2**) articular process, (**3**) dorsal border of the mandibular ramus.

Fig. 332 **TMJ Dysplasia**. The cross-sectional CT slices of the mandible of the same case reveal the position of the ankylosed tooth 46, as well as its relationship to the mandibular canal (**arrows**).

Fig. 333 **TMJ Dysplasia**. This three-dimensional surface reconstruction reveals that the right condyle and the articular fossa make no contact. Clearly visible is the hyperplastically elongated coronoid process on the right side due to compensatory forces (compare with Fig. **331**).

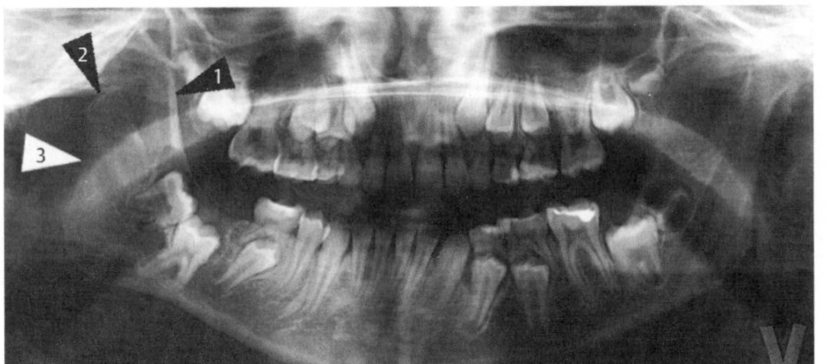

331

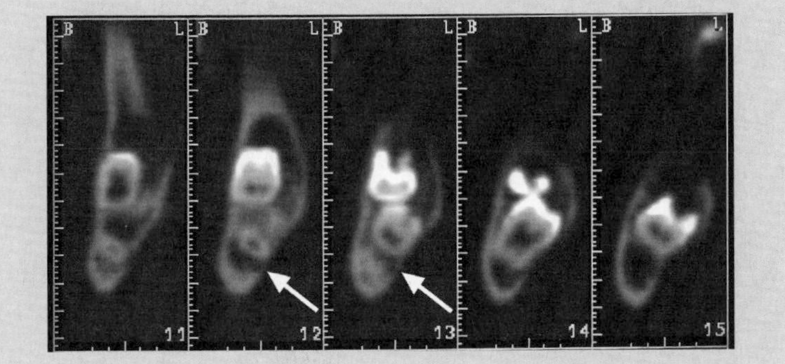

332

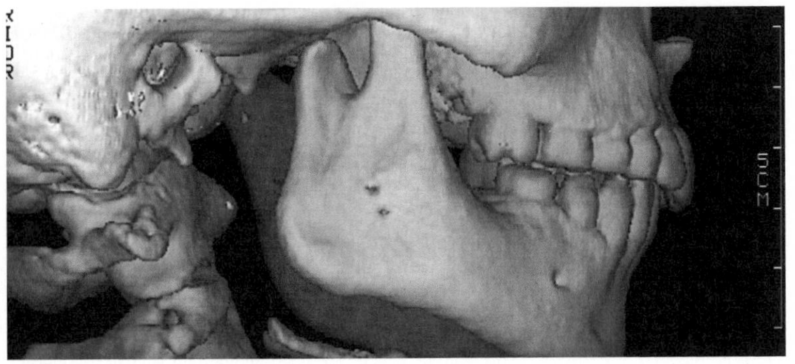

333

Hyperplasia may affect only the condyle, or may be combined with hemimandibular hyperplasia and unilateral open bite. Hyperplasias are formed in various shapes and sizes during varying phases of growth during the second decade of life, and most often lead to pronounced facial asymmetries.

Dysgenesis of the condylar process can lead to malformation of the articular process without formation of the head of the condyle, but also to symmetrical or unilateral double formation of the condyle, which can range in severity from a more or less pronounced notch in the joint surface (bifid condyle), all the way to complete gemination. The etiology of this developmental abnormality, which usually does not inhibit function or elicit pain, remains unclear.

Inflammation within the TMJ: Arthritis in the form of inflammation of the synovial membrane may affect an individual joint (monoarthritis) or several joints (polyarthritis). It is possible to differentiate clinically among acute, subacute, and chronic forms. The etiology is seldom a direct (primary) arthritis, but rather in most cases bacterial and viral infections that have spread from other sites in the body.

Inflammation of the temporomandibular joints can often be elicited by hematogenous spread of inflammation from the adjacent anatomic regions, for example otitis media, osteomyelitis of the jaw, or inflammation associated with third molars.

Fig. 334a, b Inflammation of the TMJ. Juvenile chronic polyarthritis (JcP) in a 15-year-old female. The three-dimensional surface reconstruction shows the facial skeleton laterally from the right (**a**) and the left (**b**). The chronic inflammation has led to bilateral destruction of the condylar surfaces. The remaining portions of the condyles are displaced anteriorly.

Fig. 335a, b Inflammation of the TMJ. Axial CT of the skull at the level of the condyle surfaces. In habitual occlusion, the condyles are displaced anteriorly and toward the left. With the bone window (left) and the soft tissue window (right), the axial slices reveal erosions of the cortical bone and sclerotic areas. These pathologic alterations represent the reparative processes in cases of chronic inflammation of the condyle.

Fig. 336a, b Inflammation of the TMJ. In the soft tissue window (left, circled area in the region of the lateral pterygoid muscle) the muscle density was measured. It was between 66.5 Hounsfield units (HU) to 64.8 HU; these values are elevated vis-à-vis a normal value of about 40 HU, and this increased density of the muscular tissue indicates overloading. The average density value for the entire lateral pterygoid muscle (right picture) was 39.3 HU for the first measurement and 40.6 HU for the second value.

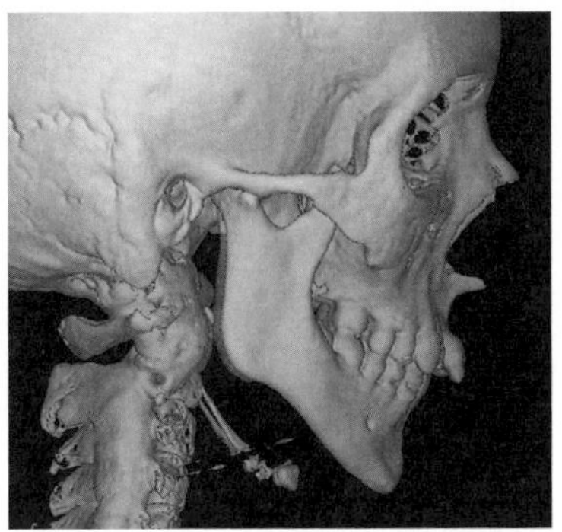

334 a

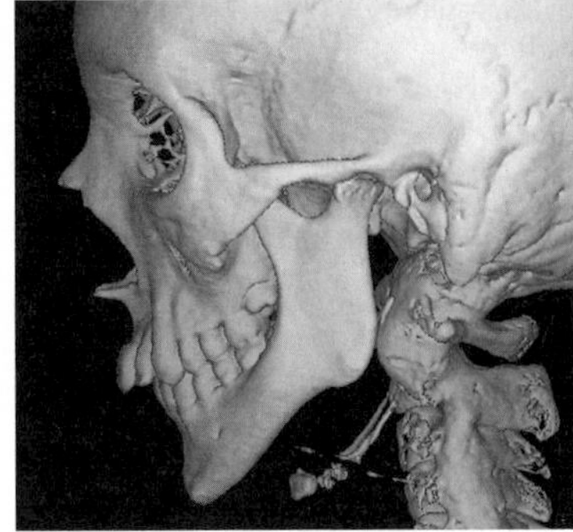

334 b

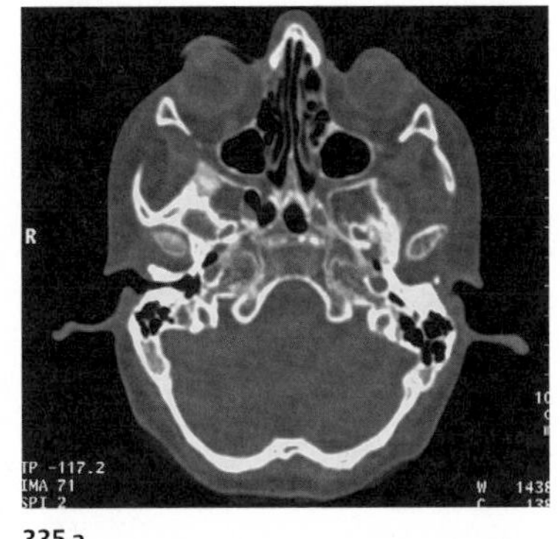

335 a

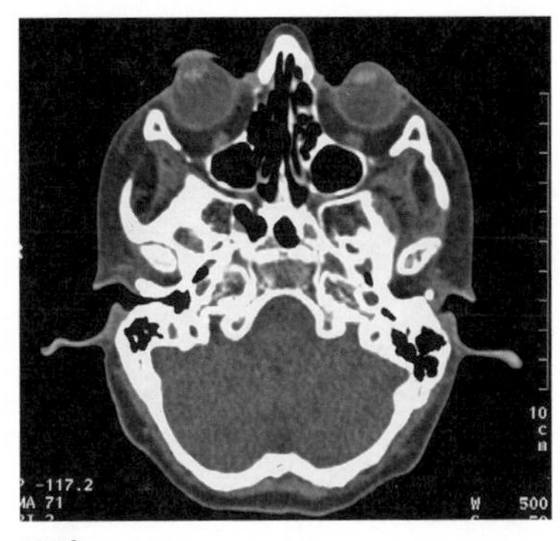

335 b

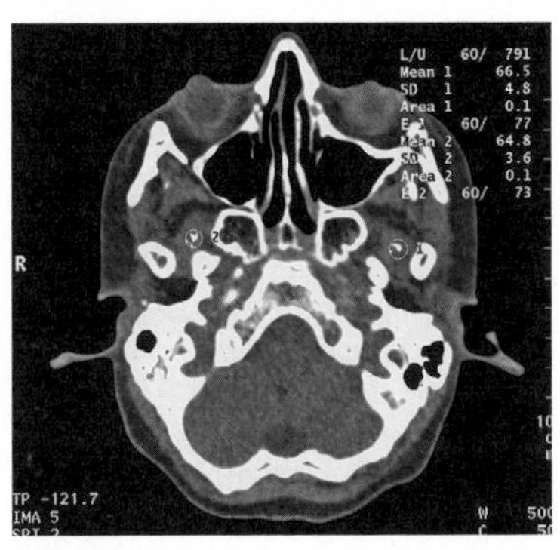

336 a

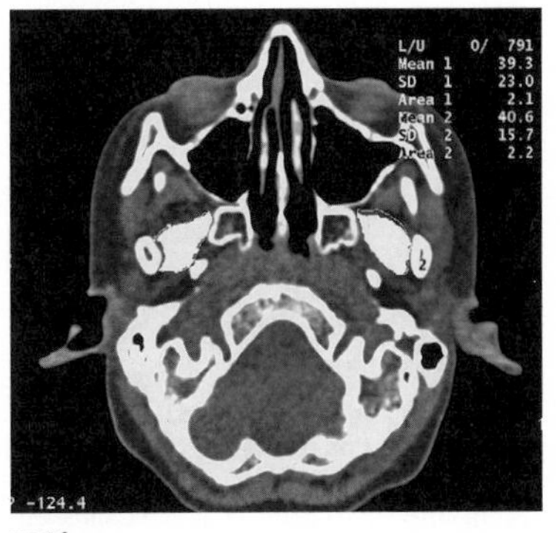

336 b

Inflammation of the TMJ may also accompany rheumatic diseases; examples include juvenile chronic polyarthritis (JcP) with forms of the Still–Chauffard syndrome in the first to third years of life, seronegative JcP in early school age (first and second decade), seropositive JcP in the second decade, primarily in females before age 16, and chronic polyarthritis of adults (cP) in a relationship of 3♀ : 1♂.

In the initial stages, no radiographic signs can be detected. The earliest radiographically diagnostic—quantitative—signs include decalcification of bone in the subchondral region. Following destruction of the joint cartilage (not visible in the radiograph) and perforation of the covering osseous lamella, the radiograph will reveal blurred contour defects near the joint. With continuing destruction and sclerosing reparative processes, there is a narrowing of the joint space as well as flattening and widening of the joint surfaces, leading to the characteristic picture of osteoarthritis, which exhibits osteophytic proliferations and fragmentations at the margin (*free TMJ bodies*) and detritus cysts; this process can end as fibrotic or (less frequently) osseous ankylosis.

Inflammation of the synovial fluid and the attendant functional disturbances may also occur following trauma or as accompanying symptoms with tumors or tumor-like lesions.

Fig. 337 Inflammation of the TMJ. On the right side of this panoramic radiograph, one observes a monoarticular (asymmetric) JcP in a 39-year-old female, which commenced in childhood. Note also the flat fossa as a sign of a pathologic condition that began in early childhood. A collagen implant had been placed in the chin region (arrow) to compensate for the retrognathia.

Fig. 338 Inflammation of the TMJ. This section from a panoramic radiograph reveals destruction of the right condyle in a 68-year-old female; the etiology could not be definitely assessed, but it was likely due to an infectious process spreading from the ankylosed and completely impacted tooth 48. Note the "washed out" appearance of the osseous structures at the angle of the mandible, which is an expression of chronic osteomyelitis; note also the compensatory hyperplasia of the coronoid process on the right side.

Fig. 339 a, b Inflammation of the TMJ. The linear tomography of the right TMJ (**a**) reveals the so-called "Bonnet" protective position of the condyle radiographically in a case of acute arthritis. The linear tomography of the left TMJ (**b**) reveals the radiographic signs of arthrosis deformans in a 42-year-old male. Typical are the sclerosed areas in the condyle near the joint, and the flatter fossa with a narrow radiographic joint space, as well as reactive osteophytic proliferations (*raven's beak*).

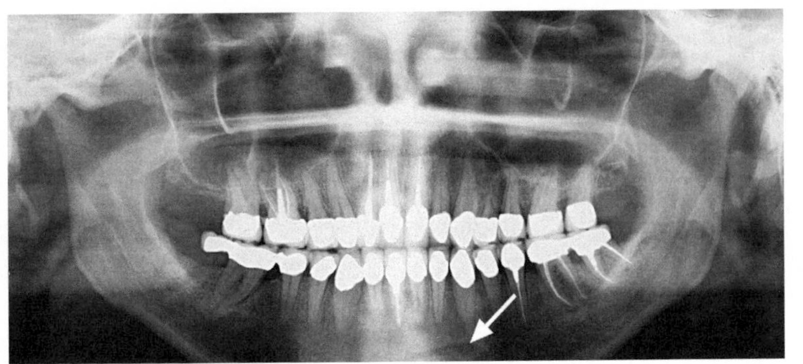

337

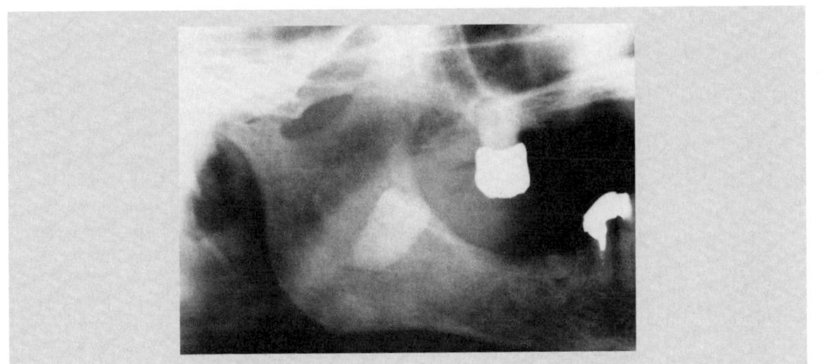

338

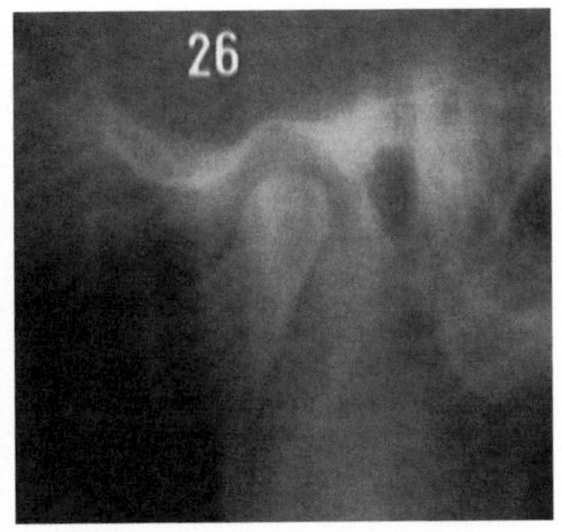

339 a

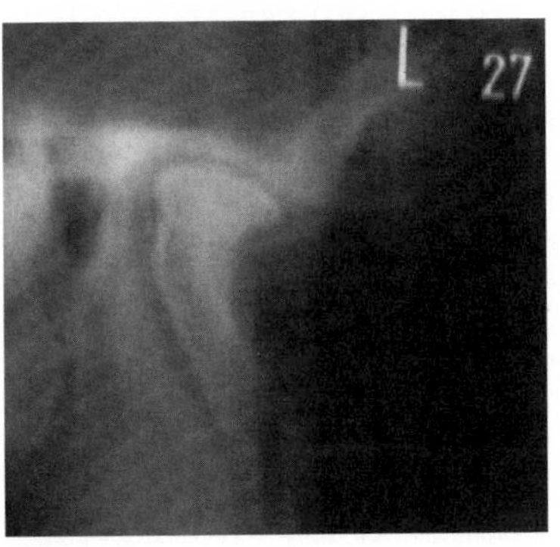

339 b

Tumors and tumor-like lesions: The most common benign neoplasms in the TMJ are the osteochondromas (see also p. **283**). These are found in the condyle near the TMJ, and evolve from developmental disturbances and inflammation during the school-age years, or from osseous metaplasia following trauma. Their early development leads to adaptation of the shape and size of the articular fossa. Especially in females, the extraordinary increase in size elicits hemimandibular, active hyperplasia with inhibition of mouth opening and facial asymmetries. These lesions may also be observed between radiolucent collagen structures and radiopaque ossifications. The osteochondroma has a tendency toward malignant transformation, whereby the enchondroma of the premaxilla occurs more frequently than on the condyle itself.

Synovial chondromatosis is sometimes observed unilaterally in the TMJ, usually in middle-aged males. Cartilaginous nodules formed metaplastically in the synovial membrane are forced into the joint space in more or less large quantities by the movements within the joint capsule; these cause jaw movement inhibitions as well as extraordinarily severe pain and inflammation in the soft tissues of the affected joint. In a panoramic radiograph these can only be visualized when they are present in large quantities and calcified, and for this reason additional examination using computed tomography (CT) or MRI is indicated. Subsequent consequences include arthrosis, which render radiographic diagnosis and differentiation much more difficult.

Fig. 340 Chondromatosis of the TMJ. In a 52-year-old male, the panoramic radiograph reveals hazy, spheroid shadowing (**arrow**) dorsal to the right condyle. The benign, tumor-like lesion is formed by the accumulation of hyaline cartilage nodules that later calcified within the synovia, and these are sloughed into the joint capsule (so-called *free joint bodies*) and lead subsequently to deforming arthrosis. This condition is attended by severe pain and functional disturbances of the affected joint. The nodules can only be visualized in a panoramic radiograph when they are calcified and in sufficient numbers.

Fig. 341 Chondromatosis of the TMJ. "Zoomed" section from an axial CT at the level of the joint surface of the right condyle of the same patient as depicted above. This soft tissue projection reveals several of the often quite numerously occurring, calcified cartilage nodules dorsal to the ventrally displaced condyle.

Fig. 342 a, b Chondromatosis of the TMJ. In a 29-year-old female, conventional tomography exhibits in two selected sections (**a** 21, **b** 24) ventral to the right TMJ (exposure performed during maximum intercuspation) the so-called "free joint bodies" (**arrows**). The late phase of this disorder also reveals pronounced arthrosis with narrowing of the joint space.

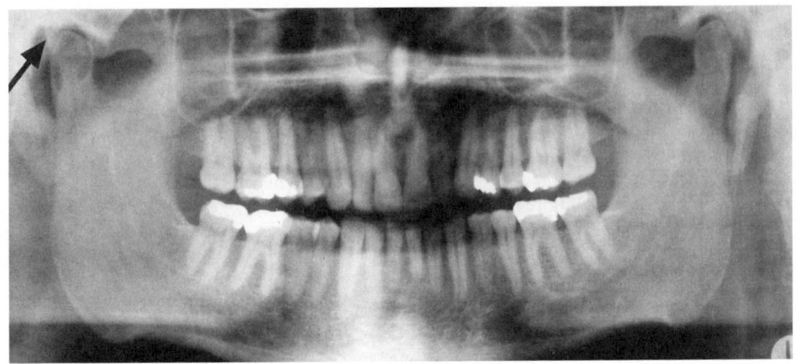

340

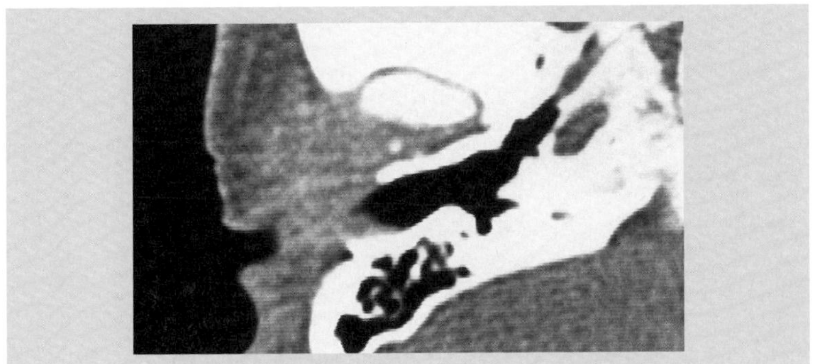

341

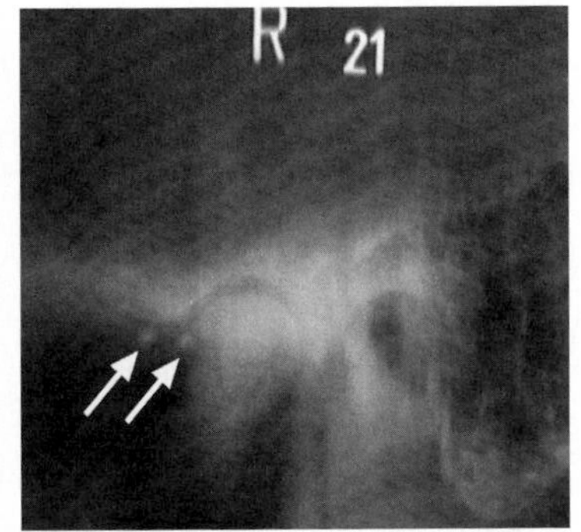

342 a

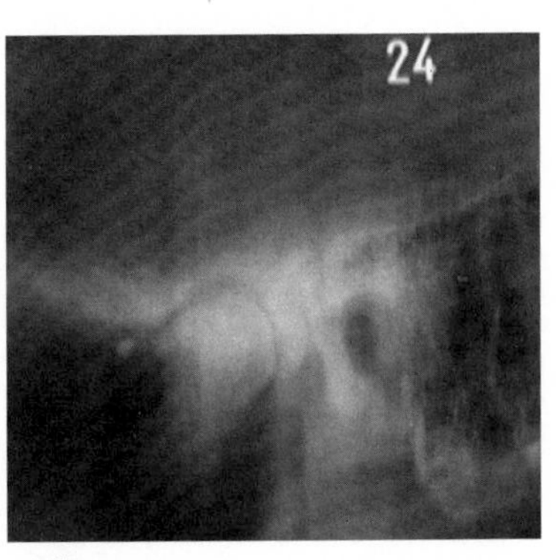

342 b

Additional (rare) benign and malignant neoplasms of the condyle include the giant cell granuloma, Langerhans cellular histiocytosis (eosinophilic granuloma), myxoma, hemangioma, as well as fibrosarcoma and synovialoma.
If the radiograph reveals spheroid radiolucencies over the fossa or in the articular tubercle, it is an indication in virtually all cases of pneumatization of the temporal bone, and this can also occur in the mastoid process.

Trauma: High fractures of the neck of the mandibular condyle or intracapsular fracture of the condyle itself often present shapes and positional alterations of the condyle that differ from the normal. The abatement of intracapsular hematomas, and fracture healing, lead surprisingly seldom to the otherwise expected functional disturbances.

Fig. 343 Osteochondroma of the condyle. The panoramic radiograph reveals an osteochondroma on the right condyle in an 84-year-old female, who exhibited no clinical symptoms. The osteocartilaginous tumor rests broadly upon the condyle and causes various radiolucencies and radiopacities. The articular fossa appears quite flat in comparison to the contralateral side (see also Fig. **423**).

Fig. 344 TMJ ankylosis. The panoramic radiograph reveals TMJ ankylosis on the left side subsequent to trauma in a 13-year-old male. Radiographic diagnosis cannot always differentiate definitively between fibrous or osseous ankylosis.

Fig. 345 Condyle fracture. This panoramic radiograph of a 60-year-old female reveals an intracapsular fracture of the left condyle. The cranial fragment of the head is displaced ventrally and is somewhat rotated. The original radiograph revealed a discrete sign of an osseous step. Note the obvious deviation of the mandibular midline toward the injured side.

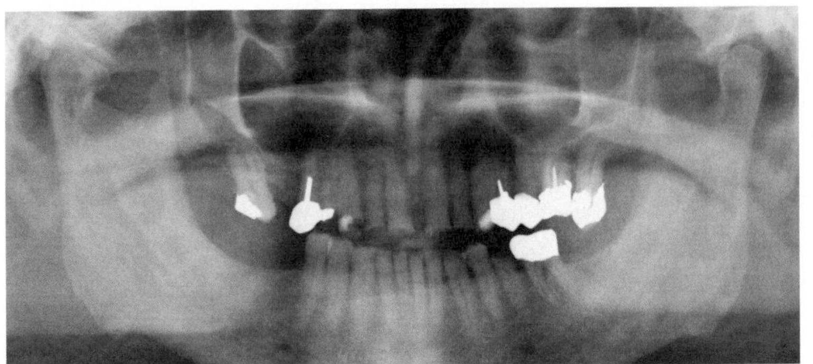

343

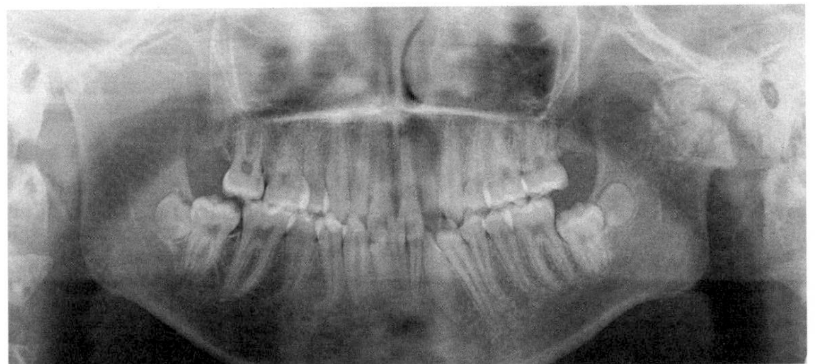

344

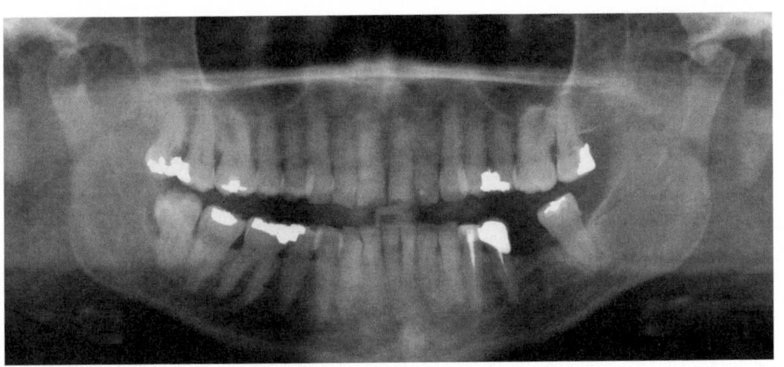

345

The term secondary arthropathy refers to disorders of the TMJ whose etiology is not found within the joint itself. In rare cases, the temporomandibular joints may also be negatively affected secondarily by spreading bacterial and viral infections, metabolic disturbances, or allergies. In over 90% of cases, however, it is the influence of the occlusal articular balance, associated with development of the masticatory apparatus that leads to more severe secondary arthropathies.

Even slight occlusal functional disturbances can traumatize the soft tissues of the temporomandibular joints and lead over the long term to discopathies and destruction of TMJ structures. Such trauma can even result from dental restorations and bridgework, etc. with premature contacts, infraocculusion and lateral movement interferences, and also by tooth loss in the supportive zones with subsequent tooth positional anomalies.

Except for depiction of malpositions of the condyles, radiographic diagnosis in initial stages will not reveal any pathologic conditions; however, a panoramic radiograph taken with the patient in habitual occlusion (see also p. **13**) can provide valuable information concerning the occlusoarticular *status quo*. This is because with the teeth in habitual occlusion the corresponding TMJ condyle position can be clearly viewed and examined in a single radiograph.

Fig. 346 TMJ disorders caused by traumatic occlusion. This panoramic radiograph taken in habitual occlusion, reveals a positional anomaly of tooth 37 in a 23-year-old female, caused by eruption force from the partially impacted tooth 38. The result was a premature contact between teeth 27 and 37, which elicited TMJ discomfort. Note also the midline shift of the mandibular anterior segment on the left side.

Fig. 347 TMJ disorders caused by traumatic occlusion. This panoramic radiograph of a 27-year-old male was taken as a diagnostic measure for TMJ discomfort. Similar case as in Fig. **346**. This projection was not taken in habitual occlusion, and therefore can provide no information concerning the positions of the condyles. In the radiographic diagnosis of TMJ discomfort, it is absolutely necessary to take the panoramic view with the patient in habitual occlusion (see p. **13**).

Fig. 348 TMJ disorders caused by traumatic occlusion. During the fabrication and seating of bridgework or removable partial dentures, the danger always exists of destabilizing the occlusoarticular balance by occlusal trauma, which can lead secondarily to temporomandibular joint injury. This panoramic radiograph of a 55-year-old female, taken in habitual occlusion, reveals a retruded position of the right condyle with distraction and anterior displacement of the left condyle, as well as compression due to infraocclusion on the left side. When taking such a radiograph it is critical that the patient's skull be positioned precisely symmetrically in the median-saggital plane in order to make possible appropriate diagnostic conclusions from examination of the image. One of the most important signs of proper positioning include symmetrical depiction of the superimpositions by the opposing jaw, as well as comparisons of the width of the left and right ascending rami (see Fig. **27**).

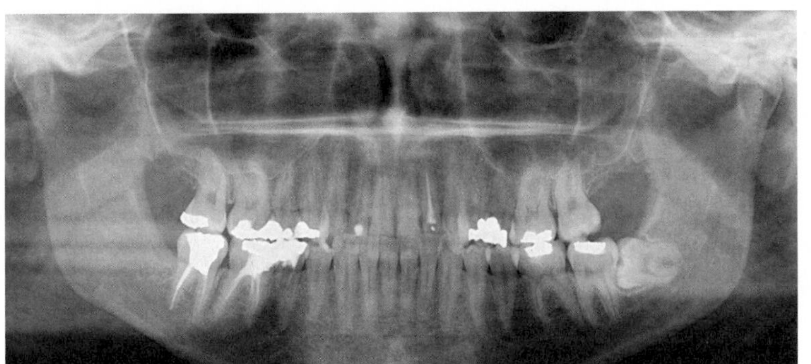

346

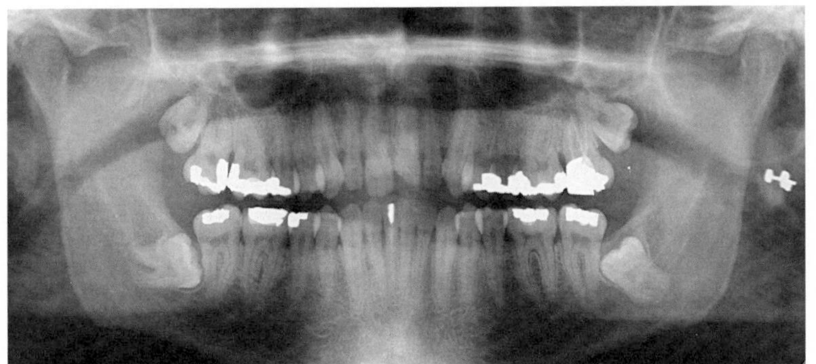

347

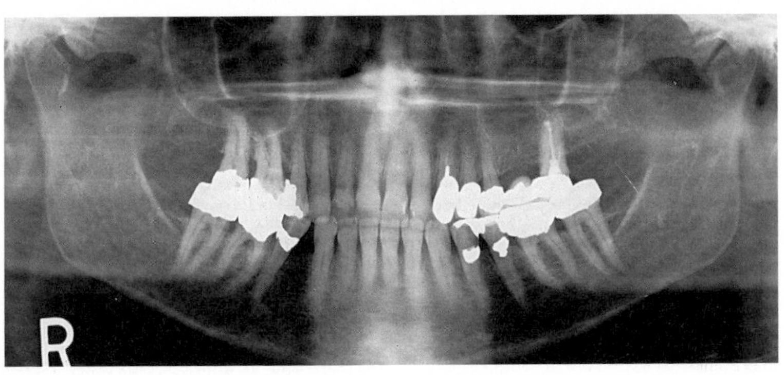

348

The panoramic radiograph depicted in Figure **349** and the lateral and frontal spiral tomographies taken in habitual occlusion clearly demonstrate that these methods can considerably enhance the clinical examination if performed with great care.

Isolated depiction of the form and morphology of the hard tissues (without simultaneous accurate depiction of tooth position) will provide better qualitative information with axial CT and the lateral and coronal slices deriving from the CT, with 3D-surface reconstructions. When the articular disk and the tendons and muscles that stabilize jaw movements are damaged by occlusal disharmonies over an extended period of time, accurate depictions must be performed either using the invasive method of double-contrast arthrotomography, or the noninvasive MRI. With either procedure, not only lateral (two-dimensional) but also frontal (coronal) sections should be depicted in order to ascertain the existence of partial medial or lateral disk displacements. Perforations of the disk or (more frequently) of its posterior ligament can only be rendered visible by injecting a contrast medium into the lower joint chamber.

If surgical procedures on the TMJ are anticipated, it is prudent to prepare preoperative three-dimensional surface reconstructions in various directions.

Fig. 349 Diagnostic value of the panoramic radiograph in functional arthropathies. In routine dental practice, a symmetrically projected panoramic radiograph taken in habitual occlusion permits an initial overview of the gross occlusal alterations caused by dental restorations with lateral displacement of the mandibular midline, and deviations of the condyle positions vis-à-vis the normal, in relation to the joint surfaces of the articular eminence. This projection makes possible an initial consideration of the morphology and also of any pathologic alterations of the condyles, and is a valuable aid in determining whether the patient should be referred to a specialist or whether proper occlusal relationships can be re-established by the general dentist. If lesions of the TMJ disk are already observable or suspected, further examination using MRI must be undertaken. This panoramic radiograph of a 45-year-old female who presented with TMJ discomfort reveals a distraction on the right side and compression of the condyle on the left side during habitual occlusion, with infraocclusion on the left side and displacement of the mandibular midline toward the right. The condyles themselves do not yet reveal any pathologic alterations. The lateral and frontal tomographies, taken subsequently, confirm the findings from the panoramic radiograph, and lead to suspicion of an anterior displacement of the articular disk.

Fig. 350 a, b Lateral spiral tomographies. The right condyle (**a**) is in a distracted position. The left condyle (**b**) is in a compression position.

Fig. 351 a, b Frontal spiral tomographies. The right condyle (**a**) is in a distracted position. The left condyle (**b**) is in a compression position. Because of the anterior displacement of the disk, the joint reveals a clearly narrowed radiographic joint space.

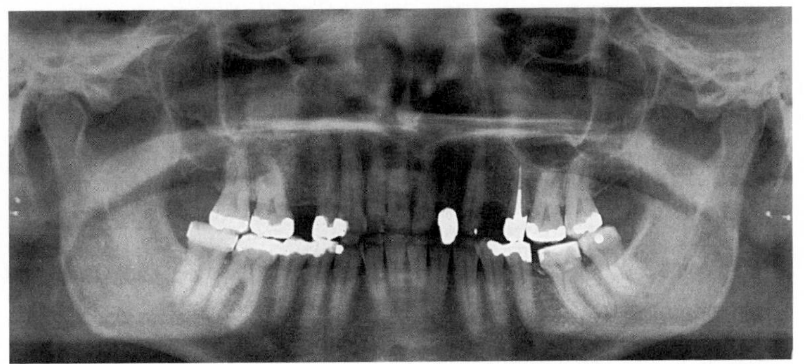

349

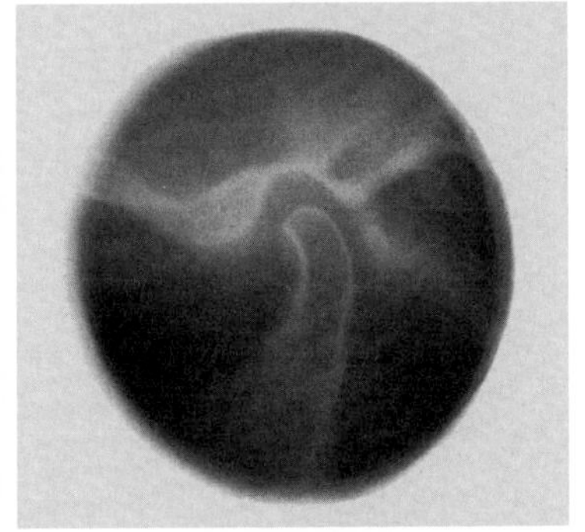

350 a

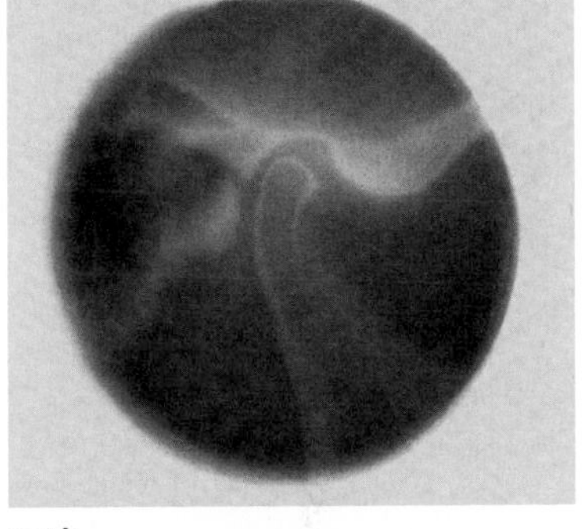

350 b

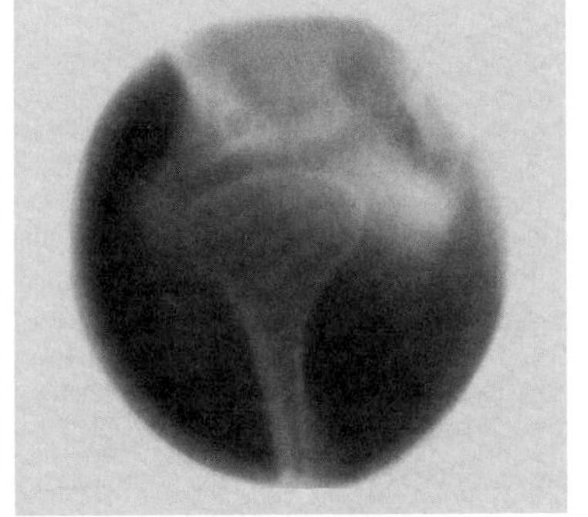

351 a

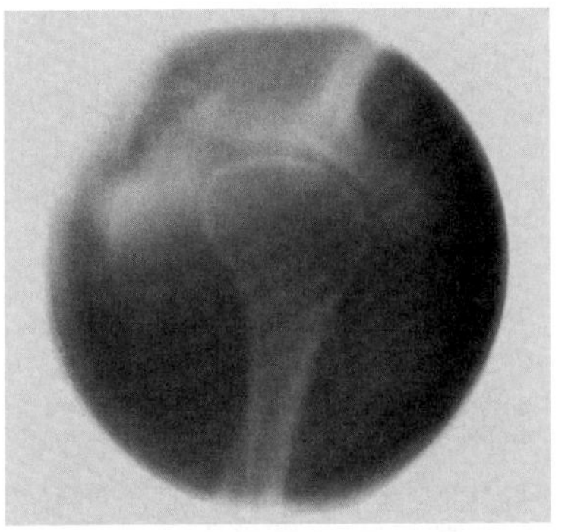

351 b

With appropriate positioning of the patient, the myriad forms of osteoarthritis can be well depicted in a panoramic radiograph, especially the anterior region of the temporomandibular joint. Typical radiographic signs include destruction and flattening of the condyle and the articular fossa, with radiopacities caused by reactive bony outgrowths (osteophytes) with rolled edges and a narrow radiographic TMJ space. Because the structural alterations in the area of the fossa and in the posterior regions of the TMJ often cannot be optimally depicted in the panoramic radiograph or in section projections using linear tomography, some cases may require the preparations of lateral and coronal CT, or even MRI, in habitual occlusion and with maximum mouth opening.

In most cases, anterior displacements of the disk can be described as either "with repositioning" (spontaneous repositioning upon jaw closure) or "without repositioning." For this reason a normal case (Fig. **352**) and two typical cases of anterior disk displacement, one with (Fig. **353**), and one without repositioning (Fig. **354**) are presented here.

Fig. 352a, b Depicting the articular disk using MRI. a The disk in its normal position, in habitual occlusion (**arrow**). **b** Disk in its normal position, maximum mouth opening (**arrow**).

Fig. 353a, b Anterior disk displacement, with repositioning. a In habitual occlusion, the condyle is in the retruded position. The disk (**arrow**) is displaced anteriorly. During the mouth-opening movement, the posterior ligament is positioned anterior to the condyle (**arrow**). **b** With increasing mouth opening, the condyle snaps onto the disk (**arrow**) causing the typical TMJ "popping."

Fig. 354a, b Anterior disk displacement, without repositioning. a In habitual occlusion, the condyle is in the retruded position. The damaged disk is displaced anteriorly (**arrow**). **b** Even during mouth opening, the disk remains fixed in its anterior position (**arrow**).

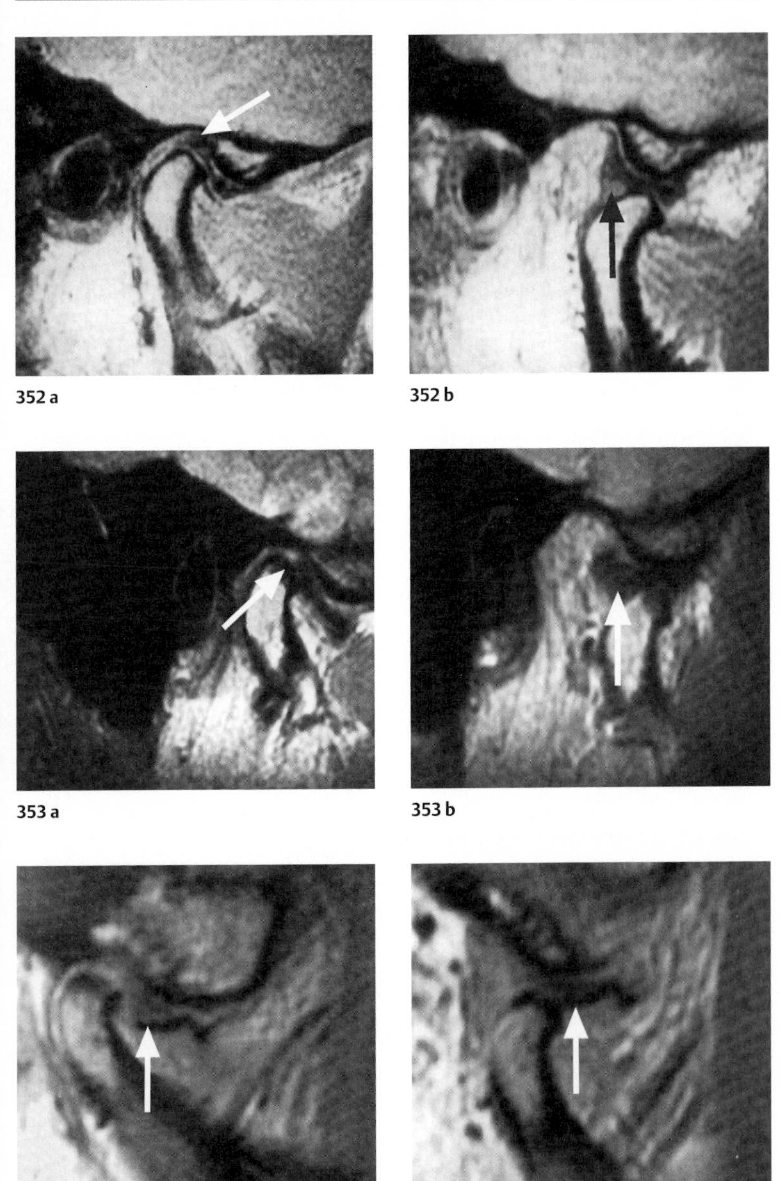

352 a

352 b

353 a

353 b

354 a

354 b

Classification of Cysts

A cyst is defined as a cavity lined with epithelium. According to the World Health Organization (WHO), cysts of the jaws are classified as either developmentally induced or inflammation-induced. Within the group of developmentally elicited cysts, various forms are differentiated according to topographic and histologic criteria into odontogenic and nonodontogenic cysts (the latter are also referred to as dysontogenetic cysts). Within the group of inflammation-elicited cysts, the radicular cysts dominate; these take their origin at the apex of a nonvital tooth. Cysts may also form within the soft tissues, but this category of pathology is not addressed in this chapter. Pseudocysts are cystoid radiolucencies that do not reflect the above-mentioned criteria, but do simulate true cysts radiographically (see pp. **279** and **281**).

Developmentally induced odontogenic cysts, such as the keratocyst or primordial cyst may develop from proliferating epithelial remnants of the dental lamella or the enamel epithelium, while follicular cysts develop from the enamel epithelium. The lateral periodontal cyst develops from epithelial remnants of the dental lamella without connection to the sulcus. Often observed in the maxilla, nonodontogenic cysts develop from epithelial remnants of the nasopalatine tract and the Hochstetter epithelial wall. Depending upon the frequency of their occurrence, inflammation-induced odontogenic cysts most often develop from radicular cysts, which in turn originated from epithelial rest cells of Malassez in the periodontal ligament space.

Radiographic signs: In the initial stage, cysts exhibit a characteristic round shape, which with increasing size may become more ovoid depending upon the resistance of the surrounding tissues, and often achieve extraordinary size. Cystic "growth" results from osmotic processes that cause increasing internal pressure; this leads to compression of soft tissues and to distention of osseous structures. The "growing" cyst exerts forces upon the surrounding bone and distends the thickened osseous boundaries, resulting in the radiographic tangential effect which renders the cyst clearly visible. Harder structures such as the teeth are much more slowly displaced, and sometimes also resorbed. Developmentally induced cysts often surround vital teeth, with maintenance of the lamina dura.

Follicular cysts, as seen in the radiograph, are always at the cementoenamel junction. The tooth crown resides within the lumen of the cyst. Large follicular cysts often do not permit radiographic visualization of this typical attachment.

Radicular cysts most often attach in the periapical zone of the root. The root apex resides within the cystic lumen and the lamina dura is not discernible.

Residual cysts of all types cannot be differentiated radiographically.

Radiographic Classification of Cysts of the Jaw:

Fig. 355 Developmentally induced odontogenic cysts:

1 Primordial cyst
2 Keratocyst
3 Follicular cyst
4 Eruption cyst
5 Lateral periodontal cyst

Fig. 356 Developmentally induced nonodontogenic cysts:

1 Nasopalatine cyst
2 Nasolabial (globulomaxillary) cyst

Fig. 357 Inflammation-induced cysts:

1 Apical radicular cyst
2 Lateral radicular cyst
3 Residual radicular cyst
4 Paradental (Craig) cyst

Pseudocysts are discussed and depicted beginning on page **278**.

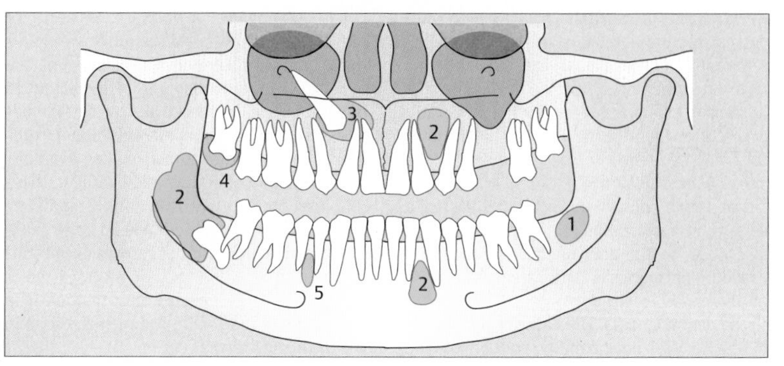

355

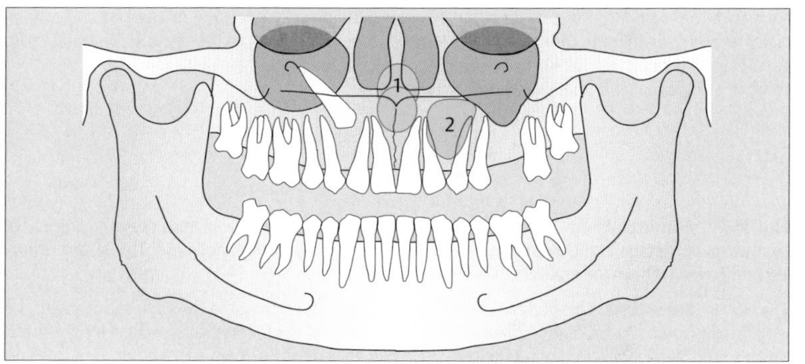

356

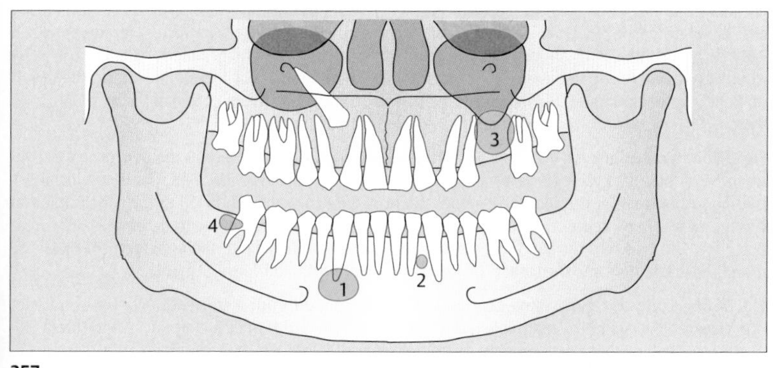

357

Keratocysts (primordial cysts): The keratocyst (primordial cyst) develops from epithelial remnants of the dental lamella and the enamel epithelium. Localized at the site of a normal or a supernumerary tooth, the keratocyst is often found at the distal end of the dental arch (frequently in the mandible) at the site of a third molar and a supernumerary molar, or may be observed within the place of a supernumerary premolar. Keratocysts can also occur in the area of the maxillary and mandibular canines or in the area of the angle of the mandible without any apparent contact to the dental lamella. The lining of the keratocyst is keratinized squamous epithelium, and the lesion may manifest in both uni- and multilocular forms. In a typical radiographic picture of the keratocyst, one often observes the formation of "satellites" or pouches that initially exhibit a round shape, and then with further progression the satellites coalesce to impart a characteristic scalloped border that is pathognomonic. For this reason, the use of radiographs almost always underestimates the expanse of keratocysts, because of the density and the overlapping of the satellites by intact bone that occur due to the summation effect in radiographic equipment common to most dental practices, for example, periapical or panoramic radiographs; these difficulties make early detection extraordinarily difficult. Affected teeth and adjacent teeth are forced apart, and root resorption often is in evidence.

The primordial cyst occurs most frequently in the second decade of life and the keratocyst in the third and fourth.

Males are significantly more frequently affected than females.

The differential diagnosis should include follicular cyst, unicystic ameloblastoma, odontogenic fibromyxoma, but also residual cysts of all etiologies.

Fig. 358 Primordial cyst. The panoramic radiograph of this 13-year-old male reveals a primordial cyst at an early stage in the location of the congenitally missing third molar, 38. This lesion almost certainly evolved from the epithelium of the dental lamella.

Fig. 359a Keratocyst. This periapical radiograph reveals a keratocyst in the right maxilla with the rare localization between teeth 12 and 13. Note that roots of the two teeth have been forced apart, and also the clearly scalloped border of the cyst. The periodontal ligament space around tooth 12 remains intact.

Fig. 359b Keratocyst. This section from a panoramic radiograph of a 44-year-old male reveals the recurrence of a keratocyst in the right mandible; initially, this lesion was interpreted as a radicular cyst emanating from tooth 46. Clearly visible is the formation of round "satellites" (**arrows**), which will become confluent upon further development of the cyst, resulting in a scalloped border. The roots of nonvital tooth 36 have begun to resorb and therefore appear to be quite short. The cyst is obviously impinging upon the mandibular canal and expanding in the direction of the mandibular ramus.

Fig. 360a Follicular cyst. This section from a panoramic radiograph reveals the pericoronal or central type of follicular cyst in the left mandible around totally impacted tooth 48. The cyst is localized, pathognomonically, at the cementoenamel junction. Clinical examination led to the conclusion that this lesion was in an acute stage and its radiographic expanse is impossible to determine with great accuracy. The crown of the tooth resides within the cystic lumen. Note the impingement upon the mandibular foramen, and the Linkow blade implant serving as a bridge abutment.

Fig. 360b Follicular cyst. Same case as above. This section from a conventional posteroanterior overview radiograph of the mandible (see p. **91**) reveals the position of the displaced and totally impacted tooth 48 within the ascending mandibular ramus. Note the sharply demarcated, arcuate lingual border of the compact bone (**arrows**). Fifty-nine-year-old male.

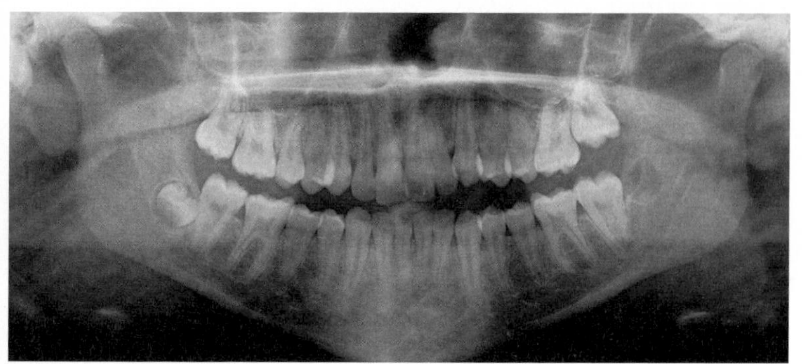

358

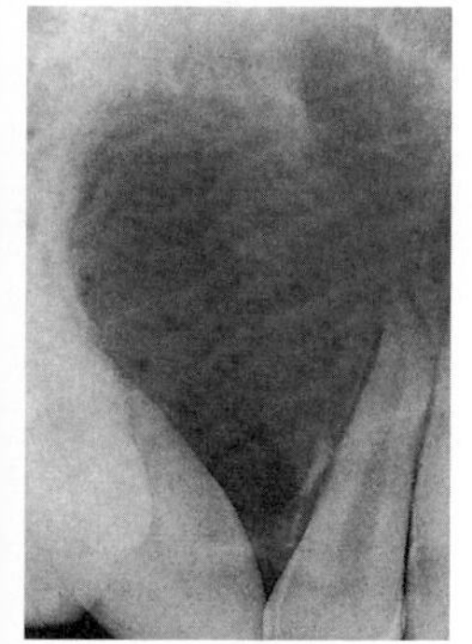

359 a

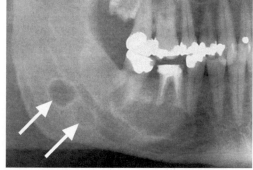

359 b

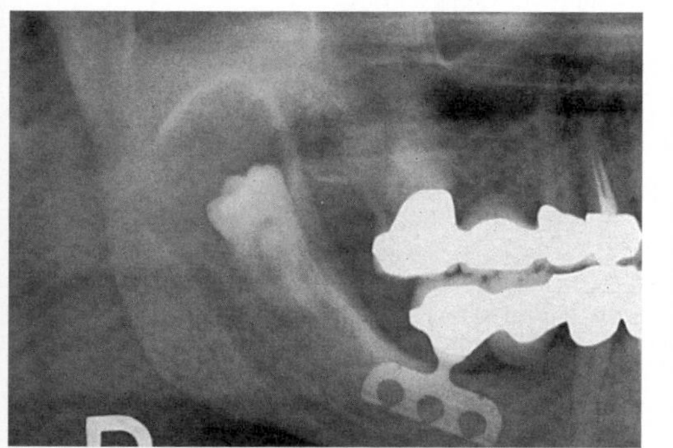

360 a

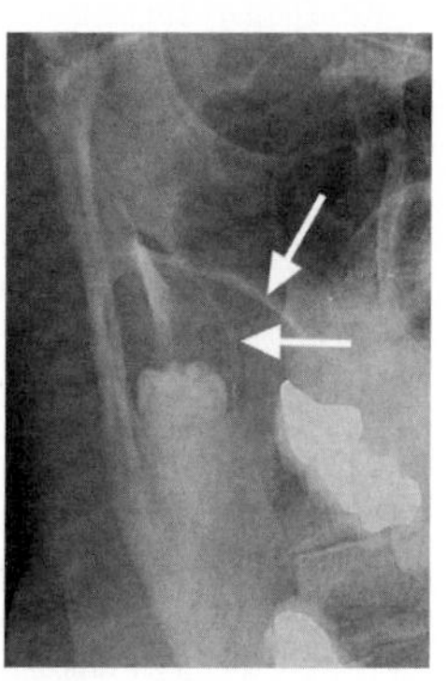

360 b

Follicular cysts: Follicular cysts develop between the layers of the enamel epithelium or between the enamel epithelium and the crown of the tooth. They expand slowly via osmotic processes and the increasing internal pressure.

Follicular cysts may develop spontaneously following various eliciting irritations in the region of the tooth crown of normal or supernumerary tooth buds. For this reason, the follicular cyst as observed radiographically is clearly evident at the cementoenamel junction and encloses the crown of the tooth. The entire tooth crown or in some cases only a portion of the crown, for example, in the case of lateral cysts, are typically observed within the radiolucency that is the cystic lumen.

As with virtually all other types of cysts, follicular cysts are expansive/expanding lesions. Through slow size increase, the cyst inhibits not only the growth of the affected tooth but also that of the structures in the immediate area, and can also lead to destructive resorption of adjacent tissues. Because of the forces exerted by the expanding cyst upon surrounding bone, the affected teeth may become impacted, are forced into extreme positions within the bone, and in some cases even undergo resorption. Because follicular cysts grow only slowly and usually without symptoms, the failure of a tooth to erupt, tipping of teeth within the dental arch, and the development of asymmetric facial swelling are frequently only noticed in the later stages. There is often compression of the mandibular canal or the maxillary sinuses.

Radiographic signs: Of importance is the width of the follicular sac observed as the radiolucency surrounding the tooth crown: If it achieves about 6 mm, it is reasonable to assume that the lesion represents a cystically altered follicular sac. A variant of the follicular cyst, which is often observed around erupting third molars, is the **eruption cyst**, which develops as a result of inflammatory irritation during tooth eruption. Follicular cysts either include the entire tooth crown (**central type**) or partially include the tooth crown (**lateral type**) and typically appear to be attached at the cementoenamel junction. In the case of cysts that develop without inhibition, the cystic lumen will exhibit a radiopaque border. During an inflammatory phase, the typical opaque border may be partially or totally lost, the transition to intact surrounding structures appears indistinct and diffuse, which may render the differential diagnosis more difficult. In the radiograph, follicular cysts usually appear as a single chamber and only rarely as multi-chambered lesions, and this fact makes the differentiation between ameloblastoma and keratocyst virtually impossible. Expansive follicular cysts frequently distend the osseous borders resulting in thinning of the compact bone. Teeth that have been displaced by an expanding follicular cyst often reside within the mandibular ramus, within the maxillary sinus, or even erupting through the basal compact bone on the inferior surface of the mandible; such teeth can therefore obviously not be captured in a conventional intraoral radiographic survey.

Fig. 361 a Eruption cyst. This section of a panoramic radiograph from a 16-year-old female reveals an eruption cyst occlusal to the erupting tooth 48 (**arrow**), which is still covered by mucosa (**arrows above**). The clinical eruption of tooth 18 has already begun, the overlying osseous lamella is completely gone, and the tooth crown is covered only by a flap of gingiva (**arrow**).

Fig. 361 b Eruption cyst. The periapical radiograph of tooth 28 reveals a very thin, distended osseous lamella (**arrow**).

Fig. 362 Follicular cyst. This panoramic radiograph of a 43-year-old male reveals a lateral follicular cyst on the partially erupted tooth 38. Visible also is pericoronitis with paracoronal pockets and reactive sclerosis surrounding the nonvital tooth 48, as well as a radicular residual cyst in the molar region of the left maxilla (**arrows**).

Fig. 363 Follicular cyst. This panoramic radiograph reveals a follicular maxillary cyst (**arrow**) emanating from tooth 23. Such cysts are often localized in the region of the maxillary canines. Noteworthy also are the small radicular cysts apical to nonvital tooth 46, and the focal sclerosing osteomyelitis emanating from nonvital tooth 36.

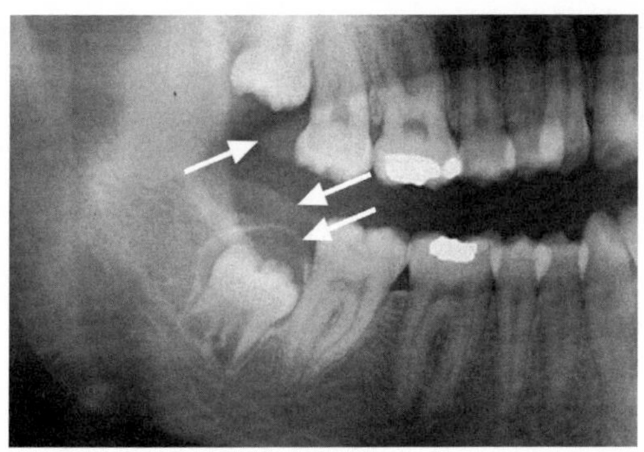

361 a

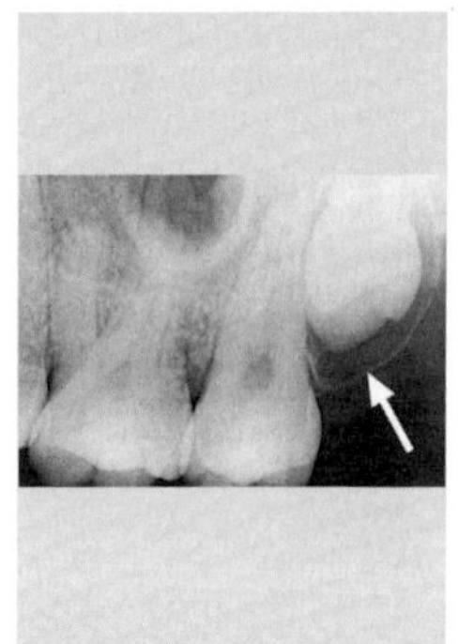

361 b

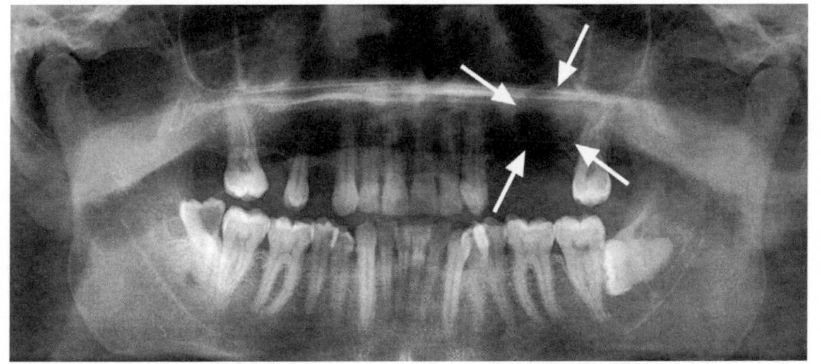

362

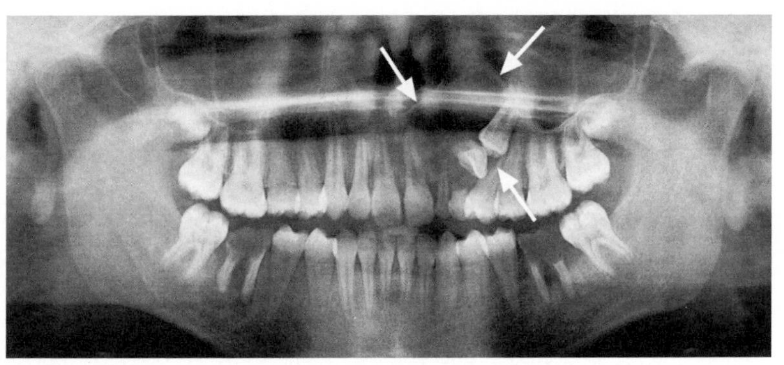

363

Differential diagnosis of follicular cysts: Radiographic equipment in most modern dental practices permits early radiographic diagnosis of follicular cysts due to the unmistakable attachment of the cystic cavity at the cementoenamel junction.

Depending upon age, gender and localization, the following entities should be included in the differential diagnosis:

- Ameloblastoma
- Ameloblastic fibroma
- Keratocyst
- Central giant cell granuloma
- Calcifying odontogenic cyst

Residual cysts of various etiologies cannot be identified radiographically within a differential diagnosis.

Radiographic technique: The overview of the jaws that is required for comprehensive examination can only be guaranteed using a panoramic radiograph. The panoramic radiograph, however, is a zonographic summation image and provides only a two-dimensional view; therefore, large follicular cysts must additionally be depicted in the third dimension, and this demands the use of modern computed tomography (CT) and/or magnetic resonance imaging (MRI).

Follicular cysts are usually localized in the mandible. Most often affected are the mandibular third molars, the maxillary canines, the maxillary third molars, and the mandibular canines, in approximately this order of frequency.

Corresponding to the growth spurt in the second decade of life, and the apical and periodontal inflammatory irritations that usually occur in the fourth and fifth decades of life, the age distribution for follicular cysts exhibits two peaks.

Lateral periodontal cyst: The lateral periodontal cyst is typically observed between the roots of vital teeth in the premolar regions of the mandible. In addition to their presence in areas of missing teeth, they can also be observed in radiographs lateral to a tooth root. This cyst exhibits no communication with the sulcus of adjacent teeth, and most likely occurs due to inflammatory irritation on the remnants of odontogenic epithelia. Statistically, these cysts are more common in males than in females, and are less common in the maxilla than in the mandible. These cysts occur most often after the age of 50 and are often diagnosed by chance. The differential diagnosis should include osteoblastoma or keratocyst, but the latter occurs much more frequently in the canine region.

Fig. 364 Follicular cyst. This panoramic radiograph of a 50-year-old male reveals a follicular cyst in the left tubercle region, that was likely elicited by the medially impacted tooth 28 (**arrows**). This example demonstrates that the “classical” attachment of a follicular cyst at the cementoenamel junction, in the case of large cysts, can no longer be discerned. This renders radiographic differential diagnosis extremely difficult, for example, differentiation between follicular cyst and ameloblastoma.

Fig. 365 Follicular cyst. The panoramic radiograph of a 23-year-old male revealed the serendipitous finding of a follicular cyst emanating from a mesiodens (**white arrow**). The cyst had developed to an extraordinary size (**black arrows**), totally symptom-free. It developed expansively left of the floor of the nose and the lateral wall of the nose toward the sinus. On the right side, the cyst completely compressed the sinus, eroded the floor of the nasal cavity and extended to the floor of the orbit. This radiograph also depicts how easily a mesiodens can remain undetected in the shadow of the cervical vertebrae.

Fig. 366 Lateral periodontal cyst. The panoramic radiograph of a 50-year-old male reveals a lateral periodontal cyst between teeth 33 and 34, which is a most frequent area of localization for this lesion. The adjacent teeth remain clinically vital.

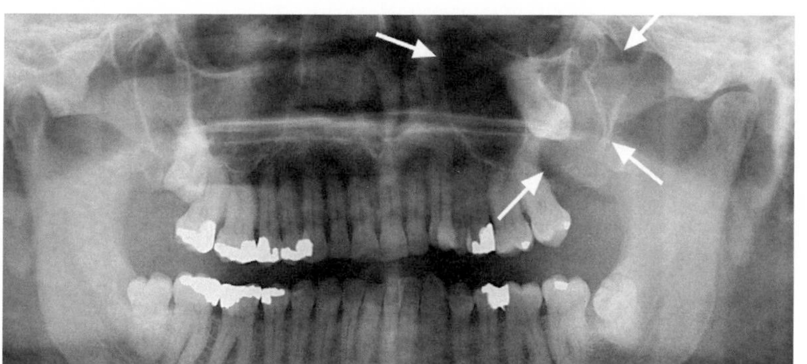

364

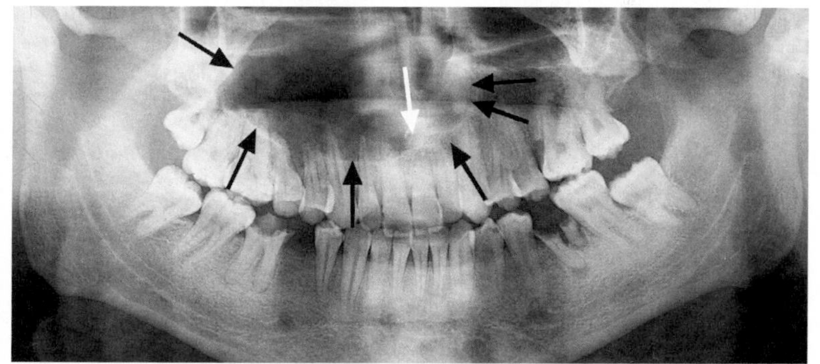

365

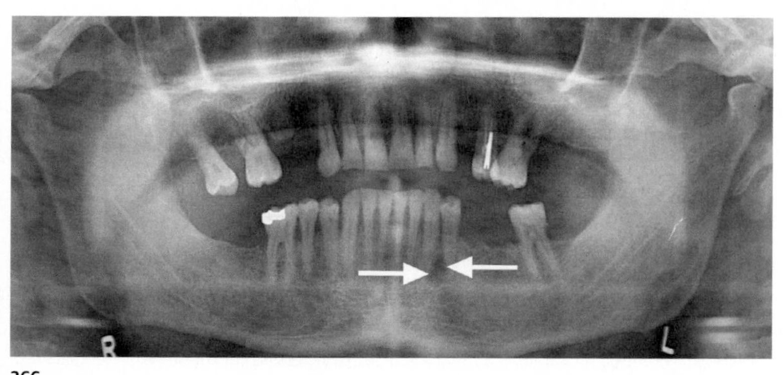

366

Nasopalatine and nasoalveolar cysts: Nasopalatine (incisive duct) cysts and nasoalveolar (globulomaxillary) cysts derive from epithelial remnants of the nasopalatine tract and the Hochstetter epithelial wall.

Nasopalatine cysts develop in the incisive canal or ventral and dorsal to it. If the cyst is positioned centrally in the canal, one observes a heart-shaped configuration, without displacement of the roots of the central incisors. If the cyst is localized ventrally, it grows between the roots of the incisors and displaces them laterally. If the cyst is expanding dorsal to the canal, the radiolucency appears in the approximate midline and is oval in shape.

Nasoalveolar cysts develop within the alveolar process between the roots of the lateral incisors and the canines, and expand in the direction of the nasal cavity and the maxillary sinus.

Radiographic signs: Small nasopalatine cysts discovered early appear in periapical radiographs superimposed upon the root tips of the central incisors. Such cysts are differentiated radiographically from true apical lesions in that the lamina dura and the periodontal ligament space around the affected roots are maintained.

In the initial stages, the radiolucency elicited by nasoalveolar cysts is a characteristic shape resembling an inverted pear between the roots of the lateral incisor and the canine.

Differential diagnosis: Nasopalatine cysts of the palate and nasoalveolar cysts were previously described as "fissural" cysts. The differential diagnosis should include residual cysts, follicular cysts from the tooth buds of supernumerary anterior teeth (see also Fig. **365**), keratocysts, the ameloblastoma, and an incomplete palatal cleft.

Radiographic technique: Clear depiction of large cysts and their borders can be difficult to differentiate from the background of air-containing spaces if the exposure settings are too high.

Fig. 367a Nasopalatine cyst. This periapical radiograph reveals a sharply demarcated "periapical" radiolucency around vital tooth 21. In contrast to a true radicular cyst, however, the periodontal ligament space is completely intact. This lesion is a nasopalatine cyst that obscures the root apex due to the subtraction effect, therefore appearing similar to a true apical cyst.

Fig. 367b Nasopalatine cyst. This occlusal radiograph reveals an incisive duct cyst with its heart-shaped configuration; it has not (yet) penetrated between the roots of adjacent teeth 11 and 21 and therefore has also not displaced these teeth laterally.

Fig. 367c Nasopalatine cyst. This occlusal radiograph reveals an oval-shaped nasopalatine cyst, which is not infrequently dorsal to the incisive canal within the hard palate. Because of their location at or near the palatal suture, such cysts were previously described as median fissural palatal cysts.

Fig. 368 Nasopalatine cyst. The panoramic radiograph reveals an incisive duct cyst in a 42-year-old male. It has invaded between the roots of teeth 11 and 22 (**black arrows**) and has begun to expand in the right maxilla distending the maxillary sinus and the floor of the nose (**white arrows**). Teeth 11, 12, 13, and 14 were clinically vital.

Fig. 369 Nasoalveolar cyst. This panoramic radiograph of a 23-year-old male reveals bilateral nasoalveolar cysts (**arrows**). Such cysts develop (also unilaterally) within the alveolar process from embryonic cell remnants between the lateral incisors and the canines of the maxilla, which expanded in the direction of the paranasal and maxillary sinuses. With increasing size, these cysts eventually lose their typical "inverted pear" shape (left). Note also the lateral follicular cyst at tooth 48.

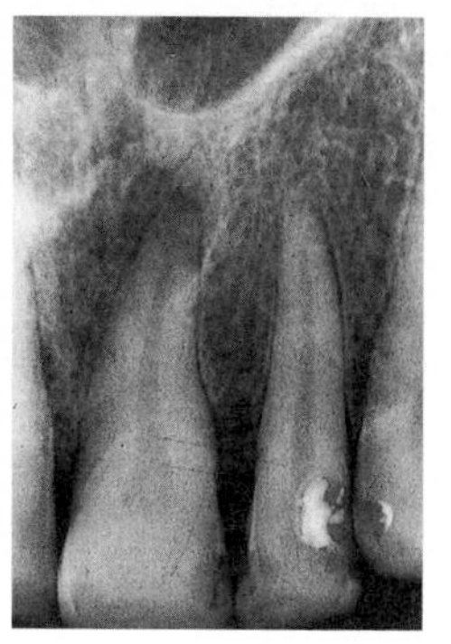

367 a

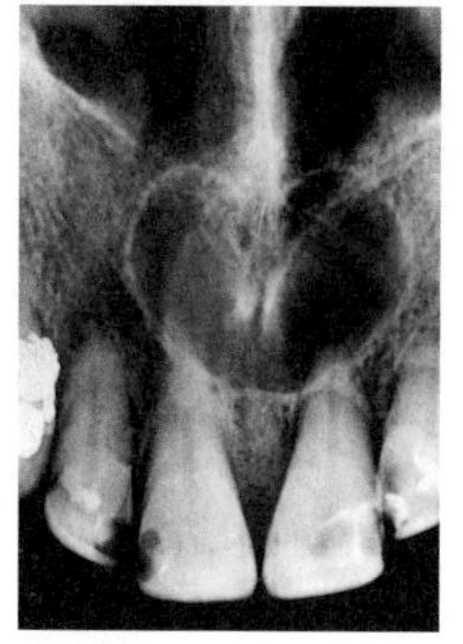

367 b

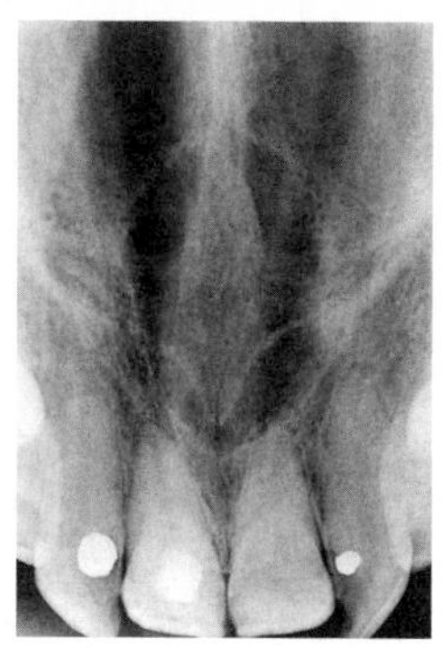

367 c

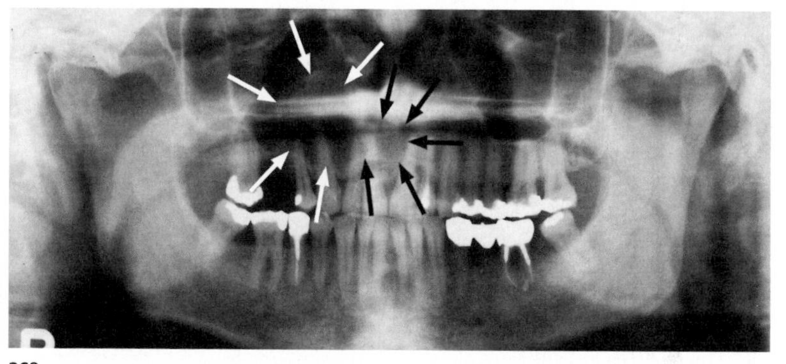

368

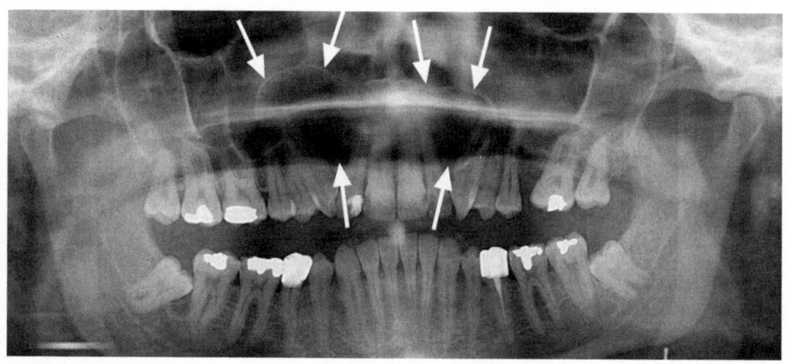

369

According to the literature, radicular cysts comprise between 80 and 90% of all odontogenic cysts.

Radicular cysts develop following pulpal necrosis caused by caries or traumatic insult, which stimulate the epithelial rest cells of Malassez in the periodontal ligament to proliferate. Radicular cysts do not develop around nonvital teeth in **all** patients; one theory seeks to explain this situation by hypothesizing a genetically based enzyme deficiency that can elevate the tendency for cyst formation. Within the center of the proliferating mass of epithelial rest cells, central cellular degeneration occurs leading eventually to cystic cavity formation, which is usually lined by squamous epithelium. The fluid content of the cyst is usually a brownish color, and contains cholesterol crystals. Osmotic forces and accumulation of metabolic products within the lumen create intracystic pressures leading to continual enlargement of the cyst and displacement of surrounding tissues. The cystic expansion caused by osmotic processes and the increasing pressure caused by accumulation of metabolic products in the lumen may be continuous and symptom-free or may proceed intermittently as a result of recurring bouts of inflammation. In the initial stages, such developments are subjective and hardly ever detectable. Radicular cysts usually expand slowly and compress the surrounding tissues in relation to their resistance; this leads in many cases to a cyst that does not exhibit the classic round shape that is generally regarded as pathognomonic for cysts. Often a typical, opaque border will form around the cyst as a result of pressure upon the osseous environment and ongoing inflammatory irritation; this border is visually enhanced by the tangential effect of the roentgen rays, and is therefore often *incorrectly* referred to as "corticalization." Furthermore, the consistency of the surrounding structures and the aggressiveness of the inflammatory processes will determine whether the tissues subjected to the increasing cystic pressure will be completely resorbed, partially resorbed, or only distended.

Fig. 370a Radicular cysts. Radiographic condition following pulpal necrosis. At this size, the radicular cyst on the clinically nonvital tooth 22 is virtually impossible to distinguish radiographically from a well-encapsulated granuloma.

Fig. 370b Radicular cysts. The radicular cyst on the clinically nonvital tooth 25 exhibits the typical radiographic signs, including open transition of the lamina dura into the cystic cavity, loss of the periodontal ligament space in the root area, and the tip of the root located within the cystic cavity. This radicular cyst is in a stage of quiescence, exhibiting a clear and well-demarcated osseous border.

Fig. 371a Radicular cysts. The radicular cyst on clinically nonvital tooth 12 shows the typical radiographic signs of an active inflammatory phase (*infected cyst*); note the blurred demarcation with apparent decalcification of surrounding bone.

Fig. 371b Radicular cysts. The apex of the clinically nonvital tooth 25 is located within a radiolucency with a blurred, poorly demarcated periphery; a typical radiographic sign of an acute stage. The sinus floor is eroded, and one notes remnants of the cystic border mesially that distend the intrasinus septum anteriorly.

Fig. 372 Radicular cysts. The panoramic radiograph of a 36-year-old male reveals in the left mandible two well-demarcated cysts on the roots of the carious and clinically nonvital tooth 36. In contrast, on the right side of the mandible one observes the radiographic signs of chronic, focal osteomyelitis in the periapical region of clinically nonvital tooth 47.

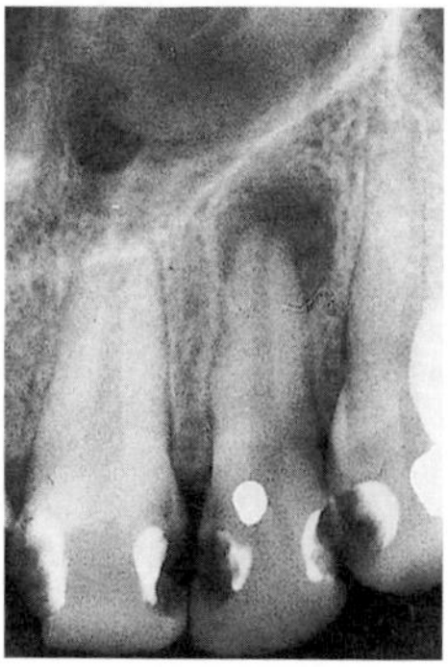

370 a

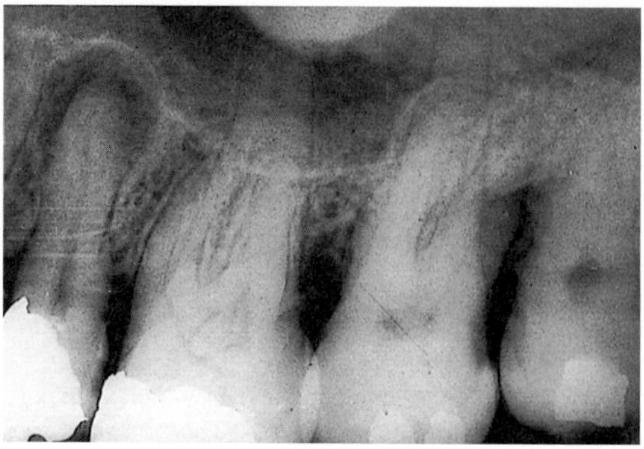

370 b

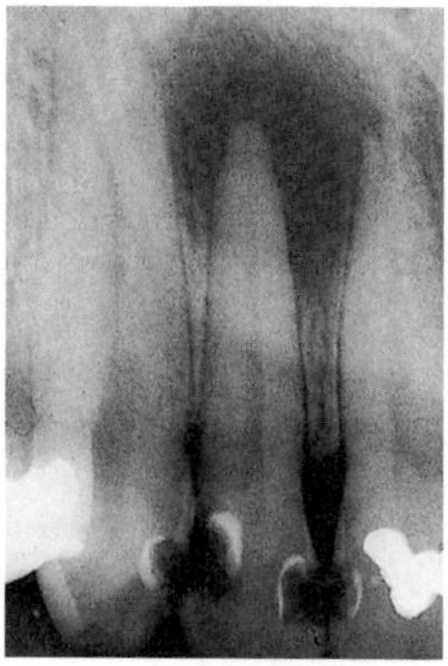

371 a

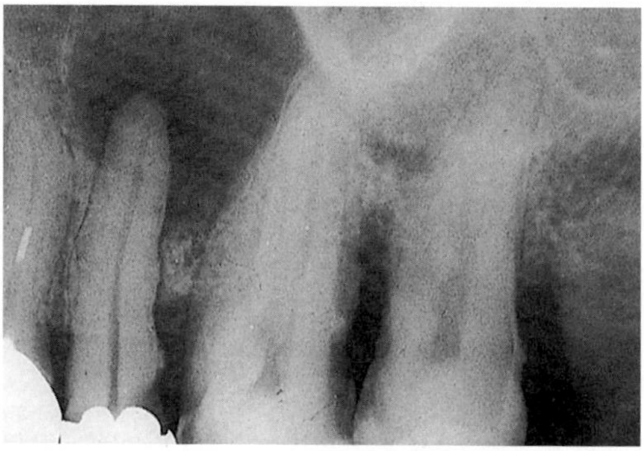

371 b

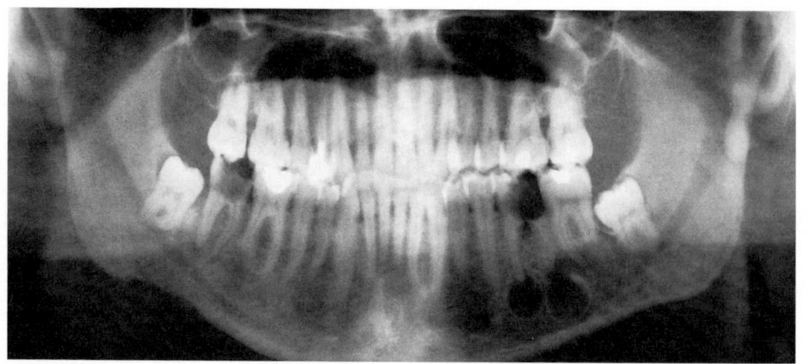

372

The overlapping (summation effect) of teeth exhibiting cysts or even adjacent teeth may lead the inexperienced observer to a diagnosis of osseous resorption caused by the "subtraction effect" as the roentgen rays traverse air-containing spaces or the cystic lumen itself.

Secondary infections and acute exacerbations during the course of the inflammatory process lead to dissolution of the opaque border and to osteolytic process in the tissues surrounding the cyst. However, such alterations occurring during an acute phase can be discerned in a radiograph only after a latent period of several days; for this reason, the clinical findings frequently do not correlate with the radiographic picture. This is also the case with expansive areas of osteomyelitis of the jaws. Because the development of radicular cysts proceeds slowly, and it often takes years until they are detected radiographically, usually serendipitously, radicular cysts of the relatively short-duration primary dentition are practically unknown.

Multi-chambered radicular cysts are also extremely rare. A radiograph may **appear** to depict a multi-chambered cyst, but this is most often due to the radiographic superimposition of several cysts upon each other, cysts that emanate from individual roots of multi-rooted teeth or an accessory apical foramen of a single rooted tooth.

Recurrent radicular cysts may develop following extraction of a tooth with an attached cyst, due to remnants of the cyst or epithelial rest cells. Recurrent cysts cannot be differentiated radiographically from residual cysts of other origins.

Radiographic signs of radicular cysts: In the radiograph, the cystic lumen appears as a round radiolucency surrounded by an opaque border which, in the case of small cysts, appears to surround the root tip centrally or laterally. In almost all cases of radicular cysts, the root apex is within the radiolucency. The epithelial rest cells of Malassez within the periodontal ligament proliferate near the anatomical apical foramen (central position) or an ectopic accessory foramen.

In all radiographs revealing periapically localized odontogenic and nonodontogenic lesions, maintenance of the lamina dura and therefore also the periodontal ligament space is a very important radiographic sign. In the case of a small radicular cyst, the lamina dura ends at the border of the cyst and appears perpendicular to the opaque margin exhibited by cysts in a quiescence stage.

Depending on the time point of the radiographic examination, infected radicular cysts in the acute stage exhibit the above-described radiographic signs only partially, or several days later not at all. The opaque border may be partially or entirely lost and the osseous structure may appear dissolved and washed out.

Fig. 373a Radicular cysts. This periapical radiograph from a 41-year-old male reveals a radicular cyst emanating from the palatal root of the clinically nonvital tooth 26. The floor of the sinus appears shadowed as a result of the subtraction effect of the radiolucency.

Fig. 373b Radicular cysts. This section from a panoramic radiograph of the same case reveals the radicular cyst (**arrows**) within the left maxillary sinus. The reactive mucosal swelling caused by sinus irritation can be discerned by right-left comparison in the image.

Fig. 374 Radicular cysts. This panoramic radiograph of a 27-year-old female exhibits a "multi-chambered" radicular cyst emanating from the clinically nonvital teeth 36 and 37; in reality this appearance resulted from two separate cysts on these teeth that were overlapped in the radiographic projection. The arrow indicates the intervening border and not a true septum.

Fig. 375 Radicular residual (recurrent) cyst. Panoramic radiograph of a 22-year-old female reveals an infected radicular recurrent cyst emanating from fragments of the cyst that were associated with tooth 36, which had been extracted. In the acute stage, the cyst has lost its typical opaque border due to decalcification. This is a large mandibular cyst, primarily oval in shape, and some distention of the basal compact bone is visible. Tooth 35 appears to be undergoing radicular resorption.

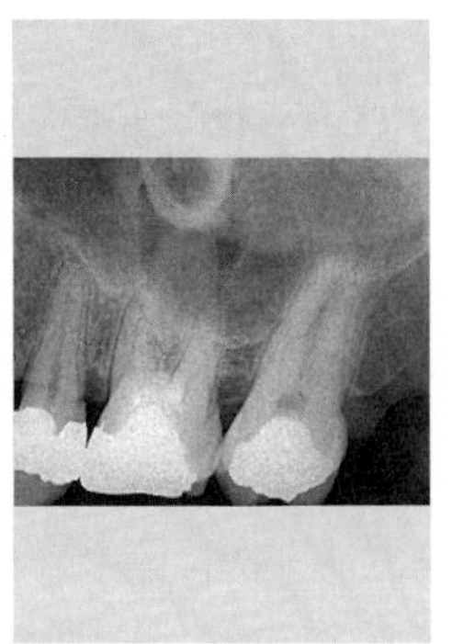

373 a

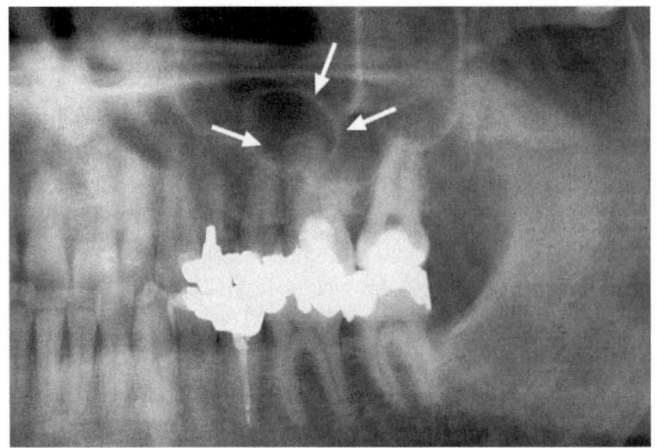

373 b

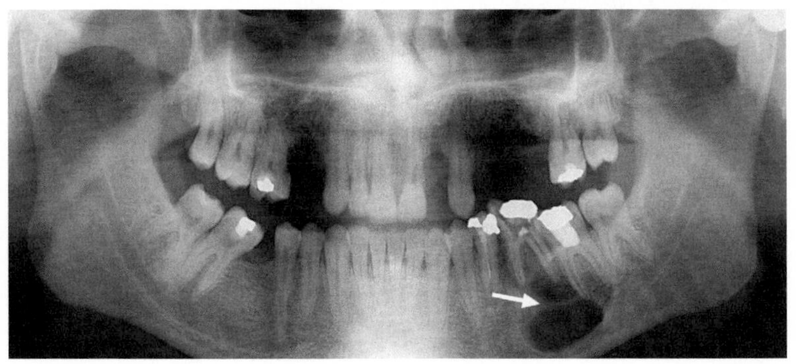

374

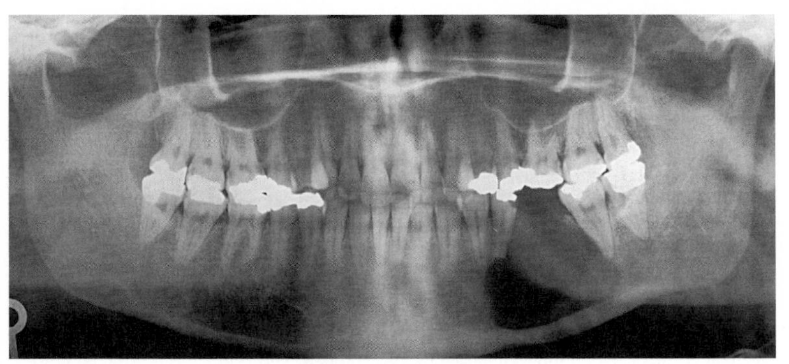

375

Radicular cysts are observed more frequently in the maxilla than in the mandible. The most common localization is the anterior dental segment. They are more common in females than in males, and the most common occurrence is during the third and fourth decades of life.

Differential diagnosis: Small radicular cysts cannot be radiographically distinguished from a well-encapsulated granuloma. According to Shear, even cystoid radiolucencies with a diameter of 1 cm can be determined histologically to be actual cysts in only 50% of cases; therefore, extreme care is clearly necessary during radiographic diagnosis. Incorrect diagnosis may also occur with the existence of periapical cemental dysplasia, as well as cemento-osseous dysplasia in the initial stages. The differential diagnosis must also include true periodontal cysts, osteoblastoma, ossifying fibroma, and well-demarcated bone marrow islands in the premolar region of the mandible.

Especially during an inflammatory phase, large residual (recurrent) cysts are difficult to differentiate from a solitary bone cyst or (especially following recurrent inflammation) from a malignant primary tumor or a metastatic lesion.

Radiographic technique: Small radicular cysts can be well depicted using periapical radiographs, but larger cysts will require a panoramic overview. These radiographs, however, reveal the cysts only in two dimensions, so it is absolutely necessary to prepare radiographs to depict the third dimension of localization. While an occlusal radiograph with proper central ray projection (see p. **58**) will be adequate in the mandible, the maxillary occlusal radiograph with the attendant projection angle will not depict the dorsal boundary of large cysts, and in many cases an axial CT will be indicated.

As a result of the relatively low resistance of the osseous structures in the region of the maxillary sinus and the lingual plate of bone in the mandible, large expansive cysts will effectively thin the adjacent osseous lamellae. These thinned lamellae will not be visible against the background of air-containing spaces if normal exposure settings are employed; in such cases, it will be necessary to reduce the exposure settings.

Paradental (Craig) cysts: Inflammation-induced cysts include also the so-called Craig cyst, which can develop distally and buccally in the radicular regions of an incompletely erupted mandibular third molar. The Craig cyst may develop from a recurrent pericoronitis, and cannot be differentiated radiographically from this lesion.

Fig. 376 Radicular residual (recurrent) cyst. The panoramic radiograph of a 40-year-old male presented the serendipitous finding of a residual radicular cyst at the extraction site of tooth 46. It is well known that, especially in elderly patients, an ameloblastoma may develop following tooth extraction; for this reason, histologic examination of the soft tissues of the cyst should be performed.

Fig. 377 Radicular residual (recurrent) cyst. The panoramic radiograph of a 57-year-old male revealed the serendipitous finding of an ossifying fibroma, which, in this localization, simulates a true residual radicular cyst. Note the typical demarcation and the displacement of the mandibular canal.

Fig. 378 Inflammation-induced paradental (Craig) cyst. This panoramic radiograph of a 44-year-old male reveals an inflammation-induced paradental cyst distal to the malpositioned tooth 48.

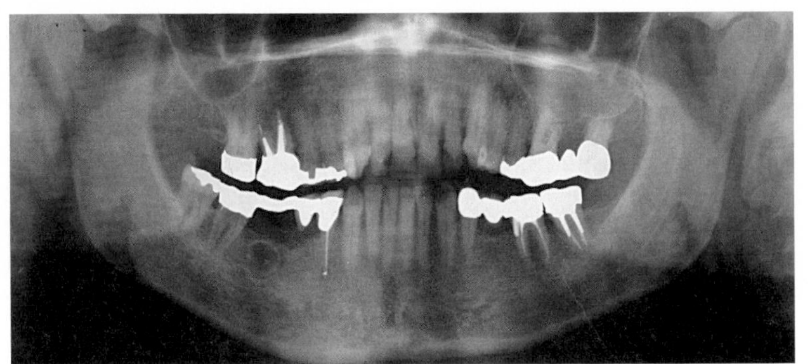

376

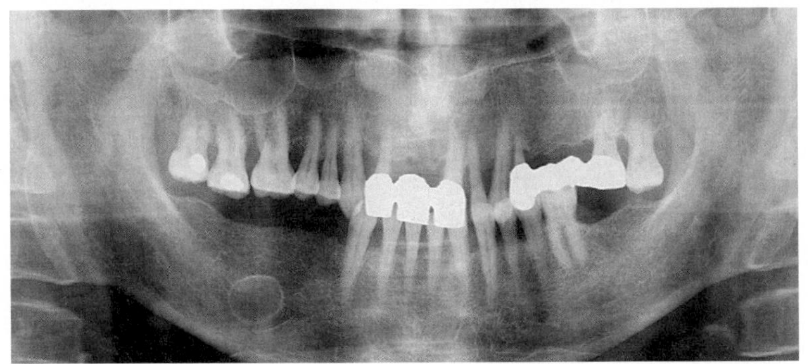

377

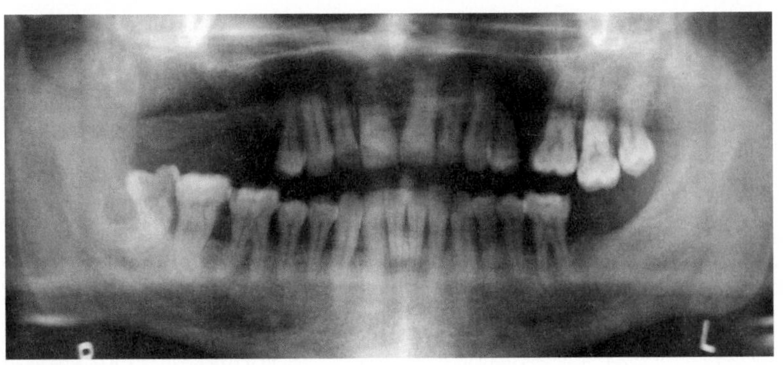

378

According to Reichart and Ries (1983) and Heikinheimo (1993) the following cell groups are involved in normal odontogenesis:

- Epithelial cells such as ameloblasts, dental lamina epithelium, and squamous epithelium from the oral mucosa
- Ectomesenchymal cells such as odontoblasts and cementoblasts
- Mesenchyme with fibrocytes, fibroblasts, lipid tissue, hemangioendothelium, osteocytes, osteoblasts, and chondrocytes
- Neuroectodermal cells such as neuroblasts, Schwann cells, and melanocytes

The new principles of classification were based on the proposal by Kramer et al. (1992) and the 1992 WHO classification of odontogenic tumors (including hamartoma and the dysplasias), and provide the framework for the presentations in this chapter, with the exception of the rare malignant tumors.

Disturbances of the interactions between and among the above-listed cell types during odontogenesis lead to malformations and neoplasia (Reichart and Ries 1983), which frequently manifest as benign odontogenic tumors and only rarely as malignant tumors. The latter may develop following recurrence as odontogenic carcinoma (e.g., the malignant ameloblastoma) or as odontogenic sarcoma (e.g., the ameloblastic fibrosarcoma). A comprehensive presentation can be found in Reichart and Philipsen (1999).

In comparison to the diagnostic possibilities offered by histopathologic techniques, the clinical and also the radiographic diagnosis often only provide empirical information and "probable" diagnoses, but no precise diagnosis. For this reason, clinical biopsy and microscopic examination of the fine tissues within the surgical specimen will be of extraordinary importance in many cases when considering further therapeutic options. Because several odontogenic cysts and tumors have the potential for recurrence, a target-oriented follow-up program is obligatory in order to avoid additional expansive surgical procedures and the danger of malignant transformation.

Fig. 379a Ameloblastoma. The surgical specimen exhibits the typical signs of a multilocular ameloblastoma. Note especially the expanse of the benign odontogenic tumor, which was visible clinically as a facial swelling; note also the large, spherical cavitated structures that could only be depicted radiographically using reduced exposure settings. In clinical practice, occlusal radiographs are often helpful. In the case of a large ameloblastoma at the angle of the mandible or (less frequently) in the maxilla, a CT must be obtained.

Fig. 379b Ameloblastoma. In this 19-year-old female, a serendipitous discovery was made of a honeycomb-like ameloblastoma in its early stage in the region of teeth 36 and 37. The multilocular radiolucencies give the appearance of root resorption due to the radiographic subtraction effect. This appearance can be confused with a hemangioma.

Fig. 380 Ameloblastoma. The panoramic radiograph of a 23-year-old male reveals a multilocular ameloblastoma with displacement of tooth 38. Note the obvious thinning and distention of the basal compact bone, with displacement of the mandibular canal (**arrow**) and distention of the mandibular ramus.

Fig. 381 Ameloblastoma. The panoramic radiograph of a 28-year-old male reveals a unilocular ameloblastoma. The missing third molars provide an indication that the lesion developed as a result of extraction of tooth 38. If the crown of a tooth is present within the radiolucency, a radiographic differential diagnosis vis-à-vis follicular cysts is often not possible.

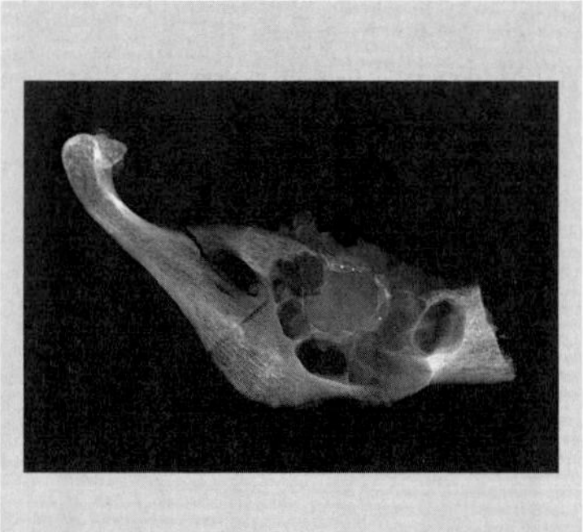

379 a

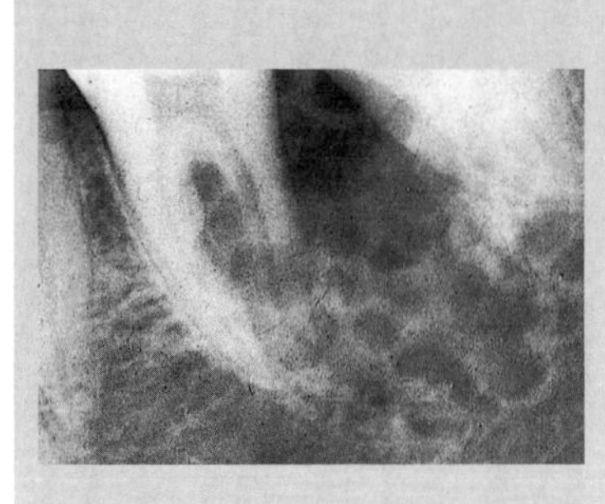

379 b

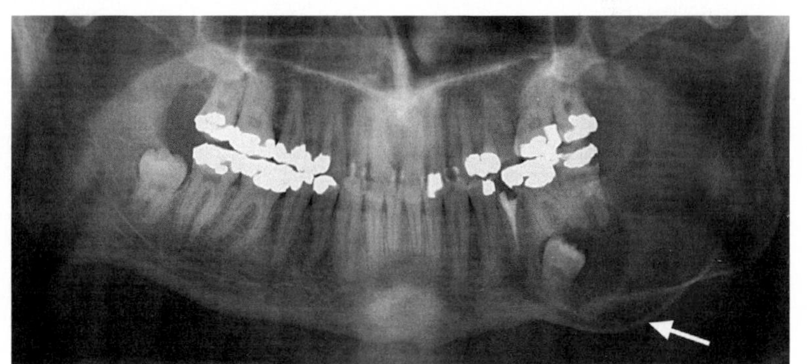

380

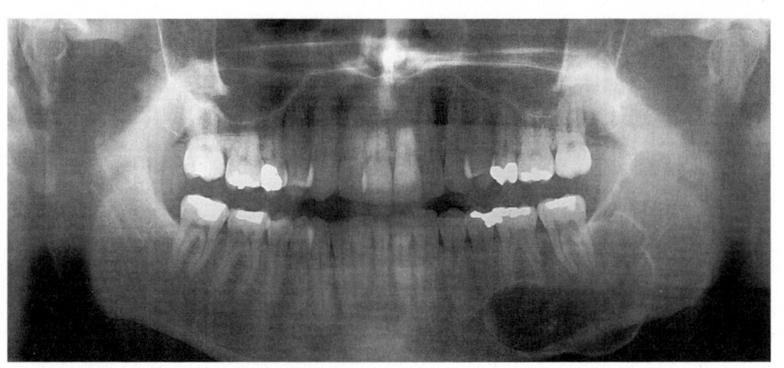

381

It is, however, very important that the dentition be carefully monitored throughout the mixed-dentition stage, both clinically and radiographically. This demands more than the routine bite-wing radiographs that are taken for early diagnosis of dental caries. Suspicious clinical findings such as missing or tipped teeth, diastemata, or painless swelling must be further investigated using panoramic radiographs in order to detect early on any expansion of odontogenic cysts and tumors not clinically apparent. This will make possible early diagnosis, and possibly spare the patient extensive surgical intervention and consequences.

Ameloblastoma

The most frequent localization is the molar region of the mandible (80%), followed by the premolar region, and (less often) the mandibular anterior region. The ameloblastoma is rare in the maxilla, and when it occurs it is usually in the molar regions.

The ameloblastoma is the most frequently encountered odontogenic tumor. Its histologic picture may vary enormously. The most common radiographic appearance is one of multilocular (multi-chambered or multi-cystic), soap bubble-like radiolucencies, compartmentalized by sharply demarcated septa. Unilocular forms are usually observed with the follicular ameloblastoma, such as those that occur during the active growth phase of the second decade of life. In many cases, an impacted tooth (usually a molar) is enclosed within the tumor. A less common variant is the honeycomb-like ameloblastoma that does not encompass teeth and whose septa are much thicker. The soap bubble-like structure usually creates a scalloped external contour. In later stages, the compact bone is distended and thinned; the dominant radiolucency demands a reduction of the normally employed exposure settings for a clear depiction of the structural details. The mandibular canal is often impinged upon, and is often no longer clearly visible within the radiolucency. In the maxilla, an ameloblastoma may impinge upon the maxillary sinuses and distend the sinus walls. The lesion grows slowly and develops with painless swelling and facial asymmetry whose etiology is frequently discerned only in very late stages. Peripheral variants of this lesion occur primarily in elderly patients, often with inclusion of oral mucosa.

Fig. 382 Ameloblastic fibroma. The panoramic radiograph of an 8-year-old male reveals an early stage ameloblastic fibroma. In contrast to a follicular cyst, the well-demarcated radiolucency sits like a hat on the occlusal surface of the displaced third molar (47) and is not attached at the cementoenamel junction of that tooth. The pericoronal follicular sac appears in this radiograph to have not communicated with the oral cavity.

Fig. 383 Ameloblastic fibroma. In this 9-year-old female, the lesion is localized on the occlusal surface of the far distally displaced second molar (37). The pericoronal follicular sac has opened. With progressive tumor expansion, and displacement of tooth 37 and germ of tooth 38, the radiographic differentiation between a unilocular ameloblastoma and a follicular cyst becomes more difficult. Note also the remnants of nonvital teeth 75, 84, and 85, which may have elicited the pericoronal inflammation and premature resorption of the follicular sacs. Tooth 22 is only observed as a “peg lateral.”

Fig. 384 Ameloblastic fibro-odontoma. The panoramic radiograph of a 20-year-old female reveals a dysplastic tooth 48 with irregular calcifications. Radiographic signs of the slow, nonaggressive expansion of the lesion include impingement of the mandibular canal and tooth 47. In contrast to the various shapes and forms of a complex odontoma, the demarcation in this case is not clearly defined around the lesion.

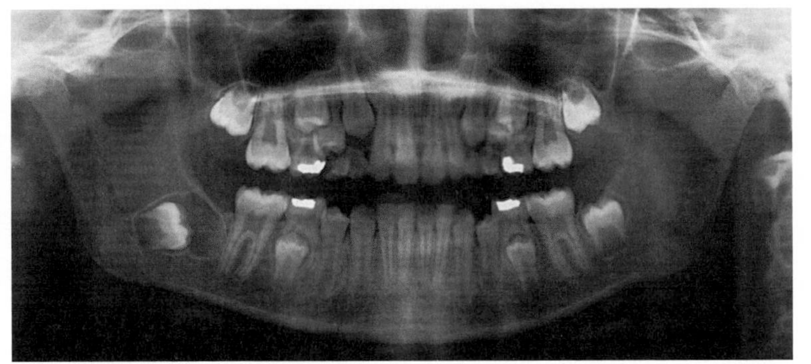

382

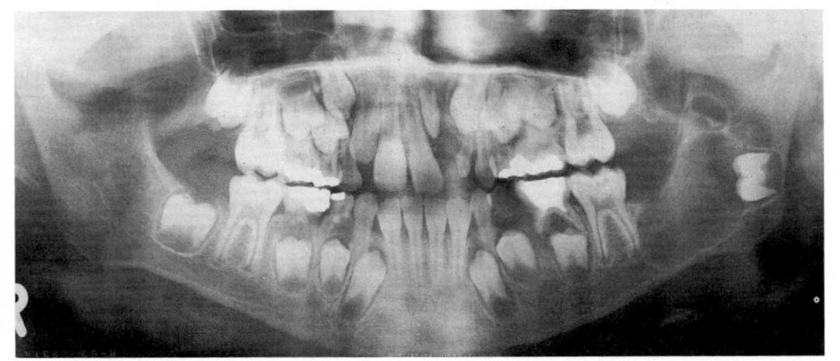

383

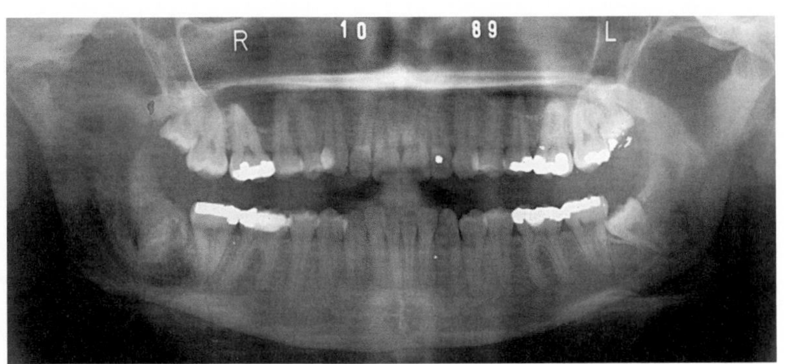

384

In older adults, following tooth extractions in the posterior segment, an ameloblastoma with a large soap bubble-like radiographic appearance can develop; this can be confused with a residual cyst. The lateral displacement of the enclosed or adjacent teeth, in combination with superimpositions by the radiolucency of the tumor, lead to subtraction effects on the roots, which in combination with radiographic overexposure can create the appearance of root resorptions.
The lesion is benign, but can recur even years later, and must therefore be removed with a relatively radical surgical procedure. Malignant ameloblastoma is extremely rare.
Presurgical spatial orientation demands computed tomography (CT).
The ameloblastoma occurs most frequently during the third and fourth decades of life. Early stages of the lesion are only seldom detected and then only serendipitously. Males and females are equally affected. The differential diagnosis should include follicular cyst, keratocyst, ameloblastic fibroma in later stages, odontogenic myxoma, or the central giant cell granuloma.

Ameloblastic Fibroma

On the basis of the proposal by Kramer et al. (1992) and upon the work by Reichart and Ries (1983), the ameloblastic fibroma and the ameloblastic fibro-odontoma are classified as benign tumors with odontogenic epithelium and odontogenic ectomesenchyme (see Reichart and Philipsen 1999).
The ameloblastic fibroma is found predominantly in the molar region of the mandible.
In its initial stages, the ameloblastic fibroma is detected upon the occlusal surface of a molar; this is in clear distinction to a follicular cyst, which is always detected at the cementoenamel junction. The ameloblastic fibroma is usually unilocular, but multi-chambered forms may be detected. Affected and adjacent teeth, as well as the mandibular canal, are often displaced. In the later stages of development, it is virtually impossible to differentiate radiographically between a follicular cyst and an ameloblastoma.

Fig. 385a Odontogenic myxoma. This section from a panoramic radiograph of a 34-year-old female reveals an odontogenic myxoma at the angle of the mandible. The sharp and irregularly distributed septa have the appearance of a torn fishing net, and can only be depicted using reduced exposure settings. Usually the marginal contour is scalloped in appearance.

Fig. 385b Odontogenic myxoma. A unilateral occlusal radiograph of the mandible, using reduced exposure settings, clearly reveals the typical structure with numerous irregular septa. Note also that the compact bone is distended laterally, and thinned, an appearance not unlike that of an ameloblastoma.

Fig. 386 Odontogenic myxoma. The panoramic radiograph of an 85-year-old female reveals the recurrence of an odontogenic myxoma. Note the destruction of the neck and the head of the mandible, as well as the thinned and distended compact bone. Expansion of a recurrent odontogenic myxoma depicts characteristically a spotty destruction of osseous structures, which extends into the right molar region of the body of the mandible.

Fig. 387 Odontogenic myxoma. The panoramic radiograph of a 13-year-old male reveals an odontogenic myxoma in the left maxilla. Teeth 26 and 27 are displaced, or inhibited from their normal eruption. Note also the cleft of the alveolar process and palate between teeth 13 and 11. Tooth 17, appears as a single-rooted taurodont (see Fig. **227**).

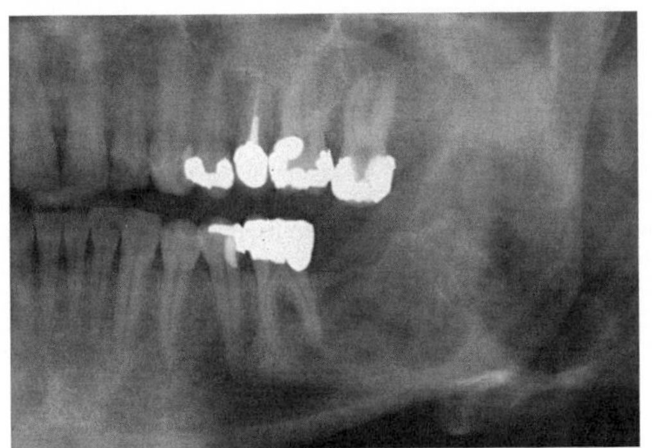

385 a

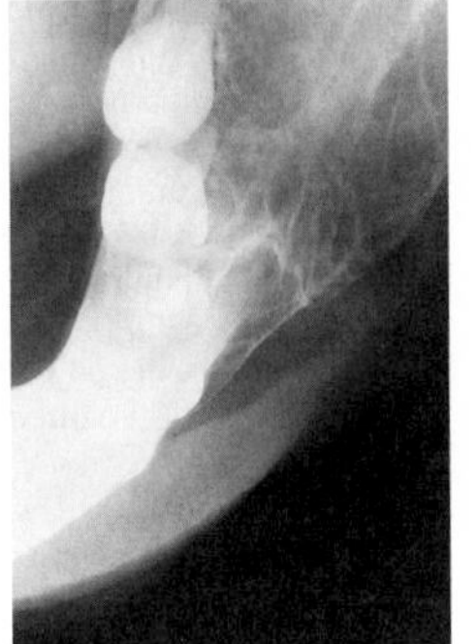

385 b

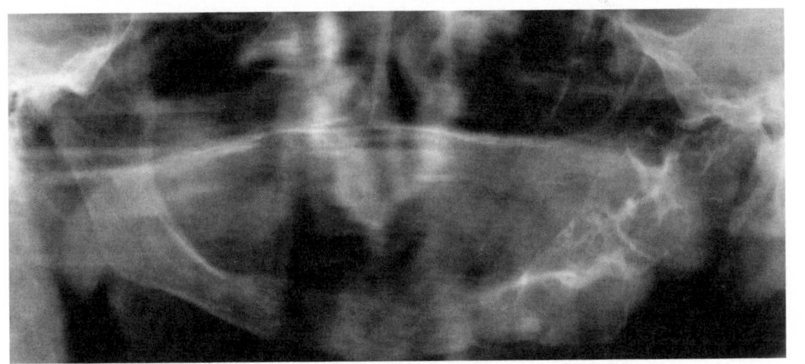

386

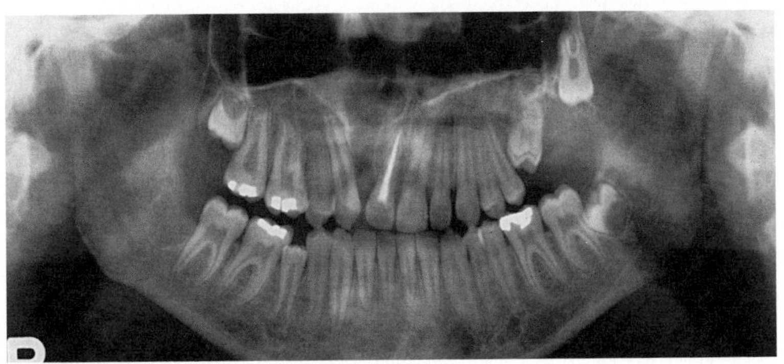

387

Following careful surgical removal, the benign tumor seldom recurs; some cases of malignant transformation have been reported, and therefore histologic examination of the excised lesion is recommended.
The most common age of occurrence is at the end of the first and the beginning of the second decade of life; for this reason children entering puberty should be examined additionally by means of a panoramic radiograph. Males are significantly more affected than females.
The differential diagnosis should include above all the follicular cyst and the ameloblastoma.

Ameloblastic Fibro-Odontoma

Philipsen et al. (1997) described and clarified the relationship of the ameloblastic fibroma to the ameloblastic fibro-odontoma and the odontomas in general.
The ameloblastic fibro-odontoma is found most frequently in the molar region of the mandible. In addition to dentin, it also contains enamel fragments. In over 80% of cases, it is combined with a retained or otherwise impacted molar. The mandibular canal is often displaced. In addition to compact radiopacities, cases may also be encountered with radiopacity surrounded by a wide band of radiolucency. It is not always possible radiographically to differentiate the similarities with a complex odontoma; often only histologic examination can lead to a precise diagnosis (see Fig. **384**). The lesion can occur even in early childhood, and the statistical peak is at 9 years of age. In most cases, males are affected.
The differential diagnosis must include the complex odontoma above all.

Ameloblastic Fibrodentinoma

This dentin-forming odontogenic tumor (WHO classification, Kramer et al. 1992) is considered to be a stage between an ameloblastic fibroma and an ameloblastic fibro-odontoma (Reichart and Philipsen 1999), and has only been documented in a very few cases.

Fig. 388a Calcifying epithelial odontogenic tumor. The lateral skull projection of a 48-year-old female, despite not being ideal, does reveal the clear demarcation and the calcifications (**arrows**). This radiograph was taken 10 years following surgical removal of a follicular cyst at tooth 28.

Fig. 388b Calcifying epithelial odontogenic tumor. This section from a panoramic radiograph of a 46-year-old female reveals a calcifying epithelial odontogenic tumor pericoronal to the completely impacted tooth 18.

Fig. 389 Calcifying epithelial odontogenic tumor. The panoramic radiograph of a 52-year-old female reveals a calcifying epithelial odontogenic tumor (**arrows**) associated with the totally impacted and dysplastic tooth 33. Note the expansive, calcified radiopacities and the thinned and distended basal compact bone. In the dental practice, the third dimension can only be depicted using an occlusal radiograph. With a lesion of this size, however, there is an indication for CT.

Fig. 390 Calcifying epithelial odontogenic tumor. The panoramic radiograph of a 40-year-old male reveals the calcified epithelial odontogenic tumor associated with the totally impacted tooth 37. Typical is the loss of visibility of the follicular sac. Note the spot-like and spherical calcifications exhibiting clear demarcations. The mandibular canal has been significantly displaced; it is partially superimposed by the radiopacities and its positional relationship to the tumor cannot be clarified in a two-dimensional panoramic radiograph. Even using CT or transversal projections, the course of the mandibular canal cannot always be depicted.

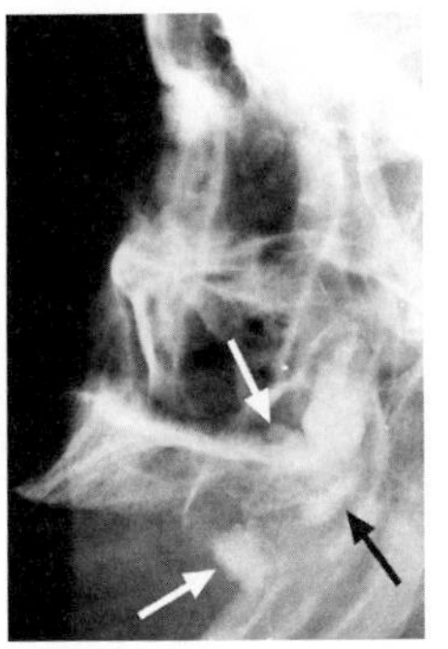
388 a

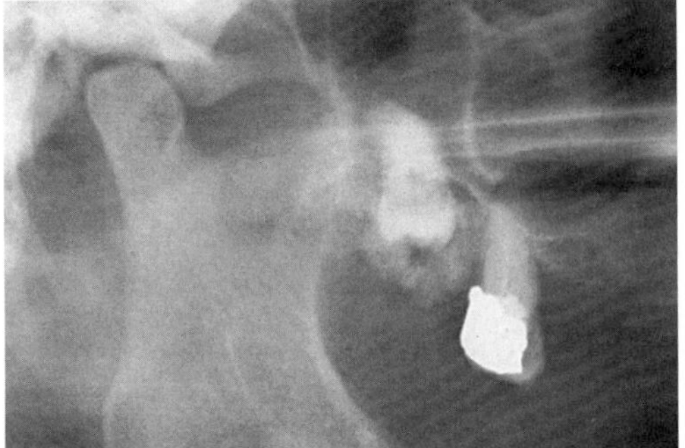
388 b

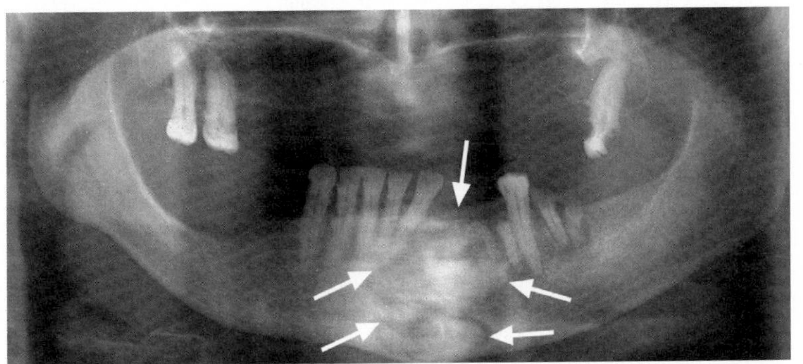
389

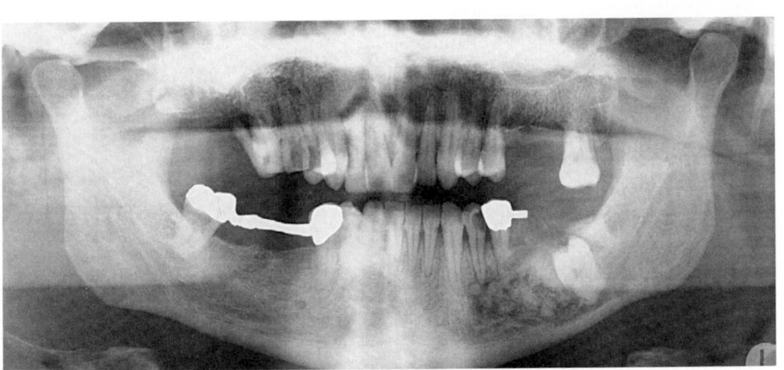
390

In radiographs, the ameloblastic fibrodentinoma appears as a mixed radiolucent and radiopaque lesion primarily detected in the mixed dentition stage of young boys.

Odontogenic Myxoma

The odontogenic myxoma develops from the ectomesenchyme. It occurs almost exclusively in the jaws, while the *skeletal* myxoma occurs only in the condylus.

The tumor grows relatively rapidly and is frequently detected in the mandible. Within the mandible, it is usually detected at the angle, within the ramus, and in the molar regions. Although this lesion is most frequently endosteal, it can also infiltrate the adjacent musculature. The lesion is usually well-demarcated but irregularly shaped and often exhibits weak radiopaque strands, and the compact bone of the mandible is distended and thinned. Rare transitions to myxosarcoma have been described. In order to achieve clear and precise depiction of the structures, it is recommended that the exposure settings be cut in half. Recurrence is relatively frequent, exhibiting small, round radiolucencies as well as wispy septa as characteristic signs of renewed and further expansion.

The age distribution spans a broad plateau including the tenth to fifth decade of life. Males and females are equally affected.

The differential diagnosis should include ameloblastoma and granulomatosis, and radiographic differentiation can be very difficult.

Calcifying Epithelial Odontogenic Tumor

This tumor derives from ectodermal cells and was first described by Pindborg (1958). It occurs primarily in the molar and premolar regions of the mandible, and less frequently in the tuberosity regions.

Radiographically it appears initially as a well-demarcated, cystoid radiolucency in which an impacted tooth is enclosed. In later stages, one observes expanding, calcified, or also spherical radiopacities. Expansive tumors often exhibit an irregular configuration and are poorly demarcated.

Fig. 391 Calcifying odontogenic cyst. The panoramic radiograph of a 13-year-old female reveals in the left mandible a sharply demarcated cystoid radiolucency that includes calcified radiopacities. Note also the displacement of the adjacent impacted teeth, and the supereruption of the left maxillary premolars and molars, as signs of a lesion that has existed for many years. The mandibular canal is also displaced.

Fig. 392a Calcifying odontogenic cyst. The periapical radiograph of a 9-year-old male reveals an expanded follicular sac around the rotated and tipped tooth 35. This is a very early stage of a calcifying odontogenic cyst, which cannot be identified as such at this stage radiographically.

Fig. 392b Calcifying odontogenic cyst. The periapical radiograph of a 15-year-old male reveals an already progressive calcifying odontogenic cyst. Above the crown of the encompassed tooth 35 one notes radiopacity, which can only be detected with reduced exposure settings. This is a typical picture of the initial stage of a calcifying odontogenic cyst.

Fig. 393 Adenomatoid odontogenic tumor. The panoramic radiograph of a 13-year-old female reveals the extrafollicular type of central adenomatoid odontogenic tumor. This lesion frequently mimics the existence of a nasoalveolar (globulomaxillary) nonodontogenic cyst, with displacement of the roots of teeth 22 and 23 and the balloon-like radiolucency (see p. **246**), or an odontogenic keratocyst (see p. **241**).

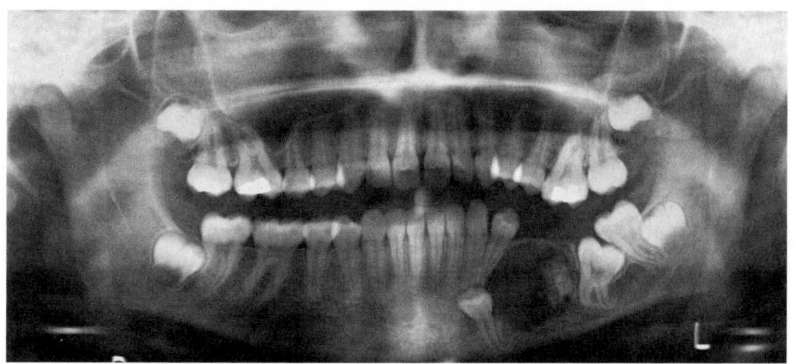

391

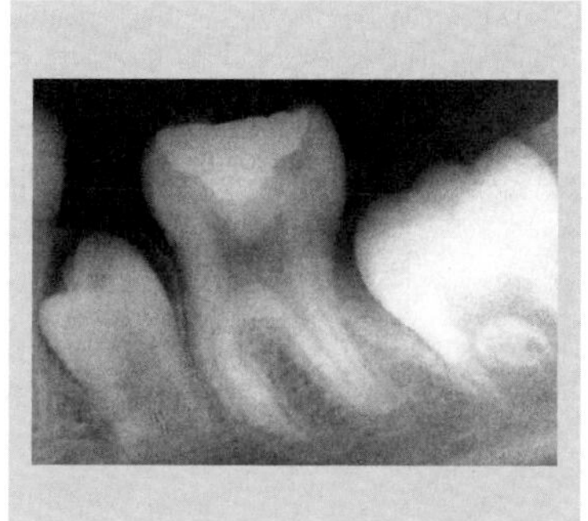

392 a

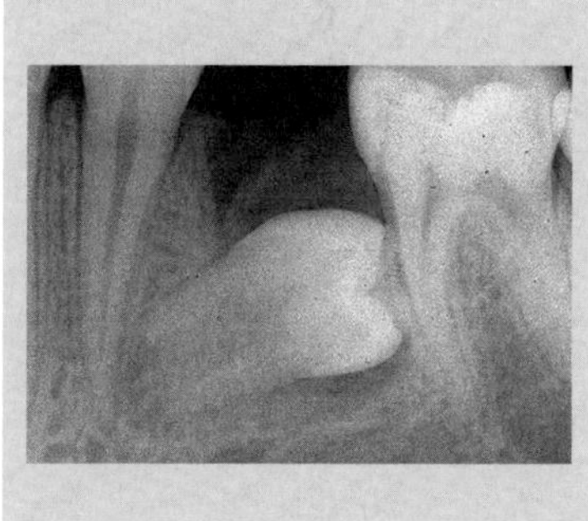

392 b

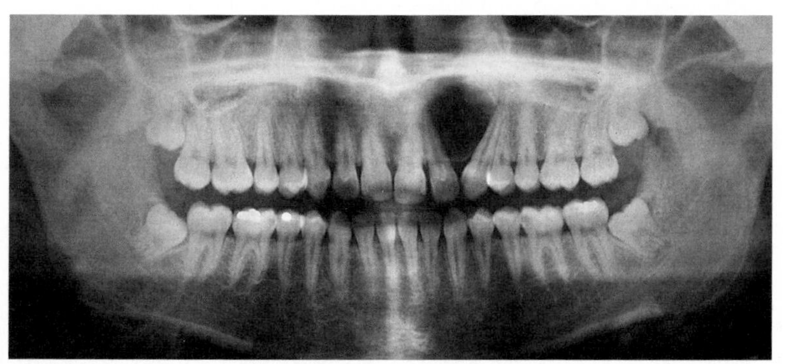

393

The compact bone and bordering lamellae of the maxilla are distended and thinned, and the mandibular canal is displaced.
This tumor can occur between ages 30 and 50. Recurrence is not infrequent many years later. Males and females are equally affected.
Depending upon the stage of development, the differential diagnosis should include ameloblastoma, ameloblastic fibroma, follicular cyst, or calcifying odontogenic cyst.

Calcifying Odontogenic Cyst

According to the WHO classification (Toida 1998), this lesion is an odontogenic cyst with epithelial lining.
This cyst may be localized in both the maxilla and the mandible. The cyst displaces and encompasses teeth, exhibits a sharp demarcation, and in later stages often exhibits calcified radiopacities of varying degree.
The cyst occurs primarily in the second decade of life.
The differential diagnosis must include the keratocyst, the ameloblastoma, and the calcifying odontogenic tumor.

Adenomatoid Odontogenic Tumor

This nomenclature derives from the publications of Philipsen and Birn (1969), Kuntz and Reichart (1986), and Philipsen and Reichart (1999). It is an extremely rare tumor.
This tumor is usually discovered centrally within the alveolar bone in the canine region of the maxilla and, less frequently, of the mandible. It is possible to distinguish between follicular types with an impacted tooth, and extrafollicular types without inclusion of a tooth.
The tumor usually occurs during the second decade of life. Females are much more often affected than males.
Because of its localization, the displacement of adjacent tooth roots and the resultant "inverted pear" shape, the differential diagnosis should include above all the nasoalveolar (globulomaxillary) cyst.

Fig. 394 a, b Compound odontoma. a The periapical radiograph of a partially luxated tooth 11 (caused by trauma) serendipitously reveals a half-moon-shaped radiolucency on the distal surface, including variously dense radiopacities. This is readily identified as a calcifying odontogenic cyst.
b Approximately 2 years later, a compound odontoma had developed, whose broad and circumscript zone of radiolucency is an indication that growth has not ceased. Note also the diastema, which is a clinical sign of expansion and growth of the odontoma.

Fig. 395 Compound odontoma. Small compound odontoma between teeth 32 and 33; the existence of this odontoma was suspected clinically because of the diastema.

Fig. 396 Compound odontoma. The panoramic radiograph of a 25-year-old male reveals a compound odontoma that has displaced tooth 35 almost to the level of the basal compact bone. This case demonstrates that clinical findings and routine periapical radiographs must often be enhanced by a panoramic view in order to glean a full overview perspective.

Fig. 397 Compound odontoma. The panoramic radiograph of a 19-year-old female exhibits in the region of the maxillary third molars, bilaterally, compound odontomas. On the right side, the odontoma is scarcely visible due to radiographic superimposition (**arrow**). A histologic examination of the odontoma on the left side revealed a conglomerate of fused dental elements; this is not an uncommon lesion in the maxilla of females.

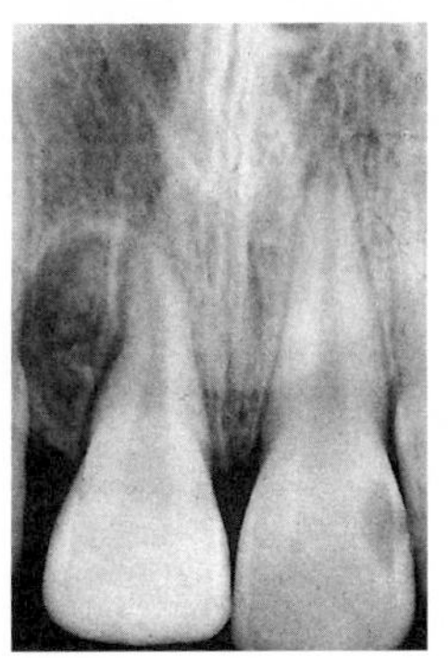

394 a

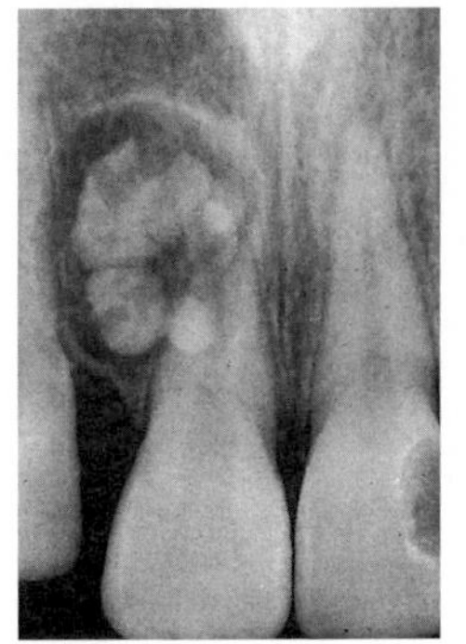

394 b

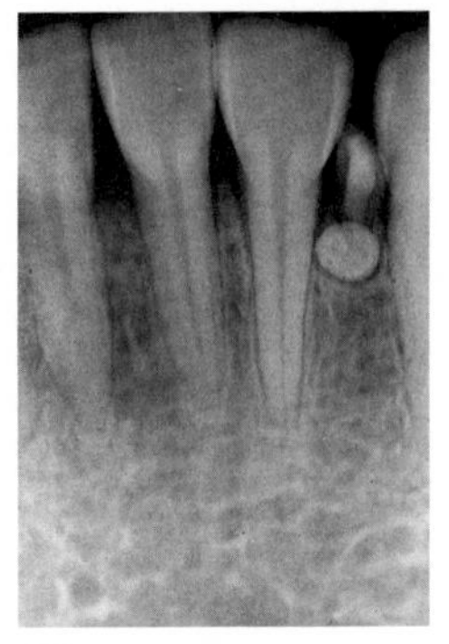

395

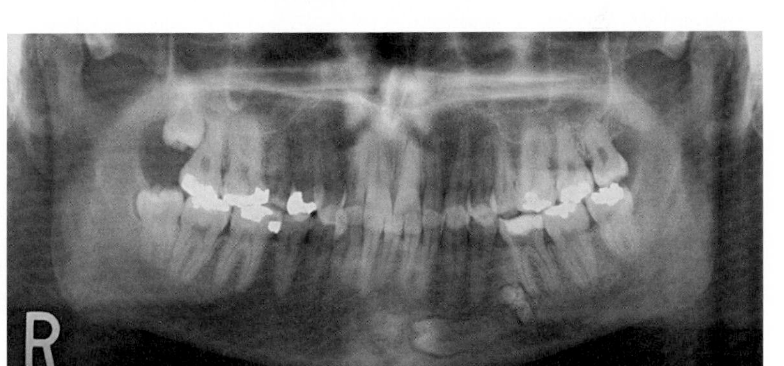

396

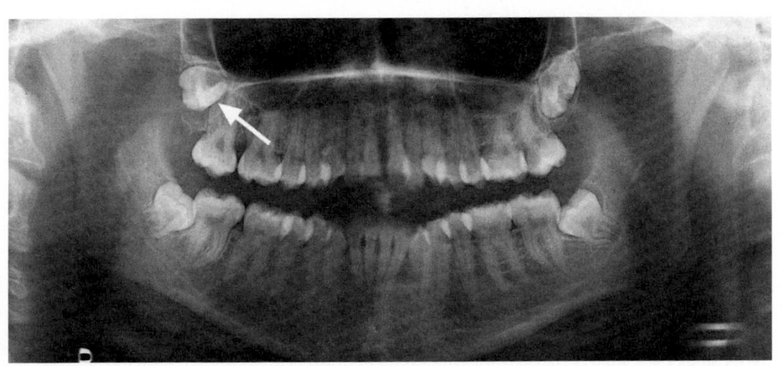

397

The **odontoma** is a developmentally induced, tumor-like malformation (**hamartoma**) of the dental lamella. Its growth is self-limiting. In a highly simplified classification, odontomas consist either of a number of more or less developed teeth, or a conglomerate of various dental tissues.

According to this classification, the lesions are termed either as *compound* or *complex* odontomas. They are most often observed in the place of a supernumerary tooth and also at the distal end of the dental arch. Depending upon the various stages of development, the radiographic signs will also vary, and are not always those typically characteristic of an odontoma.

Compound odontomas are found primarily in the anterior regions of the mandible and maxilla, and less frequently in the premolar regions. Much less frequently, they are observed in the third molar regions of both jaws. The fully developed teeth or numerous tooth fragments are quite easy to identify in a radiograph, usually near a completely developed tooth crown. Depending upon the stage of development, one observes early on a well-demarcated osteolysis, and later the slowly developing dental elements surrounded by a broad zone of radiolucency; the latter is a radiographic sign of the zone of growth. In the later stages, there remains only a narrow zone of radiolucency that is usually no longer well demarcated.

The compound odontoma develops during the second decade of life, and may be indicated clinically by the formation of diastemata or delayed tooth eruption. Females are much more often affected, especially in the maxillary molar region.

In the early developmental stages, one may also observe transparencies simulating keratocysts and paradental cysts. There is no differential diagnosis for completely developed compound odontomas.

Complex odontomas contain all of the basic elements of a tooth, but these exist as an amorphic mass.

The complex odontoma is most frequently observed at the angle of the mandible and in the area of the tuberosity. It is usually associated with a displaced or impacted third molar and is often difficult to discern in a radiograph due to the superimposition of the dense structures of the lesion.

Fig. 398 Complex odontoma. The panoramic radiograph of a 25-year-old female reveals a complex odontoma at the left mandibular angle; the tumor rests upon the impacted tooth 37 on compact bone. The irregular contour of the radiopacity is due to the partially formed and fused dental elements. The mandibular canal is almost completely displaced. A complex odontoma of this shape and size can often be differentiated from an ameloblastic fibro-odontoma only via histologic examination.

Fig. 399 Complex odontoma. The panoramic radiograph of a 14-year-old male reveals a complex odontoma at the right mandibular angle. It appears to rest upon or emanate from impacted tooth 47, which also appears to distend the basal compact bone. The well-demarcated, regular contour is an indication that the lesion consists of amorphic hard tissues of even density, in which no fully formed teeth are present.

Fig. 400 Complex odontoma. The panoramic radiograph of a 25-year-old male reveals a complex odontoma exhibiting small, "cloud-like" structures at the angle of the mandible on the left side. Such odontomas at the distal end of the dental arch in the mandible frequently "erupt" as the third molar erupts. The arrow indicates the position of the horizontally impacted tooth 38, whose crown is in intimate contact with the lesion. Note that the adjacent tooth, 37, has not been displaced. An additional, small odontoma is present mesial to tooth 28, which appears to have inhibited proper positioning of the third molar in the occlusal plane.

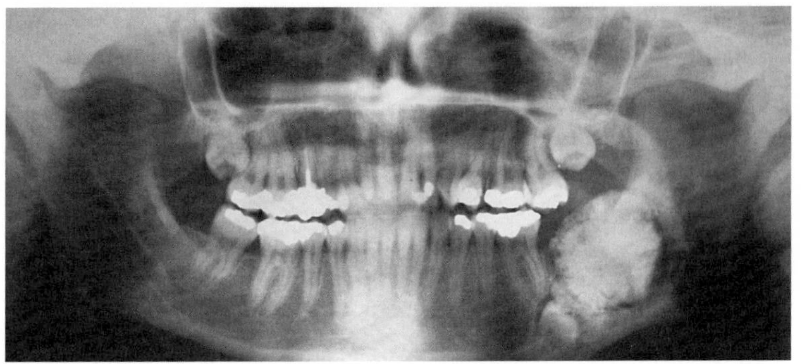

398

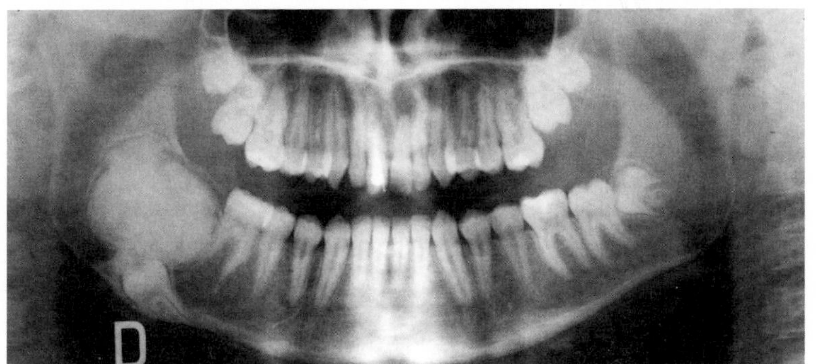

399

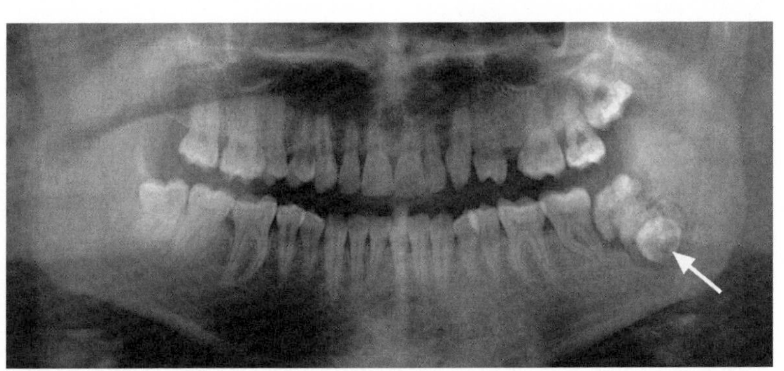

400

In addition to small, hazy radiopacities that appear to reside on the occlusal surface of a displaced molar, relatively large, spherical complex odontomas of homogeneous density are often observed surrounded by a narrow layer of well-demarcated radiolucency. Quite often, large complex odontomas are surrounded by a serrated marginal contour and a conspicuous, broad zone of radiolucency, which signals the ever-present continuing growth potential. Large complex odontomas often appear to contact the occlusal surface of a displaced molar via a peduncle. Particularly in males, there is often a tendency for such small dysplasias to "erupt," especially in the mandible. In contrast to the mandibular canal itself, the adjacent teeth are seldom displaced. Complex odontomas usually occur in the first and second decades of life, especially in females.

Radiographically, complex odontomas during stages of active growth are difficult to differentiate from the ameloblastic fibro-odontoma.

Cementum-Forming Dysplasias

According to the WHO classification of 1992, these lesions derive from the ectomesenchyme with odontogenic epithelial remnants. Included in this category are above all periapical cemental dysplasia and florid cemento-osseous dysplasia (Summerlin et al. 1994), as well as cementum-forming fibroma and the cementoblastoma.

Periapical cemental dysplasia: These lesions are most often found in the mandibular anterior region in females, but can also extend in some cases into the premolar regions.

Periapical cemental dysplasia exhibits various stages of development, and begins with a periapical fibrosis, which, as a radiolucency, may simulate chronic apical periodontitis; the latter can only be ruled out by means of a vitality test. During a second stage of development, one observes spotty depositions of cementum around the root apex; in the third stage, these coalesce to form complete radiopacities with contact to the root surface. An especially rare form of the lesion is referred to as **florid cemento-osseous dysplasia**, which is primarily observed in the black African population.

Fig. 401 a Periapical cemental dysplasia. This periapical radiograph of the mandibular anterior segment reveals periapical radiolucencies around the apices of clinically vital teeth 41, 31, and 32; note that the radiolucencies are not clearly demarcated. This is a case of periapical cemental dysplasia in the stage of osteolysis and fibrosis.

Fig. 401 b Periapical cemental dysplasia. During the second stage of development, spotty radiopacities are visible due to accumulation of cementum within the periapical radiolucencies.

Fig. 401 c Periapical cemental dysplasia. During the third stage of development, dense radiopacities can be observed periapically, and this is a sign of continuing growth, surrounded by a well-demarcated marginal radiolucency. The latter can no longer be detected in the final stages (around teeth 42 and 41). Teeth 31 and 32 exhibit this radiographic appearance following *erroneous* endodontic treatment and apicoectomy.

Fig. 402 Periapical cemental dysplasia. The panoramic radiograph of a 50-year-old female reveals multiple periapical cemental dysplasias on the anterior teeth of the mandible. This is the third stage of cementum deposition. Periapical cemental dysplasia occurs in middle-aged females, almost exclusively on the mandibular anterior teeth. Incorporation of the premolars is relatively rare.

Fig. 403 Florid cemento-osseous dysplasia. The panoramic radiograph of a 43-year-old female reveals a special variation of florid cemento-osseous dysplasia. This lesion is observed primarily in females of black-African descent, occurring as multiple lesions in the jaws, with relatively large and well-demarcated periapical alterations, depending upon the stage of development, and a clear radiopacity with embedded cementicles.

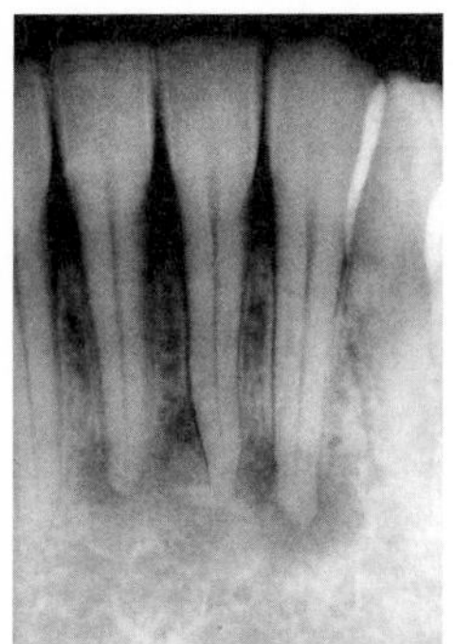

401 a

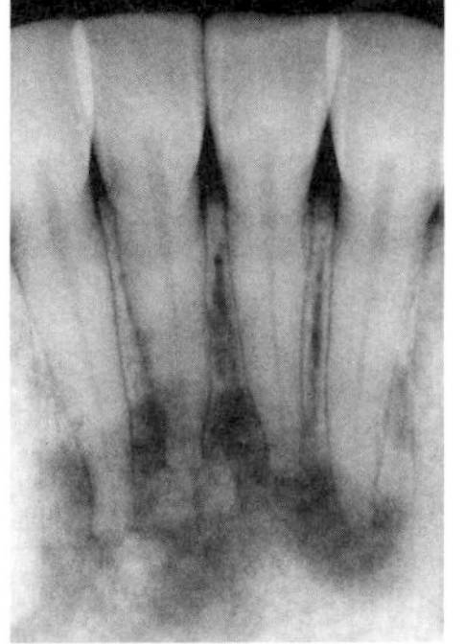

401 b

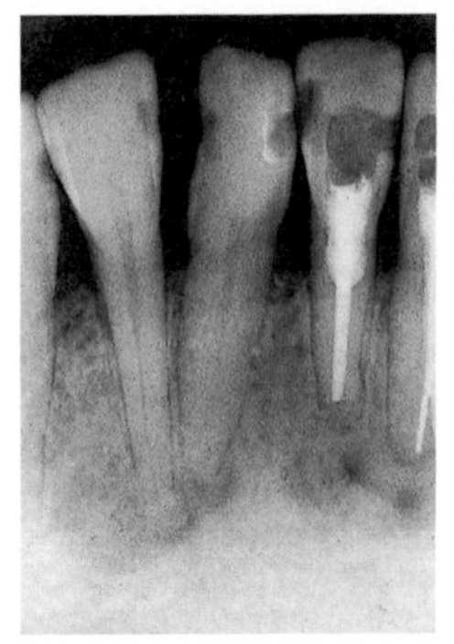

401 c

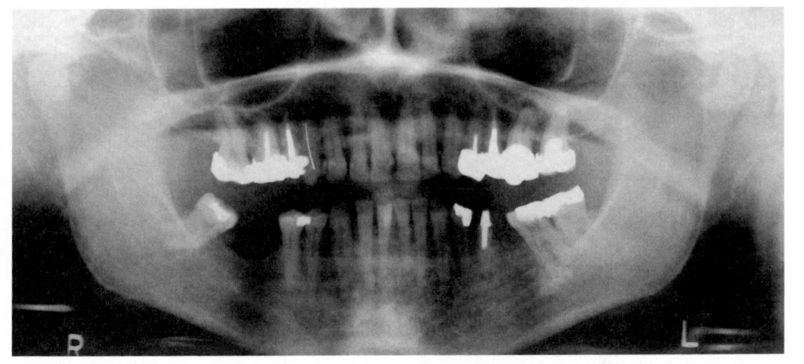

402

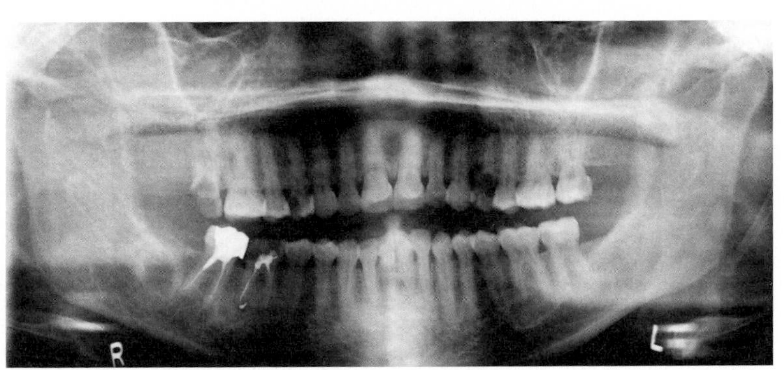

403

Because the affected teeth remain vital, periapical cemental dysplasia is almost always discovered quite late. The age peak is within the fourth decade of life. Females are almost exclusively affected.
The differential diagnosis should include apical periodontal pathology as well as cementoblastoma.

Cementoblastoma

This benign odontogenic tumor develops through deposition of cementum-like hard tissue. A nonmineralized growth zone appears as a radiolucency surrounding or traversing the radiopacity.
Cementoblastoma is primarily observed in the premolar and molar regions of the mandible. The hard tissue lesions are attached to the root(s) of the affected teeth; this renders extraction of such teeth very difficult or even impossible. In the initial stages, a difficult to differentiate periapical radiolucency may be noticed in the radiograph. Subsequent deposition of new cementum leads slowly to increasing radiopacity, which is easy to discern within the nonmineralized, spotty, or strand-like radiolucencies that surround the tumor in the growth zone. The roots of the affected teeth are only seldom resorbed but may give the impression of root resorption in the radiograph because of superimposition. It is easy to differentiate the approximately cherry-sized, dense cementoblastoma that is clearly surrounded by a zone of radiolucency from gigantiform depositions that are rich with spots or strands in the growth zones. Larger cementoblastomas lead to thinning of the compact bone and distention. The mandibular canal is impinged upon.
Cementoblastomas occur most frequently in the second decade of life and sometimes also in the third. They are more frequently observed in males.
The differential diagnosis should include calcifying epithelial odontogenic tumor as well as ossifying fibroma.

Fig. 404 Cementoblastoma. This panoramic radiograph of a 41-year-old man clearly reveals an evenly dense cementoblastoma at tooth 44. From the radiographic appearance alone it is not possible to discern whether the broad surrounding zone of radiolucency is a sign of continuing tumor growth or whether the infection emanating from the nonvital tooth 46 has elicited sequester formation.

Fig. 405 Cementoblastoma. The panoramic radiograph of a 24-year-old male reveals a benign cementoblastoma between the roots of tooth 36. The spotty radiopacities surrounded by a visible and radiolucent boundary are difficult to visualize. The apical regions of the roots are rendered virtually invisible because of the cementum deposition, as a result of the summation effect; the visual appearance is similar to that of root resorption.

Fig. 406 a, b Cementoblastoma. a This section from a panoramic radiograph of a 19-year-old male reveals a gigantiform benign cementoblastoma emanating from tooth 46. Note the obvious displacement of the mandibular canal and the adjacent teeth. Visible are the irregular radiopacities resulting from cementum deposition, and the radiolucent, nonmineralized intervening lines. The summation effect of the roentgen rays leads to superimposition of the tooth roots, and possible resorption of the distal root. **b** This unilateral occlusal radiograph was taken in a dental practice using reduced exposure settings (see Fig. **90** and Fig. **94**). Even without the use of CT, the radiograph reveals that the lesion has penetrated through the lingual compact bone.

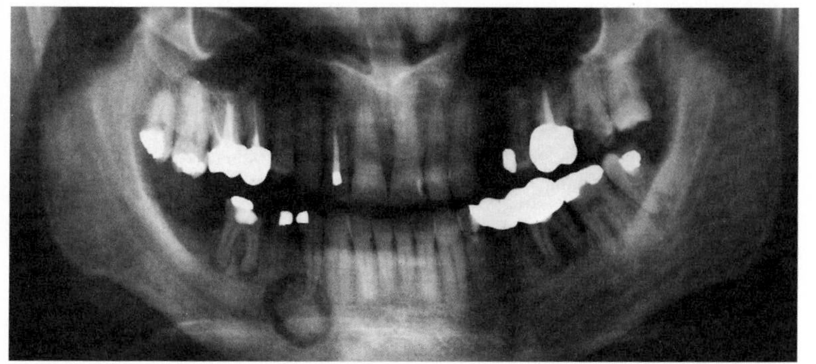

404

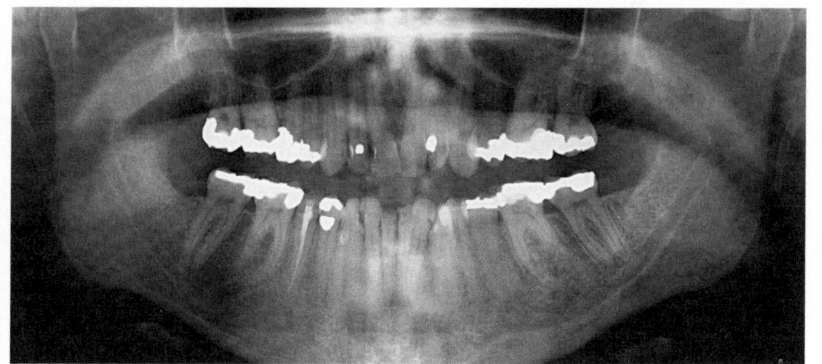

405

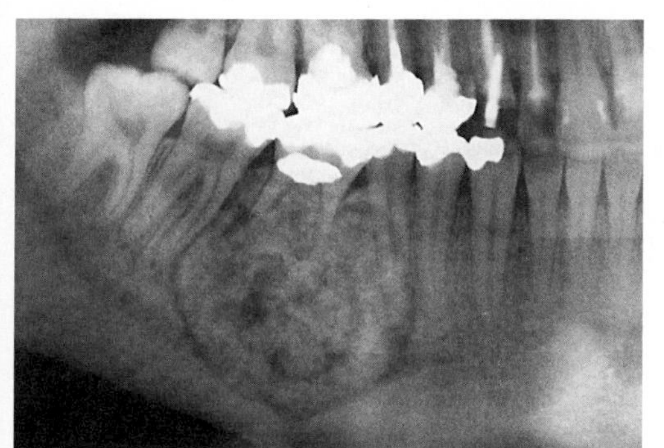

406 a

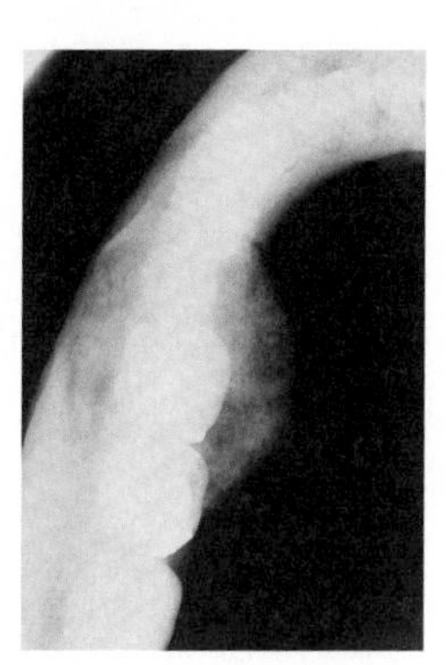

406 b

In this chapter, we will summarize several nonodontogenic pathologic alterations and anomalies, lesions that would not have been possible to observe in a dental practice in earlier times. The modern possibilities in the area of radiographic diagnosis, and the demands of our profession in oral health, permit and demand a comprehensive examination that will guarantee for the patient, but also for all dentists, the highest degree of confidence in the diagnosis.

As a consequence, one of the most important duties in the dental profession is to critically observe the dentition and jaw development in children and young adults using appropriate examination methods, and to regularly assess the condition of the jaws and teeth in adult patients. This can only be effectively accomplished using panoramic radiography, and *not* simply with the routine periapical radiographic survey because intraoral IR do not provide complete coverage of the jaws. The dose for a status with 20 intraoral radiographs is equivalent to the dose of four panoramic radiographs. Using today's modern technology, the radiation exposure for a targeted and comprehensive radiographic examination is so low that routine examination can easily be justified. Any additional, significant reduction of radiation exposure is not likely to occur solely through further development of high technology, but more likely through improvement of exposure technique involving the use of a well-considered, radiation-sparing examination strategy in order to avoid unnecessary or inappropriate ionizing radiation to the patient.

However, because overviews such as the panoramic radiograph may in some cases have to be followed by supplemental radiographic diagnostic examination procedures (even the panoramic overview provides only a two-dimensional representation complicated by system-related summation effects), additional targeted examinations may need to be referred to a specialist clinic or a radiographic institute in order to substantiate or rule out clinical findings or preliminary differential diagnoses.

Fig. 407 Fibrous dysplasia. In this 6-year-old female, the panoramic radiograph was centered on the maxilla, and revealed an expansive radiopacity in the left maxillary sinus, with impingement upon the lateral wall of the nasal cavity and deviation of the nasal septum. Note also the displacement of teeth 23–26 due to distention of the maxilla.

Fig. 408 a, b Fibrous dysplasia. a The posteroanterior Waters projection of the same case reveals again the distention of the left maxilla by the dysplastic bone. Within the hazy radiopacity, it is virtually impossible to discern the corticalized covering lamella of the maxilla, the lateral wall of the nasal cavity, and the narrowed maxillary sinus. The osseous sutures of the midface are, however, not traversed by the lesion. **b** The maxillary occlusal radiograph of the same case clearly shows the orange peel-like structure of the dysplastic bone, which in this advanced stage of the disease consists of connective tissue with osseous islands. Here also one can observe that while the osseous sutures appear compressed, they are not traversed by the lesion.

Fig. 409 Fibrous dysplasia. This panoramic radiograph of a 30-year-old male reveals the late stage of fibrous dysplasia. Noteworthy is that the symphysis of the mandible that is present even in neonates has no influence upon the expansion of the fibrous dysplasia beyond the midline of the mandible.

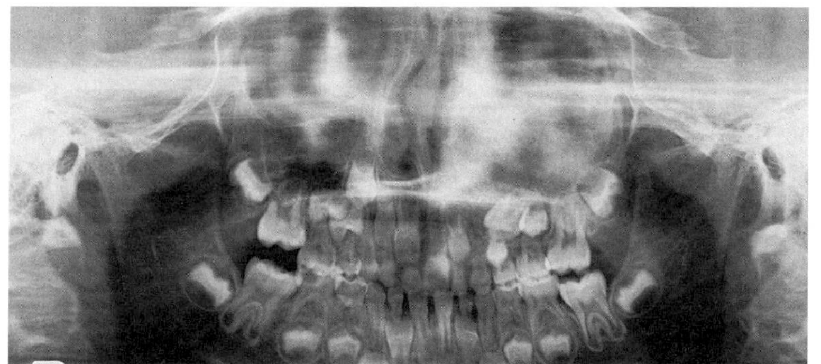

407

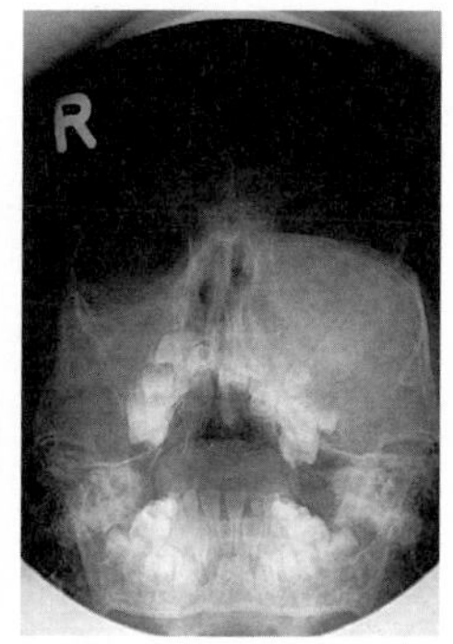

408 a

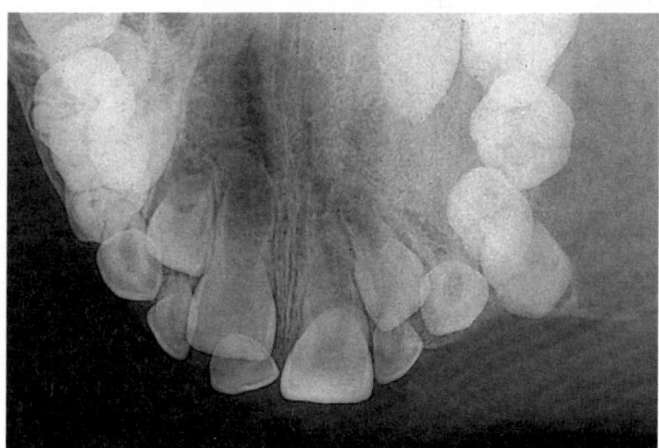

408 b

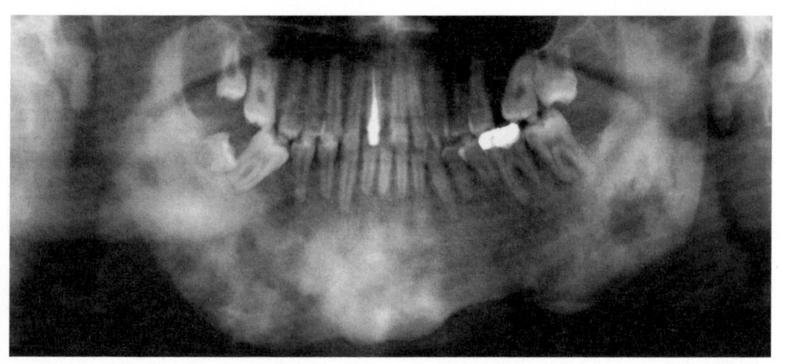

409

Fibrous dysplasia (Jaffé–Lichtenstein–Uehlinger) is a tumor-like lesion that occurs in the jaws usually in the monostotic form and exhibits relationships to other fibroblastic osseous disorders, such as the ossifying fibroma. The clinical course of fibrous dysplasia is essentially asymptomatic and is often only noted because of obvious facial asymmetries. Normal bone is replaced by fiber-rich and cell-poor connective tissue in which irregularly distributed islands of metaplastic bone are embedded. The disease is self-limiting, and usually ends after puberty. However, the osseous alterations can maintain their activity over decades, and can be discerned using radionuclide imaging. End products of fibrous dysplasia often persist throughout life in the form of cancellous or compact osteomas, which can present diagnostic difficulties.

Fibrous dysplasia that occurs in the maxilla and mandible exhibits radiographic differences vis-à-vis the pseudocystic lesions that are observed in the skeleton. It begins with a poorly demarcated radiolucency caused by fibrosis, and with further progression one may observe distention of bone with irregular transitions to healthy tissue, and hazy radiopacities with a superficial orange peel appearance. Within the distended bone, anatomic structures and bordering lamella are displaced and rendered invisible radiographically by progressive fibrosis. Osseous boundaries in the maxilla, for example the median suture, are not crossed. Late-stage lesions in the maxilla and the mandible are characterized by differing radiographic appearances. While in the maxilla a radiopacity compromising the maxillary sinus (osteoma) is often observed, in the mandible one often notes spotty, roundish radiopacities that cross over the midline; the latter can often be observed in the later stages of oligo- or polyostotic fibrotic forms of the disease. Depending upon the time of onset of the disease, displaced or otherwise malpositioned teeth may be in evidence clinically.

Fig. 410 a, b Peripheral giant cell granuloma. a The periapical radiograph of a 38-year-old female reveals a cuff-shaped radiolucency at the entrance to the alveolus of clinically vital tooth 12. A clinically diagnosable hyperplasia (epulis) proceeded along the periodontium toward the root apex.
b This section from a panoramic radiograph reveals the cup-shaped osseous defect around tooth 12. The differential diagnosis would include involutive periodontal recession.

Fig. 411 a, b Central giant cell granuloma. a The periapical radiograph of the mandibular anterior segment reveals an expansive multilocular radiolucency in the body of the mandible, with a scalloped border along the cortical bone. **b** An occlusal radiograph of the mandible reveals the expanse of the lesion and the thinning of the lingual compact bone in the third dimension. This benign giant cell granuloma can be differentiated from an aggressive giant cell tumor only by serologic tests.

Fig. 412 Central giant cell granuloma. This panoramic radiograph of a 21-year-old male was centered on the mandible, and reveals a huge and sharply demarcated radiopacity traversed by strand-like radiolucencies and a scalloped basal boundary. The large lesion was expanding in the direction of the alveolar ridge, leading to displacement/divergence of the adjacent teeth and total impaction of tooth 43. The basal compact bone was distended.

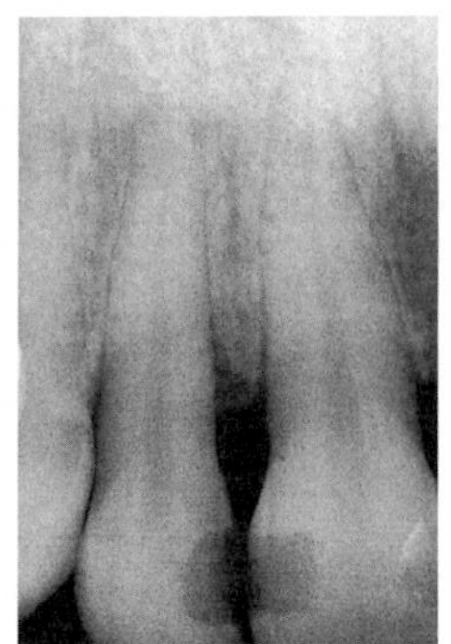

410 a

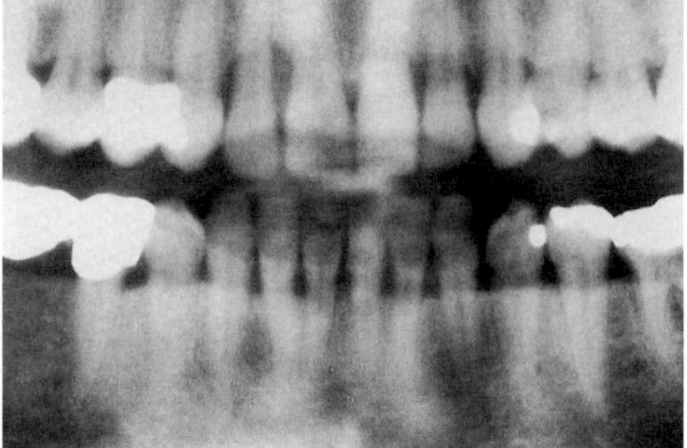

410 b

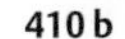

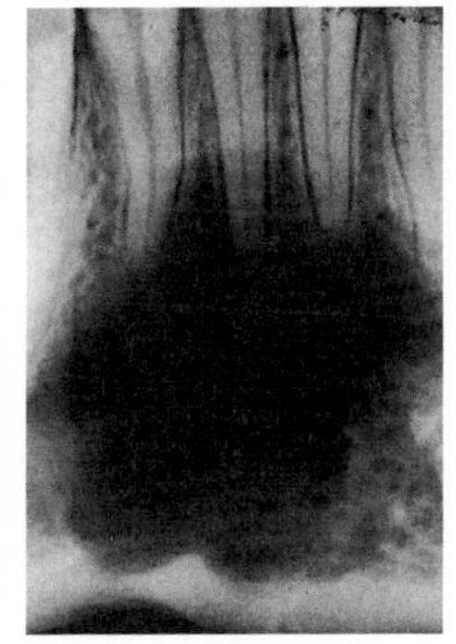

411 a

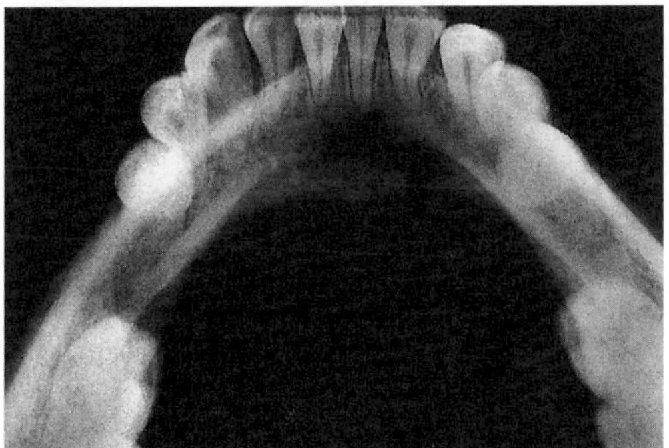

411 b

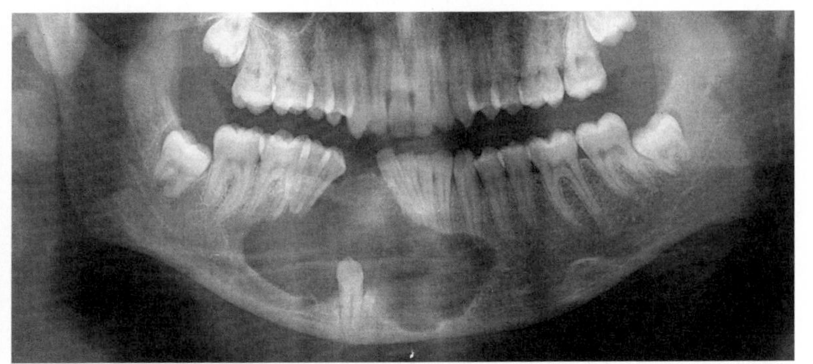

412

The lamina dura, which is normally quite easy to visualize on a two-dimensional radiograph because of the tangential effects of the roentgen rays, is often no longer apparent due to progressive osseous fibrosis; the roots of adjacent teeth may appear to be undergoing resorption.

Especially in females, fibrous dysplasia may occur in early childhood. It tends to regress spontaneously during puberty, and is only seldom observed after puberty, and then only as the radiographic sequelae.

The radiographic differential diagnosis should include particularly the fibroblastic diseases of bone as well as hyperparathyroidism (Recklinghausen disease).

Malignant transformation is exceedingly rare.

Peripheral and Central Giant Cell Granuloma

This tumor-like, benign giant cell granuloma may occur peripherally or centrally.

Because of its frequent localization at the entrance to the alveolus, the peripheral form is referred to clinically as an **epulis**. The lesion is encountered clinically as an exophytic lesion at the entrance to the alveolae of anterior teeth, and frequently in the mandible of females in the third to fifth decades of life; it may progress and invade aggressively, and may appear as a recurrence with initial cup-shaped lesions and isolated invasion of the alveolar bone.

The central giant cell granuloma is observed intraosseously, and also generally occurs in the mandible; radiographically it exhibits single and multi-chambered radiolucencies that not infrequently appear to invade toward the basal compact bone, forming a scalloped border. Distension of the bone with thinning of the compact bone, as well as displacement of adjacent teeth and root resorptions have been described.

The lesions occur most often in females in the second to fourth decade of life.

The radiographic differential diagnosis can be difficult vis-à-vis ameloblastoma, odontogenic cyst, aneurysmatic pseudocyst, and the “brown tumor” of hyperparathyroidism.

Fig. 413a Eosinophilic granuloma. This section from a panoramic radiograph of a 17-year-old male reveals an eosinophilic granuloma from the category of Langerhans-cell granulomatosis. Around the clinically vital but severely mobile teeth 48, 47, and 46, one observes radiolucencies in which the teeth appear to “hang.” In contrast to typical aggressive periodontitis, the dissolution of osseous structures begins in the apical region of the alveolar ridge.

Fig. 413b Eosinophilic granuloma. The lateral overview skull projection of an 11-year-old male reveals the typical radiographic signs of a “punched-out” lesion at the top of the skull. In advanced cases, numerous confluent defects present the typical “geographic skull” appearance.

Fig. 414a, b Eosinophilic granuloma. a The posterior periapical radiograph of a 30-year-old male reveals the pathognomonic sign of a tooth “suspended” within a radiolucency in the right molar region. When areas of osteolysis become confluent, there is often the appearance of a scalloped border at the basal aspect of the lesion, and this is accompanied by a sclerosing osseous border. **b** The premolar region of the left maxilla reveals an intra-alveolar dissolution of osseous septa and an arcuate boundary between teeth 24 and 25.

Fig. 415 Eosinophilic granuloma. The panoramic radiograph of a 66-year-old male reveals an eosinophilic granuloma in the mandibular anterior region. The severely tipped teeth appear to “swim” freely within the radiolucency. Note also the scalloped basal border with reactive sclerosis.

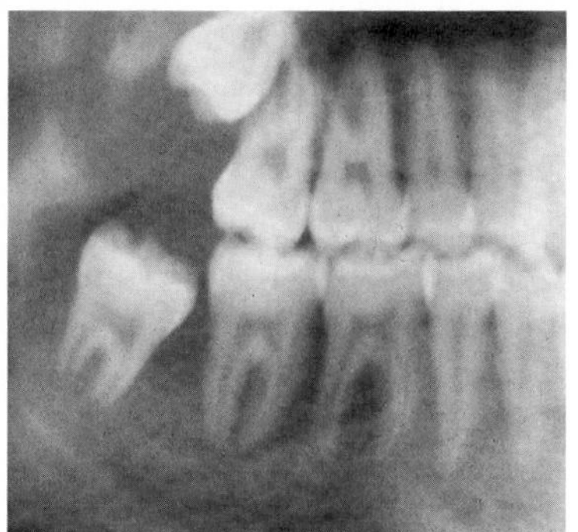
413 a

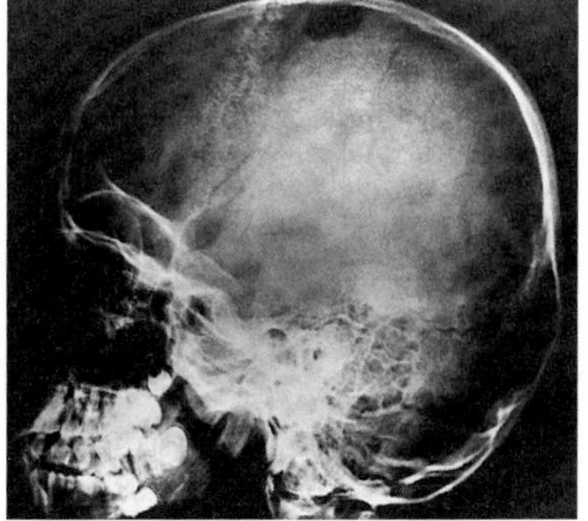
413 b

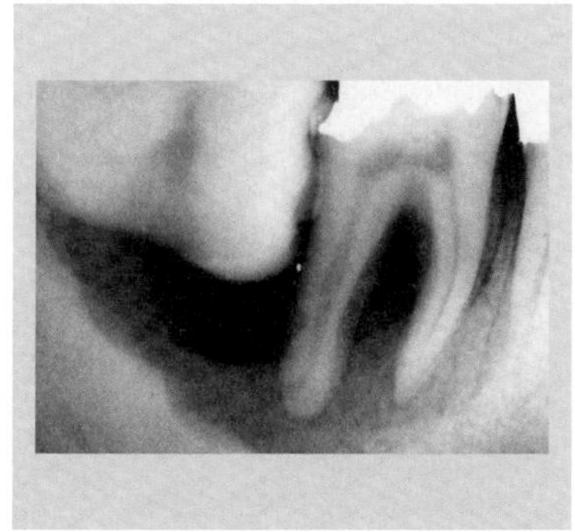
414 a

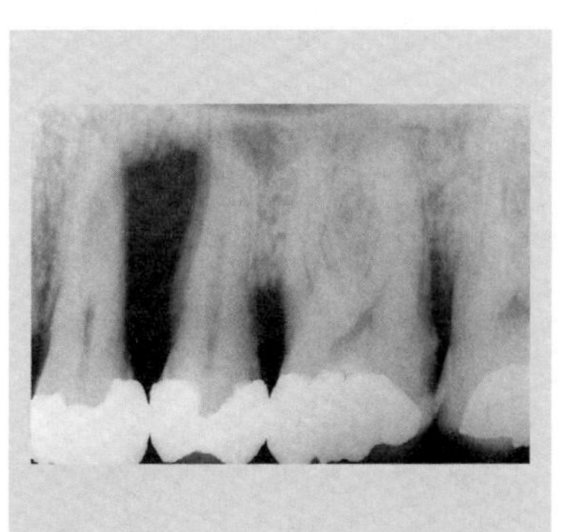
414 b

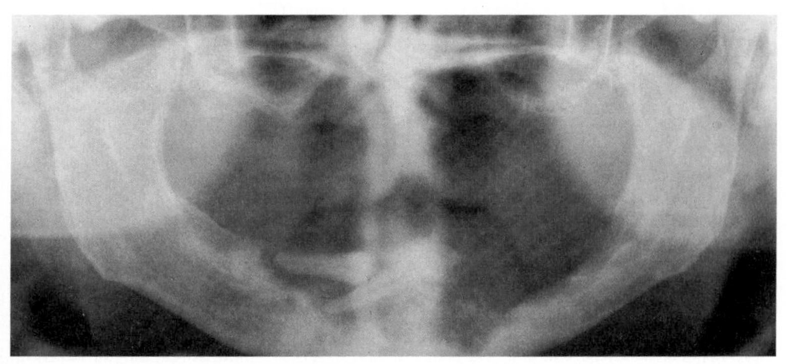
415

The **osteoclastoma** (giant cell myeloma) is a rapidly growing giant cell tumor, which is exceptionally rare.

Eosinophilic Granuloma (Langerhans-Cell Granulomatosis, Histiocytosis X)

This disease is of unknown etiology and pathogenesis, and results from the proliferation of Langerhans cells, histiocytes, macrophages, and bone marrow cells; the categorization includes three overlapping pathologic manifestations:

- The disseminated form of Abt–Letterer–Siwe syndrome, which occurs in infancy and progresses continuously
- The Hand–Schüller–Christian syndrome, which affects older children and adolescents in its disseminated form
- The mildest form, eosinophilic granuloma, is most commonly found in the jaws of adolescents, but can also affect older individuals

The eosinophilic granuloma may occur as solitary or multiple lesions in the jaws, and the ribs or flat bones such as the cranial roof may also be affected. The mandible is more often involved than the maxilla.

Radiographically, the lesion exhibits poorly demarcated and hazy areas of osteolysis; these areas may become confluent and form a scalloped border of reactive sclerosis. The eosinophilic granuloma begins at the depth of the alveolar process, destroys the interdental osseous septa, and expands over several teeth, which loose their lamina dura and appear to "hang" within the radiolucency. The eosinophilic granuloma affects primarily males. The lesion is encountered most frequently in the second decade of life, but can also be observed in men of much higher age. Following extraction of the affected teeth, spontaneous healing occurs with loss of alveolar ridge height.

Solitary and Aneurysmatic Bone Cysts

The pathogenesis of these cystoid lesions that do *not* derive from epithelium has not been completely explained or clarified; therefore, it has often been described as a pseudocyst within bone. There have been suggestions that the etiology involves disturbances of spontaneous healing of giant cell granulomas or ossifying fibromas during childhood.

Fig. 416 Solitary bone cyst. The panoramic radiograph of a 9-year-old female reveals a solitary bone cyst in the left mandible. The cystoid radiolucency is described as a pseudocyst because it does not exhibit the epithelial lining that is present in true cysts. The teeth remain clinically vital and are not displaced. The compact bone is distended and thinned. The cystic cavity, characterized on the radiograph as a cystoid radiolucency, appears to be empty.

Fig. 417 Solitary bone cyst. This section from a panoramic radiograph of a 7-year-old female reveals a solitary bone cyst in the left mandibular ramus.

Fig. 418a Aneurysmatic bone cyst. The unilateral occlusal radiograph (same case as in the following panoramic radiograph) reveals an aneurysmatic bone cyst in the right mandible of a 15-year-old female. Clearly visible is the thinning and distention of the buccal and lingual bony compact plates. Note especially the image quality: The teeth are depicted axially in the third dimension.

Fig. 418b Aneurysmatic bone cyst. Same case as in Figure **418a**. The panoramic radiograph reveals that the apices of the mandibular right posterior teeth are still surrounded by their periodontal ligament space (lamina dura) and alveolar bone. The panoramic radiograph reveals only the two-dimensional expanse of the lesion within the body of the mandible, with thinning and distention of the compact bone. In terms of a differential diagnosis, this lesion is difficult to distinguish from a central giant cell granuloma.

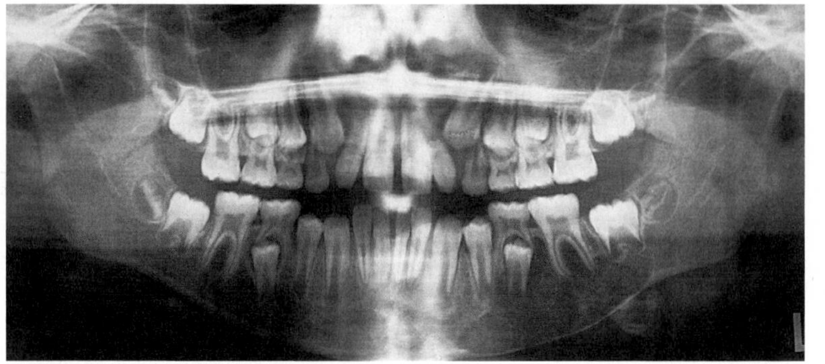

416

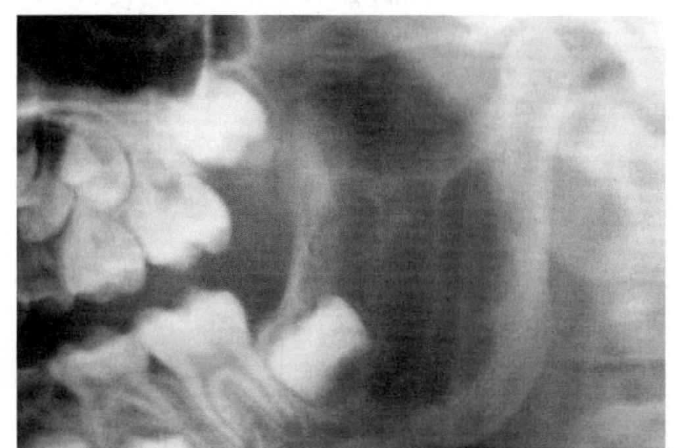

417

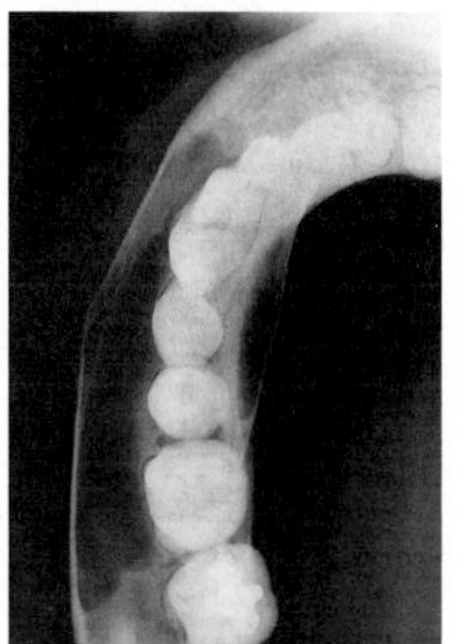

418 a

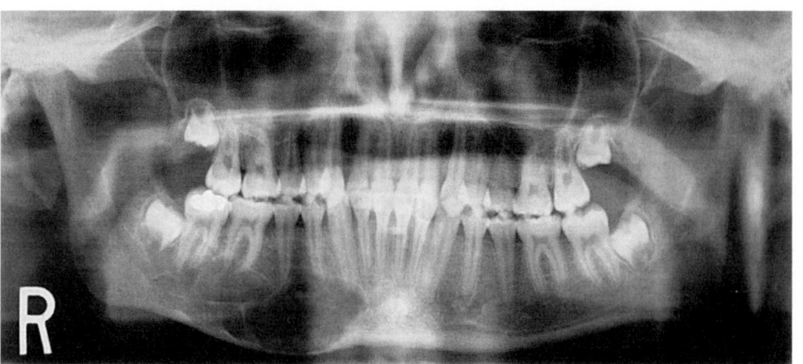

418 b

It is well known that bone resorption often occurs following injury-induced bone marrow hemorrhage, and that this leads to intraosseous cavity formation that is generally referred to as a "traumatic bone cyst"; however, these types of cavities are not lined by epithelium.

Solitary bone cysts are most frequently observed in the mandible of male children and adolescents. Following trauma, such cysts are frequently encountered in the region of the mandibular anterior teeth, which remain vital but which may eventually be displaced by growth of the lesion. Such lesions can also be found in the premolar and molar regions. The radiographic demarcation is not always as clear as that exhibited by true, symptom-free cysts; the basal compact bone may be thinned and distended. Solitary bone cysts virtually always present as single-chambered entities.

The differential diagnosis should include central giant cell granuloma, a single-chambered ameloblastoma, or a hemangioma, depending upon the shape.

The aneurysmatic bone cyst is a highly vascularized cavity filled with cavernous spaces or osteoid structures.

In the radiograph, an aneurysmatic bone cyst exhibits a scalloped border and a polycystic form traversed by irregular and expansively arranged septa. The basal compact bone is occasionally distended and thinned. The contents of an aneurysmatic bone cyst create faint radiopacities in underexposed images.

The pseudocysts are encountered almost exclusively in the mandible.

There is no gender preference for these lesions. The differential diagnosis should include central giant cell granuloma, odontogenic myxoma, mucoepidermoid tumor, or multilocular ameloblastoma.

Stafne Cyst (Latent Bone Cavity)

The cystoid radiolucency corresponding to an osseous defect exclusively in the mandible was first described by Stafne in 1942. This is a defect of embryonic origin, which is not always correctly projected in periapical radiographs of the molar region of the mandible; in a panoramic radiograph, however, it is always seen below the mandibular canal and may, in rare situations, be observed mesial to the mental foramen (Friedmann 1964, Stene and Pedersen 1977, Eversole 1978). Especially in a panoramic radiograph, the lingual depression (submandibular fovea) provides a well-demarcated radiolucency due to the elevated radiographic permeability of the bone, and the subtraction effect depicts the cystoid radiolucency. Depending upon whether the depression is expansive or only cranially located and covered by an osseous lamella, the lesion will appear to be located completely lingually or only partially so in the region of the basal compact bone.

Fig. 419 Stafne cyst (latent osseous cavity). The panoramic radiograph reveals a cystoid radiolucency in the right angle of the mandible below the mandibular canal. In addition, due to the tangential effect of the roentgen rays, the fovea in the lingual aspect of the body of the mandible appears cystoid. This was a serendipitous finding in a 41-year-old male.

Fig. 420a Stafne cyst (latent osseous cavity). The periapical radiograph reveals a well-demarcated cavity on the inferior border of the body of the mandible, and appears to be open caudally. Clearly evident is the lining with an osseous lamella.

Fig. 420b Stafne cyst (latent osseous cavity). This section from a panoramic radiograph of a 4-year-old male reveals a Stafne cyst at the left mandibular angle (see also Fig. **224**).

Fig. 421 Stafne cyst (latent osseous cavity). The panoramic radiograph of a 59-year-old male reveals, as a serendipitous finding in the right angle of the mandible, a cyst-like structure. Note also the compensatory sclerosed alveolar ridge in the right mandible, and the abnormal shape of the semilunar incisive.

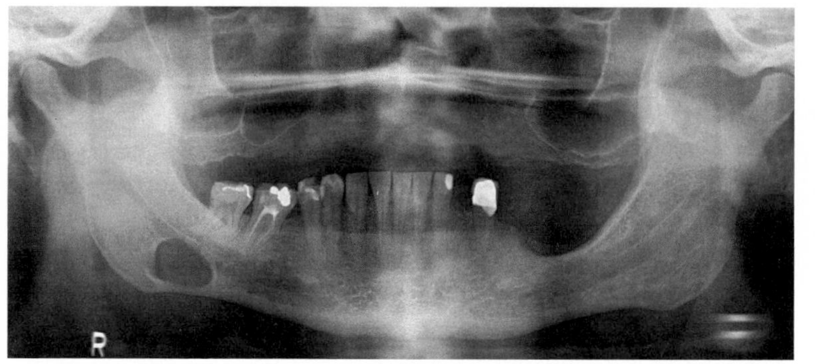

419

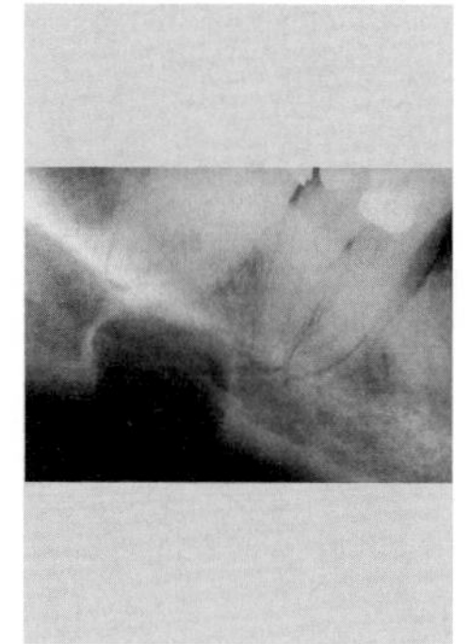

420 a

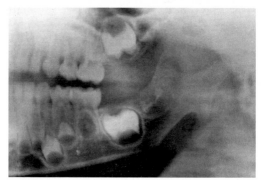

420 b

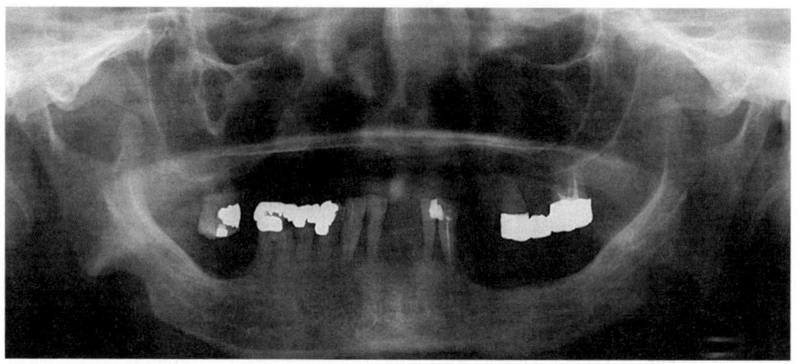

421

Chondroma, Osteochondroma

Chondroma of the jaws is rare and usually benign if only mature cartilage cells are present; however, the lesion in certain localizations, for example, in the region of the premaxilla, does have a tendency toward malignant transformation. One differentiates between the enchondroma, located centrally in the bone, and the periosteal (peripheral) chondroma.

A solitary chondroma may develop in regions where cartilage cells are present from the embryologic developmental stage. Chondroma and osteochondroma are rare in the region of the embryonic symphysis of the mandible, but more common in the region of the embryonic premaxilla and the median suture as well as the joint surfaces of the condyles. The radiographic picture of a chondroma is most often a well-demarcated radiolucency. Osteochondromas, on the other hand, exhibit within their radiolucency calcified radiopacities that appear as round calcification centers, especially in the region of the embryonic premaxilla. In this localization, a panoramic radiograph will reveal scarcely more than an unclear, poorly demarcated, and virtually indefinable radiopacity. To corroborate the initial radiographic findings, an occlusal radiograph of the maxilla can be taken in the dental office, or the patient may need to be referred for examination using computed tomography (CT). More frequently, the head of the mandible contains osseous cartilaginous exostoses (osteochondroma) of widely varying sizes. In individual cases this may lead to obvious facial asymmetries and functional disturbances. These lesions are frequently irregularly shaped and plump, with a radiographic picture of adjacent areas of radiolucency and radiopacity. The joint cavity and the articular tubercle (articular eminence) appear flattened.

Chondroma and osteochondroma grow asymptomatically; they are benign tumors that are usually first detected in middle-aged individuals. While the osteochondroma of the maxilla, a facultative malignant tumor, is most often detected in males, the rare gigantiform osteochondroma of the condyle is most frequently observed in females.

A true differential diagnosis for a suspected malignant chondrosarcoma of the maxilla can only be developed histologically.

Fig. 422a, b Chondroma, osteochondroma. a The occlusal radiograph of the maxilla of a 42-year-old female reveals an expansive enchondroma on the roof of the palate. The tumor is well-demarcated against the alveolar process. Within the tumor, one observes within the radiolucency fine, irregular and net-like trabeculi with spotty and round calcification centers. In this localization, the chondroma is a facultative malignant tumor that is difficult to differentiate radiographically from the various forms of the benign chondroma. **b** This section from a panoramic radiograph of the same case, with the patient intentionally positioned closer to the image receptor in order to provide clearer vision through the premaxilla, reveals only a clear but indefinable radiopacity.

Fig. 423 Osteochondroma of the condyle. This panoramic radiograph of a 27-year-old female reveals in the right mandibular condyle, ventrally, an osteochondroma exhibiting spotty radiolucencies. One should compare the different positions of the condyle during mouth opening, and note also the small chondroma on the compact bone beneath tooth 31. The arrow indicates a subtraction effect caused by superimposition of the left condyle upon the external auditory meatus.

Fig. 424 Osteochondroma of the condyle. The panoramic radiograph of a 35-year-old female reveals a gigantiform osteochondroma on the left mandibular condyle. This had led to corresponding functional disturbances and massive facial asymmetry.

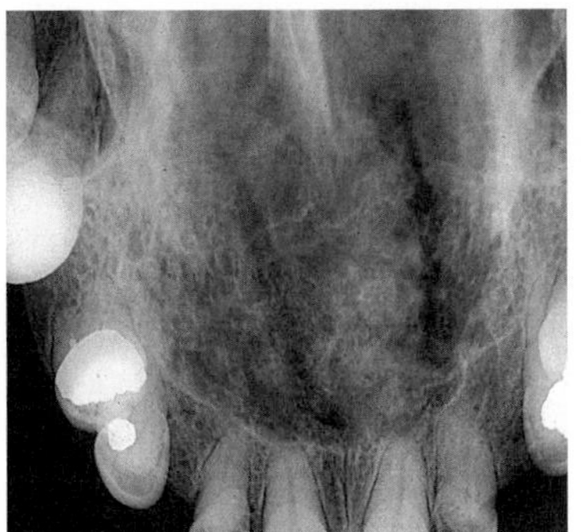
422 a

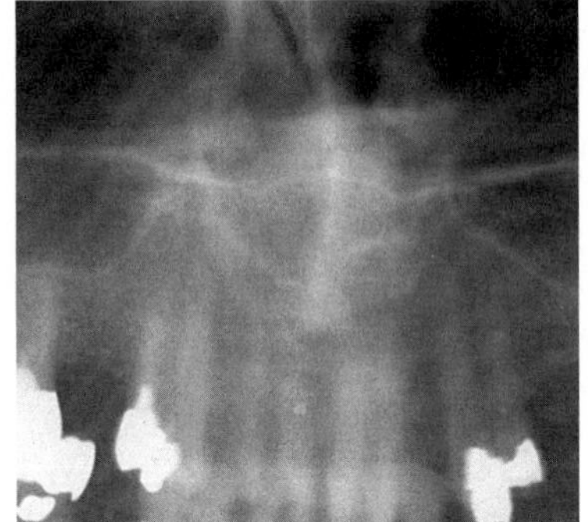
422 b

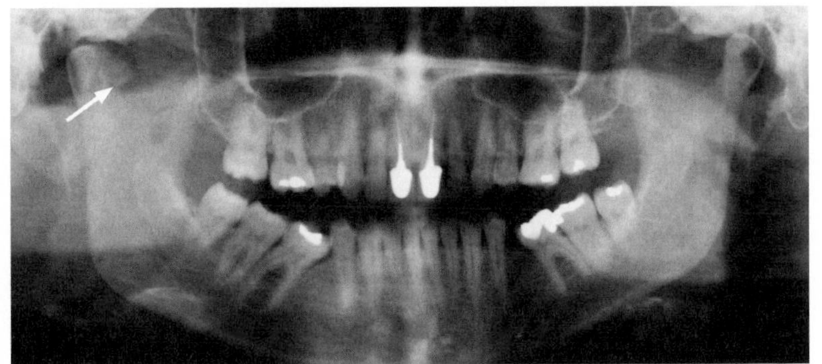
423

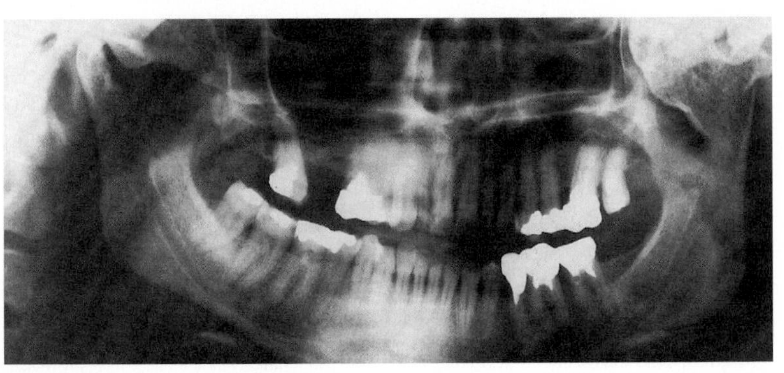
424

Ossifying Fibroma

The ossifying fibroma as a benign tumor is difficult, even histologically, to differentiate from fibrous dysplasia, which exhibits a quite similar radiographic appearance. The tumor is most often localized in the premolar-molar regions of the mandible. It can, however, also appear as a juvenile ossifying fibroma in the maxilla, where it grows asymptomatically and impinges upon the maxillary sinus. It is often detected only after the appearance of increasing facial asymmetry.

Irregular osseous trabeculae or also foci of cementum are embedded within the connective tissue stroma; the radiographic appearance is one of increasing radiopacity. The peripheral demarcation is clearly visible, especially in the mandible, and there is no encapsulation. The compact bone is distended and thinned, and there is impingement upon the mandibular canal.

The tumor grows asymptomatically and is usually only detected in the third to fifth decade of life. The juvenile form occurs primarily in the maxilla and is detected in the second decade of life. Females are affected much more frequently than males.

If the radiographic image also includes a frosted glass appearance, the differential diagnosis should include fibrous dysplasia above all.

Ossifying fibroma can recur, especially in the maxilla. Malignant transformation has been described, especially following recurrence.

Fig. 425 Ossifying fibroma. The panoramic radiograph of a 56-year-old female reveals an ossifying fibroma in the right premolar-molar region. The peripheral margin of the lesion is clearly visible. The compact bone is distended and thinned, appearing as "lobes." The body of the mandible is locally thickened. The mandibular canal is displaced, and to some extent virtually invisible because of the superimposition of calcified islands of cancellous bone.

Fig. 426 a, b Ossifying fibroma. Because this 40-year-old male presented with a painless swelling of the left side of the face, a CT examination was performed. **a** Note a well-demarcated radiolucency on the right side, which appears to fill the maxillary sinus, and which has even distended the lateral wall of the nasal cavity and the dorsal wall of the sinus and canine fossa. **b** Using the CT soft tissue window one observes irregularly distributed and calcified islands of cancellous bone. The juvenile form of ossifying fibroma depicted here usually occurs during the second decade of life.

Fig. 427 a, b Ossifying fibroma. a This section from a panoramic radiograph of a 19-year-old male reveals a cementum-forming, ossifying fibroma. The radiolucency has a frosted-glass appearance and is sharply demarcated; the basal compact bone is distended. The mesial root of tooth 46 appears to be shortened due to resorption, although the distal root has been lengthened by secondary cementum deposition. There is displacement of the mandibular canal. **b** The unilateral occlusal radiograph of the mandible reveals that the buccal and especially also the lingual compact bone are greatly distended and thinned. This occlusal radiograph was definitely indicated, and clearly reveals the irregular and spotty radiopacities.

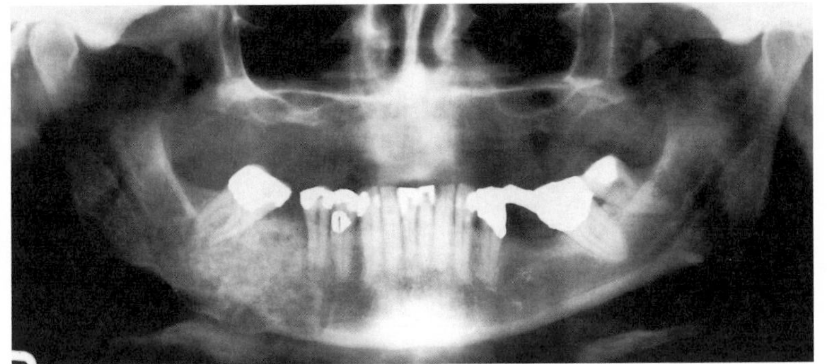

425

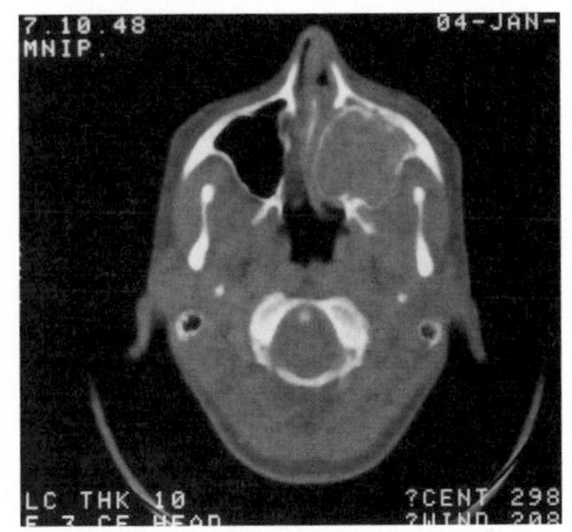

426 a

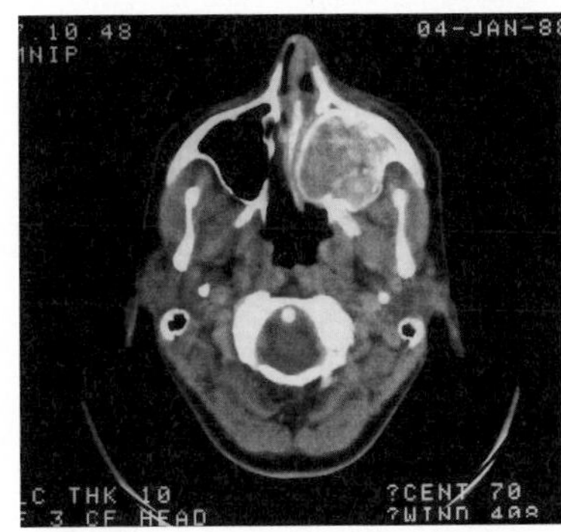

426 b

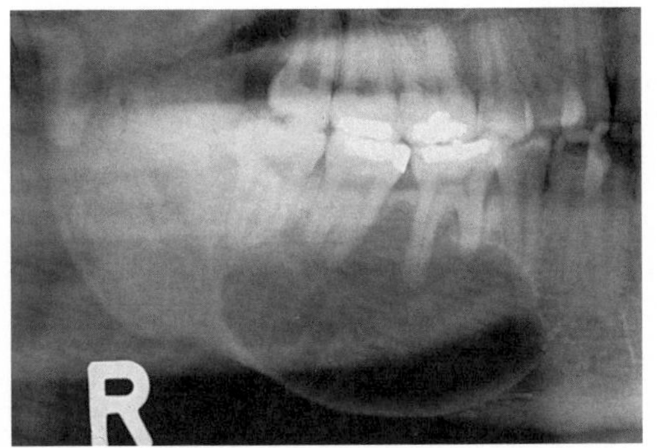

427 a

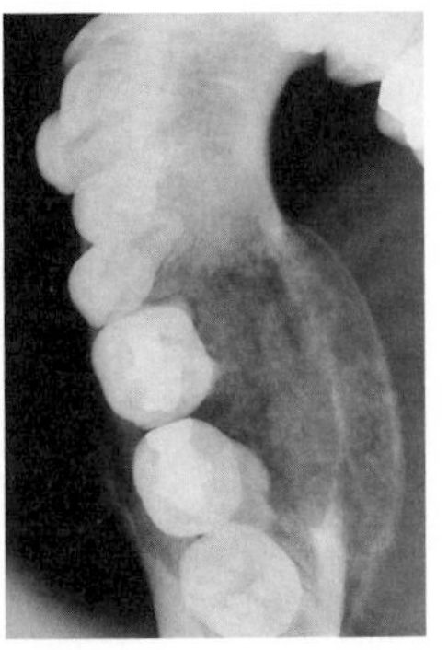

427 b

Osteoblastoma, Osteoid Osteoma

These two benign tumors are rare in the jaws; they are characterized by the laying down of osseous ground substance within a fiber-rich stroma. The two tumors cannot be distinguished from each other histopathologically.

The **osteoblastoma** is usually detected in the mandible. The initial stage is characterized by a poorly demarcated osteolysis which, depending upon its localization, is quite difficult to differentiate from the initial stages of periapical cemental dysplasia or a metastatic malignant lesion. In later stages of development one notes an irregularly formed and later ossified radiopacity in the center of the lesion, and a circumscript radiolucent border that is also surrounded by a zone of reactive sclerosis. Patients will complain of local numbness.

The **osteoid osteoma** was described in 1935 by Jaffé; this lesion is also usually found in the mandible. The radiograph reveals a nucleus with a round "nidus" and, depending upon the stage of development, a more or less broad radiolucent zone surrounded by an irregular festoon of sclerosed bone; this appearance has led to the use of the word "cockade" or "rosette" to describe the lesion in the professional literature. Patients complain of diffuse, deep osseous pain at night that responds to aspirin therapy (!). Spontaneous healing with the formation of a compact osteoma has been described.

Osteoma

This benign bone lesion grows slowly over a long period of time, and without symptoms. During the course of radiographic diagnosis of a suspected osteoma, one must also consider other osseous or ossifying alterations such as osteochondroma, osteoid osteoma, or the end product of fibrous dysplasia; however, the latter does not appear as spherical but rather expansive in the radiograph. The osteoma may also occur in patients with Gardner syndrome or Paget disease of bone.

Fig. 428 **Osteoblastoma**. The panoramic radiograph of a 70-year-old male reveals an osteoblastoma with irregular radiopacity in the center, surrounded by a zone of radiolucency in the body of the mandible on the right side. Mesial to this lesion, note also the end product of an osteoblastoma, an osteoma.

Fig. 429 **Osteoblastoma**. This section from a panoramic radiograph of a 23-year-old female reveals the lytic initial stage of an osteoblastoma, whose radiolucent figure is superimposed upon the axial third of the root of tooth 13 (**arrow**). The tooth itself remains vital.

Fig. 430 **Osteoid osteoma**. The panoramic radiograph of a 29-year-old male reveals the classic shape of an osteoid osteoma in the region of teeth 33 and 34, with a dense, central "nidus" and a circumscript zone of radiolucency that is surrounded by a rosette of irregular radiopacity. The typical configuration achieves a diameter up to 1 cm. Dental jargon is sometimes used to describe the lesion as "cockade" or "rosette."

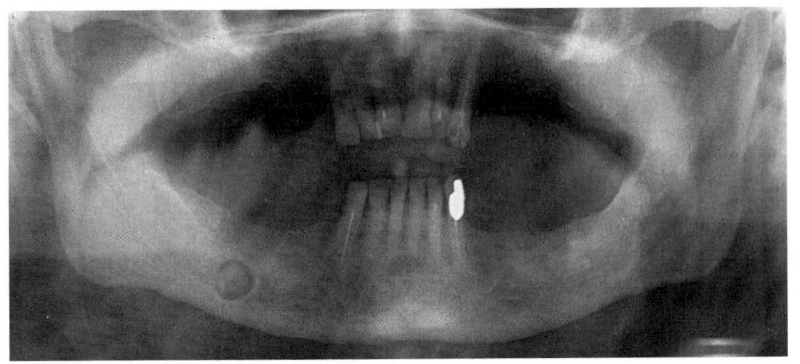

428

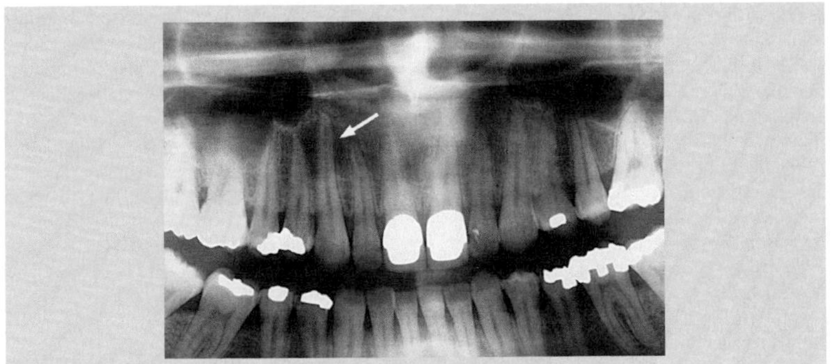

429

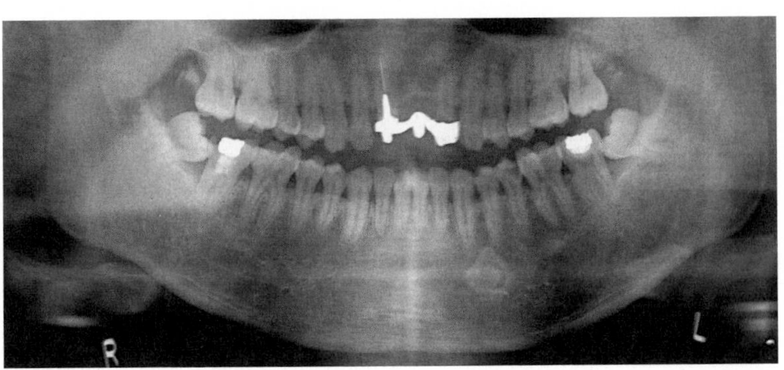

430

The osteoma may consist of compact bone exhibiting a fully mineralized osseous tissue with haversion osteons (Osteoma eburneum), or a mature layered lamellar osseous tissue. The osteoma may be located centrally within bone, or peripherally emanating from the periosteum.

The radiographic image of the osteoma usually exhibits round shapes, with the exception of the end product of fibrous dysplasia, and is more or less radiopaque depending upon the fine tissue structure.

Osteoma is more common in males, and usually occurs only after age 40 (also with the exception of fibrous dysplasia).

Osteocartilaginous Exostoses

Exostoses of the jaws are also classified as osteomas. There is a possible hereditary component. The osseous lesion may appear as a palatal torus along the median suture of the maxilla as a solitary lesion, or symmetrically as lingual tori in the premolar regions of the mandible. Exostoses are harmless, and cause problems only when partial or full dentures are necessary. A rare manifestation includes multiple exostoses on the buccal and vestibular compact bone of the mandible.

Such exostoses are often not captured by the central ray of periapical or panoramic radiographs; the lesions are usually detected clinically by inspection and palpation. If necessary, radiographic depiction with demonstration of the third dimension is possible with occlusal radiographs in the mandible.

The palatal torus is an accompanying symptom of the glossopalatal-ankylosis syndrome, and also of generalized cortical hyperostosis (Worth type).

Intestinal Polyposis (Gardner Syndrome)

Intestinal polyposis III was first described by Gardner in 1950. It is an autosomal dominant hereditary disease in which polyposis of the colon is accompanied by formation of osteomas and osteofibromas in the mandible. The intestinal polyps undergo malignant transformation in about 40% of cases, often only years after the osseous alterations in the mandible; for this reason, routine dental examination using a panoramic radiograph is of primary importance. Dentists and dental hygienists have the responsibility to refer such findings for further medical examination. The radiographic picture is one of irregular, spotty radiopacities of enostoses and exostoses that are almost always detected in the mandible. Individual dental anomalies as well as supernumerary teeth are often also observed.

This disorder is observed primarily in males in the third and fourth decades of life.

The differential diagnosis vis-à-vis Paget disease of bone or end products of fibrous dysplasia is always difficult.

Fig. 431 a, b Osteoma. a This section from a panoramic radiograph of a 60-year-old male reveals an enossal osteoma, which is scarcely discernable (**arrows**). **b** Radioisotope scanning was performed on the same patient and clearly reveals growth activity (**arrow**) in this location. Clinically, the patient experienced deep bone pain.

Fig. 432 Osteoma. This section from a panoramic radiograph of a 61-year-old male reveals a pedunculated peripheral osteoma at the right mandibular angle. With this localization, the differential diagnosis should also include a large sialolith in the bend of Wharton's duct, or a calcified lymph node.

Fig. 433 Osteoma. This panoramic radiograph of a 25-year-old male was centered on the maxilla, and reveals a pedunculated peripheral osteoma on the posterior (dorsal) recess of the left maxillary sinus.

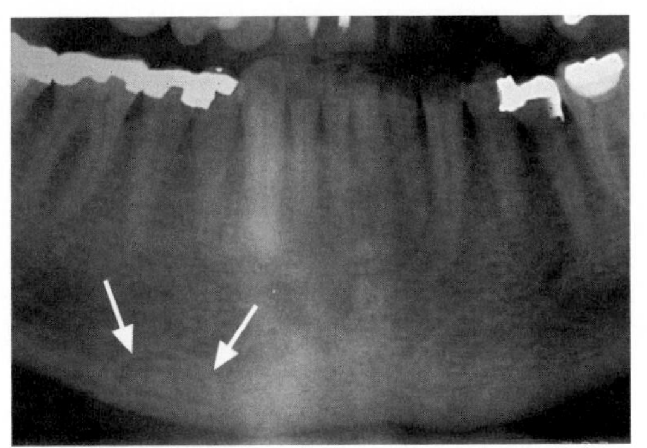

431 a

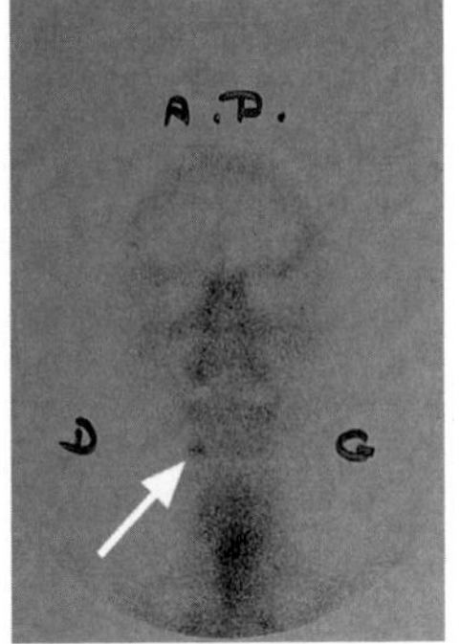

431 b

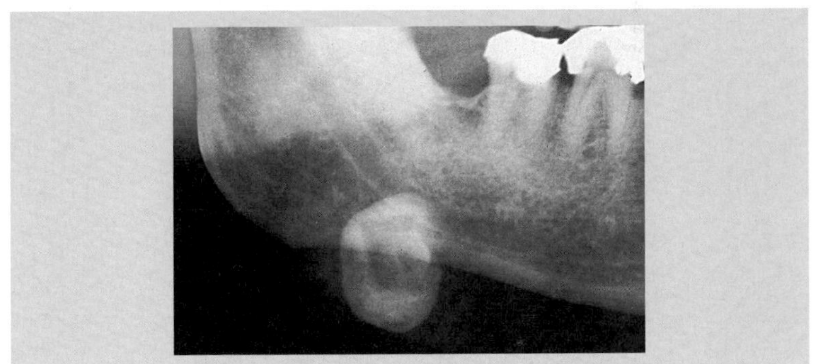

432

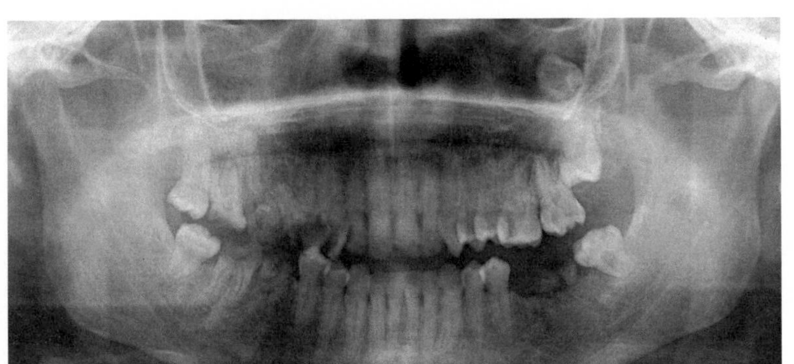

433

Paget Disease of Bone (Osteodystrophia deformans)

Paget disease of bone begins with very few symptoms but is later associated with significant rheumatoid pain; this disease affects primarily elderly males. The etiology remains unclarified. Paget disease of bone is characterized by dramatic osseous remodeling. In addition to thickening and deformation of the overall skeleton, there is an enlargement and coarsening of the skull and facial skeleton, affecting the jaws and particularly the maxilla. The enlargement and flattening of the maxilla leads to the formation of diastemata, the teeth become mobile and often must be extracted. Denture wearers complain that the maxillary prosthesis no longer fits and has "become too small."

In radiographs, the teeth of the frequently affected maxilla exhibit hypercementosis and the root apices appear widened, often giving the impression of root resorption. Within bone, one observes poorly demarcated radiolucencies due to osseous resorption, adjacent to irregular, cloudy radiopacities resulting from osseous apposition (*cotton wool* effect), and in a few cases one may observe well-demarcated osteomas. The normal structure of the bone is no longer evident, and even the periodontal ligament space of clinically mobile teeth is no longer radiographically discernable. This disease occurs primarily in males after age 50. The differential diagnosis should include chronic forms of osteomyelitis and hypo- or hyperparathyroidism; radiographic differentiation is often difficult. Malignant transformation to osteosarcoma has been described in about 1% of cases.

Fig. 434a Exostoses. In a 19-year-old male, a mandibular occlusal radiograph was taken to enhance the suspected findings from a panoramic radiograph. The occlusal projection reveals numerous hyperostoses lateral to the mental protuberance in the third dimension.

Fig. 434b Exostoses. The occlusal radiograph of the mandible clearly reveals lingually localized exostoses (tori); such exostoses are also often observed in the region of the mid-palatal suture as palatal tori. Neither vestibular nor lingual nor even palatal exostoses can be adequately depicted in a two-dimensional panoramic radiograph; these lesions are easily detected by clinical inspection and palpation.

Fig. 435 Gardner syndrome. This section of a panoramic radiograph reveals multiple enostoses or exostoses (third dimension!) and osteomas in both maxilla and mandible of an elderly male. Such manifestations in the jaws represent an early dental radiographic sign of an existing intestinal polyposis III; such findings may play a significant role, especially for early diagnosis of the autosomal dominant inherited mesenchymal dysplasia. Malignant transformation can be expected to occur in about 50% of cases.

Fig. 436a–c Paget disease of bone. These three maxillary periapical radiographs of a 69-year-old male reveal Paget disease of bone, which occurs in the entire skeleton but also in the jaws, primarily in the maxilla. These typical radiographic signs exhibit on the one hand poorly demarcated resorption lacunae as radiolucencies, and on the other hand irregular and dense radiopacities with the so-called "cotton wool effect." Such radiographic signs signal the chaotic stages of bone remodeling. The clearest and most common accompanying clinical symptoms include enlargement of the circumference of the skull and flattening and broadening of the maxilla.

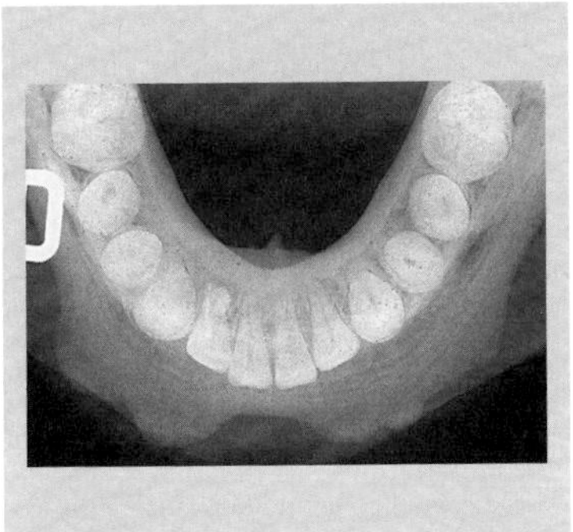

434 a

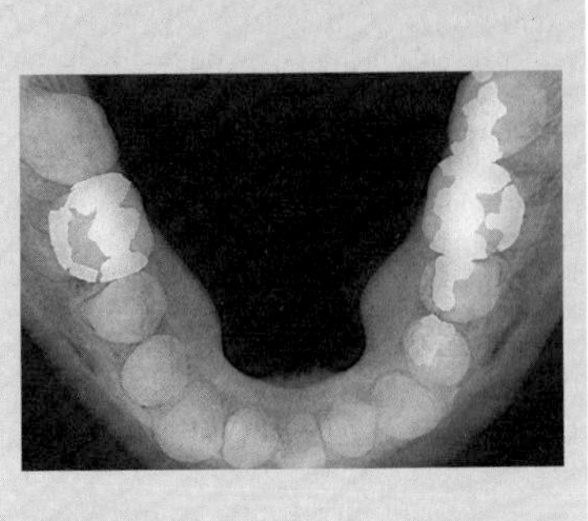

434 b

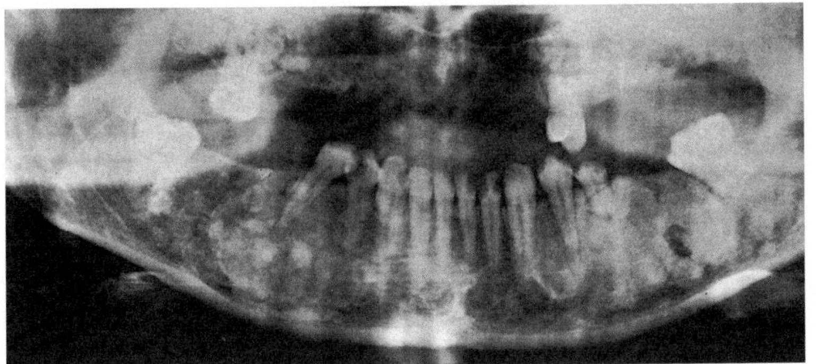

435

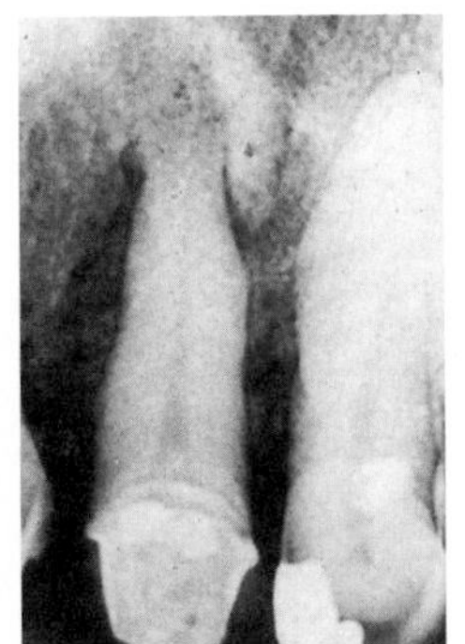

436 a

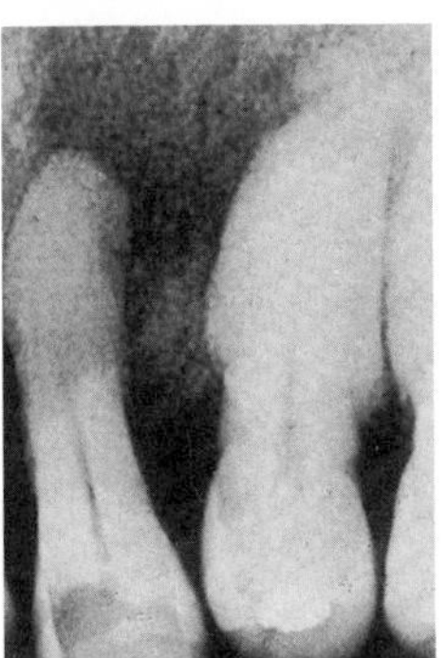

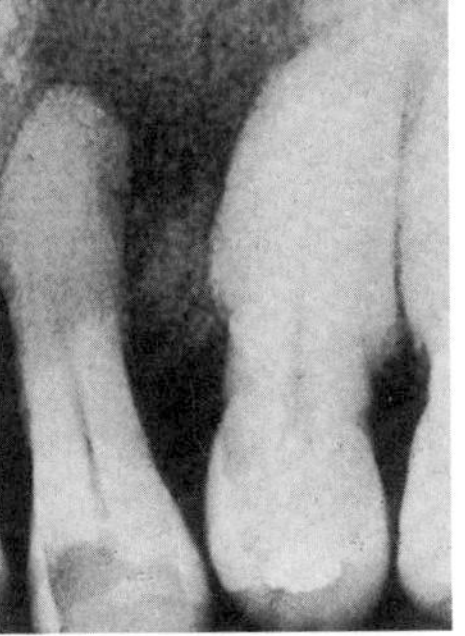

436 b

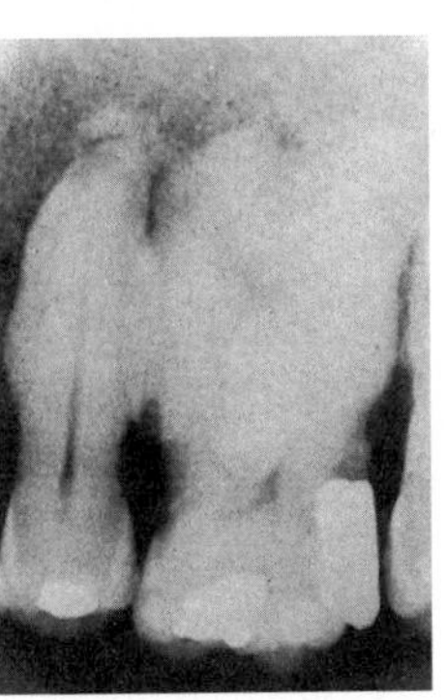

436 c

Osteogenesis imperfecta tarda

Osteogenesis imperfecta tarda (Lobstein syndrome, van-der-Hoeve syndrome) is a disease with varying hereditary etiologies and various symptoms, which derive from a general mesenchymal impairment. The clinical classification includes four basic types, all of which frequently manifest with dentogenesis imperfecta. From the dental/oral point-of-view, types I, III, and IV are of significance because the carrier may live beyond childhood and the dentogenic infections can lead to progressive forms of osteomyelitis.

The radiograph reveals thin and fragile jaw bones. The types of dentogenesis imperfecta associated with the disease lead to retention/impaction of teeth as well as damage to both dentin and enamel. The lamina dura is often not discernible in the radiograph and the cancellous bone appears resorbed and radiolucent.

In early childhood there is a danger of osseous fracture, a danger which reduces with increasing age.

Osteoporosis

The decrease in estrogen levels following menopause leads to a reduction of total osseous tissue in women.

In a panoramic radiograph the loss of bone density can be observed not only in the jaws but also in the cervical vertebrae. The oblique line of the mandible and the covering lamella of the cervical vertebrae become more radiopaque, and this effect is increased by the tangential effect of the roentgen rays.

Osteopetrosis

Osteopetrosis can occur due to functional disturbance of osteoclast function in the face of maintained osseous apposition (Albers–Schönberg syndrome) resulting in various forms of this disease, which are inherited as either autosomal recessive or dominant traits. This disease process is occasionally detected in routine dental practice radiographs as a serendipitous finding, usually in the stage of late manifestations with a radiographic picture of homogenous radiopacity and obliteration of normal marrow spaces. There is a loss of the usually dense radiopacity with a transition into the no longer well-demarcated compact bone. Delayed wound healing following tooth extraction has been reported.

Fig. 437 Osteogenesis imperfecta tarda. This panoramic radiograph of a 7-year-old female reveals osteogenesis imperfecta tarda (Lobstein's syndrome, type I; van-der-Hoeve syndrome) with associated dentinogenesis imperfecta. Clearly obvious are the thin and underdeveloped jaws, the dental dysplasias with pulpal obliteration and enamel defects, as well as numerous tooth impactions/retentions.

Fig. 438 Osteoporosis. This panoramic radiograph of a 93-year-old female reveals senile osteoporosis. Clearly obvious is the elevated radiolucency of the jaws, with loss of indications of osseous trabeculi and thinning of the compact bone of the mandible; note also, however, the dominant radiopacity of the oblique line and the pronounced appearance of the deck plates of the otherwise radiolucent cervical vertebrae.

Fig. 439 Osteopetrosis. The panoramic radiograph reveals a functional disturbance of osteoclasts and reduced resorption of the pre-formed bone. The broadened compact bone and the density of the marrow spaces are indications of the Albers–Schönberg syndrome of the *osteopetrosis tarda* type, which is usually detected serendipitously during the course of a comprehensive examination of the masticatory apparatus.

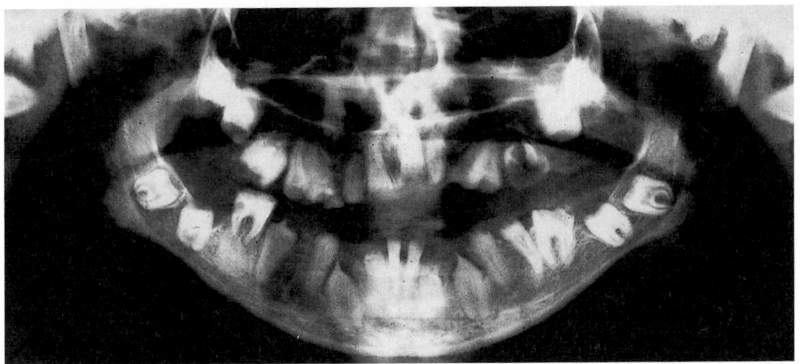

437

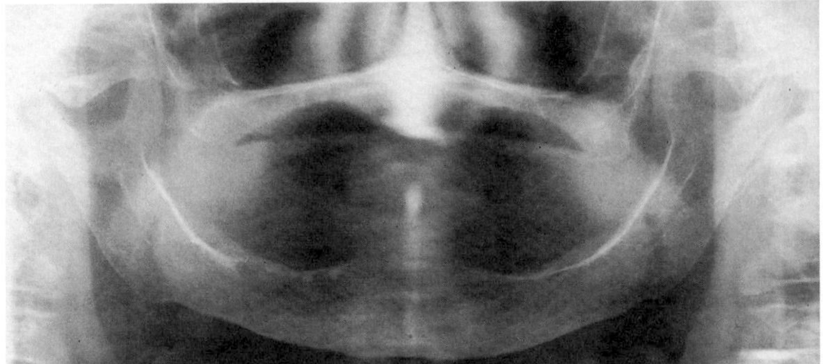

438

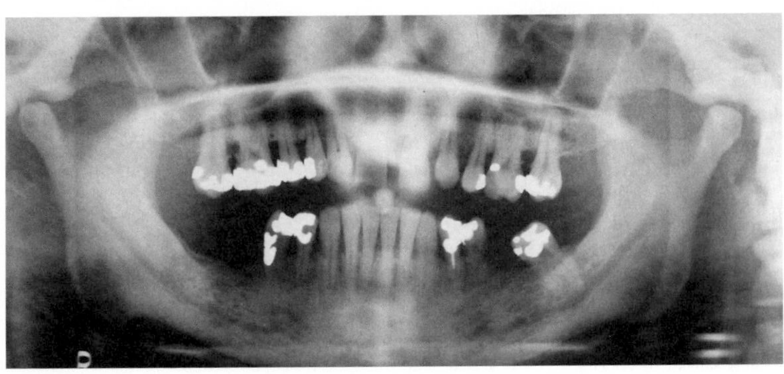

439

Hyperparathyroidism

Hyperparathyroidism is classified as a metabolic osteopathy in which osteoclast function is stimulated and enhanced by an overproduction of parathyroid hormone; this leads to acceleration of calcium metabolism, which elicits various osseous manifestations. The metabolic disturbance can be caused primarily by adrenal adenoma, hyperplasia, or carcinoma leading to radiographic signs of generalized fibrous osteodystrophy (Recklinghausen disease), or secondarily by renal insufficiency, hypercalcemia, and also other etiologic factors.

Dental/oral radiographs reveal premature loss of the lamina dura as well as "washed out" osseous structure exhibiting a frosted glass appearance with poorly demarcated radiolucencies; for this reason, the compact bone and other osseous lamella can no longer be clearly discerned on the film. The poorly demarcated and poorly visible radiolucencies indicate the existence of the so-called "brown tumors" containing hemosiderin that are associated with Recklinghausen disease (1891) of bone.

Hemangioma

The central (enossal) hemangioma is a benign tumor of the blood vasculature that is relatively rare, but which presents significant diagnostic difficulties. The appearance of this lesion is extraordinarily variable: In addition to sunburst-like radiopacities indicative of osteosarcoma, one may also encounter poorly definable radiolucencies, strand-like alterations of trabecular bone, small and large "soap bubble" appearance reminiscent of ameloblastoma, and distention of the jaw with extraosseous phleboliths. This myriad of appearances makes any attempt at radiographic diagnosis extraordinarily difficult. The most common site of occurrence for hemangioma in the head-neck region is the mandible of young females. Clinical manifestations such as supereruption, tooth migration, and tooth mobility indicate the dangers that might be associated with tooth extraction. Massive hemorrhage may occur, which can only be staunched with immediate reimplantation of the tooth and compression. Immediate referral to an appropriate specialist is obligatory!

Fig. 440 Hyperparathyroidism. This panoramic radiograph is indicative of secondary hyperparathyroidism elicited by renal insufficiency. The typical radiographic signs include the frosted glass and vague depiction of the trabecular structures, with loss of normal bordering lamellae of the nasal sinuses. Note especially the individual lamina dura and widening of the periodontal ligament space. In advanced cases one may observe spotty and poorly demarcated radiolucencies (Recklinghausen disease of bone), which are often referred to as "brown tumors" because of their hemosiderin content.

Fig. 441 Hemangioma. This periapical radiograph of the left maxillary premolar region of a 21-year-old female reveals an intraosseous hemangioma that has effectively destroyed the osseous structure between teeth 24 and 25. The round radiolucencies are reminiscent of the honeycomb-type lesions of ameloblastoma (see Fig. **379b**). Elevated mobility of both teeth was ascertained clinically.

Fig. 442 Hemangioma. A comparison of the healthy left side of the mandible in the panoramic radiograph reveals on the right side an irregular, strand-like structure that extends from about tooth 33 and into the mandibular ramus up to the semilunar notch on the right side. Clearly visible are numerous phleboliths (**arrow**), and the mandibular canal can only be observed along parts of its course. It is important to remember that an intraosseous hemangioma can manifest itself in extraordinarily variable images, ranging from strand-like radiopacities all the way to poorly demarcated radiolucencies.

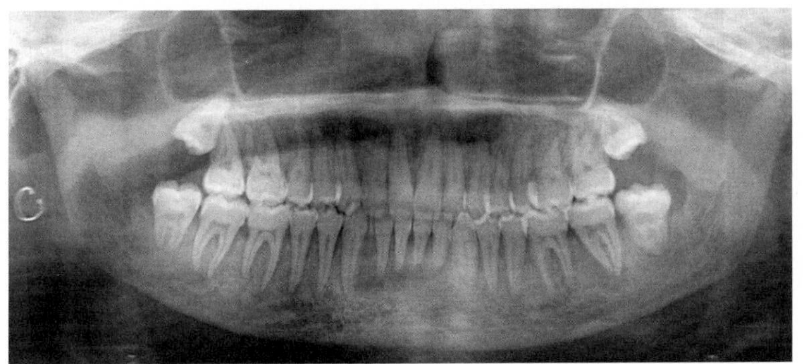

440

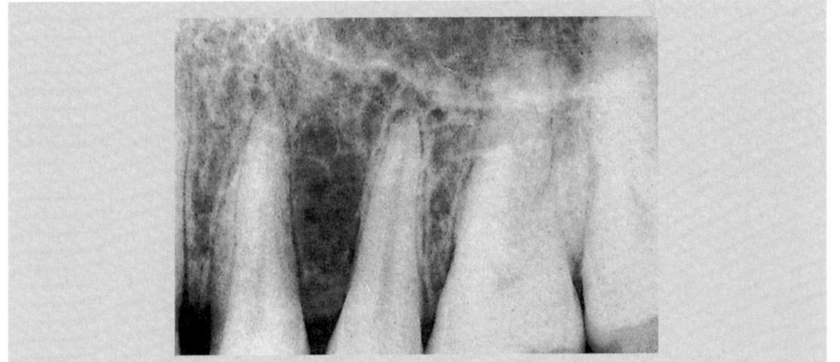

441

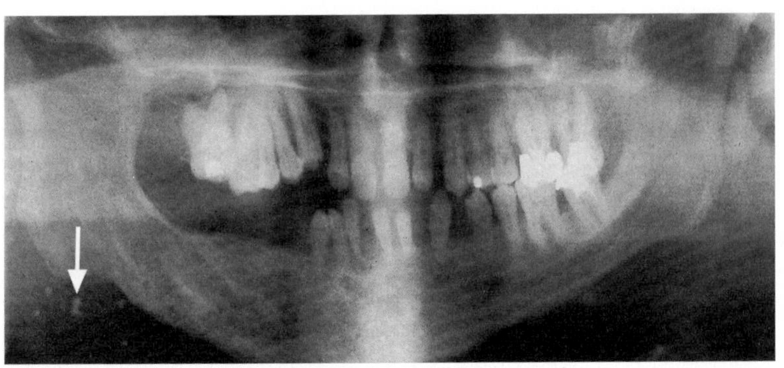

442

Infiltrating Carcinoma

Carcinoma of the oral mucosa is the most frequent malignant tumor of the oral cavity. This lesion can develop as an intraepithelial carcinoma, for example in the mucosa of the floor of the mouth, and it frequently also emanates from white and flat leukoplakia (precancerous lesions). This intraepithelial carcinoma consequently infiltrates into the adjacent bone of the lingual mandibular wall.

With the use of typical dental radiographic examination methods, the lesions are usually detected only in later stages because the summation effect of the roentgen rays renders invisible the very early distribution of areas of radiolucency that are only of millimeter size. Only in later stages of development can one observe undermining, moth-eaten like osteolysis, which eliminate the lamina dura of nondisplaced teeth and destroy the mandibular canal (paresthesia!).

Most patients will be smokers of advanced age.

Much later in its development course, the carcinoma may be discovered in the mucosa of the maxillary sinuses, but this usually only occurs following significant clinical symptoms or penetration into the oral cavity.

The recommended methods for examination include thin-layer projections with CT or magnetic resonance imaging (MRI).

Sarcoma

The undifferentiated and highly malignant Ewing sarcoma originates in bone and is a rapidly growing tumor that metastasizes early and is most often observed at the angle of the mandible. In its initial stages, the extremely pressure-sensitive and painful lesion is accompanied by high fever and may simulate the clinical appearance of acute osteomyelitis. The radiographic appearance is one that exhibits (with delay) destruction of osseous architecture and radiolucencies, as well as onion-like distention of compact bone and the formation of spicules (calcified bone spicules) that appear in the radiographs as a “sunburst” effect.

Most often affected are children and adolescents in the first and second decades of life.

The examination method of choice is MRI.

Fig. 443 Carcinoma. The panoramic radiograph of a 74-year-old male reveals in the left mandible an infiltrating carcinoma of the oral mucosa. In the premolar-molar regions one observes a moth-eaten area of osteolysis that begins distal to tooth 32 and extends into the mandibular ramus with apparent destruction of the mandibular canal and exhibiting spotty radiolucencies and irregular radiopacities.

Fig. 444 Ewing sarcoma. The panoramic radiograph of a 7-year-old male reveals a highly malignant Ewing sarcoma on the right side of the mandible. This tumor is always accompanied by severe clinical manifestations. It is characterized radiographically by irregular radiolucencies including periosteal reactions and typical “sunburst effects” (**arrows**). The affected jaw is distended, and the teeth are often displaced. Without complete knowledge of the clinical situation, radiographic differential diagnosis vis-à-vis osteosarcoma and some variation of intraosseous hemangioma is exceedingly difficult.

Fig. 445 Osteosarcoma. The panoramic radiograph of a 29-year-old female reveals, at the extraction site of tooth 37, irregular new bone formation with zones of radiolucency; such lesions are difficult to diagnosis radiographically. Only a histopathologic examination can clarify noncalcified osteoids, cartilaginous tissue, or fibroblastic tissue components.

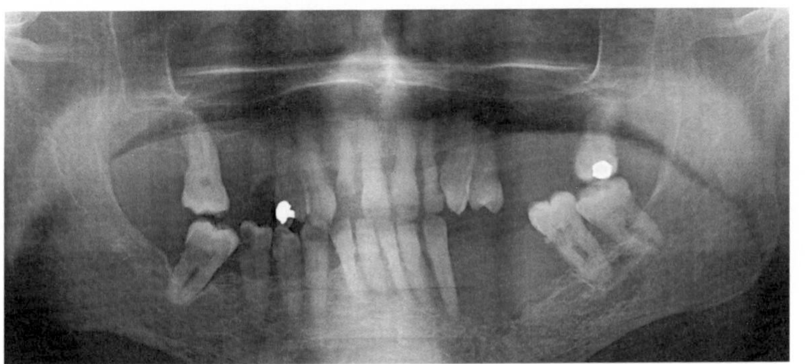

443

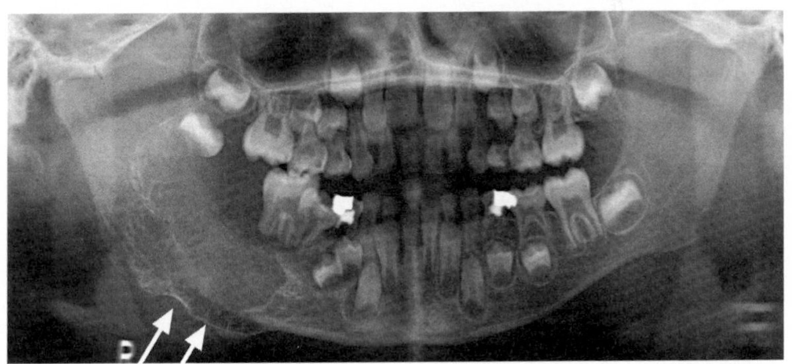

444

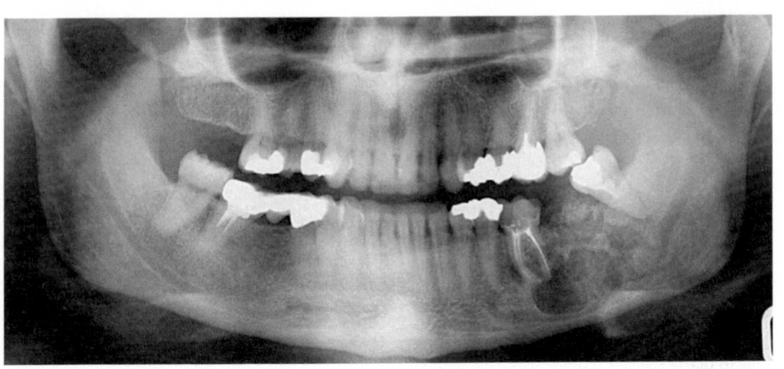

445

The **osteosarcoma** is a primary mesenchymal tumor that may be dominated by osteoblastic, chondroblastic, and/or fibroblastic cell types.

The radiographic appearance may include both osteolytic and osteoblastic alterations, and because of the myriad of cell compositions the radiographic picture can vary enormously, but osteolytic processes usually prevail. If the lesion is dominated by osteoblastic cells, the radiographic picture will be one of "sunburst" (spicules); the periodontal ligament space may be both widened and obliterated.

Osseous trauma and tooth extraction may precede such tumor formation. The osteosarcoma is a lesion that appears most frequently in the second and third decades of life (exception: malignant transformation of Paget disease of bone).

Chondroblastic osteosarcoma can derive from malignant transformation of an osteochondroma (see Fig. **422**).

The tumor is usually located in the region of the embryonic premaxilla.

The radiographic picture reveals destruction of the normal osseous structures, with irregular, even chaotic-appearing radiolucencies and radiopacities. This tumor cannot be satisfactorily depicted with a panoramic radiograph. Enhancing visualization can be achieved using a cephalometric radiograph, occlusal projections, or CT and MRI.

The lesions are most often observed in males in the fourth and fifth decades of life.

Fibroblastic osteosarcoma is an extremely rare malignant osseous tumor, and in about 10% of cases is located in the skull, including the jaws.

The radiograph reveals a poorly demarcated osteolysis that penetrates the bordering osseous lamellae and can also penetrate the surrounding soft tissues. Such osteosarcomas are difficult to differentiate from metastases of other malignant tumors.

The fibrosarcoma may occur in both genders and at virtually any age. The age peak resides in the 2nd–4th decades of life.

Fig. 446 Osteosarcoma. The panoramic radiograph of a 40-year-old male reveals an osteosarcoma that has developed, as is often the case, from the base of an osteochondroma with its typical localization and shape. The pathognomonic radiographic signs include the loss of depiction of the anterior nasal spine, the piriform aperture at the entrance to the nasal cavity, the median suture of the maxilla in its anterior region, and the incisal foramen with the incisal canal. In a panoramic radiograph, one usually only observes a round, diffuse radiopacity (**arrows**); this necessitates additional, supplemental radiographs with differing central ray projections.

Fig. 447 a, b Osteosarcoma. a The lateral cephalometric radiograph of the same case reveals a round radiolucency in the region of the premaxilla (**arrows**) and loss of the normally visible osseous structures. **b** The corresponding occlusal radiograph exhibits the diffuse, spotty radiopacity and a moth-eaten radiolucency. The anterior nasal spine, the median suture, and the incisal canal with the incisal foramen are no longer discernible in the radiograph.

Fig. 448 Ameloblastic fibrosarcoma. The panoramic radiograph of a 16-year-old female reveals in the right maxilla an ameloblastic fibrosarcoma. The tumor has expanded beyond the bordering lamellae of the maxillary sinus. Tooth 18 is included within the lesion, the periodontal ligament space of the apparently supererupted tooth 16 cannot be discerned as it transitions to tooth 15.

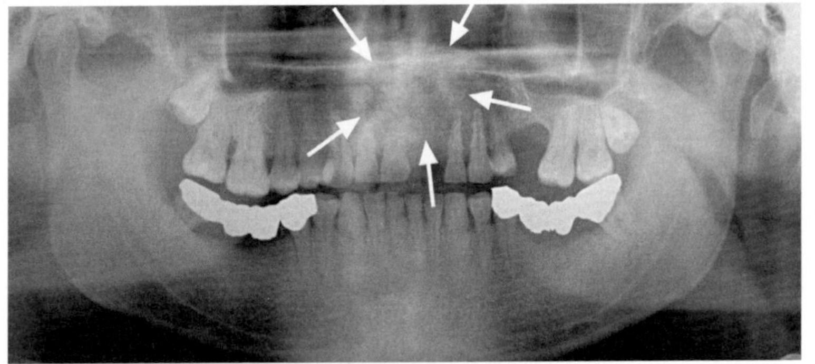

446

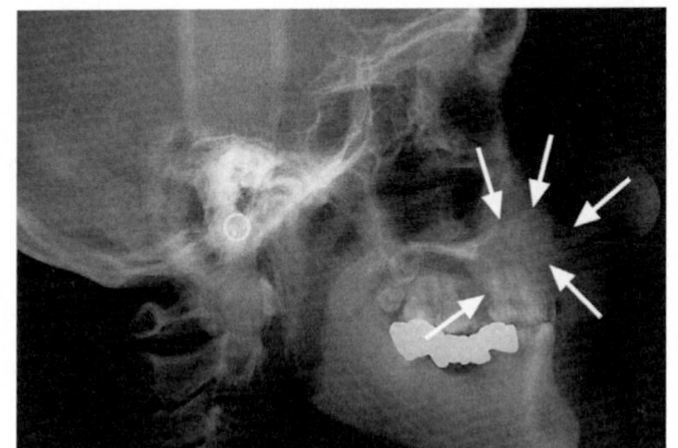

447 a

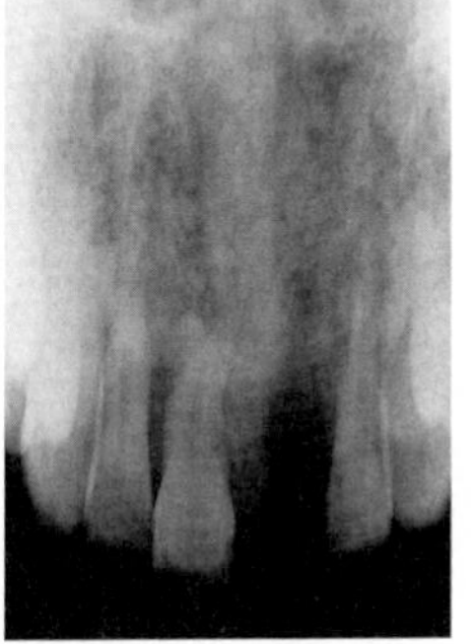

447 b

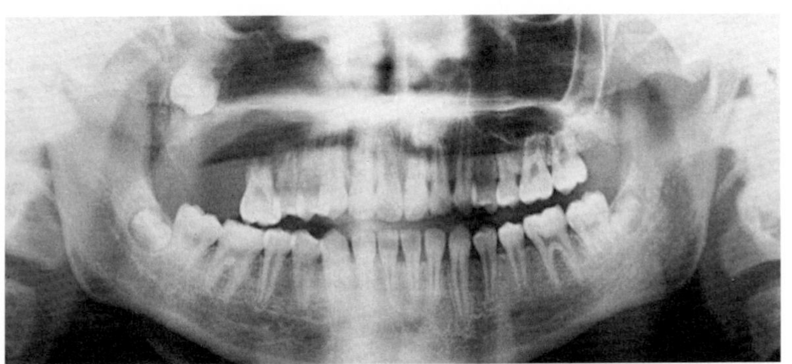

448

The metastasis is a satellite of a primary tumor; despite its varying localization within the body, the metastasis exhibits histologic fine tissue structure that is identical to the primary tumor. Within the jaws, metastases from sarcomas are less common than from carcinomas; metastasis to the mandible can occur relatively early, and virtually always via the blood vascular system.

The most important primary tumors are:

- Mammary carcinoma
- Bronchial carcinoma
- Thyroid carcinoma
- Prostate carcinoma

Unfortunately, when medical specialists are searching for metastases, the jaws are seldom included as possible targets; therefore, metastases within the jaws are usually detected only serendipitously.

The most important clinical symptoms that may accompany metastasis in the mandible, and which therefore provide a clue as to the existence of a primary tumor include:

- Deep bone pain
- Unexplained tooth mobility
- Paresthesia of the lower lip
- Spontaneous fracture of the mandible

If the results of clinical and/or radiographic diagnosis raise suspicion about the possibility of metastasis, radioisotope scanning can be used as an enhancing diagnostic method to clarify the diagnosis.

Fig. 449 Metastases. This panoramic radiograph of a 69-year-old male reveals the presence of metastasis from his prostate carcinoma, on the right side of the edentulous mandible. Within the poorly demarcated radiolucency, one observes the moth-eaten and undermined cancellous bone structure, which are in direct contact with the compact basal bone. Both the roof and the floor of the mandibular canal have been destroyed.

Fig. 450 Metastases. The panoramic radiograph reveals metastasis from a colon carcinoma in the right ascending mandibular ramus. The arrows indicate the expansion of the tumor at this relatively early stage; a superficial inspection would not identify the spotty radiolucencies with poorly demarcated borders. Structural alterations can also be observed in the region of the mandibular canal. The observer should compare this region with that of the left angle of the mandible.

Fig. 451 a, b Metastases. Radioisotope scanning was performed on the same patient; note the obvious zones of activity in the right ascending ramus. **a** Posteroanterior radioisotope scanning revealing elevated activity in the right ramus extending to the neck of the mandible. **b** Lateral radioisotope scanning reveals enhanced activity high in the right mandibular ramus.

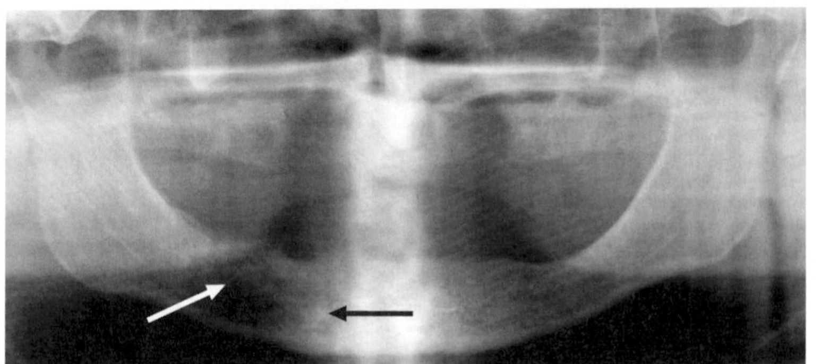

449

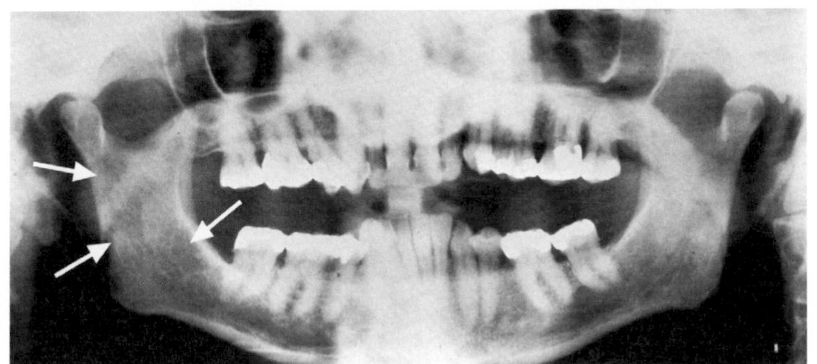

450

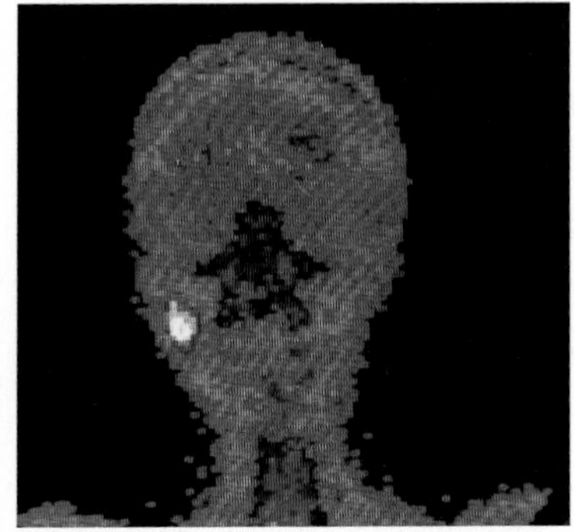

451 a

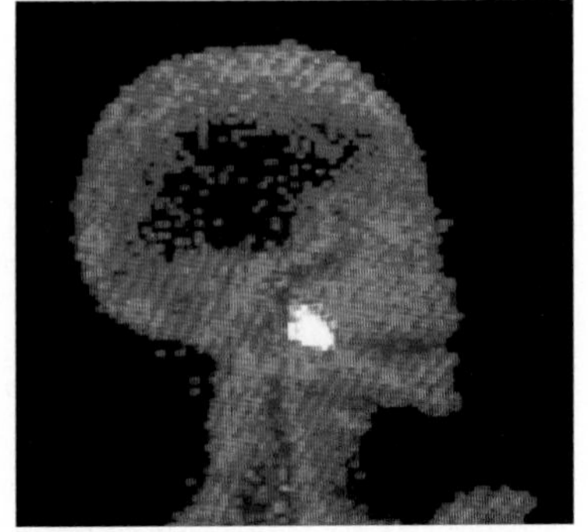

451 b

In the discipline of traumatology, the radiograph plays a very special role and must also fulfill various demands, because it serves not only as one aspect of data collection but also as **documentation** for the patient, the caregiver, and even for the insurance company. Radiography must adhere in all cases to the medical guidelines for preventing radiation overdose, but the radiograph will continue to find important applications in forensic dentistry and forensic pathology.

In dental practice, this aspect is important even for apparently minor accidents and injuries, because even apparently banal events are frequently followed by unexpected consequences, which demand a detailed report to governmental agencies or insurance companies. It is always important to keep in mind that fracture lines at any localization can only be diagnosed with certainty when the central ray courses parallel to the fracture line; this is also the case for clear depiction of hard tissue dislocations. Even if radiographs do not provide unequivocal evidence for the *existence* of a fracture, the presence of a fracture cannot absolutely be ruled out. Especially in children, even following dental injuries that appear clinically uncomplicated, it is prudent for the dentist to take a panoramic radiograph in order to document "greenstick fractures" and fractures of the neck of the mandible that are difficult to detect clinically, again for possible forensic reasons. This extra step in case documentation will also help to avoid incorrect conclusions that may lead later to tooth loss or growth disturbances.

Fig. 452 Depiction of tooth fractures: The schematic diagrams illustrate a transverse fracture and an oblique fracture of the maxillary anterior teeth, with lateral radiographic projection. **Left:** Only when the central ray is precisely parallel to the fracture line will the fracture be clearly depicted. **Middle:** If the central ray is directed obliquely to the fracture line, the radiograph will depict several fracture lines, simulating a complex fracture. **Right:** Oblique fractures often exhibit no clear radiographic signs. Using magnifying loupes, one may observe a tiny step-formation along the mesial or distal root surface and/or a poorly discernible addition effect created by the superimposition of the displaced root fragments.

Fig. 453 a, b Depicting the fracture line: a Normal projection of the maxillary anterior region; one can observe several fine fracture lines in teeth 11 and 21. **b** Using a more horizontal projection (note the apparent lengthening of the teeth), the central ray traverses parallel through the fracture line, depicting it in its true shape and localization.

Fig. 454 Radiographic depiction of tooth luxation: As a result of facial trauma, teeth 21 and 22 were luxated palatally. The fundus of the alveoli are obvious. Both the vestibular alveolar wall and the interdental septum are fractured.

Fig. 455 Depiction of tooth luxations: The schematic diagrams depict three types of tooth luxations in the maxilla, with lateral radiographic projections. **Left:** If a facial injury has luxated the tooth and its crown vestibularly, the radiograph usually does not provide any clear signs of such luxation. **Middle:** If the facial trauma luxates the tooth crown palatally, such luxation is visible in the radiograph as a radiolucency at the fundus of the alveolus. **Right:** If the trauma causes the tooth to be forced apically into its alveolus, the apex of the root will appear *above* the apices of the adjacent teeth. The periodontal ligament space or the lamina dura will no longer be discernible.

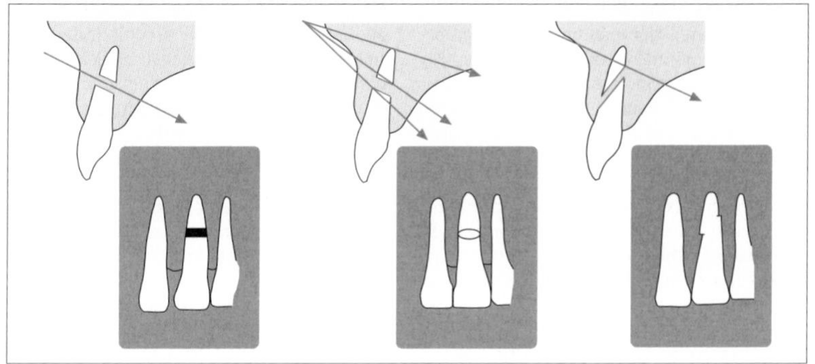

452

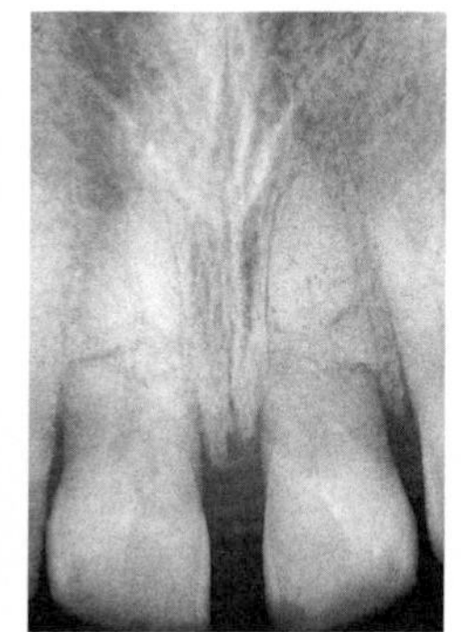

453 a

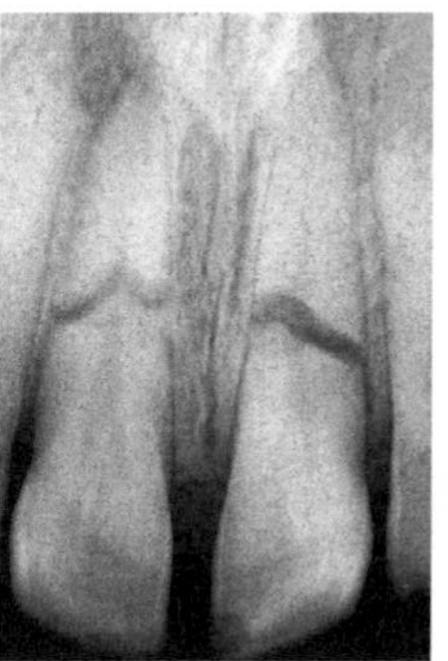

453 b

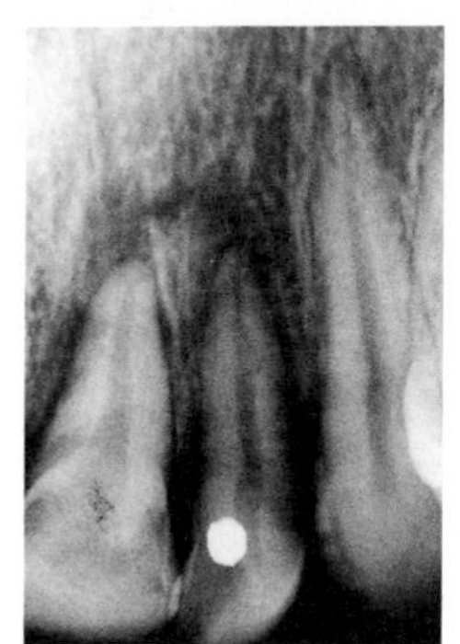

454

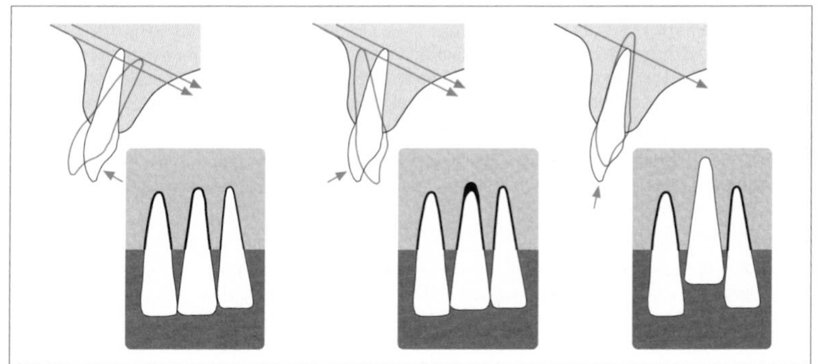

455

In most cases where there is suspicion of osseous fracture, the panoramic radiograph taken in the normal position and with a bite plane can be used to detect fractures of teeth, the jaws, and the condyles; however, a radiograph taken in habitual occlusion (see p. **13**) should be also taken if there is suspicion of osseous dislocations. It is reasonable to **expect** dislocations resulting primarily from the trauma itself but also secondarily due to muscle tension, especially in the mandible, and such dislocations will not always be visible in the third dimension due to the effects of superimpositions of hard structures in the panoramic radiograph. Because two-dimensional radiographic procedures usually cannot answer questions concerning the third dimension, additional radiographs taken with varying central ray projection are in most cases obligatory. Clinical vitality testing of all injured teeth must be performed regularly for at least 6 months following the accident in order to ascertain and document any subsequent consequences in a timely manner.

Today, traffic accidents are all too common and lead not infrequently to complicated multiple injuries. Conventional clinical procedures for triage and initial examination of traumatized or unconscious patients may not provide adequate information concerning accurate jaw/tooth positions, and therefore it is not uncommon that subsequent examination procedures are necessary later. Therefore, despite elevated radiation exposure, multiple injuries of the facial skeleton should be approached from the very beginning via computed tomography (CT) examinations.
The CT, which permits secondary tomography and three-dimensional surface reconstructions in any desired plane, is absolutely necessary for all surgical planning in cases of severe midface injuries; in addition, the CT and CBCT (cone beam computed tomography) techniques provide a single examination procedure that precludes additional radiation exposure for the patient.

Fig. 456 Tooth fractures: This panoramic radiograph of a 20-year-old male, and the inserted periapical radiograph of the maxillary anterior region, reveal crown fractures of teeth 12 and 22, as well as root fractures of teeth 11 and 21. The overall osseous structures are without pathologic findings. The two black arrows indicate apparent fracture lines. These are sometimes caused by marginal radiopacities due to the superimposition of various anatomic planes; this is described as the Mach-effect (Ernst Mach, physicist). In the case depicted here, the situation is one of bilateral superimposition of the coronoid process by the caudal end of the lateral lamina of the pterygoid process of the sphenoid bone.

Fig. 457 Tooth trauma with radicular cyst: The panoramic radiograph of a 31-year-old male, and the inserted periapical radiograph of the maxillary anterior region, reveal a radicular cyst emanating from the traumatized tooth 11, which was clinically nonvital and which exhibited obliteration of the pulp canal. The surrounding osseous structures do not exhibit pathologic findings.

Fig. 458 Ramus, collum, and alveolar ridge fractures: This panoramic radiograph of a 21-year-old male exhibits, in addition to crown fractures of teeth 21 and 22, an oblique ramus fracture with dislocation on the right side and a fracture of the neck of the mandible (white arrows) with dislocation of a small fragment laterally (it is smaller and sharply demarcated, and therefore is located nearer to the image receptor). The **black arrows** indicate a fracture line in the maxilla that is scarcely visible in the radiograph; this signals a maxillary alveolar ridge fracture.

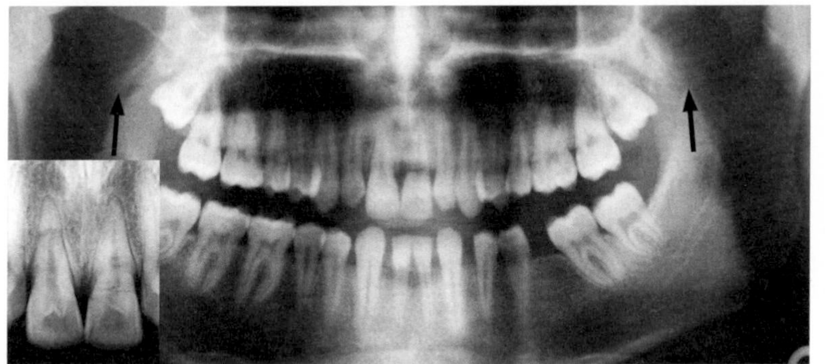

456

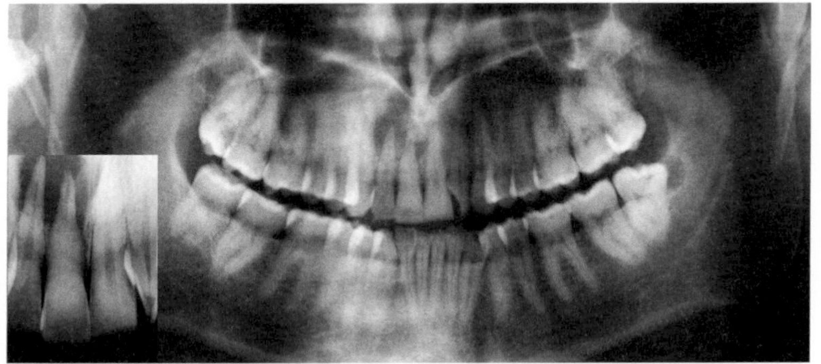

457

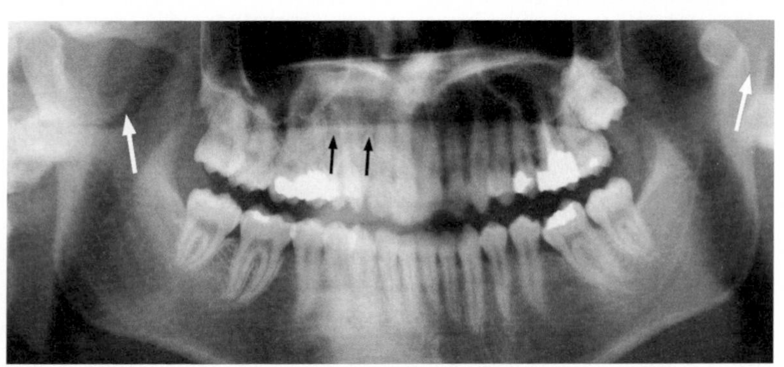

458

Radiographic indications of fractures: In addition to the various types of dental injuries, the dentist must always differentiate between fractures caused by injury and spontaneous fractures, i.e., pathologically initiated fractures. "*Iatrogenic*" fractures comprise an important group, with particular forensic significance.

In terms of **dental injuries**, one can make a basic differentiation between crown and root fractures vis-à-vis tooth luxation, and these can be further categorized as traumatic, pathologic, and/or iatrogenic dental injuries. The most important types of dental fractures include horizontal, oblique, and axial fractures of the tooth crown, the tooth root, or the entire tooth. Tooth luxation can be grossly categorized as complete or incomplete luxation, with or without damage to the alveolus.

The radiographic diagnostic image possibilities for tooth fracture and tooth luxation are relatively limited because they are dependent upon the spatial orientation of the fracture line within the tooth or the luxated tooth to the selected projection of the central ray (exception: total luxation). Only those fracture lines that are directly targeted by the central ray will be discernibly depicted in the radiograph. If the central ray is projected obliquely upon the fracture line, the result will be only a blurred picture of the actual fracture. This means that the quality of depiction of the fracture is dependent almost completely upon the alignment of the central ray with the fracture line; the result is that any *clinical* classification on the basis of radiographs will be, in many cases, questionable.

Fig. 459 Mandibular fractures: The panoramic radiograph of a 21-year-old male reveals a transverse fracture of the mandible on the right side and a fracture of the mandibular angle on the left side. The fracture line in both localizations goes through the alveoli of teeth 43 and 38. This situation is one of a fresh and sharply demarcated fracture open to the oral cavity and therefore presenting an entryway for infection. On the right side, one can clearly observe a step between teeth 43 and 42, and an additional step on the basal compact bone. At the angle of the mandible, likely also as a result of muscle tension, steps indicating dislocations are visible. The small radiopacities near the fracture line at the angle of the mandible do not represent osseous sequester, rather these are the result of a radiographic addition effect of overlapping fragments.

Fig. 460 Iatrogenic fracture at the angle of the mandible: The panoramic radiograph of a 63-year-old female reveals her condition 20 months following improperly performed extraction of tooth 38. Note especially the location of the partially impacted tooth 48, which does not exhibit a contiguous periodontal ligament space. The fracture line does not exhibit any formation of lamellar, calcified bone, the fragments are either only connective tissue or connected with woven (primitive) bone, and not yet consolidated, a situation which cannot always be clearly defined radiographically. Note also the abnormal shape and position of the fragments.

Fig. 461 Artifact resembling a fracture: This panoramic radiograph of a 6-year-old male reveals what appears to be a "step" (**arrow**) at the basal compact bone in the body of the mandible. The double-projection of tooth 46 and teeth 16 and 17 indicate that the suspected step-formation is actually an artifact caused by horizontal head movement during the radiographic exposure. Noteworthy is the vertical double formation which becomes visible due to the movement of the entire head above the image height.

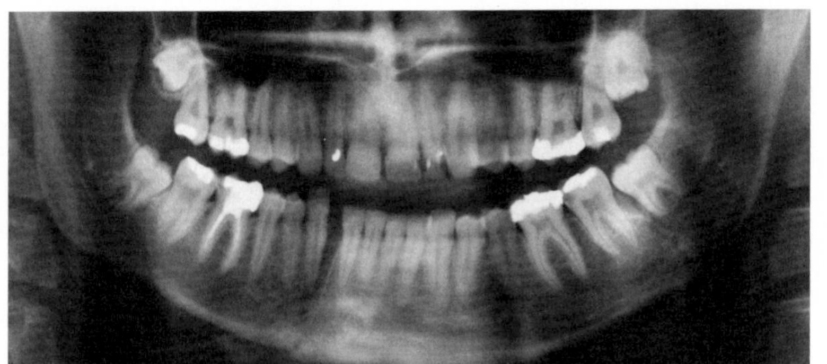

459

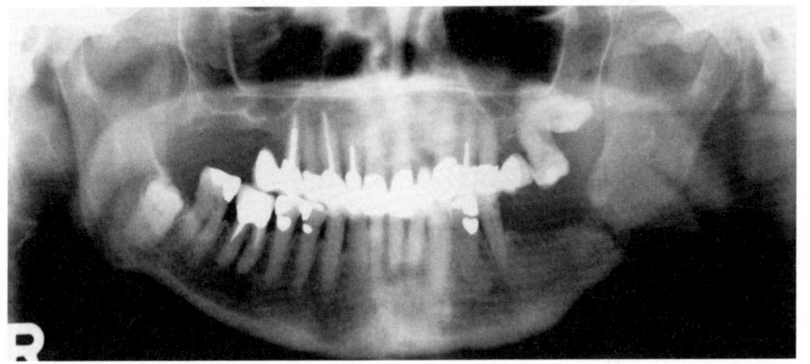

460

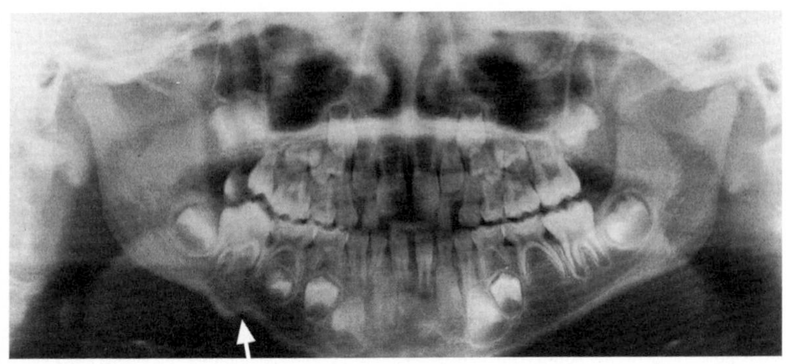

461

Furthermore, if traumatic compression causes an oblique fracture of the anterior teeth and the fragments overlap, it will be virtually impossible to discern any radiographic evidence of a continuous transverse fracture line; at best (using loupes or digital zoom) one may be able to radiographically detect a tiny step around the tooth at the site of the fracture.

The same principle applies accordingly for incomplete luxations in which the direction of luxation of the affected tooth and the projection angle of the central ray will be the determining factors with regard to diagnostic value of the radiograph. If the force causing the luxation of anterior teeth is high, it may also cause fractures of the alveolar ridge and the thin vestibular wall of the alveolus.

Fractures of premolars and molars often occur as a result of forces of mastication upon large restorations exhibiting premature contacts.

Iatrogenic **tooth fracture** can occur from use of excessive force in seating a post-and-core restoration, as well as during the extraction of multi-rooted teeth.

Fractures of the jaw frequently occur in a susceptible mandible in the form of transverse fracture of the body of the mandible, oblique or vertical fractures of the ascending ramus, deep or high collum fractures, and less frequently fractures of the coronoid process. In children and adolescents, jaw fractures frequently occur at predilection sites such as near the mandibular third molars (fracture at the angle of the mandible) or along the periodontal ligament space of tooth buds, which weaken the developing jaw.

Pathologic fractures (spontaneous fractures) may occur in the presence of any space-creating pathologic alteration of the jaws, such as cysts of all types, osteomyelitis, osteoporosis, age atrophy, or osteoradionecrosis. If one suspects fracture of the body of the mandible, both the panoramic radiograph and occlusal radiographs (see p. **58**) should be employed in order to depict all bone fragments in the third dimension. For the observation of fractures of the angle of the mandible, the ascending ramus, and the collum, conventional overview radiographs taken with maximum mouth opening (see p. **91**) are generally sufficient; in some special cases CT may be indicated.

Fig. 462 Fracture of the maxillary alveolar ridge: The panoramic radiograph of a 56-year-old male reveals fracture of the alveolar ridge with dislocation of the fragments and total luxation of tooth 22. The **arrows** pointing up indicate the fracture line; the **arrows** pointing down indicate the fundus of the alveoli of teeth 14, 13, 12, 11, and 21, which were luxated with the bone fragment. Nondislocated alveolar ridge fractures in the maxilla are often difficult to discern in a panoramic radiograph; for this reason, occlusal radiographs or CT should be employed.

Fig. 463 Mandibular fractures: The panoramic radiograph of a 58-year-old male depicts the condition following an accident. Note the transverse fracture through the body of the mandible distal to tooth 43; the root of the tooth resides in the fracture line. Note also the oblique vertical fracture of the left ascending ramus of the mandible. The wire-loop technique described by Hauptmeyer was selected for immobilization, in order to prevent movement of the fragments using intermaxillary rubber bands.

Fig. 464 Fracture of the zygomatic arch: The panoramic radiograph of a 31-year-old male reveals the zygomatic arch fracture on the left side (**right arrow**). The **left arrow** does **not** indicate a fracture line but rather a somewhat widened zygomaticotemporal suture resulting from the dislocation of the small osseous fragment. Lateral view of the slightly dislocated small fragments. An impression fracture of the zygoma cannot be ruled out using this radiographic technique; therefore a conventional axial skull projection (Grashey–Schinz, see p. **87**) or an axial CT is indicated.

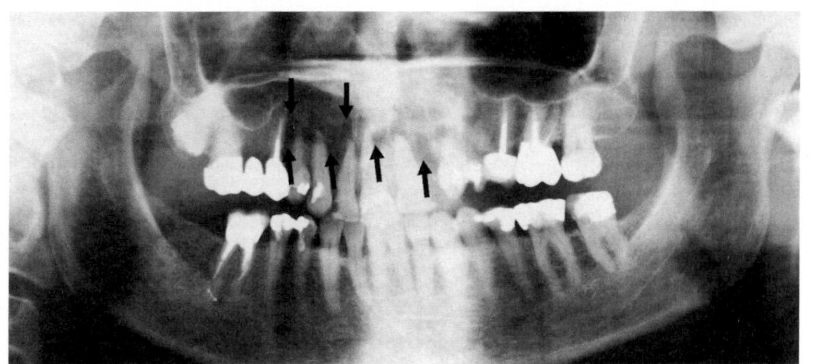
462

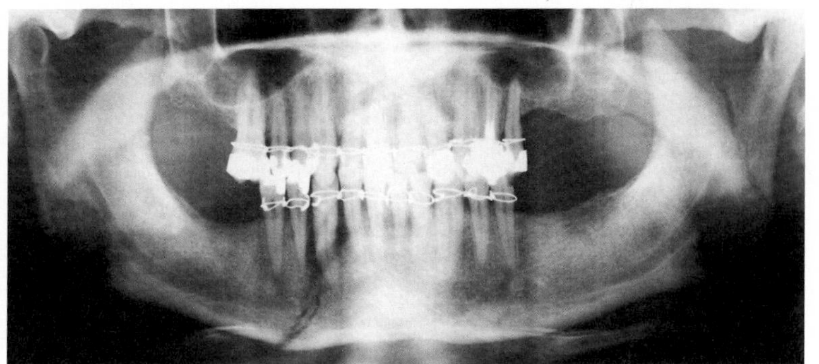
463

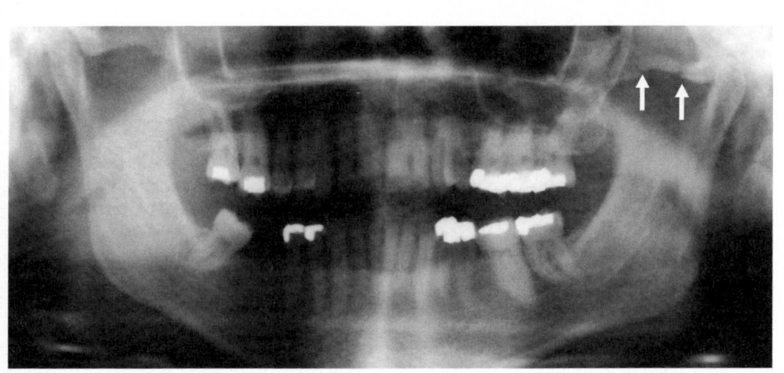
464

Maxillary fractures are less common, and usually observed as tooth fracture with accompanying fracture of the alveolar ridge. In most cases, an occlusal radiograph will adequately depict the third dimension, but only obliquely (see p. **58**).

Fresh fractures can be diagnosed radiographically because they are sharply demarcated. The exceptions to this general rule are fractures with dislocations whereby the bone fragments are superimposed upon each other. In such cases, one seldom sees a true fracture line in the radiograph, but rather enhanced radiopacity due to the addition effect.

In infractions (greenstick fractures in children) in which the periosteum is not severed and there is no dislocation, osseous fragments can completely heal without callus formation through direct contact of the fracture surfaces following neovascularization and activation of osteons. With larger dislocation of the fracture surfaces, hematoma formation is followed by progressive decalcification of bone near the fracture line, visible radiographically as poorly demarcated margins. A connective tissue callus forms, which becomes radiographically visible because of the laying down of woven bone and deposition of calcium salts. Finally, definitive healing occurs with the formation of lamellar bone.

The healing process may be delayed by unstable immobilization and by fracture line osteomyelitis. This will be radiographically visible as osseous resorptions, reactive sclerosis, and finally the formation of pseudoarthroses. An erupted tooth whose root resides within the fracture space provides an entry point for infection.

Fractures within the temporomandibular joint (TMJ) may appear as either deep or high collum fractures, but also as an intracapsular shearing fracture of the condyle. In the dental office, a normal panoramic radiograph using a bite plane projects the condyle well. Radiographs taken in habitual occlusion reveal the relationship of the condyle to the fossa somewhat better. If the fragment does not appear enlarged, the condyle is within the plane of focus. If it does appear to be enlarged that means that it is medially displaced; if it appears reduced in size it is dislocated laterally.

In earlier times, the technique described by Parma (1929) was considered important, but it is no longer used today for various reasons. The Schüller projection (1907) has for the most part been replaced in fracture diagnosis by the axial CT, which is adequate for treatment planning because three-dimensional surface reconstructions can be generated from the CT data.

Fig. 465 Pathologic (spontaneous) fracture: The panoramic radiograph of a 67-year-old male reveals a pathologic fracture (spontaneous fracture resulting from pathologic alterations) in the right mandible (**arrow**). The mandible exhibits extreme age-related atrophy that began as bone loss due to periodontitis.

Fig. 466a Pathologic fracture: The periapical radiograph reveals chronic apical periodontitis following transverse fracture of the distal root of tooth 47, as well as pulpal necrosis. The patient was unable to provide any history that would account for the fracture.

Fig. 466b Iatrogenic tooth fracture: The periapical radiograph reveals an oblique axial fracture of tooth 35, caused by improper seating of a post and core which cracked the root. Note also the area of osteolysis with reactive osteosclerosis emanating from the fracture line.

Fig. 467 Iatrogenic tooth fracture: The panoramic radiograph reveals a root fragment in the dorsal wall of the right maxillary sinus (**arrow**). The root fracture occurred during extraction of tooth 16, whose root tip was in intimate contact with the floor of the maxillary sinus. During the attempt to remove the root fragment, it was forced into the sinus.

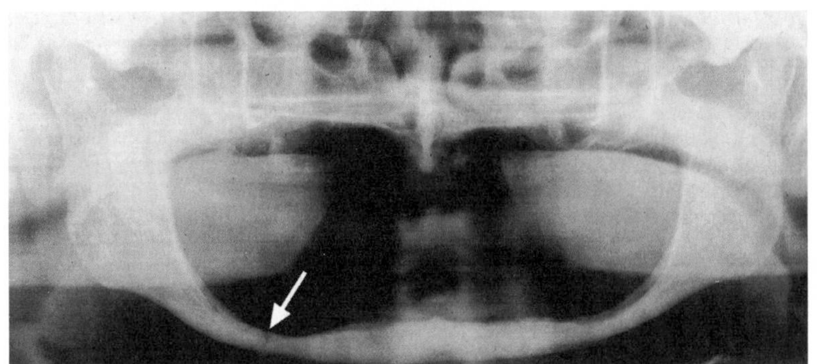

465

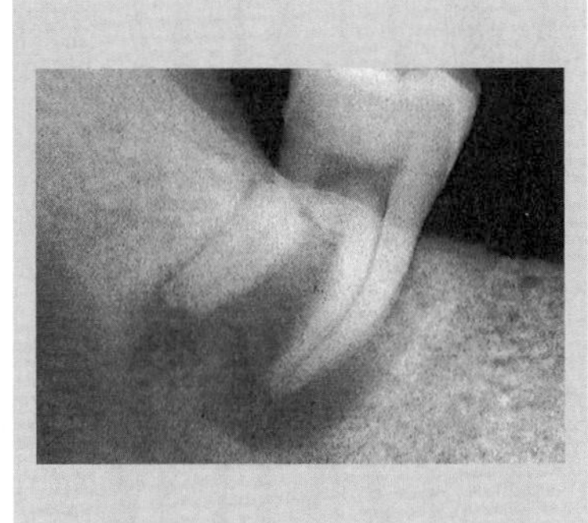

466a

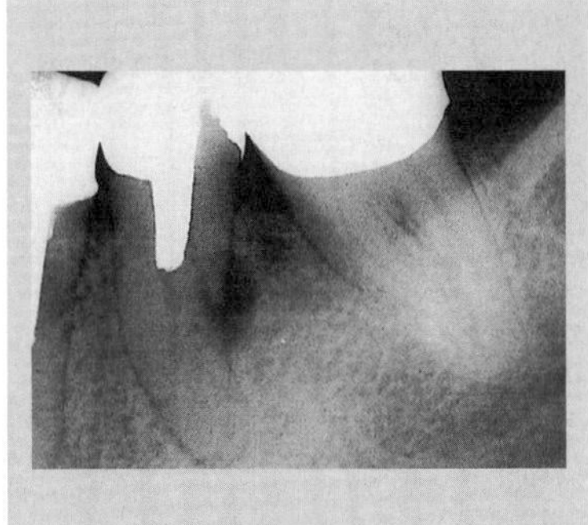

466b

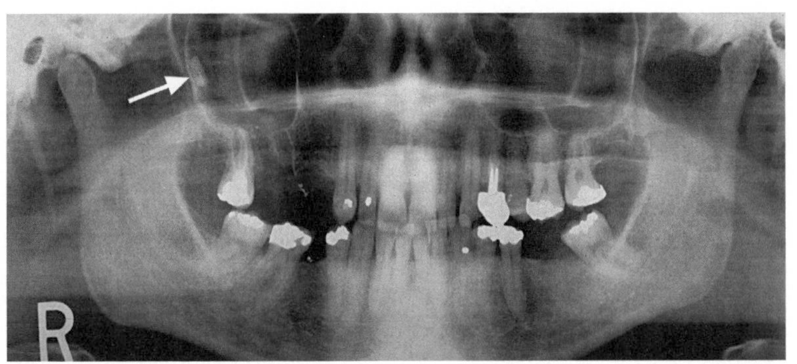

467

Luxations within the TMJ can be documented using panoramic radiography. There are some clinical manifestations of TMJ luxation that only seldom even require radiographic examination, for example following trauma or in the cases of discopathy.

TMJ luxation, unilaterally or bilaterally, may occur because of looseness or "play" within the joint capsule; such luxations can usually be clinically repositioned by hand. TMJ luxations may also be observed in cases of mandibulo-acroteric dysplasia or the Hajdu–Cheney Syndrome, both of which are associated with looseness within the joint capsule. TMJ luxations in which the condyle (with or without the disk) becomes ventrally displaced over the articular eminence can usually not be successfully examined in the dental practice because the disk itself can only be successfully visualized using magnetic resonance imaging and not by means of conventional radiography. Central luxations are only rarely observed, usually in cases of severe compression fractures; these must be examined using CT or MRI.

Fig. 468 Multiple facial skeletal fractures: The panoramic radiograph depicts multiple injuries to the facial skeleton, resulting from a traffic accident. Visible even in this image are bilateral collum fractures, an oblique and a transverse fracture of the body of the mandible on the right side, depressed fractures right and left of the zygomatic bone, midface fractures in the region of the nose, the nasal sinuses and the floor of the orbit, maxillary fracture on the right side and numerous tooth fractures. The **arrows** indicate those fracture lines that could be detected despite the summation effects associated with panoramic radiography.

Fig. 469 Selected axial slices from the CT: Same patient as Fig. **468**. **Left:** The axial CT at the level of the palatal vault shows particularly well the maxillary fracture on the right side, the fractures through the right maxillary sinus and the bilateral hematosinus. **Right:** This axial slice reveals the numerous fractures in the depth of the midface in the third dimension; conventional spiral tomography cannot depict such lesions with this degree of overview and clarity.

Fig. 470 Selected coronal reconstructions: Same case as above. These coronal reconstructions reveal: **Left:** Deep collum fracture on the right and collum fracture on the left with displacement of the small fragments medially (in a panoramic radiograph, the condyle lying medial and distant to the image receptor would appear enlarged) (see Fig. **468**). **Right:** The coronal CT reveals the numerous fractures within the depth of the midface, and a massive hematoma in the nasal cavity and in the paranasal sinuses. The maxillary fracture at the palatal vault is clearly visible from this view in the frontal plane.

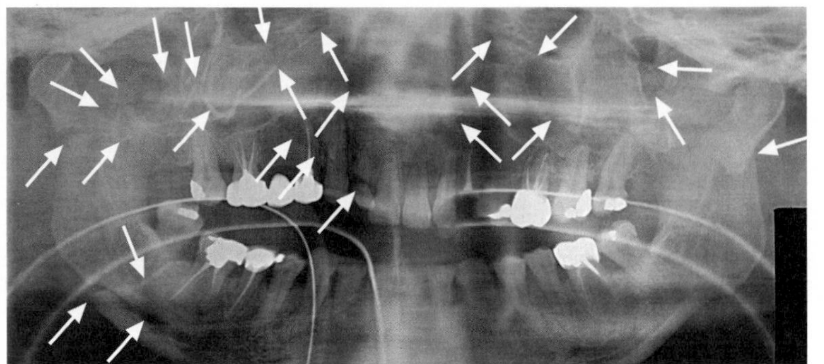

468

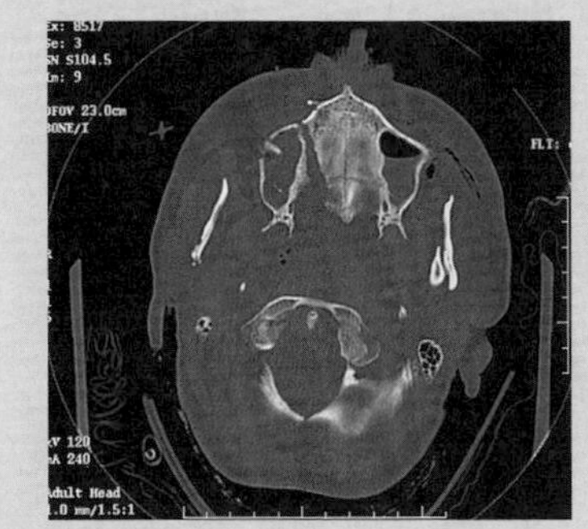
Se: 3
SN S104.5
FLT:

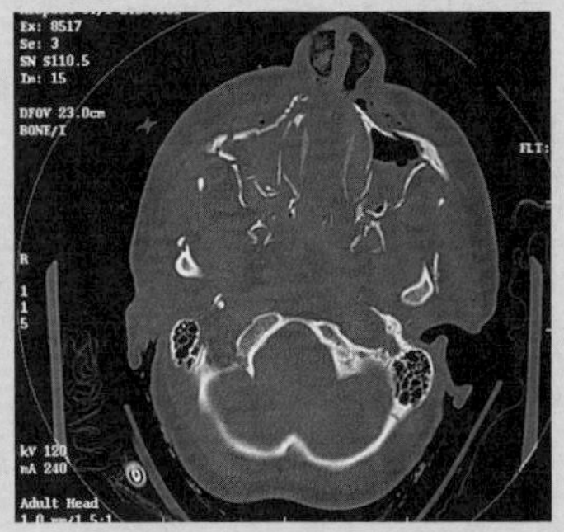
Ex: 8517
Se: 3
SN S110.5
Im: 15
DFOV 23.0cm
BONE/I
FLT:
R
kV 120
mA 240
Adult Head

469

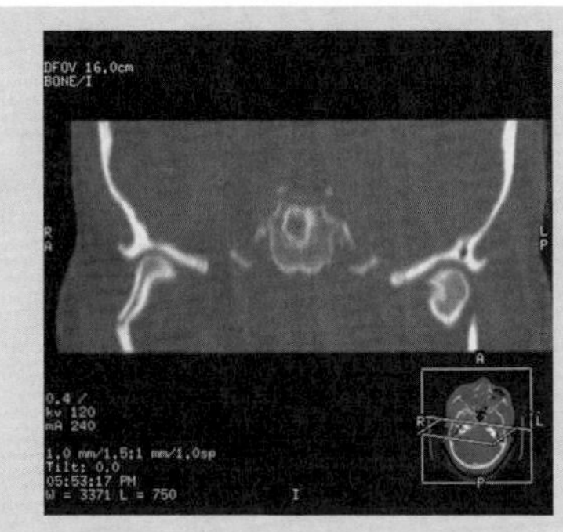
DFOV 16.0cm
BONE/I
kv 120
mA 240
1.0 mm/1.5:1 mm/1.0sp
Tilt: 0.0
05:53:17 PM
W = 3371 L = 750

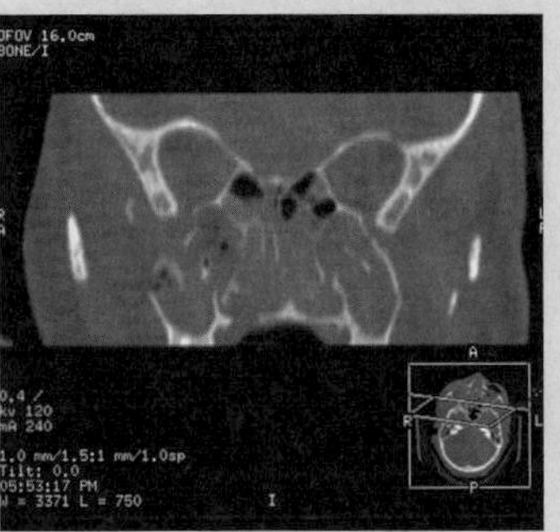
kv 120
mA 240
1.0 mm/1.5:1 mm/1.0sp
Tilt: 0.0
05:53:17 PM
W = 3371 L = 750

470

Radiographs will often reveal foreign bodies that have become lodged in bone or in surrounding soft tissues as a result of work, sport-related, or other accidents. More often one observes dental materials or instrument fragments that have become lodged in the jaws or the teeth as a result of iatrogenic errors or untoward events during dental treatment. Less frequently one may observe materials that have been placed into the jaws or facial soft tissues for cosmetic or radiotherapeutic purposes. Radiographic interpretation may also be impaired by a patient's jewelry or sections of the protective lead vest that may be projected onto the radiograph; such problems were discussed in the chapter on radiographic errors.

When preparing this chapter, it seemed reasonable to combine the often extraordinary depiction of foreign bodies with some of the more frequent therapeutic errors in order to underscore the potential *forensic* significance of radiography, and to enunciate the very basic necessity for radiographic perfection from the point-of-view of quality assurance. On the other hand, it was not possible in this short chapter to completely describe and illustrate this very important area and therefore the selection of cases is intended to stimulate additional curiosity on the part of the reader, and makes no claim to completeness.

The quality and comprehensiveness of the initial patient examination, and therewith the most basic documentation of the status quo play very important roles in quality assurance and radiation protection in the dental practice arena, a role that is equal in importance even to the well-considered selection of necessary radiographs during the individual treatment phases. A well-thought-out radiographic examination, i.e., an examination strategy, reduces not only the radiation exposure dose for the patient, but reduces also the costs, while reducing unnecessary work load in the dental practice.

Fig. 471 Foreign body: The panoramic radiograph reveals root canal filling material that extruded during endodontic treatment of teeth 25 and 26 and which was forced into the maxillary sinus where it wandered into the craniodorsal recess of the sinus (**arrow**); this also led to the development of aspergillosis (see also Fig. **327**). Note also the depiction of impacted teeth 38 and 48. The appearance is a view along the tooth long axis of these third molars, indicating that both are horizontally impacted beneath the retromolar trigone (cf. Fig. **175a**).

Fig. 472 Foreign bodies: Because of overfilling of the mesial root of tooth 48 during endodontic therapy, filling material was forced through the roof of the mandibular canal; the patient experienced paresthesia. Note also the compound odontoma with microdonts in the retromolar regions 19 (!) and 29 (!).

Fig. 473a Foreign body: This section from a panoramic radiograph reveals radiopaque root canal filling material on the floor of the left maxillary sinus; it emanated from overfilling the root canal of tooth 25.

Fig. 473b Foreign body: Following inferior alveolar nerve block anesthesia, the dentist first extracted tooth 38 and then seated a crown on tooth 37; unfortunately a large mass of cement flowed into the empty alveolus. This radiograph, taken several weeks later, clearly shows the signs of bone resorption and the simultaneous osseous reaction with delayed wound healing.

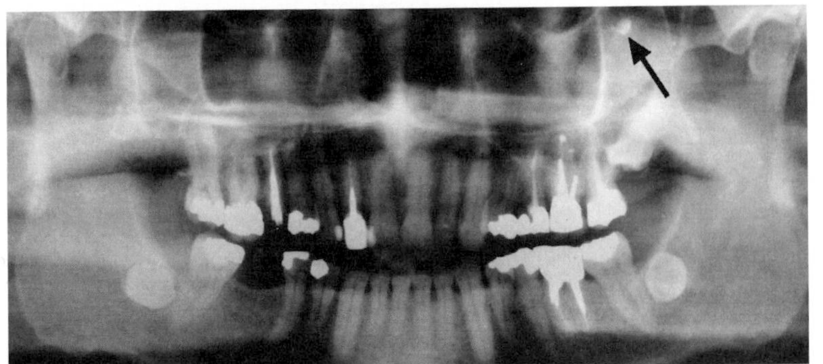

471

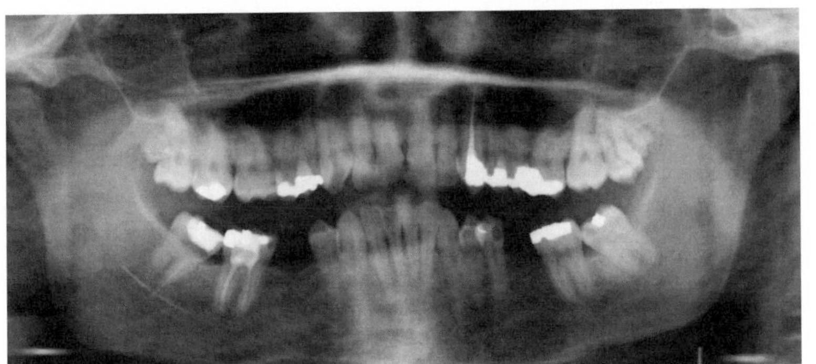

472

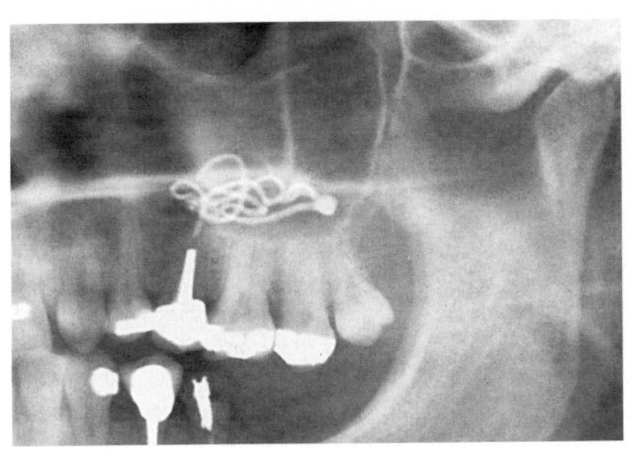

473 a

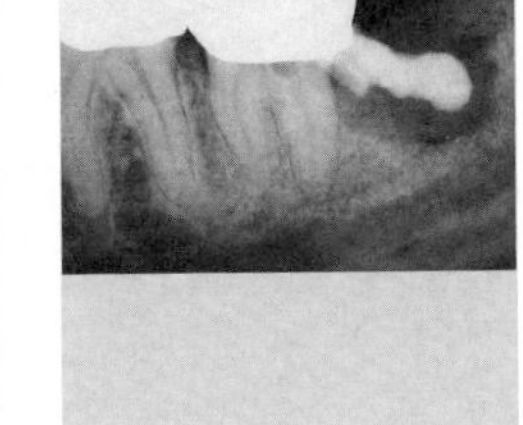

473 b

The optimization of the exposure settings necessary for diagnosis and therapy will be achieved only through proper indication and perfect and wherever possible *standardized* radiographic technique; such technique must be regularly checked and corrected through self-critical control radiographs in order to consistently achieve the highest image quality. In addition to the potentially serious problem of prevention of excess radiation exposure, and with regard for statutory responsibilities and quality assurance, the dentist should also be cognizant of the right of each patient to see and consider all entries in his/her patient chart. Patients are effectively lay persons in terms of knowledge of dental treatment methods and above all the possibilities for complications; patients require information which, when provided effectively, will increase trust in the treatment plan while simultaneously motivating the patient toward full cooperation. In the area of radiographic diagnosis, the old adage "a picture is worth a thousand words" takes on enhanced meaning when the patient is seated in front of the computer screen (digital radiographs) or the viewbox (conventional films) to truly understand the oral/dental problems at hand.

For various reasons—some obvious—the radiographs depicted in this chapter are not accompanied any clinical or personal data.

Additional examples in the area of "foreign bodies" can be found in the chapter dealing with technical errors when taking panoramic or intraoral radiographs.

Fig. 474 **Foreign bodies:** Subperiosteal implant with bone resorption on the left side of the mandible. Note also the arch-shaped radiopacity that was caused by the patient's necklace.

Fig. 475 **Foreign bodies:** Rare (bizarre!) form of subperiosteal implants from the early days of dental implantology, clearly exhibiting bone resorption in the maxilla.

Fig. 476 **Foreign bodies:** Subperiosteal implant in the anterior segment of the mandible, with obvious bone resorption around the vertical pillars; clinically, the patient had noticed paresthesia on the left side (mental foramen!).

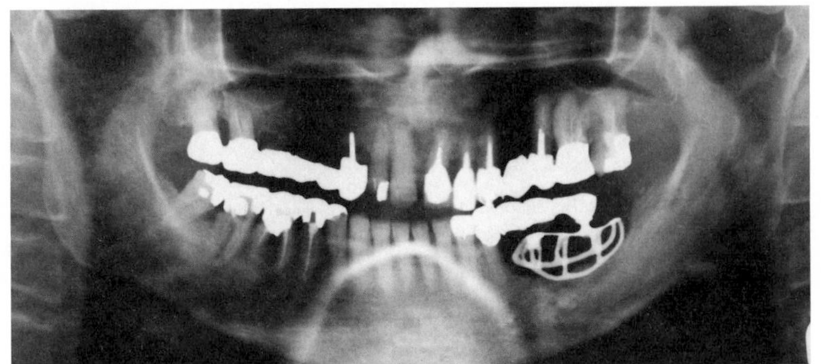

474

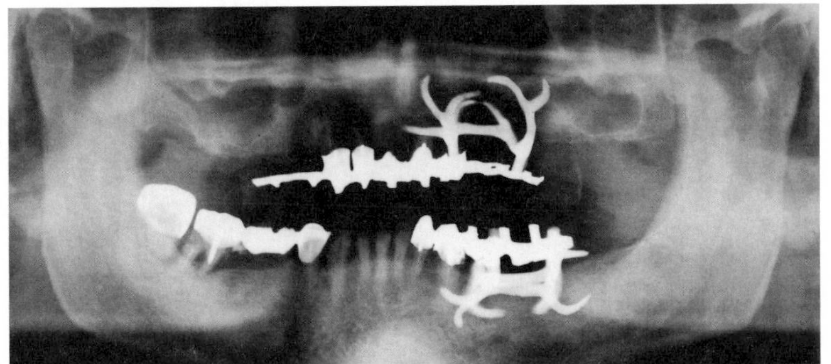

475

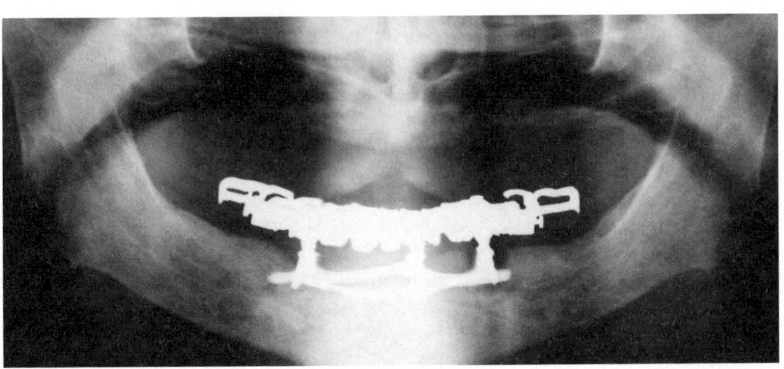

476

Fig. 477 **Foreign bodies:** Implants with transdental fixations; note resorptions of the abutment roots, additional pin implants, and a bar-type construction to support a partial denture.

Fig. 478 a, b **Foreign bodies:** The section from a panoramic radiograph (**a**) and the supplemental occlusal view of the chin region (**b**) reveal the transosseous implants and bone screws; these types of screws are usually employed for fixation of bone fragments in the extremities. Noteworthy is a chronic sclerosing osteomyelitis with osseous resorption and formation of a sequester. Mounted on the screws are custom metal crowns connected by a bar to retain a partial denture.

Fig. 479 **Foreign bodies:** The panoramic radiograph reveals a poorly constructed wire loop osteosynthesis attempt that was made following an accident that caused a depressed fracture of the zygoma as well as fracture of the zygomatic arch on the right side.

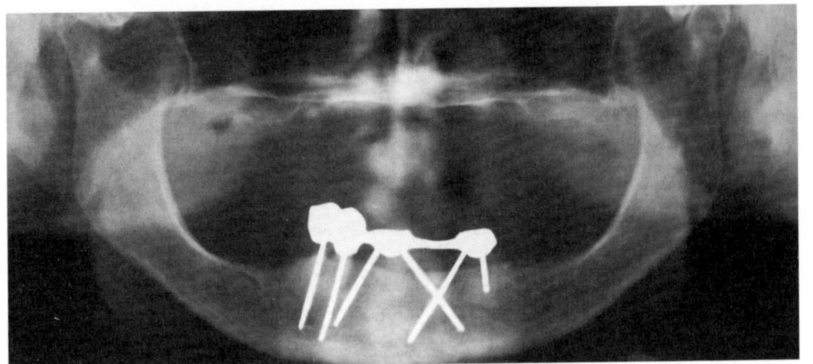

477

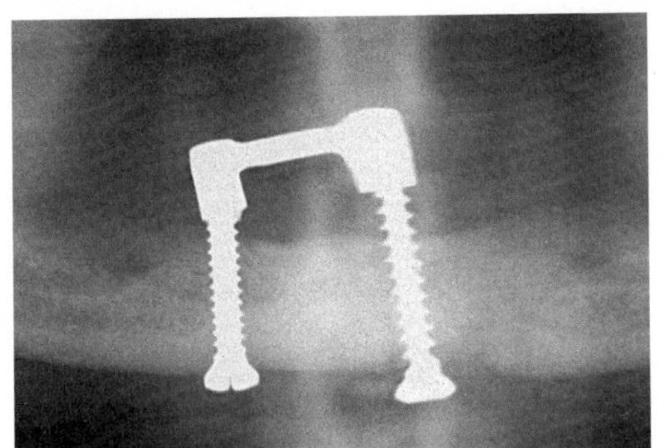

478 a

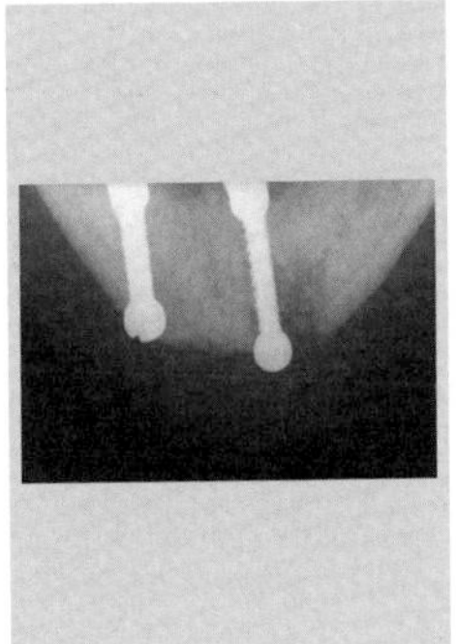

478 b

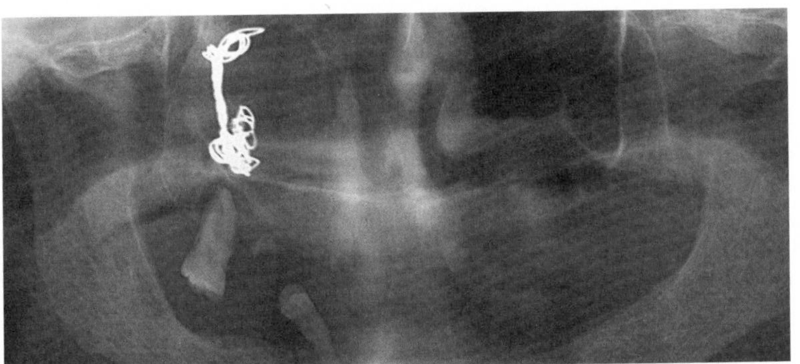

479

Fig. 480a Foreign bodies: This periapical radiograph was taken immediately after placing an amalgam restoration in tooth 34 and shows amalgam particles that were in the oral vestibulum. Because of the radiographic summation effect the amalgam appears to be within the alveolar bone.

Fig. 480b Foreign bodies: This section from a panoramic radiograph reveals an amalgam particle within the body of the mandible; the particle is surrounded by a radiolucent zone and a zone of reactive sclerosis. This situation resulted from the extraction of tooth 46 years previously when a particle of amalgam from the restoration lodged in the mesial alveolus and remained there without clinical symptoms.

Fig. 481a Foreign bodies: This section from a conventional chest radiograph clearly shows that during an oral intubation procedure an anterior bridge was dislodged and subsequently aspirated (**arrow**).

Fig. 481b Foreign bodies: The periapical radiograph shows the endodontically treated tooth 22 with a periapical radiolucency, and also the post-and-core restoration that was seated altogether improperly, so that the post protruded into the alveolar bone where an osteomyelitis was occasioned.

Fig. 482a Foreign bodies: This section from a conventional radiograph of the lumbar vertebrae reveals a swallowed root canal instrument (**arrow**). There are reports that eating sauerkraut or asparagus will enhance passage of such a foreign body through the intestinal tract!

Fig. 482b Foreign bodies: The periapical radiograph reveals a root canal file “searching for” the root canal in the distal root of tooth 47!

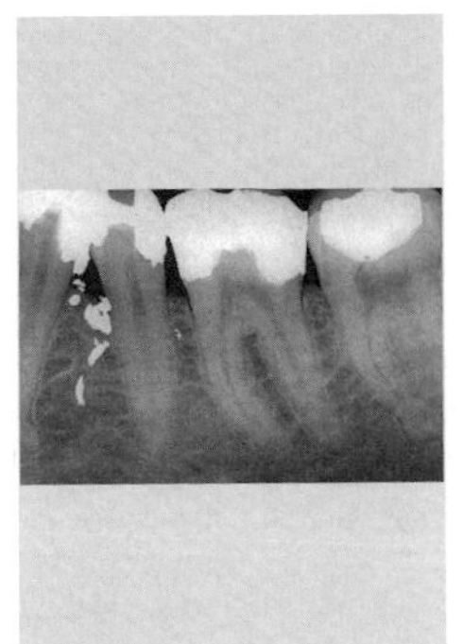

480 a

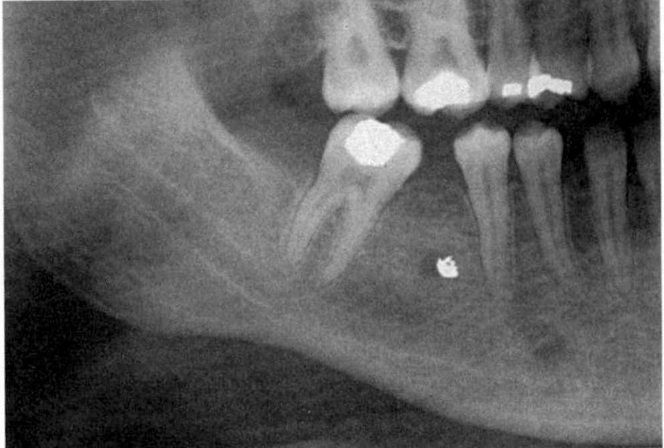

480 b

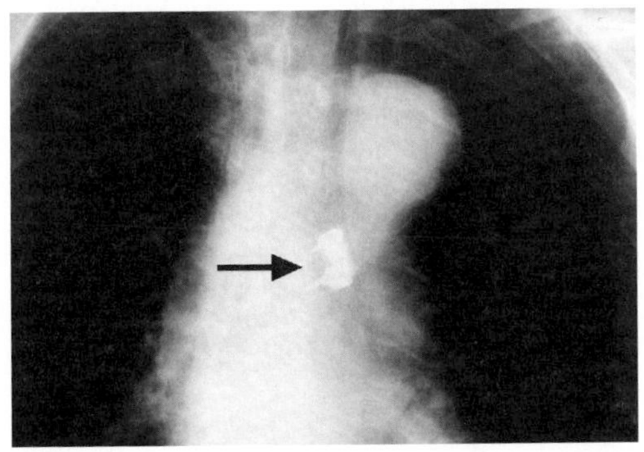

481 a

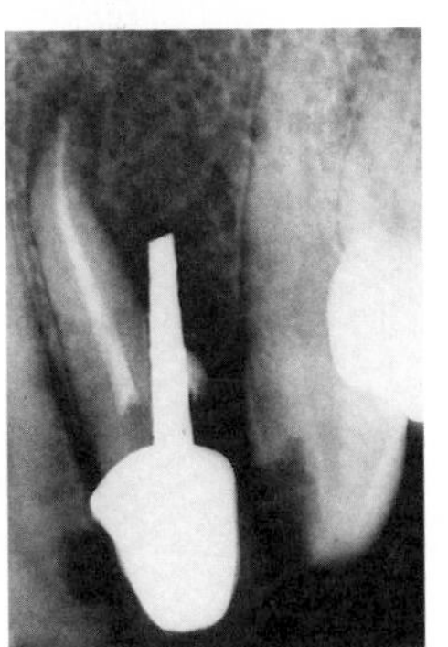

481 b

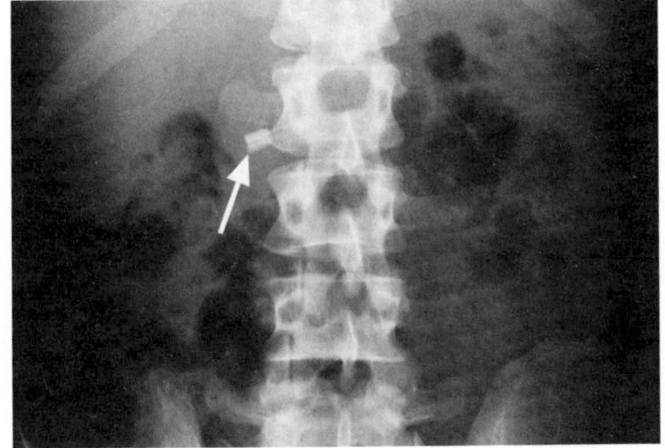

482 a

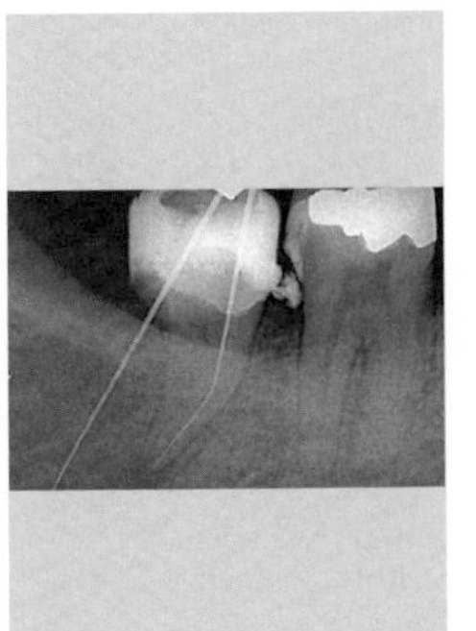

482 b

Fig. 483 Foreign bodies: This panoramic radiograph of a 17-year-old female reveals root fragments of deciduous teeth 75 and 85, with persisting deciduous teeth 55 and 65, as well as delayed eruption of teeth 17, 15, 13, 23, 25, 27, 37, and 47.

Fig. 484 Foreign bodies: This panoramic radiograph reveals the condition following a hunting accident shotgun blast. The metal spheres imbedded in the right half of the face do not appear enlarged and are sharply demarcated, which indicates that they are close to the image receptor and therefore within the soft tissues. No dental injuries can be noted.

Fig. 485 a Foreign bodies: This section from a panoramic radiograph reveals radium needles (usually radium 226), which were placed to provide radiation therapy for a malignant tumor of the parotid gland.

Fig. 485 b Foreign bodies: The periapical radiograph shows an amalgam build-up restoration incorporating parapulpal pins on tooth 46. The mesial pin penetrated the tooth at the cementoenamel junction and elicited an iatrogenic marginal periodontitis with a bony pocket and reactive sclerosis of the alveolar bone.

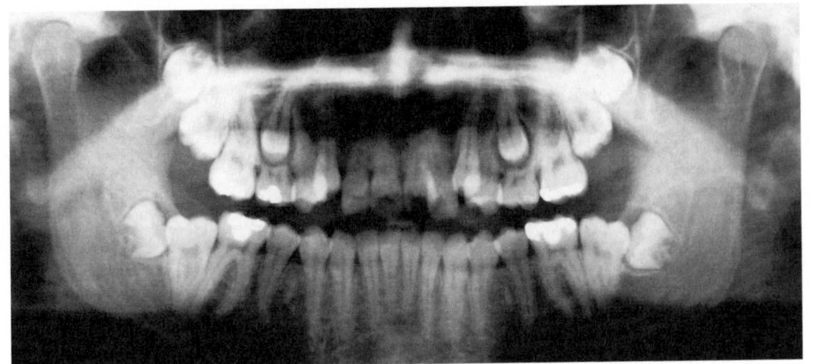

483

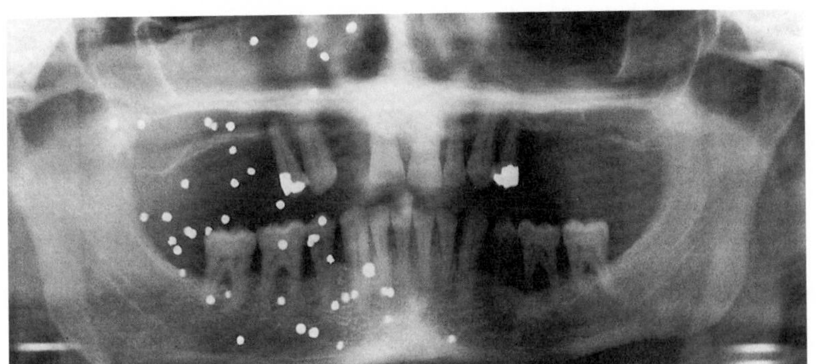

484

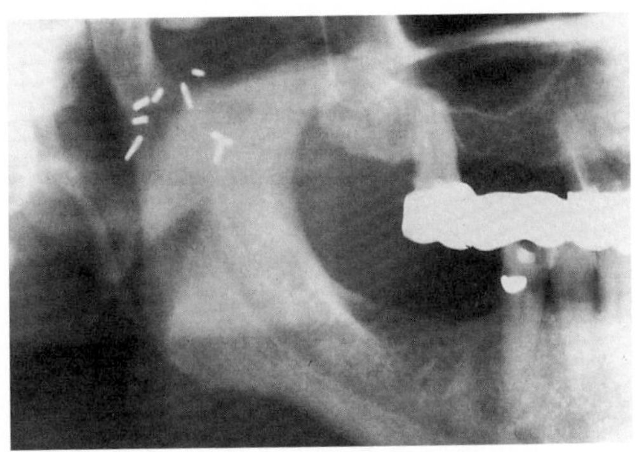

485 a

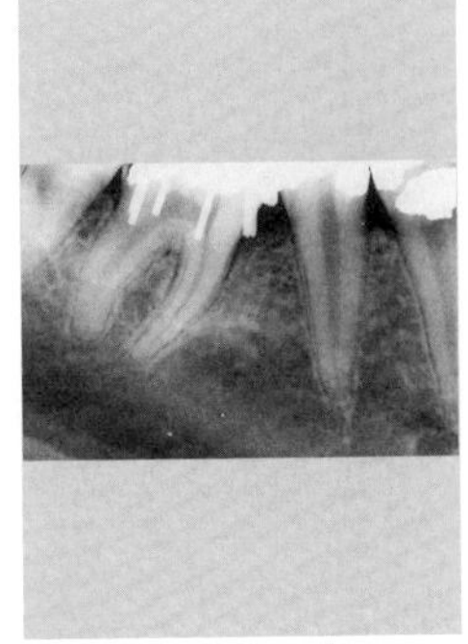

485 b

A

Abrahams JJ, Kalyanpur A. Dental implants and dental CT software programs. *Semin Ultrasound CT MR*. 1995;16:468–486.

Adam G, Drobnitzky M, Nolte-Ernsting CCA,Günther RW. Optimizing joint imaging: MR imaging techniques. *Eur Radiol*. 1996;6:882–889.

Agence Nationale D'Accréditation et d'Evaluation en Santé (ANAES). Information des patients: recommandations destinées aux médecins. *Rev Prat Med Gen*. 2000;14:1053–1055.

Akesson L, Rohlin M, Hakansson J. Marginal bone in periodontal disease: an evaluation of image quality in panoramic and intra-oral radiography. *Dentomaxillofac Radiol*. 1989;18:105.

American Academy of Oral and Maxillofacial Radiology. Radiology Practice Committee. Updated quality assurance self-assessment exercise in intraoral and panoramic radiography. *Oral Surg Oral Med Oral Pathol*. 2000;89:369–374.

Andersen L, Fejerskov O, Philipsen HP. Oral giant cell granulomas. *Acta Pathol Microbiol Scand*. 1973;81:606–616.

Arai Y, Tammisalo E, Iwai K, Hashimoto K, Shinoda K. Development of a compact computer tomographic apparatus for dental use. 1999;28:245–248.

Araki K, Matsuda Y, Okano T, Webber RL, Ojanperä J. Tomographic slice thickness of a prototype (Ortho TACT), X-ray system. In: Lemke HU, Vannier MW, Inamura K, Farman A, eds. Computer assisted radiology CARS '99. Amsterdam: Elsevier; 1999:972–976.

Aroua A, Vader J-P, Burnand B, Valley J-F. Enquête sur l'exposition de la population suisse par le radiodiagnostic. *Méd Hyg*. 2000;58:1480–1481.

B

Beck-Mannagetta J, Zischka A, Kiesler J, Ienberger T. Benigne und maligne neoplastische Veränderungen im Bereich des Kiefergelenks. *Acta Chir Austriaca*. ISSN 0001-544-X. 1997.

Beir V. Health effects of exposure to low level ionizing radiation. National Research Council, Committee on the Biological Effects of Ionizing Radiation. Washington, D. C.: National Academy Press; 1990.

Bergmann F, Krug R. Esthetic Implantology: Spezialaufbauten und Planung sind Voraussetzung. *Frialog*. 1999;11:1–3.

Bertrand P, Dechaume M, Lacronique G. *Radiographie Bucco-Dentaire*. Paris: Editions Masson; 1950.

Beyer D, Herzog M, Zanella FE, Bohndorf K, Walter E, Hüls A. *Röntgendiagnostik von Zahn- und Kiefererkrankungen*. Berlin: Springer; 1987.

Blankestijn J, Panders AK, Vermey A, Scherpbier AJJA. Synovial chondromatosis of the temporomandibular joint. *J Maxillofac Surg*. 1985;13:32.

Bohner P, Holler C, Haßfeld S. Operation planning in craniomaxillo-facial surgery. *Comput Aided Surg*. 1997;2:153–161.

Borchers J. Dokumentationssysteme. In: Ewen K, ed. *Moderne Bildgebung. Physic, Gerätetechnik, Bildbearbeitung und -kommunikation, Strahlenschutz, Qualitätskontrolle*. Stuttgart: Thieme; 1998a:223–234.

Borchers J. Grundbegriffe der Medizininformatik. In: Ewen K, ed. *Moderne Bildgebung. Physic, Gerätetechnik, Bildbearbeitung und -kommunikation, Strahlenschutz, Qualitätskontrolle*. Stuttgart: Thieme; 1998b: 235–246.

Bredemeier S. *Untersuchungen zur Strahlenexposition des Patienten bei konventionellen und digitalen Panorama-Schichtaufnahmen* [dissertation]. Göttingen; 1999.

Brochhagen HG, Lazar F, Zaika Z, et al. Dental-CT des Unterkiefers bei retinierten Weisheitszähnen – Lokalisation des Canalis mandibularis und postoperative Komplikationen am Nervus alveolaris inferior nach Zahnextraktion. *Fortschr Röntgenstr*. 1999;170:34–35.

Bschorer R, Fuhrmann A, Gehrke G, Keese E, Uffelmann U. Die Darstellung des Canalis mandibulae mit der Unterkieferquerschnitt-Panoramaschichttechnik. *Dtsch Zahnärztl Z*. 1993;48:786.

Bukal J, Schwenzer N, Oswald J, Remagen W, Prein J. Fibröse Dysplasie – ossifizierendes Fibrom. In: Pfeifer G, Schwenzer N, eds. *Fortschritte der Kiefer- und Gesichts-Chirurgie*. Vol 31. Stuttgart: Thieme; 1986.

C

Cavézian R, Pasquet G. Techniques de radiologie dentaire. Éditions Techniques. *Encycl Med Chir.* Paris. Radiodiagnostic Squelette normal. 1992;30850 A10:18.

Cavézian R, Pasquet G, Thibierge M, Cabanis EA. Justice et imagerie en Odonto-stomatologie. De la responsabilité médicale à la radiologie maxillo-dentaire. *Actual Odonto-Stomat*. 1993;182: 291–311.

Cavézian R, Pasquet G, Bell G, Baller G. Imagerie dento-maxillaire. 2nd ed. Paris: Masson; 2001.

Chen SK, Hollender L. Frequency domain analysis of cross-sectional images of the posterior mandible. *Oral Surg Oral Med Oral Pathol*. 1994;77:290.

Cieszyński A. Zahnärztliche Röntgenologie. 2nd ed. Leipzig: JA Barth; 1926.

Cohnen M, Cohnen B, Koch JA, et al. Möglichkeiten der Dosisreduktion bei koronarer Spiral-CT des Mittelgesichts. *Aktuelle Radiol*. 1998;8:34–39.

Conover GL, Hildebolt CF, Yokoyama-Crothers N. Comparison of linear measurements made from storage phosphor and dental radiographs. 1996;25:268–273.

Conseil d'état. Rapport public 1998: jurisprudence et avis de 1997. Réflexions sur le droit et la santé.

Coonar H. Primary intraosseous carcinoma of maxilla. *Br Dent J*. 1979;147:47.

Costen JB. Syndrome of ear and sinus symptoms dependent upon disturbed function of the temporomandibular joint. *Ann Oto Rhino Laryngol*. 1934;43:1–15.

D

Dammann F, Momingo-Traserra E, Remy C, et al. Strahlenexposition bei der Spiral-CT der Nasennebenhöhlen. *Fortschr Röntgenstr.* 2000;172:232–237.

Dammert S, Funke M, Neumann D, Merten A, Grabbe E. Optimierung der Aufnahme- und Rekonstruktionsparameter in der Mehrschicht Spiral-CT zur Untersuchung des knöchernen Mittelgesichts. *Fortschr Röntgenstr.* 2000;172:153.

Danforth RA, Clark DE. Effective dose from radiation absorbed during a panoramic examination with a new generation machine. *Oral Surg Oral Med Oral Pathol*. 2000;89:236–243.

Dayan D, Buchner A, Gosky M, Harel-Raviv M. The peripheral odontogenic keratocyst. *Int J Oral Maxillofac Surg*. 1988;17:81–83.

Décret n° 98-1186 du 24 décembre 1998 modifiant le décret n° 86-1103 du 2 octobre 1986 modifié relatif à la protection des travailleurs contre les dangers des rayonnements ionisants. *J Officiel de la République Française*. 1998;229:19555. (see: http://admin.net/jo/19981226/).

Dermaut LR, Demunck A. Apical root resorption on upper incisors caused by intrusive tooth movement: a radiographic study:. *Am J Orthod Dentofac Orthop*. 1986;90:321–326.

Dolwick MF, Katzberg RW, Helms CA. Internal derangements of the temporomandibular joint: Fact or fiction? *J Prosthet Dent*. 1983;49:415–418.

Drace JE, Enzmann DR. Defining the normal temporomandibular joint: closed-, partially open-, and open-mouth MR imaging of asymptomatic subjects. *Radiology*. 1990;177:67–71.

Düker J. Röntgendiagnostik mit der Panoramaschichtaufnahme. 2nd ed. Heidelberg: Hüthig; 2000.

E

Eickholz P, Riess T, Lenhard M, Hassfeld S, Staehle HJ. Digital radiography of interproximal bone loss: validity of different filters. *J Clin Periodontal*. 1999;26:294–300.

Ekestubbe A, Gröndahl K, Ekholm S, Johansson PE, Grondahl HG. Low-dose tomographic techniques for dental implant planning. *Int J Oral Maxillofac Implants*. 1996;11:650–659.

Ekestubbe A. Conventional spiral and low-dose computed mandibular tomography for dental implant planning. *Swed Dent J Suppl.* 1999;138:1–82.

Ekestubbe A, Thilander A, Gröndahl HG. Absorbed doses and energy imparted from tomography for dental implant installation. Spiral tomography using the Scanora technique compared with hypocycloidal tomography. *Dentomaxillofac Radiol.* 1992;21:65–69.

Ekestubbe A, Thilander A, Gröndahl K, Gröndahl HG. Absorbed doses from computed tomography for dental implant surgery: comparison with conventional tomography. *Dentomaxillofac Radiol.* 1993;22:13–17.

Evans Jr FO et al. Sinusitis of the maxillary antrum. *N Engl J Med.* 1975;293:735.

Eversole LR. *Clinical Outline of Oral Pathology.* Philadelphia: Lea & Febiger; 1984.

F

Faculty of General Dental Practitioner (UK), The Royal College of Surgeons of England. *Selection Criteria for Dental Radiography.* Nottingham: Penn Advertising & Marketing; 1998.

Farman AG, Farman TT. RVG-ui. A sensor to rival direct-exposure intra-oral X-ray film. *Int J Comput Dent.* 1999;2:183–196.

Farman AG, Farman TT. Evaluation of a new F speed dental x-ray film. The effect of processing solutions and a comparison with D and E speed films. *Dentomaxillofac Radiol.* 2000;29:41–45.

Favre-Dauvergne E, Auriol M, Le Charpentier Y. Kystes des maxillaires. *Encycl. Med. Chir., Editions Techniques.* Paris; 1994. Stomatologie 1. 22–062–G10.6p.

Favre-Dauvergne E, Auriol M, Le Charpentier Y. Tumeurs odontogéniques. *Encycl. Med. Chir., Editions Techniques.* Paris; 1995. Stomatologie 1. 22–062–F10.10p.

Favre-Dauvergne E, Auriol M, Fleuridas G, Le Charpentier Y. Tumeurs et pseudo-tumeurs non odontogéniques bénignes des maxillaires. *Encycl. Med. Chir., Éditions Techniques.* Paris; 1995. Stomatologie 1. 22–062–H10.11p.

Fireman SM, Noyek AM. Dental anatomy and radiology of the maxillary sinus. Symposium on the maxillary sinus. *Otolaryngol Clin Am.* 1976;9:83.

Fischbach R, Lin Y, Heindel W, Friedrich R, Brochhagen HG. Vergleich der Kernspintomographie und der Funkionsarthrographie bei Patienten mit Kiefergelenkgeräuschen. *Zentralbl Radiol.* 1993;147:830.

Freyschmidt J. *Knochenerkrankungen im Erwachsenenalter.* Berlin: Springer; 1986a.

Freyschmidt J. *Skeletterkrankungen.* 2nd ed. Berlin: Springer; 1997.

Friedlander AH, Friedlander IK. Panoramic dental radiography: An aid in detecting individuals prone to stroke. *Br Dent J.* 1996;181:1.

Fuhrmann A, Rother U. Improved cross-sectional images with rotational panoramic radiography (Siemens Orthophos) [abstract]. *5th European Congress on Dental and Maxillo-facial Radiology.* November 1995.

Fuhrmann A, Bücker A, Diedrich P. Radiologisch-mikroskopische Interpretation des horizontalen Knochenabbaus. *Dtsch Zahnärztl Z.* 1995a;50:594–598.

Fuhrmann A, Klein HM, Wehrbein H, Günther RW, Diedrich P. Hochauflösende Computertomographie fazialer und oraler Knochendehiszenzen. *Dtsch Zahnärztl Z.* 1993;48:242–246.

Fuhrmann RAW, Schnappauf A, Diedrich PR. Three-dimensional imaging of craniomaxillofacial structures with a standard personal comp. *Dentomaxillofac Radiol.* 1995b;24:260–263.

G

Gahleitner A, Nasel C, Schick S, et al. Dentale Magnetresonanztomographie (Dental-MRT) als Verfahren zur Darstellung des maxillomandibulären Zahnhalteapparates. *Fortschr Röntgenstr.* 1998;169:424–428.

Gahleitner A, Solar P, Nasel C, et al. Die Magnetresonanztomographie in der Dentalradiologie (Dental-MRT). *Radiologe.* 1999;39:1044–1050.

Gardner EJ. A genetic and clinical study of intestinal polyposis, a predisposing factor for carcinoma of the colon and rectum. *Am J Hum Genet* 1951;3:167–176.

Ghanem N, Altehoefer C, Högerle S, Moser E, Langer M. Vergleichende diagnostische Wertigkeit der MRT und Knochenmarkszintigraphie bei ossären Metastasen von soliden Tumoren. *Fortschr Röntgenstr.* 2000;172:59.

Gher ME, Richardson AC. The accuracy of dental radiographic techniques used for evaluation of implant fixture placement. *Int J Periodontics Restor Dent.* 1995;15:268–283.

Gibiliso JA. *Stafne's Oral Radiographic Diagnosis*. Philadelphia: Saunders; 1985.

Giedion A. Konstitutionell-genetische Skeletterkrankungen. In: Frommhold W, Dihlmann W, Stender H-St, Thurn P, Schinz HR, eds. *Radiologische Diagnostik.* Vol VI/2. Stuttgart: Thieme; 1991.

Goaz PW, White SC. *Oral Radiology*. St. Louis: Mosby; 1987.

Gorlin RJ, et al. The multiple basal-cell nevi syndrome. *Cancer.* 1965;18:89.

Gorlin RJ, Cohen MM, Levin LS. Syndrome of the Head and Neck. 3rd ed. London: Oxford University Press; 1990.

Gorlin RJ. Nevoid basal cell carcinoma syndrome. *Derm Clin.* 1995;13:1.

Grobovschek M, Schurich H, Pilz P. Osteoidfibrom. *Fortschr Röntgenstr.* 1982;136:171.

Gröndahl K, Ekestubbe A, Gröndahl HG. *Radiography in Oral Endosseous Prosthetics*. Göteborg: Nobel Biocare AB; 1996.

H

Hallikainen D, Gröndahl HG, Kanerva H, Tammisalo E. *Optimized Sequential Dentomaxillofacial Radiography. The Scanora® Concept.* Helsinki: Yliopistopaino; 1992.

Hallikainen D, Linqvist C, Iizuka T, Mikkonen P, Paukku P. Cross-sectional tomography in evaluation of the patient undergoing sagittal split osteotomy. *Dentomaxillofac Radiol.* 1991;20:181 (Abstr).

Hardt N, Hofer B. *Szintigraphie der Kiefer- und Gesichtsschädel-Erkrankungen*. Berlin: Quintessenz; 1988.

Haßfeld S, Ziegler C, Mühling J. Kann die digitale Panoramaschichtröntgentechnik das filmbasierte Verfahren ersetzen? *Zahnärztl Welt.* 1997;106:510–514.

Haßfeld S, Streib S, Sahl H, Stratmann U, Fehrentz D, Zöller J. Low-dose Computertomographie des Kieferknochens in der präimplantologischen Diagnostik. Grenzen der Dosisreduzierung und Genauigkeit von Längenmessungen. *Mund Kiefer Gesichtschir.* 1998;2:188–193.

Haßfeld S, Zöller J, Albert FK, Wirtz CR, Knauth M, Mühling J. Preoperative planning and intraoperative navigation in skull base surgery. *J Craniomaxillofac Surg.* 1998;26:220–225.

Haßfeld S, Stein W. Dreidimensionale Planung für die dentale Implantologie anhand computertomographischer Daten. *Dtsch Zahnärztl Z.* 2000;55:313–325.

Haßfeld S, Zöller J, Dupont F, Mühling J. Die Darstellung der Frontzahnregion mit Hilfe des Orthophos/P12-Programms. *Zahnärztl Praxis.* 1994;45:191–195.

Heckmann K. Die Röntgenperspektive und ihre Umwandlung durch eine Aufnahmetechnik. *Fortschr Röntgenstr.* 1939;60:144.

Hidajat N, Schröder RJ, Wolf M, et al. Meßgrößen zur Charakterisierung der Patientenexposition in der Computertomographie und ihre Bedeutung für die Risikoabschätzung. *Radiologe.* 1997;37:464–469.

Hirsch E, Visser H, Graf HL. Präimplantäre Röntgendiagnostik. Informationsbedarf versus Strahlenbelastung. *Implantologie.* 2002;10:291.

Hirschfelder U. *Dreidimensionale computertomographische Analyse von Kiefer-, Gesichts- und Schädelanomalien. Die klinische Anwendung der CT in der Kieferorthopädie.* Munich: Hanser; 1991.

Hirschfelder U, Hirschfelder H. 3-D-Rekonstruktion zur Beurteilung der Morphologie kraniofazialer Strukturen. *Dtsch Zahnärztl Z.* 1989;44:187.

Hirschfelder U, Hirschfelder H. Einsatz neuer CT-Techniken für Kieferorthopädische Fragestellungen. *Dtsch Zahnärztl Z.* 1993;48:128–133.

Horbaschek H, Chabbal J, Solzbach Z. Flachbild Detektor. In: Schmidt T, Stieve FE, eds. *Digitale Bildgebung in der diagnostichen Radiologie*. Berlin: H. Hoffmann Verlag; 1996; 139–146.

Hounsfield GN. Computerized transverse axial scanning (tomography). Part 1. Description of system. *Br J Radiol*. 1973;46:1016.

I

ICRU 54. Medical Imaging – The Assessment of Image Quality. ICRU Report 54. Bethesda, Ma: International Commission on Radiation Units and Measurements; 1996.

Imhof K. Dental-CT: Ein neues Programm zur Planung und Überprüfung von Kieferimplantaten. *Elektromedica*. 1992;60:26–29.

Isberg A, Stenstrom B, Isacsson G. Frequency of bilateral temporomandibular joint disc displacement in patients with unilateral symptoms: A 5-year follow-up of the asymptomatic joint. A clinical and arthrotomographic study. *Dentomaxillofac Radiol*. 1991;20:73–76.

K

Kahle W, Leonhard H, Platzer W. *Taschenatlas der Anatomie*. Vol 1. Stuttgart: Thieme; 1999.

Kalender W. Computertomographie – Technische Entwicklung. In: Rosenbusch G, Oudkerk M, Amman E, eds. *Radiologie in der medizinischen Diagnostik*. Berlin: Blackwell; 1994.

Kalender WA et al. Grundlagen der Spiral-CT: Prinzipien von Aufnahme und Rekonstruktion. *Z Med Phys*. 1997;7:231–240.

Kalender WA et al. Grundlagen der Spiral-CT: Bildqualität. *Z Med Phys*. 1998;8:7–18.

Kaeppler G, Axmann-Krcmar D, Gomez-Roman G, Schulte W. Die Genauigkeit verschiedener Panoramaschichtaufnahmen und transversaler Schichtaufnahmen für die präimplantologische Planung. *Z Zahnärztl Implantol*. 1995;11:209–220.

Kaeppler G, Axmann-Krcmar D, Schwenzer N. Anwendungsbereich transversaler Schichtaufnahmen (Scanora) in der zahnärztlichen Implantologie. *Z Zahnärztl Implantol*. 1997;13:18–26.

Kaeppler G. New radiographic programs for transverse conventional tomograms in the dentomaxillofacial region. *Quintessence Int*. 1999;30:541–549.

Kaeppler G. Conventional cross-sectional tomographic evaluation of mandibular third molars. *Quintessence Int*. 2000;31:49–56.

Kaeppler G, Axmann-Krcmar D, Reuter I, Meyle J, Gomez-Roman G. A clinical evaluation of some factors affecting image quality in panoramic radiography. *Dentomaxillofac Radiol*. 2000;29:81–84.

Kalifa G. Radiologiste ou radioprotectioniste? Entretiens de Jérôme Pellissier Tanon. *Radioprotection*. 1999;34:95–97.

Katzberg RW, Westesson PL. *Diagnosis of the Temporomandibular Joint*. Philadelphia: Saunders; 1994.

Kornas M, Haßfeld S, Mende U, Zöller J. Metrische Genauigkeit der CT-Analyse vor enossaler Implantation. *Dtsch Zahnärztl Z*. 1998:53;120–126.

Kramer IRH, Pindborg JJ, Shear M. The WHO histological typing of odontogenic tumours: a commentary on the second edition. *Cancer*. 1992;70:2988–2994.

Kullendorff B, Nilsson M. Diagnostic accuracy of direct digital dental radiography for the detection of periapical bone lesions. II. Effects on diagnostic accuracy after application of image processing. *Oral Surg Oral Med Oral Pathol Oral Radiol Endod*. 1996;82:585–589.

Kühnisch J., Pasler F.A., Bücher K., Hickel R., Heinrich-Weltzien R. Triangular-shaped radiolucencies leading to false positive caries diagnoses from bitewing radiographs. 8th congress of the European Academy of Paediatric Dentistry, Amsterdam, 8–11th June 2006.

L

Langlais RP, Langland OE, Nortje CJ. *Diagnostic Imaging of the Jaws*. Baltimore: Williams and Wilkins; 1995.

Laudenbach P, Bonneau E, Korach G. *Radiographie panoramique dentaire et maxillofacial.* Paris: Masson; 1977.

Lazzerini F, Minorati D, Nessi R, Gagliani M, Uslenghi CM. The measurement parameters in dental radiography: a comparison between traditional and digital technics [in Italian]. *Radiol Med Torino.* 1996;91:364–369.

Lenglinger FX, Muhr T, Krennmair G. Dental-CT: Untersuchungstechnik, Strahlenbelastung und Anatomie. *Radiologe.* 1999;39:1027–1034.

Lichtenstein L. Histiocytosis X intergration of eosinophilic granuloma of bone. Letterer-Siwe disease and Schüller-Christian disease as related manifestations of a single nosologic entity. *Arch Pathol.* 1953;56:84–102.

Lopez AJ, Cavézian R, Iba-Zizen MT. Imagerie par résonance magnétique des articulations temporomandibulaires. *Actual Odonto-Stomatol.* 1993;182:291–311.

Ludlow JB, Abreu Jr M. Performance of film, desktop monitor and laptop displays in caries detection. *Dentomaxillofac Radiol.* 1999;28:26–30.

M

MacDonal-Jankowski DS. The synchrondrosis between the greater horn and the body of the hyoid bone: a radiological assessment. *Dentomaxillofac Radiol.* 1990;19:171–172.

Makek M. Clinical *Pathology of Fibro-Osteo-Cemental Lesions in the Cranio-Facial and Jaw Bones.* Basel: Karger; 1983.

Makek M, Lello G. Benign cementoblastoma. Case report and literature review. *J Maxillofac Surg.* 1982;10:182.

Marroquin BB, Willershausen-Zönnchen B, Pistorius A, Göller M. Zuverlässigket apikaler Röntgenaufnahmen bei der Diagnostik von Unterkiefer-Knochenläsionen. *Schweiz Monatschr Zahnmed.* 1995;105:9.

Martin-Duverneuil N, Chiras J. *Imagerie maxillofaciale.* Paris: Médicine-Sciences, Flammarion; 1997.

Mittermayer C. *Oralpathologie – Erkrankungen der Mundregion. Lehrbuch für Zahnmedizin, Mund- und Kieferheilkunde.* Stuttgart: Schattauer; 1993.

Möbes O, Becker J, Schnelle C, Ewen K, Kemper J, Cohnen M. Strahlenexposition bei der digitalen Volumentomographie, Panoramaschichtaufnahme und Computertomographie. *Dtsch Zahnärztl Z.* 2000;55:336–339.

Molander B, Ahquist M, Grödahl HG, Hollender L. Agreement between panoramic and intra-oral radiography in the assessment of marginal bone height. *Dentomaxillofac Radiol.* 1991; 20: 155.

Mongini F. *Headache and Facial Pain.* New York: Thieme; 1999.

Mozzo P, Procacci C, Tacconi A, Tinazzi Martini P, Bergamo Andreis IA. A new volumetric CT machine for dental imaging based on the cone-beam technique: preliminary results. *Eur Radiol.* 1998;8:1558–1564.

Musgrove BT, Moody GH. Synovial chondromatosis of the temporomandibular joint. *Int J Oral Maxillofac Surg.* 1991;20:93.

N

Neitzel U. Grundlagen der digitalen Bildgebung. In: Ewen K, ed. *Moderne Bildgebung, Physik, Gerätetechnik, Bildbearbeitung und -kommunikation, Strahlenschutz, Qualitätskontrolle.* Stuttgart: Thieme; 1998:63–76.

Nitzan DW, Marmary Y. Osteomyelitis of the mandible in a patient with osteopetrosis. *J Oral Maxillofac Surg.* 1982;40:377.

NRPB. Risk of radiation-induced cancer at low doses and low dose rates for radiation protection purposes. Documents of the NRPB. Vol 6. No 1. Chilton, Didcot, Oxon, UK: National Radiological Protection Board. United Kingdom 1995.

O

O'Mara RE. Role of bone scanning in dental and maxillofacial disorders. In: Freemann LM, Weissmann HS, eds. *Nuclear Medicine Annual*. New York: Raven Press; 1985:265–284.

O'Neil DW, Koch MG, Lowe JW. Regional odontodysplasia: report of case. *J Dent Child*. 1990;57:6, 459–461.

O'Riordan B. Phleboliths and salivary calculi. *Br J Oral Surg*. 1974;12:119.

P

Paatero YV. A new tomographic method for radiographing curved outer surfaces. *Acta Radiol*. 1949;32:177.

Paatero YV. Orthoradial jaw pantomography. *Ann Med Int Feun (Suppl 28)*. 1958;48:222, 227.

Paatero YV. Pantomography and orthopantomography. *Oral Surg*. 1961;14:947–953.

Parma Č. *Röntgenographie der Zähne und der Kiefer*. Berlin/Vienna: Urban & Schwarzenberg; 1936.

Pasler FA. *Manuel de radiologie dentaire et maxillofacial*. Paris: Payot & Doin; 1987.

Pasler FA, Stöckli PW. Röntgenuntersuchung. In: Stöckli PW, Ben-Zur ED, eds. *Zahnmedizin bei Kindern und Jugendlichen*. Stuttgart: Thieme; 1984.

Pasler FA. *Atlas de Médicine dentaire*. Paris: Médicine-Sciences, Flammarion; 1999.

Pasler FA, Visser H. *Zahnmedizinische Radiologie – Bildgebende Verfahren*. 2nd ed. (Farbatlanten der Zahnmedizin. Vol 5) Stuttgart: Thieme; 2000.

Pasler FA, Visser H. Qualitätssicherung bei Panoramaschichtaufnahmen. *ZWR*. 2001;110(7–8): 505–513.

Pasler FA. *Zahnärztliche Radiologie*. 4th ed. Stuttgart: Thieme; 2003.

Pasler F.A., Kühnisch J., Bücher K., Hickel R., Heinrich-Weltzien R. Triangular-shaped radiolucencies leading to false positive caries diagnoses from bitewing radiographs. 8th congress of the European Academy of Paediatric Dentistry, Amsterdam, 8–11th June 2006.

Pellerin Y. Difficultés en radiologie dentaire rétro-alvéolaire classique au cours de la réalisation des cliches. *Revue d'Odonto-Stomatol*. 1992;21(6):401–409.

Philipsen HP, Ormiston IW, Reichart PA. The desmo- and osteoplastic ameloblastoma. Histologic variant or clinicopathologic entity? Case reports. *J Oral Maxillofac Surg*. 1992;21:352–357.

Philipsen HP, Reichart PA. Squamous odontogenic tumor (SQT): a benign neoplasm of the periodontium. A review of 36 reported cases. *J Clin Periodontol*. 1986;23:922–926.

Philipsen HP, Reichart PA. The adenomatoid odontogenic tumour: ultrastructure of tumour cells and non-calcified amorphous masses. *J Oral Pathol Med*. 1996;25:491–496.

Philipsen HP, Reichart PA. The unicystic ameloblastom – a review of 193 cases from the literature. *Oral Oncol*. 1998;34:317–325.

Philipsen HP, Reichart PA, Praetorius F. Mixed odontogenic tumours and odontomas. Considerations on interrelationship. Review of the literature and presentation of 134 new cases of odontomas. *Oral Oncol*. 1997;33:86–89.

Philipsen HP, Samman N, Ormiston IW, Wu PC, Reichart PA. Variants of the adenomatoid odontogenic tumor with a note on tumor origin. *J Oral Pathol Med*. 1992;21:348–352.

Pilling E, Päßler L. Computergestützte Implantationsplanung mit dem Tomographiegerät COMMCAT. *Quintessenz*. 1998;49:709–711.

Pindborg JJ. A calcifying epithelial odontogenic tumor. *Cancer*. 1958;11:838.

Pindborg JJ, Hjørting-Hansen E. *Atlas of Diseases of the Jaws*. Copenhagen: Munksgaard; 1974.

Pindborg JJ, Kramer IRH, Torloni H. *Histological typing of odontogenic tumours, jaw cysts and allied lesions. International histological classification of tumours No. 5*. Geneva: WHO; 1971.

Pinna V, Marchi MD, Puzzuoli A, Bernardi L, Clauser L, Nordera P. La tomografia computerizzata tridimensionale nella patologia maxillo-facciale. *Rivista di Neuroradiol*. 1993;6:19–34.

Pistorius A, Treinen J, Mildenberger P, Willershausen-Zönnchen B. Diagnostik und Anwendungsbereiche der Computertomographie in der Parodontologie. *Acta Med Dent Helv*. 1997;2:2.

Poyton HG. *Oral Radiology*. Baltimore: Williams and Wilkins; 1982.

Preece JW. Isn't it time we changed our perception of diagnostic radiation risks? *Oral Surg Oral Med Oral Pathol.* 1997; 84:329.

R

Ramm B, Nunnemann A. *Röntgenqualitätsprüfungen und Strahlenschutz.* Stuttgart: Enke; 1992.

Reichart PA, Dornow H. Gingivo-periodontal manifestations in chronic benign neutropenia. *J Clin Periodontal.* 1978;5:74–80.

Reichart PA, Philipsen HP. *Oralpathologie. Farbatlanten der Zahnmedizin.* Vol 14. Stuttgart: Thieme; 1999.

Reichart PA, Philipsen HP, Sonners S. Ameloblastoma: biological profile of 3677 cases. *Oral Oncol. Eur J Cancer.* 1995;2:86–99.

Reichart PA, Ries P. Considerations on the classification of odontogenic tumours. *Int J Oral Surg.* 1983:12(5)323–323.

Reichart PA, Schulz P, Walz C, et al. *Früherkennung von Neubildungen im Kiefer-Gesichtsbereich durch den praktizierenden Zahnarzt.* Bonn: Deutsche Krebshilfe; 1991.

Reichart PA, Zobl H. Transformation of ameloblastic fibroma to fibrosarcoma. *Int J Oral Surg.* 1978;7:503–507.

Reiser M, Semmler W. *Magnetresonanztomographie.* 2nd ed. Berlin: Springer; 1997.

Rötig T. Untersuchungen zur Strahlenexposition des Patienten bei Spezialröntgenaufnahmen im Zahn-Mund-Kieferbereich [dissertation]. Göttingen; 1998.

Rossman K. The effect of some physical factors on radiographic image quality. *Radiology.* 1965;84:123–124.

Rustemeyer P, Hohn HP, Streubühr U, et al. Low dose Dental-CT. *Fortschr Röntgenstr.* 1999;170:34.

S

Sanderink G, Huiskens R, van der Stelt P, Welander U, Stheemann S. Image quality of direct digital intraoral x-ray sensors in assessing root canal length. Oral Surg Oral Med Pathol. 1994; 78:125.

Sargos P. Information et consentement du patient. *Bulletin de l'Ordre des médecins.* 1999;1:10–11.

Schlegel W, Bille J, eds. *Medizinische Physik.* Berlin: Springer; 2002.

Schmidt G. *Ultraschall-Kursbuch.* 2nd ed. Stuttgart: Thieme; 1996.

Schmidt-Westhausen A, Philipsen HP, Reichart PA. Das ameloblastische Fibrom – ein odontogener Tumor in Wachstumsalter. *Dtsch Zahnärztl Z.* 1991;46:66.

Schorn C, Visser H, Hermann KP, Alamo L, Funke M, Grabbe E. Dental CT: Bildqualität und Strahlenexposition in Abhängigkeit von den Scanparametern. *Fortschr Röntgenstr.* 1999;170: 137–144.

Schramm A, Gellrich NC, Randelzhofer P, Schneider U, Gläser R, Schmelzeisen R. *Use and abuse of navigational surgery in oral implantation. Proc 14th Int Cong and Exhi CARS 2000.* San Francisco. Amsterdam: Elsevier; 2000.

Seifert G, Miehlke A, Hauberich J, Chilla R. Speicheldrüsenkrankheiten. Stuttgart: Thieme; 1984.

Shear M. *Cysts of the Oral Regions.* 3rd ed. Oxford: Wright; 1992.

Sicher H, Trandler J. *Anatomie für Zahnärzte.* Berlin: Springer; 1928.

Sitzmann F, ed. *Zahn-, Mund- und Kiefererkrankungen.* Urban und Fischer; 2000.

Spiekermann H. *Implantologie. Farbatlanten der Zahnmedizin.* Vol 10. Stuttgart: Thieme; 1994.

Steinhardt G. Untersuchungen über Beanspruchung der Kiefergelenke und ihre geweblichen Folgen. *Dtsch Zahnheilkd.* 1934;91:1.

Stieve FE, Stargardt A, Stender H-St. *Strahlenschutz.* Berlin: Hoffmann; 1996.

Stöckli PW, Ben-Zur ED. Zahnmedizin bei Kindern und Jugendlichen. Stuttgart: Thieme; 1994.

Sundn S, Gröndahl K, Gröndahl HG. Accuracy and precision in the radiographic diagnosis of clinical instability in Branemark dental implants. *Clin Oral Implants Res.* 1995;6:220–226.

T

Tal H, Moses O. A comparison of panoramic radiography with computed tomography in the planning of implant surgery. *Dentomaxillofac Radiol.* 1991;20:40–42.

Tammisalo EH, Hallikainen D, Kanerva H, Tammisalo T. Comprehensive oral x-ray diagnosis: Scanora® multimodal radiography. *Dentomaxillofac Radiol.* 1992;21:9.

Tammisalo E, Tammisalo T. Multimodal radiography: a new imaging technique and system for oral diagnosis. *Proc Finn Dent Soc.* 1991;87:259–270.

Tasaki MM, Westesson PL. Temporomandibular joint diagnostic accuracy with sagittal and coronal MR imaging. *Radiology.* 1993;186:723–730.

Tetsch P, Tetsch J. *Fortschritte der zahnärztlichen Implantologie – Ein Atlas.* Munich: Hanser; 1996: 17–18.

Thibierge M, Fournier L, Cabanis EA. Principes de responsabilité médicale et exercice en imagerie médicale. *J Radiol.* 1999;80:701–707.

Thiel H-J, Haßfeld S. *Schnittbilddiagnostik in MKG-Chirurgie und Zahnmedizin.* Stuttgart: Thieme; 2001.

Treil J, Escude B, Cavézian R, Pasquet G. L'imagerie en coupes en implantologie: tomodensitométrie avec logiciel spécifique. *Actualités Odonto-Stomatol.* 1993;181:73–89.

U

Uehlinger E. Fibröse Dysplasie (Jaffé-Lichtenstein): Osteofibrosis deformans juvenilis (Uehlinger); Albrightsches Syndrom. In: Schinz HR, Baensch WE, Frommhold W, Glauner R, Uehlinger E, Wellauer J, eds. *Lehrbuch der Röntgendiagnostik.* Vol II/1. Stuttgart: Thieme; 1979.

UNSCEAR 93. *Sources and Effects of Ionizing Radiation. United Nations Scientific Committee on the Effects of Atomic Radiation.* UNSCEAR 1993 Report to the General Assembly, with Scientific Annexes. New York: United Nations; 1993.

V

Valachovic RW, Douglass CW, Reiskin AB, Channcey HH, McNeil BJ. The use of panoramic radiography in the evaluation of asymptomatic adult dental patients. *Oral Surg Oral Med Pathol.* 1986;61:289.

Valvassori GE, Potter GD, Hanafee WN, Carter BL, Buckingham RA. Radiologie in der Hals-Nasen-Ohren-Heilkunde. Stuttgart: Thieme; 1984.

Van Aken J. Untersuchungen zum Indikationsbereich von Panoramaaufnahmen. In: Jung T. *Panoramaröntgenographie. Symposium Hannover.* Heidelberg: Hüthig; 1982.

Van der Waal I. *Diseases of the Jaws. Diagnosis and Treatment. Textbook and Atlas.* Copenhagen: Munskgaard; 1991.

van Waes JM, Stöckli P. *Farbatlas der Kinderzahnmedizin.* Stuttgart: Thieme; 2001.

Verdun FR, Aroua A, Valley J-V. Evaluation der Strahlenbelastung von Patienten in der Zahnärztlichen Radiologie. Lausanne: IRA; 2004.

Verordnung über den Schutz vor Schäden durch ionisierende Strahlen (Strahlenschutzverordnung), in der Fassung der Bekanntmachung vom 30.6.1989 (BGB1 I S 1321, 1926), geändert durch Vierte Änderungsverordnung vom 18. August 1997 (BGB1 I, S 2113), Neufassung verabschiedet am 20.7.2001 (GMBI T.1), G5702 N. 38 (26.7.2001).

Visser H. Ein einfaches Verfahren zur Digitalisierung von Zahnfilmen. *Zahnärztl Welt.* 1994;103:282–287.

Visser H. *Untersuchungen zur Optimierung der parodontologischen Röntgendiagnostik.* Berlin: Quintessenz; 2000.

Visser H, Böhm O. Parodontitis und Erkrankungen der Nasennebenhöhlen. *Parodontologie.* 2003;14:31.

Visser H, Hermann KP, Köhler B. Phantomuntersuchungen zur Strahlenexposition des Patienten bei der intraoralen zahnärztlichen Diagnostik mit digitalen Röntgensystemen. In: Schmidt R. Medizinische Physik 1997. Hamburg: Deutsche Gesellschaft für Medizinische Physik; 1997c:177–178.

Visser H, Hermann KP, Schorn C, Krüger W. Doses to critical organs from computed tomography (CT). In: Farman AG, Ruprecht A, Gibbs SJ, Scarfe WC. *Advances in Maxillofacial Imaging.* Amsterdam: Elsevier; 1997b:401–406.

Visser H, Krüger W. Can dentists recognize manipulated digital radiographs? *Dentomaxillofac Radiol.* 1997;26:67–69.

Visser H, Lewandowski P, Krüger W. Comparison of storage phosphor and conventional radiography for periodontal diagnosis. *J Dent Res.* 1999;78:209 (Abstr 824).

Visser H, Matheis B, Richter B, Hermann PK, Harder D, Krüger W. Zahnfilmstatus und Panorama-Schichtaufnahme – Ergebniss einer klinisch-dosimetrischen Untersuchung. *Dtsch Zahnärztl Z.* 1997a;52:492–494.

Völke H. *Rayonnement ionisant et risques sanitaires.* Actes du 5e Colloque transfrontalier CLUSE: University of Geneva, 21–22 September; 2000.

W

Wächter R, Remagen W, Stoll P. Kann man zwischen Odonto-Ameloblastom und ameloblastischem Fibro-Odontom unterscheiden? *Dtsch Zahnärztl Z.* 1991;46:74.

Wambersie A. Radiologie et radioprotection en médecine dentaire. Première partie: Effets biologiques résultant d'une exposition aux rayonnements ionisants. *Rev Belge Méd Dent.* 1991;46:9–29.

Webber RL. The future of dental imaging. Where do we go from here? *Dentomaxillofac Radiol.* 1999;28:5.

Wehrbein H, Harhoff R, Dietrich P. Wurzelresorptionsrate bei orthodontisch bewegten, parodontal geschädigten und gesunden Zähnen. *Dtsch Zahnärztl Z.* 1990;45:176–178.

Wesely RK, Cullen CL, Bloom WS. Gardner's syndrome with bilateral osteomas of coronoid process resulting in limited opening. *Pediat Dent.* 1987;9:53–57.

Westesson PL. Diagnostic imaging of oral malignancies. *Oral Maxillofac Surg N Am.* 1993;5:2.

White SC. 1992 assessment of radiation risk from dental radiography. *Dentomaxillofac Radiol.* 1992;21:118–126.

White SC, Pharoah MJ, eds. *Oral Radiology: Principles and interpretation.* 4th ed. St. Louis: Mosby; 1999: 622–635.

White St. C, Pharoah MJ. *Oral Radiology.* St. Louis: Mosby; 2000.

Witkowski R, Prokop O, Ullrich E. *Lexikon der Syndrome und Fehlbildungen.* Berlin: Springer; 1995.

Wood NK, Goaz PW. *Differential Diagnosis of Oral and Maxillofacial Lesions.* 5th ed. St. Louis: Mosby: 1997.

Worth HM. *Principles and Practice of Oral Radiologic Interpretation.* Chicago: Yearbook Med Pub Inc; 1969.

Y

Yamamoto K, Farman AG, Webber RL, Horton RA, Kuroyanagi K. Effect of number of projections on accuracy of depth discrimination using tuned-aperture computed tomography for 3-dimensional dentoalveolar imaging of low-contrast details. *Oral Surg Oral Med Oral Pathol Oral Radiol Endod.* 1999; 88:100–105.

Yanagisawa K, Friedmann CD, Vining EM, et al. DentaScan imaging of the mandible and maxilla. *Head Neck.* 1993;15:1–7.

Yang J, Cavalcanti MG, Ruprecht A, Vannier MW. 2-D and 3-D reconstructions of spiral computed tomography in localization of the inferior alveolar canal for dental implants. *Oral Surg Oral Med Oral Pathol Oral Radiol Endod.* 1999;87:369–374.

Z

Zebedin D Fotter R, Preidler KW, Mache C, Szolar DH. Chronisch rekurrierende multifokale Osteomyelitis des Unterkiefers. *Fortschr Röntgenstr.* 1998;551–554.

Ziedses des Plantes BGA. *Planigraphie en Subtractie. Röntgenographische differentiatie methoden* [thesis]. Utrecht: Kemnik en Zoon NV; 1934.

Ziegler CM, Haßfeld S, Heil U, Tigör B, Mühling J. Transversale Schichtaufnahmen der Kiefer. *ZWR.* 1999;108:91–96.

Zilkha A. Computed tomography in facial trauma. *Radiology.* 1982;144:545–548.

Index

Page numbers in *italics* refer to illustrations.

A

B

C

D

E

F

G

H

I

J

K

L

M

N

O

P

R

S

T

Index

T

V

W

Z